IOC MANUAL OF SPORTS CARDIOLOGY

EDITED BY

MATHEW G. WILSON
ASPETAR, Qatar Orthopaedic and Sports Medicine Hospital, Doha, Qatar

JONATHAN A. DREZNER
University of Washington, Seattle, WA, USA

SANJAY SHARMA
St George's University of London, London, UK

WILEY Blackwell

Library of Congress Cataloging-in-Publication Data

Names: Wilson, Mathew G., editor. | Drezner, Jonathan A., editor. | Sharma, Sanjay (Professor of inherited cardiac diseases), editor. |
    International Olympic Committee, issuing body.
Title: IOC manual of sports cardiology / edited by Mathew G. Wilson, Jonathan A. Drezner, Sanjay Sharma.
Other titles: International Olympic Committee manual of sports cardiology | Manual of sports cardiology
Description: Oxford ; Ames, Iowa : John Wiley & Sons, Inc., 2016. | Includes bibliographical references and index.
Identifiers: LCCN 2016017737 (print) | LCCN 2016018440 (ebook) | ISBN 9781119046868 (pbk.) | ISBN 9781119046882 (pdf) |
    ISBN 9781119046875 (epub)
Subjects: | MESH: Death, Sudden, Cardiac | Athletes | Cardiovascular Diseases | Diagnostic Techniques, Cardiovascular |
    Sports Medicine–methods
Classification: LCC RB150.S84 (print) | LCC RB150.S84 (ebook) | NLM WG 214 | DDC 617.1/027–dc23
LC record available at https://lccn.loc.gov/2016017737

A catalogue record for this book is available from the British Library.

Wiley also publishes its books in a variety of electronic formats. Some content that appears in print may not be available in electronic books.

Cover images: © International Olympic Committee

Set in 9.5/11.5 pt Plantin by SPi Global, Pondicherry, India
Printed and bound in Singapore by Markono Print Media Pte Ltd

1   2017

Contents

Contributors

Ramy S. Abdelfattah
Stanford Cardiology Sports Medicine Clinic, Stanford University, Stanford, CA, USA

Michael J. Ackerman
Departments of Medicine, Pediatrics, and Molecular Pharmacology & Experimental Therapeutics, Divisions of Cardiovascular Diseases and Pediatric Cardiology, Windland Smith Rice Sudden Death Genomics Laboratory, Mayo Clinic, Rochester, MN, USA

Maria-Carmen Adamuz
Department of Sports Medicine, ASPETAR, Qatar Orthopaedic and Sports Medicine Hospital, Doha, Qatar

Juan Manuel Alonso
Department of Sports Medicine, ASPETAR, Qatar Orthopaedic and Sports Medicine Hospital, Doha, Qatar

Peter J. Angell
School of Health Sciences, Liverpool Hope University, Liverpool, UK

Elena Arbelo
Department of Cardiology, Thorax Institute, Hospital Clinic Barcelona, University of Barcelona, Barcelona, Spain

Euan Ashley
Falk Cardiovascular Research Center, Stanford, CA, USA

Irfan M. Asif
Department of Family Medicine, Greenville Health System, University of South Carolina Greenville School of Medicine, Greenville, SC, USA

Aaron L. Baggish
Cardiovascular Performance Program, Massachusetts General Hospital, Boston, MA, USA

Cristina Basso
Cardiovascular Pathology Unit, Department of Cardiac, Thoracic and Vascular Sciences, University of Padua Medical School, Padua, Italy

Elijah R. Behr
Cardiac Research Centre, St George's University of London, London, UK

Mats Börjesson
Åstrand Laboratory, Swedish School of Sport and Exercise Sciences (GIH) and Department of Cardiology, Karolinska University Hospital, Stockholm, Sweden

Martin Botha
Division of Emergency Medicine, Faculty of Health Sciences, University of the Witwatersrand, Johannesburg, South Africa

Josep Brugada
Department of Cardiology, Thorax Institute, Hospital Clinic Barcelona, University of Barcelona, Barcelona, Spain

John P. Buckley
Institute of Medicine, University Centre Shrewsbury and University of Chester, Chester, UK

N. Tim Cable
Department of Sport Science, Aspire Academy, Doha, Qatar and Research Institute for Sport and Exercise Sciences, Liverpool John Moores University, Liverpool, UK

Colleen Caleshu
Falk Cardiovascular Research Center, Stanford, CA, USA

Cindy J. Chang
Department of Orthopaedic Medicine, Divisions of Sports Medicine and Pediatric Orthopaedic Medicine, Department of Family and Community Medicine, University of California, San Francisco, CA, USA

Anne H. Child
Cardiovascular and Cell Sciences Research Institute, St George's University of London, London, UK

Guido Claessen
Department of Cardiovascular Medicine, University Hospitals Leuven, Leuven, Belgium

Domenico Corrado
Department of Cardiac, Thoracic and Vascular Sciences, University of Padua Medical School, Padua, Italy

Bethan Davies
Cardiovascular and Cell Sciences Research Institute, St George's University of London, London, UK

Mikael Dellborg
Department of Molecular and Clinical Medicine/Östra, Institute of Medicine, Sahlgrenska Academy, University of Gothenburg and Adult Congenital Heart Unit, Sahlgrenska University Hospital/Östra, Gothenburg, Sweden

Paul Dijkstra
Department of Sports Medicine, ASPETAR, Qatar Orthopaedic and Sports Medicine Hospital, Doha, Qatar

Jonathan A. Drezner
Department of Family Medicine, University of Washington, Seattle, WA, USA

Andrew D'Silva
St George's University Hospital Foundation NHS Trust, St George's University of London, London, UK

Gherardo Finocchiaro
Cardiovascular and Cell Sciences Research Centre, St George's University of London, London, UK

Victor Froelicher
Palo Alto Veterans Affairs Health Care System and Stanford University, Stanford, CA, USA

Sabiha Gati
Department of Cardiovascular Sciences, St George's University of London, London, UK

Keith P. George
Research Institute for Sport and Exercise Sciences, Liverpool John Moores University, Liverpool, UK

Eduard Guasch
Unitat de Fibril·lació Auricular, Hospital Clinic, University of Barcelona, Barcelona, Catalonia, Spain

Kimberly G. Harmon
University of Washington, Seattle, WA, USA

Hein Heidbuchel
Hasselt University and Heart Center, Jessa Hospital, Hasselt, Belgium

Kathleen E. Kearney
Division of Cardiology, University of Washington School of Medicine, Seattle, WA, USA

Tracey Keteepe-Arachi
St George's University of London, London, UK

Suzy Kim
St. Jude Centers for Rehabilitation & Wellness, Brea, CA, USA

Efraim Kramer
Division of Emergency Medicine, Faculty of Health Sciences, University of the Witwatersrand, Johannesburg, South Africa

André La Gerche
Baker IDI Heart and Diabetes Institute, Melbourne, Victoria, Australia

Mark S. Link
Tufts Medical Center, Boston, MA, USA

Christopher Madias
Tufts Medical Center, Boston, MA, USA

Aneil Malhotra
Department of Cardiovascular Sciences, St George's University of London, London, UK

Greg Mellor
Cardiac Research Centre, St George's University of London, London, UK

Lluis Mont
Institut d'Investigacions Biomédiques August Pi i Sunyer (IDIBAPS), Barcelona, Catalonia, Spain

Jonathan Myers
Palo Alto Veterans Affairs Health Care System and Stanford University, Stanford, CA, USA

Rory O'Hanlon
Centre for Cardiovascular Magnetic Resonance, Blackrock Clinic, Dublin, Ireland

Catherine M. Otto
Division of Cardiology, University of Washington School of Medicine, Seattle, WA, USA

David S. Owens
Division of Cardiology, University of Washington, Seattle, WA, USA

David Oxborough
Research Institute for Sports and Exercise Sciences, Liverpool John Moores University, Liverpool, UK

Michael Papadakis
Cardiovascular and Cell Sciences Research Centre, St George's University of London, London, UK

Antonio Pelliccia
Institute of Sport Medicine and Science, Rome, Italy

Julien D. Périard
Athlete Health and Performance Research Centre, ASPETAR, Qatar Orthopaedic and Sports Medicine Hospital, Doha, Qatar

Stéphane Perrey
Movement to Health, Euromov, University of Montpellier, Montpellier, France

Guido E. Pieles
National Institute for Health Research (NIHR) Cardiovascular Biomedical Research Unit, Congenital Heart Unit, Bristol Royal Hospital for Children and Bristol Heart Institute, Bristol, UK

Jordan Prutkin
Division of Cardiology, Section of Electrophysiology, Center for Sports Cardiology, University of Washington, Seattle, WA, USA

Sébastien Racinais
Athlete Health and Performance Research Centre, ASPETAR, Qatar Orthopaedic and Sports Medicine Hospital, Doha, Qatar

Nathan Riding
Athlete Health and Performance Research Centre, ASPETAR, Qatar Orthopaedic and Sports Medicine Hospital, Doha, Qatar

Jack C. Salerno
University of Washington School of Medicine, Seattle Children's Hospital, Seattle, WA, USA

Yorck O. Schumacher
Department of Sports Medicine, ASPETAR, Qatar Orthopaedic and Sports Medicine Hospital, Doha, Qatar

Sanjay Sharma
Department of Cardiovascular Sciences, St George's University of London, London, UK

Nabeel Sheikh
St George's University of London, London, UK

Mary N. Sheppard
Department of Cardiovascular Pathology, St George's University of London, London, UK

A. Graham Stuart
Congenital Heart Unit, Bristol Royal Hospital for Children and Bristol Heart Institute, Bristol, UK

David J. Tester
Departments of Medicine, Pediatrics, and Molecular Pharmacology & Experimental Therapeutics, Divisions of Cardiovascular Diseases and Pediatric Cardiology, Windland Smith Rice Sudden Death Genomics Laboratory, Mayo Clinic, Rochester, MN, USA

Gaetano Thiene
Cardiovascular Pathology Unit, Department of Cardiac, Thoracic and Vascular Sciences, University of Padua Medical School, Padua, Italy

Jeffrey A. Towbin
The Heart Institute, University of Tennessee Health Science Center, Le Bonheur Children's Hospital and St Jude Children's Research Hospital, Memphis, TN, USA

Meagan M. Wasfy
Cardiovascular Performance Program, Massachusetts General Hospital, Boston, MA, USA

Victoria Watt
Department of Sports Medicine, ASPETAR, Qatar Orthopaedic and Sports Medicine Hospital, Doha, Qatar

Mathew G. Wilson
Department of Sports Medicine, ASPETAR, Qatar Orthopaedic and Sports Medicine Hospital, Doha, Qatar
Research Institute of Sport and Exercise Sciences, Liverpool John Moores University, Liverpool, UK
Research Institute of Sport and Exercise Sciences, University of Canberra, Canberra, ACT, Australia

Leonie C.H. Wong
Cardiovascular and Cell Sciences Research Institute, St George's University of London, London, UK

Alessandro Zorzi
Department of Cardiac, Thoracic and Vascular Sciences, University of Padua Medical School, Padua, Italy

Foreword

As an Olympian, I know that all the athletes are grateful to the IOC Medical and Scientific Commission and the research it supports, like this invaluable book.

This manual is a comprehensive and authoritative work on the cardiovascular system during its acute responses to individual bouts of exercise (both in training and during competition) and its chronic adaptations to long-term conditioning exercise. The target audience is sports medicine physicians, cardiologists, primary care physicians, emergency room physicians, physical therapists, athletics coaches, nurse practitioners and physicians' assistants. But ultimately, this book and this research support the athletes in their training and competition.

To produce this remarkable work, a team of contributing authors was recruited comprising outstanding clinicians and scientists who, through their research and publications, have provided the foundations of knowledge regarding the functioning of the heart relating to sports performance. Following a presentation of basic information on cardiac function, this manual presents detailed discussions regarding the cardiovascular management and screening of athletes, the provision of emergency care and the prevention of sudden death.

This manual constitutes a major contribution to international literature on cardiology. It joins the impressive list of publications presented by the IOC Medical and Scientific Commission, with the objective of improving the health and welfare of athletes participating at all levels of competition.

Thomas Bach
IOC President

Preface

In 1901, Dr W. Collier submitted a paper to the *British Medical Journal* entitled, 'The Effects of Severe Muscular Exertion, Sudden and Prolonged, in Young Adolescents' [1]. This early article demonstrated the predicament faced by physicians when dealing with athletes suspected of, or diagnosed with, a cardiovascular disease (CVD). Collier describes the case of an Oxford University mile runner who was performing poorly and presented for medical consultation. Physical examination at rest was normal, but upon mild exercise, the athlete demonstrated a very distinct systolic murmur. Rightly or wrongly, Collier stated that he 'had no doubt that it was over-dilation of the right ventricle' and disqualified the athlete from competition [1]. He even sent the athlete on a sea voyage, where the temptation to exercise was effectively removed. Despite much medical, academic and technological advancement in the 100 years after Collier's initial insights, many sports medicine physicians who undertake cardiovascular pre-participation screening may argue that following the diagnosis of an inherited cardiac disease, the limited ability to adequately risk-stratify and provide evidence-based exercise recommendations and disqualification criteria for athletes indicates our management remains just as inadequate and imprecise.

Athletes are perceived as the epitome of health, owing to their unique lifestyle and physical achievements. However, a small proportion of athletes die suddenly from a pathologic heart condition: so-called 'sudden cardiac death' (SCD). Most deaths in athletes under 35 years of age are attributed to inherited or congenital disorders of the heart that predispose to malignant ventricular arrhythmias. Due to the steady trickle of SCDs in young athletes, several major sport governing bodies, including the International Olympic Committee (IOC) and Fédération Internationale de Football Association (FIFA), have 'recommended' the implementation of systematic cardiac screening programmes – a trend increasingly being adopted by such bodies worldwide. Despite differences in screening methodology, both the American College of Cardiology (ACC)/American Heart Association (AHA) and the European Society of Cardiology (ESC) agree that there is compelling justification for cardiovascular pre-participation screening on medical, ethical and legal grounds [2, 3].

The purpose of pre-participation cardiovascular screening appears to be well intentioned: to promote athlete safety and provide medical clearance for participation in sport through the systematic evaluation of athletes, aimed at identifying pre-existing cardiovascular abnormalities and thereby reducing the potential for adverse events and sudden death. However, athletes who exhibit an abnormal finding on their screening evaluation may face a barrage of complex medical, psychological, ethical, financial and legal conundrums. In turn, the attending sports medicine or cardiology physician faces an equally challenging management situation, for which little evidence-based guidance is offered. As more sporting federations promote cardiovascular pre-participation screening, it is a statistical inevitability that an increased number of high-level athletes will be diagnosed with a cardiac disease associated with SCD, and an even higher number will be evaluated and monitored under suspicion of having an inherited cardiac disease.

If one assumes the resting 12-lead electrocardiogram (ECG) to be part of the standard screening process as endorsed by the IOC then it is important to consider what constitutes appropriate management following the recognition of a particularly abnormal or bizarre ECG in an otherwise healthy, asymptomatic athlete. The problem facing cardiologists and sports physicians is that the risk stratification of patients harbouring the most common diseases associated with SCD in sport is poorly described. Our limited understanding suggests risk is exacerbated when intense training and competition are imposed on a disease carrier. Guidelines from both the ACC's 36th Bethesda Conference and the ESC recommend that athletes with an 'unequivocal' or highly 'probable' diagnosis of cardiac disease should abstain from competitive sport and vigorous training, with the exception of low-intensity activities [4, 5]. Yet, the precise risk of SCD related to continued sports participation for an athlete with an inherited cardiac disease is not clearly established, and new paradigms are emerging which emphasise individualised medical management, risk reduction and informed decision-making in the consideration of continued sports participation.

One of the weaknesses of this highly specialised area is the lack of centralised information for the clinician charged with the management of athletes with an inherited or congenital cardiac condition. Both the ACC and the ESC have dedicated sports cardiology sections. However, whilst both organisations provide consensus statements/documents for a variety of conditions and situations, many of the basic scientific underpinnings that are required to fully comprehend and apply these statements are often lacking. This ultimately means sports medicine and cardiology physicians are unable to find appropriate and up-to-date answers to the majority of their questions in a single resource.

The Medical Commission of the IOC has consistently appreciated the importance of sports cardiology in protecting the health of its athletes. In choosing to commission the *IOC Manual of Sports Cardiology*, the IOC recognises the great number of challenges team physicians face when examining the cardiac health of athletes. The *IOC Manual of Sports Cardiology* provides extensive coverage of a wide array of sports cardiology topics, ranging from exercise physiology to exercise recommendations in athletes with established cardiac pathology. Most chapters are structured with a common central theme, examining the prevalence of a particular cardiac disease, its contribution to SCD, its diagnostic criteria, clinical presentation and evaluation, risk stratification and disease management, as well as considerations in the context of exercise and physical activity recommendations.

Whether Collier in 1901 was right to disqualify his Oxford University mile runner due to apparent overdilation of the right ventricle and to impose a sea voyage on him in an attempt to limit his exercise is not for debate [1]. What is for discussion is that Collier reached his diagnosis by identifying abnormal signs, symptoms and cardiovascular features, which in his view, based on the existing literature of his era, suggested that in order to prevent an adverse cardiac event, exclusion from competitive exercise was the appropriate course of action. Ultimately, it is anticipated that with our evolving understanding of inherited cardiac diseases and their potential risk for adverse cardiac events associated with intensive sport, the sports medicine and sports cardiology community will be able to reduce the number of athletes entering the 'physiological versus pathological' grey zone. Such measures should effectively mitigate the risk of SCD in athletes with confirmed pathologic cardiac disorders through improved risk stratification, targeted management and evidence-driven recommendations for physical activity. It is our hope that this *IOC Manual of Sports Cardiology* becomes the reference textbook to support the centralisation of both scientific information and appropriate management pathways.

We thank the Medical Commission of the IOC for recognising the importance of sports cardiology and affording us the opportunity to produce this manual for the benefit of the international sports medicine community. We thank all expert contributing authors, without whom this manual would not have been possible. Finally, we thank those authors and publishers who generously gave us permission to reproduce figures or data, the sources of which are acknowledged in the legends.

Mathew G. Wilson
Jonathan A. Drezner
Sanjay Sharma

References

1 Collier, W. The effects of severe muscular exertion, sudden and prolonged, in young adolescents. *Br Med J* 1901; **1**(2094): 383–6.
2 Corrado, D., Pelliccia, A., Bjornstad, H.H. et al. Cardiovascular pre-participation screening of young competitive athletes for prevention of sudden death: proposal for a common European protocol. Consensus Statement of the Study Group of Sport Cardiology of the Working Group of Cardiac Rehabilitation and Exercise Physiology and the Working Group of Myocardial and Pericardial Diseases of the European Society of Cardiology. *Eur Heart J* 2005; **26**(5): 516–24.
3 Maron, B.J., Friedman, R.A., Kligfield, P. et al. Assessment of the 12-lead electrocardiogram as a screening test for detection of cardiovascular disease in healthy general populations of young people (12–25 years of age): a scientific statement from the American Heart Association and the American College of Cardiology. *J Am Coll Cardiol* 2014; **64**(14): 1479–514.
4 Pelliccia, A., Fagard, R., Bjornstad, H.H. et al. Recommendations for competitive sports participation in athletes with cardiovascular disease: a consensus document from the Study Group of Sports Cardiology of the Working Group of Cardiac Rehabilitation and Exercise Physiology and the Working Group of Myocardial and Pericardial Diseases of the European Society of Cardiology. *Eur Heart J* 2005; **26**(14): 1422–45.
5 Maron, B.J. and Zipes, D.P. Introduction: eligibility recommendations for competitive athletes with cardiovascular abnormalities-general considerations. *J Am Coll Cardiol* 2005; **45**(8): 1318–21.

Part 1
The Cardiovascular System

1 Anatomy and Physiology of the Heart

Keith P. George[1] and Nathan Riding[2]

[1]*Research Institute for Sport and Exercise Sciences, Liverpool John Moores University, Liverpool, UK*
[2]*Athlete Health and Performance Research Centre, ASPETAR, Qatar Orthopaedic and Sports Medicine Hospital, Doha, Qatar*

Introduction

Scientists, clinicians and the lay public have long been intrigued by the heart. As early as the 4th century BC, Aristotle suggested that the heart was the origin of intelligence in man. Our understanding has advanced from this speculation, and in this chapter we seek to summarise our current understanding of the heart's anatomy and how it links to its function. Fundamentally, this chapter serves to provide 'baseline' knowledge upon which key issues related to cardiac assessment, health, disease, adaptation and clinical decision-making may be placed in context.

Gross Cardiac Anatomy

The heart is a muscular organ roughly the size of clenched fist. As a muscle, it is in continuous motion, beating on average 2.5 billion times in a lifetime. Its primary role is to pump blood into the pulmonary circulation (from the right side of the heart) and the systemic circulation (from the left side of the heart) in order to deliver oxygen and nutrients to metabolically active tissue. Consequently, the heart is a 'double pump' of cardiac muscle (cardiomyocytes) surrounding four chambers, with other anatomic features including valves, electrical conduction pathways, major blood vessels and its own circulatory system. The heart is located within the mediastinum in the thoracic cavity, in between the lungs. The base (top) of the heart lies behind the sternum, whilst the apex (bottom) can be palpated in the left chest wall (normally on the midclavicular line around the fifth intercostal space). As well as this lateral–longitudinal orientation from base to apex, the heart is also rotated with its right side lying anteriorly. On average, the overall mass of the heart is circa 250 g in females and 300 g in males. It is important to note, however, that the position, size and shape of the heart may vary significantly from person to person.

Chambers, Walls and Valves

The heart consists of four chambers, with the left and right atria located above the left and right ventricles, respectively (Figure 1.1). Whilst anatomically and mechanically different, both left and right sides of the heart contract at the same time and produce approximately the same output or flow. Separating the two sides are the interatrial and interventricular septa. In order to prevent regurgitation or backflow of blood between chambers and to ensure flow down pressure gradients (atria to ventricles; ventricles to major arteries), there are four unidirectional valves, namely the mitral, tricuspid, pulmonary and aortic valves.

Atria serve as both reservoirs and pumps. The right atrium is a thin-walled chamber that is between 29 and 45 mm along its long axis. It receives 'oxygen-depleted' blood from the superior and inferior vena cava (systemic circulation) and the coronary sinus (from the coronary circulation). It consists of both a smooth

IOC Manual of Sports Cardiology, First Edition. Edited by Mathew G. Wilson, Jonathan A. Drezner and Sanjay Sharma.
© 2017 International Olympic Committee. Published 2017 by John Wiley & Sons, Ltd.

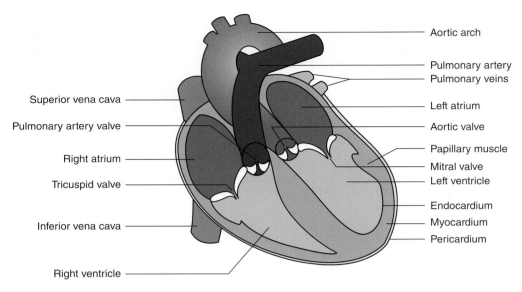

Figure 1.1 Schematic detailing the structural anatomy of the heart in the frontal plane

(posterior wall) and a rough (anterior wall) interior surface. The posterior wall receives both vena cava and contains the sinoatrial node (SA node). The anterior surface is rough due to the presence of the pectinate muscle ridges, which can act as a volume reserve. A flap-shaped auricle extending out from the anterior surface also permits an increase in atrial volume. The interatrial septum separates the right and left atria. A remnant from foetal development is the presence of a depression within the interatrial septum called the fossa ovalis. In the foetal state, this is open and allows blood to travel freely between the right and left atria, bypassing the nonfunctioning lungs; this normally closes soon after birth, but in up to 30% of adults a small opening may persist, in the form of a patent foramen ovale.

Blood flows from the right atrium into the right ventricle through the right atrioventricular orifice, which contains the tricuspid valve. The tricuspid valve comprises the annulus, three leaflets, three papillary muscles and three sets of chordae tendinae. The tricuspid valve opens when a positive pressure gradient exists between the right atrium and the right ventricle. During right ventricular contraction, with the assistance of papillary muscles and chordae tendinae, the valve prevents blood flow back into the right atrium. The three leaflets (anterior, posterior and septal) consist of sheets of dense connective tissue.

The right ventricle has a complex geometry, appearing triangular when viewed in the frontal plane and crescent-shaped when viewed transversely. Under normal loading conditions, the septum arches into the right ventricle due to the higher pressure in the left side of the heart. The right ventricle pumps into the low-pressure pulmonary system, and is thus required to do less work to achieve the same output. Consequently, right ventricular mass is approximately one-quarter that of the left ventricle, with the right ventricular free wall being 3–5 mm in thickness. The walls of the right ventricle are characterised by the presence of a series of irregular ridges called trabeculae carneae. The moderator band, a single specialised trabeculae from the anterior papillary muscle to the interventricular septum, acts as the primary conduction pathway of the right bundle branch. Blood leaves the right ventricle via the outflow tract through the unidirectional pulmonary artery valve, at a pressure of around 25 mmHg.

Reoxygenated blood returns to the heart via four pulmonary veins that drain into the left atrium. The left atrium also contains an auricle, high up in the atrial chamber and in close proximity to the free wall of the left ventricle. Whilst internally the atrial surface is smooth, the left atrial appendage is lined by pectinate muscles. The left atrium opens into the left ventricle through the mitral orifice and the mitral valve. The mitral valve contains two leaflets and is, again, a passive unidirectional valve that opens when there is a positive pressure gradient from the left atrium to the left ventricle. During left ventricular contraction, the mitral valve, chordae tendinae and two papillary muscles prevent backflow of blood into the left atrium. The left ventricle is bullet-shaped, being almost circular at the mitral valve and rapidly tapering at the apex. The interventricular septum separates the two ventricles and is as thick as the left ventricular free wall. Left ventricular wall thickness (normal range 6–12 mm) is larger than that of the right ventricle due to the higher pressures and the greater work that is undertaken to generate the same flow. Near the level of the aortic valve orifice, however, the septal wall thins. This section, called the septum membranaceum, is fibrous and encases the atrioventricular conduction bundle. The left ventricle contains a network of trabeculae in the lower third of the chamber; the presence of excessive and deep intertrabecular recesses is termed left ventricular hypertrabeculation. Blood is ejected from the left ventricle through the three-cusped unidirectional aortic valve (positioned in the aortic root) into the ascending aorta. The aortic root also includes the sinuses of Valsalva and the sinotubular junction. There are three sinuses of Valsalva, with the coronary arteries arising from the left and right sinuses. Externally, the ventricles are separated by the anterior and posterior interventricular sulci, which are shallow grooves on the surface of the heart.

Tissue Layers

The mass of the heart is often referred to simply as the 'myocardium', but this is an oversimplification of the layers of muscle and connective tissues. The outer layer consists of connective tissue and is called the pericardium. This is a thin fibroserous sac enclosing the heart and has two main parts: the fibrous pericardium and the serous pericardium. The serous pericardium consists of two membranes, in between which is a small amount of serous fluid, which helps lubricate them. The pericardium serves to afford some protection and stability to the heart. The next level is the epicardium, which contains a layer of mesothelial cells, beneath which is connective and adipose tissue. Whilst adhering to the heart, it also acts as the deeper serous layer of the pericardium, often referred to as the 'visceral pericardium'. The next layer is the myocardium, which contains most of the cardiomyocyte mass (95%) and is thus responsible for the pumping action of the heart. Fibre architecture in the myocardium plays a fundamental role in the complex mechanical activation that underpins cardiac function. Cardiac fibres are organised in a spiral or helical formation around the cardiac chambers. Lining the interior of the heart is the endocardium, which consists of subendothelial connective tissue and a thin layer of epithelium. This is continuous with the epithelium of the great blood vessels.

Coronary Circulation

The left and right coronary arteries arise from the left and right sinuses of Valsalva and lie upon the heart's surface as epicardial coronary vessels. The left main coronary artery soon branches into the left anterior descending (LAD) artery and the circumflex artery. The LAD artery appears to be a direct continuation of the left main artery and lies within the anterior interventricular sulcus, running down towards the apex. It supplies oxygenated blood to the interventricular septum, most of the right and left bundle branches and the anterior walls of both ventricles. The circumflex artery travels left around the posterior surface of the heart, supplying blood to the left atrium and the posterior aspect of the left ventricle. These arteries divide into increasingly smaller arteries, which then progress inwards to penetrate the epicardium and supply blood to the myocardium. Arising from the right coronary sinus of Valsalva, the right coronary artery runs along the right atrioventricular groove, which then arches down towards the inferior surface of the heart. It branches off into the posterior descending artery and the right marginal artery, serving the right atrium, the right ventricle and the inferior part of the left ventricle.

Coronary blood flow occurs mainly during myocardial relaxation (diastole) as a result of the increased resistance to flow in compressed arteries during myocardial contraction (systole). The myocardium extracts the greatest volume of oxygen of any given muscle bed in the human body. Following the distribution of oxygen and nutrients to the cardiac muscle, the now deoxygenated blood returns to the heart through the coronary veins. Three main tributaries (great cardiac vein, middle cardiac vein, small cardiac vein) connect to the coronary sinus, travelling along the posterior aspect of the coronary sulcus and emptying into the right atrium. Anterior veins, which drain the right ventricle, bypass the coronary sinus and directly attach to the right atrium.

Electrical Conduction in the Heart

Action Potentials and Pacemaker Cells

Cardiomyocytes require an electrical action potential (Figure 1.2) to initiate mechanical events. The onset of a heartbeat, or cardiac cycle, normally begins via the SA node in the upper right wall of the right atrium. The SA node contains pacemaker cells that uniquely self-depolarise and set off an electrical signal that is propagated across the entire myocardium. The SA node does not have a flat resting membrane potential; rather, this increases slowly, before reaching a threshold of depolarisation (Figure 1.2). Nonpacemaker cells have a stable resting membrane potential. For example, an atrial cardiomyocyte has a resting membrane potential of about -90 mV. When activated, an initial rapid depolarisation to 10 mV occurs, largely due to a change in membrane permeability and a rapid influx of Na^+. There then follows a short, small repolarisation and a plateau (near 0 mV) that last for 200–300 ms. The action potential concludes with a rapid repolarisation back to resting membrane potential.

Whilst the SA node can self-depolarise without any external neural control, in the healthy heart nerve endings innervate it via sympathetic and parasympathetic branches of the autonomic nervous system. The heart rate slows at rest under the influence of the parasympathetic vagal nerve activity; it increases (e.g. during exercise) when the vagal 'break' is withdrawn and sympathetic 'accelerator' activity to the SA node increases. Whilst there are other pacemaker cells in the heart, notably at the atrioventricular (AV) node, if the SA node is functioning properly this will initiate a standard pathway of depolarisation around the heart that underpins optimal mechanical activation and blood flow (so called sinus rhythm).

Conduction

The initial action potentials in the SA node rapidly spread to the surrounding atrial cardiomyocytes via gap junctions and atrial conductance pathways (Figure 1.3) to initiate atrial contraction. Importantly, in the healthy heart, electrical activity is prevented from travelling from the atria straight to the ventricles by atrioventricular collagen rings. Electrical activity eventually reaches the AV node in the inferior aspect of the interatrial septum. There is a brief delay in electrical propagation and mechanical activation to enable the complete filling of the ventricles.

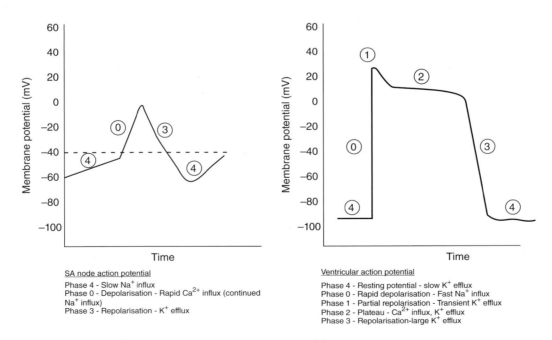

SA node action potential
Phase 4 - Slow Na^+ influx
Phase 0 - Depolarisation - Rapid Ca^{2+} influx (continued Na^+ influx)
Phase 3 - Repolarisation - K^+ efflux

Ventricular action potential
Phase 4 - Resting potential - slow K^+ efflux
Phase 0 - Rapid depolarisation - Fast Na^+ influx
Phase 1 - Partial repolarisation - Transient K^+ efflux
Phase 2 - Plateau - Ca^{2+} influx, K^+ efflux
Phase 3 - Repolarisation-large K^+ efflux

Figure 1.2 Schematic of SA node and ventricular action potentials

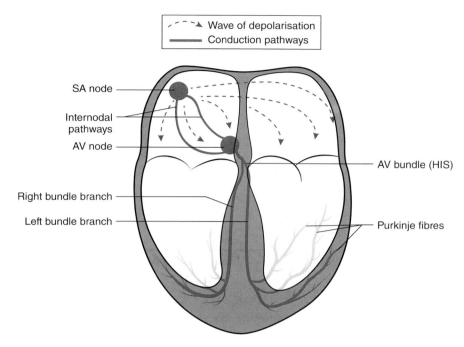

Figure 1.3 Schematic detailing the electrical conductance pathway of the heart from the SA node to the Purkinje fibres

Cell-to-cell electrical progression cannot happen quickly enough for depolarisation and mechanical activation to occur in synchrony in the larger mass of the ventricles, so a conduction system facilitates this process, ensuring the normal and effective contraction of the heart. From the AV node, the action potential travels through the atrioventricular bundle (bundle of His) and splits into the left and right bundle branches, extending down the interventricular septum towards the apex. At this point, these branches become Purkinje fibres, curving around the right and left ventricles back towards the atria along the ventricular walls. The Purkinje fibres facilitate the fastest electrical conductance in the heart to ensure the larger ventricular myocyte mass depolarises and contracts together. Ventricular action potentials are very similar to those in the atria.

12-Lead ECG

Given that every single cardiomyocyte is recruited every heartbeat, this electrical activity can be recorded on the surface of the chest wall, via an electrocardiogram (ECG). A single-lead ECG has a well-recognised pattern and nomenclature (Figure 1.4). The P-wave reflects the summation of all the atrial myocyte action potentials. Its magnitude is small, due to the smaller myocardial mass in the atria, and the duration is circa 100 ms, reflecting quite slow cell-to-cell propagation. From the end of the P-wave to the onset of the QRS, complex electrical activity is absent, reflecting slow propagation of electrical activity through the AV node. The QRS complex is the summation of both ventricle action potentials. The duration is circa 100 ms, but the magnitude is much greater than in the atria, reflecting greater myocardial mass. Consequently, the QRS complex reflects a much more rapid spread of electrical depolarisation due to the speed of the ventricular conduction pathways. After the QRS, there is another isoelectric phase, the ST segment. Finally, the T-wave represents ventricular repolarisation and is longer in duration but lower in peak magnitude than depolarisation. The repolarisation of the atria is lost within the QRS complex. Alterations in the magnitude, duration and/ or orientation of any PQRST component may reflect physiological and/or pathological changes in cardiac structure, function or neural control; this will be discussed in Chapters 10, 11, 12 and 40.

The 12-lead ECG is generated from 10 electrodes, providing a comprehensive electrical overview of the heart. Six limb leads are generated from four electrodes placed on the left and right wrists and the left and right ankles. These leads reflect electrical activity in the frontal plane, with I, II and III being bipolar and aVR, aVL and aVF unipolar. The remaining six leads reflect specific locations around the sternum and left

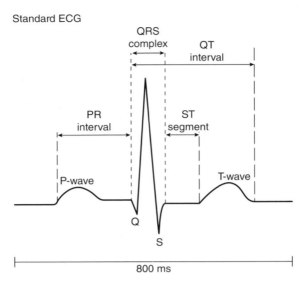

Figure 1.4 Schematic of a single-lead ECG with PQRST, and intervals notated

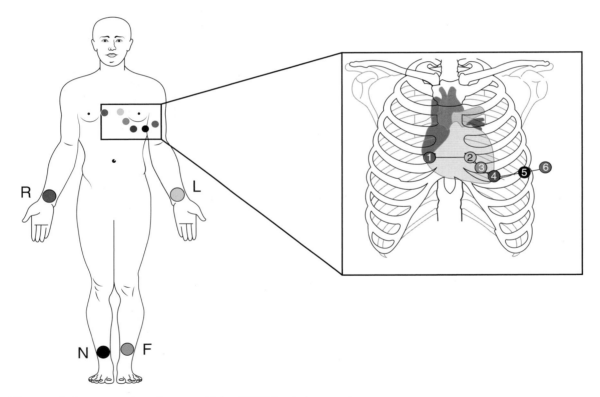

Figure 1.5 Demonstration of correct 12-lead ECG lead placement

side of the chest wall. These leads are unipolar, reflect activity in the horizontal plane and cover electrical activity originating from the right (V1 and V2) across to the left (V5 and V6) sides of the heart (Figure 1.5).

Structure of the Cardiomyocyte

Cardiomyocytes make up the vast majority of the tissue mass in the myocardium. As muscle cells, their primary role is to transform an electrical signal into mechanical contraction. In comparison to smooth and skeletal muscle cells, cardiomyocytes are shorter, normally have only one centrally located nuclei and have significant branching. Branching of the cardiomyocytes allows them to adjoin at their ends to form a network of fibres, which are tightly connected via specialised junctions called intercalated disks. These are irregular thickenings of the sarcolemma and contain desmosomes, which are responsible for cell-to-cell adhesion and gap junctions, permitting the rapid and low-resistance spread of electrical activity from one cell to another. The fibres are wrapped and bound together by connective tissue.

Like skeletal muscle, the sarcomere is the contractile unit of the cardiomyocyte. It contains long strands of (thick) myosin and interdigitated (thin) actin filaments, in addition to troponin and tropomyosin. The contraction of the sarcomere occurs between the Z-lines via a complex set of chemical and mechanical events referred to as the 'sliding filament theory'. In essence, in the presence of an electrical signal, Ca^{2+} is released from the sarcoplasmic reticulum into the intracellular space and chemically links actin and myosin via crossbridges. Repetitive coupling and uncoupling of these crossbridges, powered chemically by the hydrolysis of adenosine triphosphate, results in the movement of the actin strands towards the centre of the sarcomere. The result is a shortening of the cardiomyocyte and tension development.

Cardiac Function

Cardiac Cycle

After each cardiomyocyte receives the electrical signal being propagated cell to cell and via conduction pathways, it generates its own action potential, which sets off the metabolic and mechanical cascade of contraction coupling and tension development. Each cell has a refractory period (both absolute and relative) in which further electrical stimulation will not result in signal transduction and cell contraction, preventing the heart muscle from tetanizing. The rapid and coordinated electrical signal transduction that produces the ECG ensures that contractile function and relaxation also occur in a coordinated and synchronous fashion. The transfer from electrical signal through cellular tension development to organ contraction and relaxation is quite complex, but results in controlled, regulated and matched (left to right ventricle) outflow. The parameters of interest to overall cardiac function are electrical signal, tension development, pressure change and gradient and, finally, flow. All of these are described together very neatly in the cardiac cycle represented in Figure 1.6.

We will describe briefly events in the left side of the heart. The time course of events is the same in the right side, but pressure changes are lower. Starting at the left of Figure 1.6, the primary stimulus for the cascade

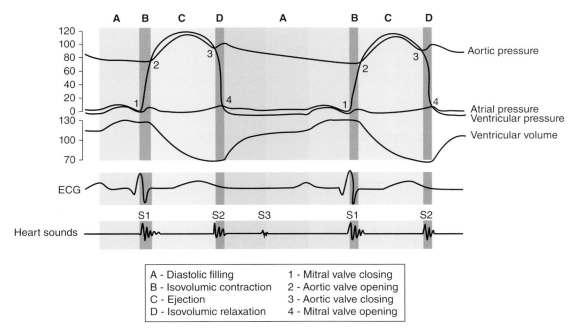

Figure 1.6 Schematic of the cardiac cycle in the left ventricle

of events in the cardiac cycle is the electrical action potential that makes up the ECG, and here we start at the P-wave. The P-wave is the summation of action potentials in the atria and leads to a small pressure rise in the atria. This pressure rise results in a positive pressure gradient between the left atrium and left ventricle, causing blood flow into the left ventricle. This effectively 'tops up' left ventricular volume. Flow into the left ventricle as a result of atrial contraction is partially related to atrial contractility, and also to compliance of the ventricle. The short PR interval, in which electrical activity slows in the AV node and no cellular contraction occurs, allows this ventricular filling to finish before the signal for ventricular contraction (the QRS) occurs. The onset of the QRS complex and ventricular contraction is regarded as the end of diastole (the filling period) and the onset of systole (the contraction period). Rapid electrical conductance in the ventricles sees a rapid rise in ventricular pressure. Initially, this takes ventricular pressure above atrial pressure and the mitral valve closes. The rapid rise now occurs in a closed chamber, so it is called isovolumic contraction. This period ends when ventricular pressure overtakes aortic pressure and the pressure gradient opens the aortic valve. Pressure continues to rise in the ventricle and aorta as there is a large and rapid ejection of blood into the aorta and ventricular volume drops. After hitting a peak pressure (~120 mmHg at rest), both ventricular and aortic pressure begin to drop as the ventricular myocyte enters repolarisation and relaxation. The end of the ejection phase comes when ventricular pressure dips below the aortic pressure and the aortic valve closes. This represents the end of systole and the beginning of diastole. Now ventricular pressure is dropping rapidly, but in a closed chamber, and this period is called isovolumic relaxation. It is not until the ventricular pressure falls below atrial pressure that the pressure gradient allows the mitral valve to open. At this point, a rapid (early) filling of the ventricle occurs as the ventricle untwists, lengthens and radially expands. The rebound relaxation from the prior contraction causes a suction effect and the ventricular volume rises rapidly. After this early filling, the ventricle enters a short period of diastasis, in which little blood flows across the mitral valve as pressure equalises in the atria and ventricles. This period is noticeable at rest but is lost quite quickly during any increase in heart rate, as diastole is preferentially shortened over systole. At the end of diastasis, we get another P-wave and the whole cycle starts again.

Heart Sounds

One of the interesting and important clinical phenomena associated with the cardiac cycle is the development of heart sounds (Figure 1.6). Sound in the heart is generated by movement and friction but is largely insulated from the outside environment. The characteristic heart sounds associated with the cardiac cycle are biphasic and are referred to globally as 'lup-dup', which reflects a low-pitched first sound and a higher-pitched, quicker second sound. The first sound occurs at the onset of systole and is associated with mitral and triscuspid valve closure and then the rapid acceleration of blood flow out of the ventricles with contraction. The second heart sound occurs at the beginning of diastole as the aortic and pulmonary artery valves shut. Valve closures occur a matter of milliseconds later in the right side of the heart, but occasionally subtle splitting of the first and second heart sounds can be detected. Third and fourth heart sounds can be heard in some cases during rapid early ventricular filling and atrial contraction, respectively. See Chapter 36 for further discussion of cardiac murmurs.

Intrinsic and Extrinsic Regulation of Cardiac Function

As well as implicit contractile properties resulting directly from electrical activation, the myocardium also possesses elastic properties that influence tension and subsequent contractility. When the myocardium is lengthened during filling, it is said to have a level of 'preload' present. Increasing preload stretches the myocardium and increases tension. An increase in tension will result in an increase in contractile force, and thus a greater output of flow (stroke volume). This has been referred to as the 'Starling law' after one of the authors of the original concept that within physiological ranges contractility or force produced by the myocardium is increased if a stretch is placed in the myocardium beforehand. Later work deduced that this length–tension relationship is also apparent for the right ventricle.

Whilst there can be some effect of heart rate on cardiomyocyte contractility (e.g. a brief increase in contractility with increased rate or a brief increase in contractility after a heart-rate pause), these effects are normally small and temporary. A second key determinant of cardiac contractility is afterload: the resistance against which the heart has to work in order to generate flow or output. If systemic blood pressure rises then ventricular pressure must rise further to generate a pressure gradient between the ventricle and aorta and so allow outflow (stroke volume). With increased systemic arterial blood pressure comes a longer, potentially slower pressure rise to aortic valve opening (isovolumic contraction) and thus a smaller ejection time, limiting stroke volume.

It is important to remember that intrinsic control of cardiac contractility and function cannot be easily 'divorced' from extrinsic regulatory processes. Together, intrinsic and extrinsic factors exert an exquisite level of control and moderation over cardiac function that allows humans to meet their circulatory needs and maintain physiological homeostasis. Extrinsic input to the heart comes in the form of neural and hormonal factors, of which neural control is the more important because of the immediacy of feedback and response. The autonomic nervous system, through its components the parasympathetic and sympathetic systems, is a key neural agent of change in the heart. Both the parasympathetic and the sympathetic system arise in the medulla in the brain, but they have polemic effects. The parasympathetic system, via the vagal nerve, innervates the SA node with increased neural activity, serving to slow heart rate. At rest, most humans are under dominant vagal tone; as intrinsic SA-node discharge will result in a heart rate of about 100 beats. min^{-1}. The sympathetic nervous system also innervates the SA node, and increased neural activity – along with vagal withdrawal – serves to increase heart rate, which is important in circumstances such as exercise. The sympathetic nervous system, however, also innervates cardiomyocytes in the atria and ventricles and can exert effects outside of a change in heart rate. Specifically, sympathetic stimulation will increase contractility. The same thing occurs with an increase in circulating catecholamines. Alterations in contractility (or inotropic state) are likely caused by changes in the rate of Ca^{2+} binding to the contractile proteins.

Pressure–Volume Relationships and the Law of Laplace

When dealing with the functional role of the heart, many are interested simply in cardiac output ($\dot{Q}$) and its direct determinants (stroke volume × heart rate). This makes intuitive sense, as flow or output is the most important end point of cardiac structure and function. It is clear from this chapter, however, that cardiac structure, function and control are complicated and that any representation of cardiac activity should also reflect changes in preload, afterload and contractility. The work the heart does in producing flow against a significant pressure resistance has led to the adoption of rate pressure product (RPP; heart rate × mean arterial pressure (MAP)) as an indirect assessment of myocardial oxygen use. Other scientists and clinicians calculate cardiac power as a measure of cardiac work: $\dot{Q}$ × MAP.

Stroke work of the heart is often represented by a pressure–volume loop (Figure 1.7). In a pressure–volume loop, the entire cardiac cycle is represented, as are the maximum and minimum volumes and pressures.

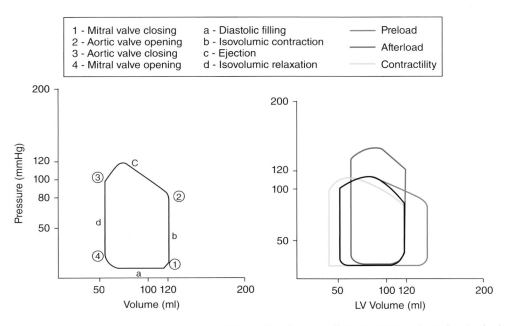

Figure 1.7 Schematic of cardiac pressure–volume loops, showing the effect of changes in preload, afterload and contractility

The area inside the loop is directly representative of the work performed by the heart. Such loops have been constructed in healthy humans, as have a range of cardiovascular pathologies, in an attempt to fully describe and understand the functional consequences of the disease processes at play, and also potentially the value of drug or device interventions.

Finally, the law of Laplace has relevance to vascular and cardiac biology, based upon observations deduced from cylinders and vessels. Simply put, the adapted law of Laplace for cardiac chambers states that wall stress (tension) is the product of transmural pressure (intra- versus extraventricular pressure) and the radius of the chamber, all divided by the thickness of the cardiac chamber wall. In endurance athletes, acute exercise-related increases in preload and thus chamber radius may be a stimulus for chamber dilation, which, according to the law of Laplace, will lead to an increase in 'end-diastolic wall stress'. To offset this increase in wall stress, the ventricular wall of the athlete likely increases in thickness in direct proportion to the increase in chamber dimension.

Conclusion

This chapter serves to summarise the basic cardiac structure, electrical activation, function and control in order to allow later chapters to advance discussion of both physiological adaptations to physical activity and pathological manifestations induced by inherited, congenital or acquired heart disease.

2 The Vascular System

N. Tim Cable

Department of Sport Science, Aspire Academy, Doha, Qatar and Research Institute for Sport and Exercise Sciences, Liverpool John Moores University, Liverpool, UK

Introduction

This chapter provides an overview of the circulatory system by reviewing key structures and processes in the vascular and lymphatic systems. The extrinsic and intrinsic control of vascular resistance are discussed, and the physiology of the endothelial control of vasodilation is outlined. The chapter concludes with a synopsis of the integrated control of blood flow and pressure. These topics are fundamental to the understanding of cardiovascular adaptation to physiology stressors such as exercise and the changes that occur with pathology.

The Circulatory Systems

The circulatory system, also called the cardiovascular system, is a closed organ system that permits blood to circulate and transport nutrients, oxygen, carbon dioxide and blood cells to and from the tissues of the body in order to maintain homeostasis. The circulatory system comprises two separate systems: the cardiovascular and lymphatic systems, which distribute blood and circulate lymph, respectively. The cardiovascular system consists of the heart, blood vessels and blood and the lymphatic system of lymph, lymph nodes and lymph vessels. The primary function of the cardiovascular system is the support of metabolism, immune-protection and, through an integration of cardiac output and peripheral resistance, blood pressure. The lymphatic system acts as a reservoir for the return of filtered blood plasma to the blood following the process of capillary filtration. An accessory function is that of immune function, as, like the blood, lymph fluid contains many white blood cells.

The Systemic Circulation

The systemic circulation consists of the arterial circulation, which carries oxygenated blood away from the heart towards the tissues, and the venous circulation, which transports deoxygenated blood back to the heart (Figure 2.1). Blood leaves the heart via the aorta and travels to the tissue via conduit vessels and smaller resistance vessels before reaching the capillaries to allow for gaseous and nutrient exchange. Waste products and carbon dioxide diffuse out of the cells into the microcirculation and, via venous capillaries, venules and venae cavae, the blood re-enters the right atrium of the heart.

Blood leaves the left ventricle of the heart via the aorta, which along its length is classified as the ascending, aortic arch, thoracic and abdominal aorta. The aorta is an elastic artery that is quite distensible, and as such is capable of propagating a pulse wave along its length via the cardiac cycle. The outer layer of the aorta contains a network of tiny blood vessels, the vasa vasorum, and the middle layer (tunica media) contains a mix of smooth-muscle cells and elastic matrix; together, these structures occupy the large majority of the vessel wall. The smooth muscle does not operate to alter the radius of the vessel, but rather, along with the

IOC Manual of Sports Cardiology, First Edition. Edited by Mathew G. Wilson, Jonathan A. Drezner and Sanjay Sharma.
© 2017 International Olympic Committee. Published 2017 by John Wiley & Sons, Ltd.

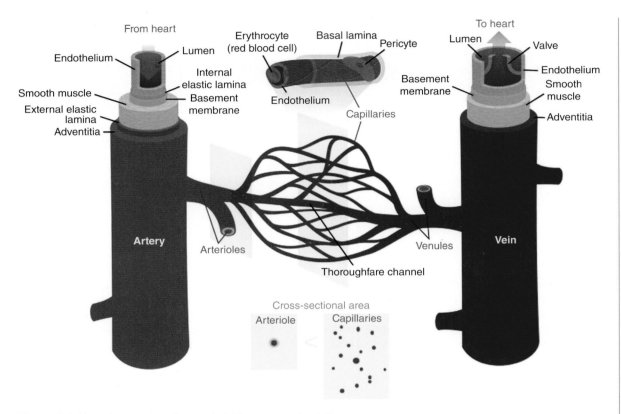

Figure 2.1 Vascular structure from arterial to venous circulation

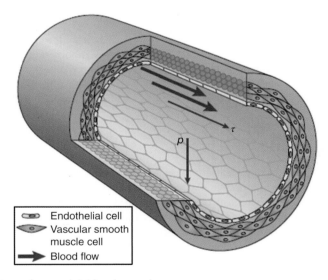

Figure 2.2 Outline structure of a conduit blood vessel

elastic matrix, serves to increase the stiffness of the wall when activated. On average, the intraluminal diameter of the aorta is of the order of 30 mm in females and 35 mm in males.

Nutrient-rich blood is supplied to the peripheral vascular beds through large conduit arteries (Figure 2.2). These elastic vessels split into smaller muscular conduit arteries and then resistance vessels (or arterioles), before splitting into capillaries. Conduit arteries vary in size, from the large carotid artery (5–7 cm) to the relatively small radial artery (2–3 cm). These arteries are made up of three distinct layers: the tunica adventitia (outer layer), the tunica media (middle layer) and the tunica intima (inner layer). The adventitia is made entirely of connective tissue and contains the neural supply to the vessels. The tunica media is composed mainly of smooth-muscle cells arranged in a circular pattern. The contraction or relaxation of this layer controls the calibre of the vessels, which in turn determines the resistance to blood flow. The tunica intima comprises a single layer of squamous cells, known as the endothelium. This monolayer coats the entire vascular tree and is the direct interface between hemodynamic flow and the vessel wall. Due to its location, the endothelium is directly exposed to changes in blood flow and shear stress.

Further down the arterial tree, conduit vessels branch to become arterioles, which have muscular walls consisting of only a few layers of smooth muscle. Given their diameter and their response to neural and humoural stimulation, these vessels are the primary site of vascular resistance. They give rise to the capillaries, which connect the arterioles to the venules. Capillaries are the smallest blood vessels in the body, with a diameter of 5–10 μm, and are therefore perfectly structured for the exchange of gases, nutrients and metabolites between the blood and the tissues.

Blood leaving the capillary networks enters the venous circulation via the venules (7–50 μm diameter). Venules are structured with an inner lining of endothelial cells, a middle layer of poorly developed muscle tissue and an outer layer of fibrous connective tissue, which is the thickest structure in veins. The middle layer is very porous, such that fluid and blood cells can migrate through its walls. Venules unite to form veins, which ultimately function to return blood from the tissues and organs to the heart. Whilst the veins process larger diameters then venules, they are structurally the same, with a thin middle layer of muscular tissues (tunica media), which collapses when the vessels are not filled with blood. Given the low density of smooth muscle, these vessels do not have a significant contractile function, and as a consequence can become engorged with blood. Indeed, the veins can contain up to 60% of total blood volume during times of extended standing or sitting or on exposure to passive heating. The return of blood to the heart is facilitated by activation of the skeletal muscle pump and by the respiratory pump as a consequence of the work of breathing. Both these mechanisms advance the column of blood forward to the right atrium of the heart, and any back flow of blood is inhibited by the existence of intraluminal values that close during the period of diastole. The veins in the upper body give rise to the superior vena cava, and those of the lower body to the inferior vena cava. Both transport blood directly into the right atrium of the heart.

The Lymphatic System

Like to the vascular system, the lymphatic system consists of a network of lymphatic vessels that carry lymph fluid directionally towards the heart. As the blood circulates through the porous capillary networks or pools within porous veins, plasma and cells 'leak' out into the extravascular spaces to form the interstitial fluid. Each day, approximately 20 l of blood undergoes capillary filtration, a process that removes plasma whilst leaving the blood cells contained in the blood vessels. Of the 20 l of filtered plasma, around 17 l is directly reabsorbed into the blood vessels, leaving 3 l in the interstitial fluid. When this interstitial fluid enters the initial lymphatic vessels of the lymphatic system, lymph is formed. The lymph fluid moves along the lymphatic network by intrinsic vessel contraction or external compression via muscle contractions, and ultimately the lymph vessels empty into the lymphatic ducts, which drain into the subclavian veins near their junction with the jugular vein. In this manner, the 3 l of filtered plasma is returned to the vascular circulation, replacing fluid that was previously lost in the periphery. As in the venous circulation, unidirectional flow is ensured by a series of intraluminal valves. Lymph circulates via lymph nodes, which are major sites of lymphocyte concentration and act to trap foreign particles and filter the lymph before the return of the fluid to the blood circulation. The lymphatic system also plays a major role in immune function, but that is beyond the focus of this chapter.

Control of Blood Flow

Regional blood flow is adjusted according to changes in the resistance to flow through blood vessels, which in turn is dependent on the diameter of the vessel, the physical characteristics of the blood (viscosity, laminar versus turbulent flow) and extravascular forces acting upon the vasculature. Of these, changes in vessel diameter are quantitatively the most important for the regulation of flow, since resistance to flow varies with the fourth power of the radius of the vessel. Consequently, very small changes in the diameter of a resistance vessel can initiate dramatic fluctuations in blood flow to the dependent tissues.

Depending on their functional requirements, tissues have varying ranges of blood flow. The rate of flow through organs such as the brain and liver remains relatively constant, even under conditions of pronounced

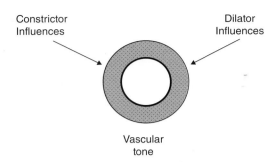

Vasoconstrictor and vasodilator influences
acting on arteries and veins determine their
state of vascular tone, which is the balance
between constrictor and dilator influences.

Figure 2.3 Vascular tone as the product of vasodilator and vasoconstrictor influences

changes in both arterial pressure and cardiac output. In more compliant vascular beds, such as the skeletal muscle, skin and splanchnic regions (gastrointestinal tract (GIT) and spleen), rates of perfusion can vary markedly depending upon the prevailing physiological conditions.

The regulation of vessel diameter, the vascular tone, is governed by the relative degree of vasoconstrictor (smooth-muscle contraction) and vasodilator (smooth-muscle relaxation) tone and the net balance between the two (see Figure 2.3). There are many factors that mediate vasoconstrictor and dilator tone, which can be broadly classified as those local (intrinsic) to the blood vessel and those extrinsic (largely neural and humoural) to it.

Neural Regulation

The sympathetic nervous system influences vasomotor tone in a number of vascular beds. All blood vessels except capillaries are innervated, with the result that stimulation is dependent upon the distribution and density of the various subclasses of adrenoceptors. The small arteries and arterioles of the skin, kidney and splanchnic regions receive a dense supply of sympathetic noradrenergic vasoconstrictor fibres, whereas those of skeletal muscle and the brain have a relatively sparse supply of these fibres. When stimulated, noradrenaline is released from postganglionic fibres, which combine with α-adrenoceptors to initiate constriction of the smooth muscle surrounding the lumen of the vessel, leading to increased resistance to blood flow and thereby reduced tissue perfusion.

The skeletal muscle and the splanchnic, renal and cutaneous vascular beds are the major determinants of changes in systematic vascular resistance, which is under sympathetic noradrenergic control. If sympathetic activity to resting limb muscles is completely abolished, there is a two- to threefold increase in blood flow; conversely, when noradrenergic activity is maximal, resting blood flow is reduced by 75%. During times of high sympathetic output, any vasoconstrictor activity in skeletal muscle mediated through less densely populated α-adrenoceptors may actually be modulated by the release of local factors from active skeletal muscle. Adenosine, adenine, nucleotides, potassium, hydrogen ions and extracellular osmolarity may directly inhibit smooth muscle-cell contraction by interrupting the vasoconstrictor impulses of sympathetic nerves.

The resistance vessels in the arterial circulation of skeletal muscle possess β-adrenoceptors, which have a high affinity for circulating adrenaline. As the exercise effort increases in duration and intensity, adrenaline concentration increases. This increase leads to stimulation of β-receptors, causing relaxation of the smooth muscles and a reduction of vascular resistance in skeletal muscle, and therefore an increase in flow.

Controversy still exists as to the contribution of the cholinergic vasodilator pathway to exercise hyperaemia. Although reflex cholinergic vasodilator responses have been observed in humans during severe mental stress, it remains unclear whether such a mechanism exerts an influence on muscle blood flow during exercise. Cholinergic activity is thought to increase muscle blood flow during the initial 10 seconds of exercise, existing primarily as an anticipatory response to exercise initiated by the cholinergic vasodilatory pathway in the motor cortex.

Local Regulating Mechanisms

Local autoregulation of the tone of peripheral blood vessel is achieved by a combination of factors. These relate to myogenic mechanisms, local metabolic factors and the release of paracrine hormones from the endothelium.

In small arteries and arterioles, the myogenic mechanism is intrinsic to the smooth muscle. An increase in transmural pressure (the difference in pressure across the vessel wall) due to a sudden increase in blood pressure causes a stretch of the smooth muscle. This results in the opening of ion channels, which causes a depolarisation, leading to smooth-muscle contraction. The consequent decrease in lumen diameter ultimately causes a reduction in blood flow. The reverse is true when the smooth muscle relaxes: the same ion channels close, leading to a vasodilation. This intrinsic mechanism operates in an attempt to maintain a constancy of blood flow in a particular vessel, with vessels in the splanchnic and renal circulations particularly sensitive to this type of control.

There are various substances either required for cellular metabolism or produced as a consequence of it that have a direct effect on the diameter of blood vessels and therefore constitute the metabolic autoregulation of peripheral blood flow. This autoreulatory control is of great significance as it allows the precise matching of local blood flow to momentary nutritive requirements of the tissue. These local responses can completely override any background neurogenic constrictor effects that are mediated by the autonomic nervous system.

Vasodilation is evoked by a fall in the partial pressure of oxygen (pO_2) in the local vascular bed. Thus, when the pO_2 decreases as metabolic activity in the region accelerates, smooth-muscle relaxation occurs and a vasodilator response is initiated. Various mechanisms have been proposed to explain this process, including a direct effect of oxygen on the vascular smooth muscle. In addition, as metabolism increases, there are local increases in the partial pressure of carbon dioxide (pCO_2) and the concentration of hydrogen ions (H^+), both of which cause a vasodilator response (the cerebral circulation being particularly responsive to these changes). In the skeletal muscle, vasodilation is associated with the accumulation of lactate, but this effect is probably mediated indirectly by changes in plasma pH. It remains unclear how these metabolites promote vasodilation, but their release during muscle contraction has a similar time course to the release of adenosine and its nucleotides, which are known to be potent vasodilator substances. Potassium is also a powerful vasodilatory substrate that is released during muscle contraction and has been shown to evoke skeletal muscle hypaemia. However, the precise mechanism by which changes in these factors mediate vasodilation and the exact time course of their action remain to be elucidated.

One possible mechanism of action is that these metabolites and ions mediate their response through a direct effect on the innermost layer of an artery. Endothelial cells are located at the interface between the blood and the vascular wall, and surprisingly they were once considered a passive layer of static cells. It is now well established that the endothelium serves as a dynamically active modulator of vasomotor tone and atherogenic development through the secretion of a number of paracine substances (substances that are released and act only locally) that play a key role in regulating vascular tone, cell growth, platelet and leukocyte inhibition, vasoregulation and vasoprotection. Indeed, endothelial dysfunction is associated with a number of lifestyle-related pathologies and increased risk of cardiovascular disease (CVD). The corollary is that the endothelium plays a key role in the healthy vascular adaptations associated with increased physical activity and exercise training.

In response to various stimuli, the endothelium produces a number of paracrine substances that have marked vasomotor effects. The three most important of these are nitric oxide (NO), endothelin (ET-1) and prostacyclin ($PG1_2$). NO and $PG1_2$ promote smooth-muscle relaxation and a vasodilatory response, whereas endothelin causes smooth-muscle contraction and vasoconstriction.

Nitric Oxide

It was first demonstrated in the 1980s that the endothelium is essential for vasodilation, when it was observed that acetylcholine (ACh) stimulated the endothelium to release an agent that relaxed the vascular smooth muscle. When this was repeated in blood vessels with the endothelium removed, the response to ACh was a constriction. In time, it was discovered that this effect was mediated by a labile factor known as endothelium-derived relaxing factor (EDRF), which required an intact endothelium; EDRF was later identified as the inorganic molecule NO. Furthermore, it was demonstrated that vascular endothelial cells synthesise NO from arginine, using the enzyme complex nitric oxide synthase (eNOS), located in the endothelium (Figure 2.4).

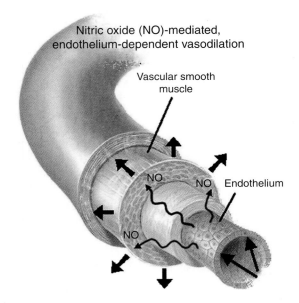

Figure 2.4 Endothelial release of NO and diffusion into smooth muscle

The importance of NO release to the endothelium was confirmed by studies that inhibited the eNOS complex. In the absence of NO, baseline blood flow was reduced by 50% and resistance to blood flow through the tissue was markedly increased. These observations demonstrated the importance of NO as an essential factor released from the endothelium, allowing for tonic vasomotor control and vasodilation in humans. It is also now recognised that arterial remodelling is shear stress- and NO-dependent and acts in a manner that homeostatically regulates wall shear stress. This provides direct evidence that the dilator action of endothelium-derived NO contributes to the control of basal and stimulated regional blood flow in humans, and therefore suggests that an impairment of NO production might account for the abnormalities in vascular reactivity that characterise a wide variety of disease states.

Mechanisms that Mediate Vasodilator Function

Endothelial shear stress is created by the frictional flow of blood on the endothelial surface of the arterial wall. The nature of flow through a vessel is dependent on the velocity of flow and on any obstructions. Flow is usually characterised as either laminar or turbulent, with 'laminar flow' referring to a smooth, undisturbed flow. Turbulent blood flow occurs at sites of vessel bifurcation, where there is vascular damage or where blood-flow velocities are high. The cardiac cycle, and therefore the pulsatile nature of arterial blood flow, provokes constant changes in the direction and magnitude of flow. Usually, in straight arterial segments, shear stress is pulsatile and unidirectional and creates a constant mechanical deformation of the vessel wall. In contrast, in regions where disturbed laminar flow occurs, pulsatile flow generates an oscillatory shear stress, creating a greater deformation.

The mechanical deformation resulting from shear stress and from the strain associated with stretch of the vessel wall is detected by a mechanosensor, which allows the influx of extracellular Ca^{2+} and Na^+ ions into the endothelial cell through the opening of ion gates. This initiates a variety of signalling systems, which are responsible for triggering the functional responses. As a result, intracellular Ca^{2+} ion concentration increases, activating eNOS and leading to the production of NO from arginine (Figure 2.5). Once formed, NO diffuses across the cell membrane and stimulates an increase in guanylyl cyclase (GC) concentration, resulting in an increase of cyclic guanosine monophosphate (cGMP) levels. cGMP is derived from guanosine triphosphate (GTP) via the catalysis of NO on soluble guanylate cyclase. It acts as a secondary messenger, and its likely mechanism of action is activation of intracellular protein kinases in response to the binding of membrane-impermeable peptide hormones to the external cell surface. Additionally, cGMP inhibits the influx of extracellular Ca^{2+}, decreases inositol triphosphate (IP^3) levels and increases vasorelaxation. Once cGMP is produced, it has the potential to provide protective effects against the

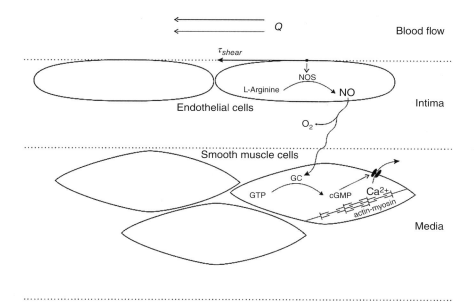

Figure 2.5 Mechanisms of shear-stress activation of eNOS and relaxation of vascular smooth muscle

development of atherosclerosis by reducing the influx of calcium through L-type calcium channels and stimulating a cGMP-sensitive phosphodiesterase, which in turn reduces the concentration of cGMP.

The importance of the endothelium in detecting increases in flow and promoting flow-mediated dilation is evidenced by studies that have either removed the endothelium or altered the pattern of shear stress. In the former, flow-mediated dilation was abolished. In the latter, when exercise training was conducted with reduced patterns of shear stress, the usual training-induced upregulation of NO release and consequent vascular remodelling did not occur.

Haemodynamics

Having discussed the structural anatomy and physiology of the vasculature system, it is pertinent to discuss the physical factors that govern the flow of blood in the circulation. These factors are based on a fundamental law of physics, Ohm's law, which states that current (I) equals the difference in voltage (ΔV) divided by resistance (R). In the context of the circulation, the voltage difference is the pressure difference between points in the circulation (ΔP; the driving pressure, perfusion pressure or pressure gradient) and the resistance is the resistance to blood flow due to the radius of a particular blood vessel. The current in Ohm's law becomes *flow* in the circulation:

$$\text{Ohm's law } I = \frac{\Delta V}{R} \quad \text{becomes} \quad F = \frac{\Delta P}{R} = \frac{P_A - P_V}{R} \qquad \text{(Equation 2.1)}$$

Equation 2.1 shows that flow through any vessel is dependent on the pressure gradient between any two points in the vessel, divided by the prevailing resistance to flow. Flow is usually measured across an organ, muscle or tissue, where ΔP is the difference between arterial (P_A) and venous (P_V) pressure. Furthermore, this concept can be extended to derive an equation for the circulation as a whole:

$$F = \frac{\Delta P}{R} \quad \text{becomes} \quad Q = \frac{MAP}{SVR} \qquad \text{(Equation 2.2)}$$

where Q = cardiac output, MAP = mean arterial pressure, SVR = systemic vascular resistance.

When described in this manner, whole-body flow (or cardiac output) is determined by the driving force (mean arterial pressure) divided by the resistance (systemic vascular resistance) against which this force must operate. The systemic vascular resistance, in turn, is a product of all the resistances offered by the calibre of each blood vessel in the body. SVR is therefore critically dependent on the vascular tone (contraction or relaxation) of the resistance vessels. In Equation 2.2, the change in pressure from the aorta to the vena cava as it enters the right atrium is given as MAP. Given that the central venous pressure at this point is close to zero, the pressure change across the circulation is therefore generally assumed to be the mean arterial pressure across the cardiac cycle (SBP − (SBP − DBP)/3).

This equation can be rearranged to give:

$$MAP = Q \times SVR$$
(Equation 2.3)

The mean arterial pressure becomes the product of cardiac output (driving force) and the total resistance to flow. Mean arterial pressure is a tightly controlled variable and the subject of negative feedback control. Arterial pressure is regulated within a narrow range and usually has an operating point around 90 mmHg in healthy adults. Regulation is maintained on a beat-to-beat basis by the baroreflex. The baroreflex operates by measuring pressure through pressure sensors located in the carotid sinus and the aortic arch. These sensors have their nerve endings located in the vessel walls and respond to changes in wall stretch. For example, if blood pressure increases, there is increased stretch in the carotid sinus and aortic arch, the nerve endings of the baroreceptors fire and neural signals are sent to the cardiovascular control centre in the brain stem. The increase is pressure is detected at the cardiovascular control centre and a reflex reduction in sympathetic activity and an increase in parasympathetic activity are initiated. This change in autonomic activity results in a decrease in cardiac output (via decreased heart rate) and a decreased contractility in blood vessels, resulting in a decreased resistance to flow. The attendant reduction in Q and SVR results in a lowering of pressure, hence resolving the pressure increase.

Although baroreceptors respond to increases and decreases in pressure, they mainly exist to correct for sudden reductions in pressure. For example, on standing, there is pooling of blood in the lower limbs due to the effect of gravity. This creates an instantaneous fall in MAP that is detected by the baroreceptors and resolved by an increase in sympathetic activity (as well as a decrease in parasympathetic activity), which increases heart rate and constricts the smooth muscle of the blood vessels, thereby increasing Q and SVR and immediately correcting MAP upwards. In this manner, the driving force for brain blood flow is preserved.

Another example of a reduced pressure signal is at the onset of exercise. As muscle contraction occurs, there are marked changes in metabolism and marked increases in some factors (e.g. adenosine, potassium, etc.) that cause relaxation in the blood vessel of skeletal muscle. This vasodilation causes a decrease in resistance, which increases flow. The increase in flow itself will increase shear stress on the endothelium and activates the release of NO, causing a further decrease in resistance. On the onset of whole-body exercise, SVR reduces markedly, causing a precipitous fall in MAP. This is detected by the baroreceptors and results in a marked increase in sympathetic activity, which increases both Q and vasoconstrictor activity and so increases resistance to flow through compliant circulation (such as in the skin and GIT). In this manner, MAP is preserved and slightly increased during dynamic exercise. In addition, during exercise, cardiac output is maintained by an increase in preload, as venous return is augmented by the activity of the muscle pump.

Conclusion

This chapter summarises the basic structure and function of the vasculature and provides an explanation of the control of blood flow and cardiovascular regulation of blood pressure. This discussion provides the necessary platform from which to discuss the acute and chronic adaptations that occur in the cardiovascular system with exercise and training and in response to the development of pathology.

3 Energy Production Pathways During Exercise

Sébastien Racinais[1] and Stéphane Perrey[2]

[1]Athlete Health and Performance Research Centre, ASPETAR, Qatar Orthopaedic and Sports Medicine Hospital, Doha, Qatar
[2]Movement to Health, Euromov, University of Montpellier, Montpellier, France

Introduction

Despite centuries of research, our understanding of exercise metabolism is still evolving. In 1777, Lavoisier described energy production as a combustion process producing heat and carbon dioxide, whilst in 1859, by measuring blood temperature, Claude Bernard showed that this process did not occur in the lung but rather in several other organs, including the skeletal muscles. Even as late as 1985, George Brooks demonstrated that lactate did not cause muscle acidosis, but was a substrate rather than an end product. This chapter presents a summary of our current understanding of energy-production pathways during exercise of varying intensities.

Primary Sources of Energy in the Human Body

Basal Metabolic Rate and Energy Storage

The basal metabolic rate (BMR) corresponds to the absolute (i.e. $kJ.h^{-1}$ or day) or relative (i.e. $kJ.h^{-1}.kg^{-1}$) rate of energy expenditure at rest, in a thermoneutral environment. It is mainly related to the energy expenditure of the liver (~27%), brain (~19%), skeletal muscles (~18%), kidneys (~10%), heart (~7%) and other organs (~19%). BMR is dependent on the metabolism, which is regulated by the hypothalamus via control of the autonomic nervous system, emotional status, body temperature and food intake.

Several equations (e.g. the Harris–Benedict equation) have been developed to estimate BMR based on sex, age, body mass and height (i.e. an index of body surface area). More recent equations (e.g. the Katch–McArdle equation) are based on lean body mass, in order to take into account the difference in metabolic activity between lean mass and body fat, and to negate the effect of sex. BMR can also be directly measured at complete rest by analysis of the expired gasses, averaging ~$6300kJ.day^{-1}$ with large inter-individual differences (between ~4300 and ~$10\,500\ kJ.day^{-1}$) [1]. BMR represents the majority of an individual's total energy expenditure, followed by the specific and additional requirements for physical activity, thermogenesis and food digestion. Daily calorie needs might therefore range from ~1.2 to 2.0 times the BMR, but of course vary considerably depending upon the duration and intensity of physical activity. For example, a 100 m run requires ~130 kJ, a 400 m run ~370 kJ and a 10 000 m run ~3350 kJ. In comparison, the available energy stores for a 70 kg man with ~25 kg muscle mass are approximately:

- 5 kJ from adenosine triphosphate (ATP) + 20 kJ from phosphocreatine (PCr)
- 400 kJ from substrates in the blood circulation (e.g. glucose)
- 600 kJ from liver glycogen
- 4000 kJ from muscle glycogen
- 80 000 kJ from protein (e.g. free amino acid)
- 450 000 kJ from lipid (e.g. triglyceride)

IOC Manual of Sports Cardiology, First Edition. Edited by Mathew G. Wilson, Jonathan A. Drezner and Sanjay Sharma.
© 2017 International Olympic Committee. Published 2017 by John Wiley & Sons, Ltd.

Notably, muscle storage of ATP and PCr is not sufficient to cover even a 100 m run. ATP has therefore to be continuously resynthesised from other substrates.

Energy Sources for Muscle Contraction

Adenosine Triphosphate (ATP)

Whilst ATP has several roles in cell structure and signalling, it is the only molecule (i.e. chemical energy) that can be used by the muscle to produce a contraction (i.e. mechanical energy). ATP is composed of an adenosine nucleotide (a monomer of RNA, comprising an adenine base and a five-carbon ribose sugar) and three phosphate groups (triphosphate). The chemical bonds of the two terminal phosphate groups store large amounts of energy, with the breakage of these bonds providing the energy required for muscular contraction. The removal of these phosphate groups converts ATP into adenosine diphosphate (ADP) and adenosine monophosphate (AMP).

Approximately 5 g of ATP is used at any one time for various cellular functions, representing around 50–75 kg of ATP (i.e. 100–150 moles) per day. However, ATP stores are small (0.2–0.5 mole, representing 100–250 g), with ATP having to be continuously recycled from ADP and AMP using energy sourced from other substrates. The substrates necessary for ATP recycling are provided by the alimentation. Proteins are broken down into amino acids (by proteolytic enzymes), fat into simple lipids (by lipases) and carbohydrate into glucose. These amino acids, simple lipids and glucose can be transformed into pyruvate and then an acetyl coenzyme A (acetyl-CoA) to enter the citric acid cycle before oxidative phosphorylation takes place (Figure 3.1). ATP production can occur with or without oxygen (O_2), but much more ATP is produced per mole of substrate in the presence of O_2.

Glycolysis

Glycolysis is the first stage of both aerobic and anaerobic respiration. It allows the transformation of the smallest form of carbohydrate that the digestive system can produce (i.e. six-carbon glucose) into two three-carbon pyruvate molecules. The main intermediate molecules in this process are successively: glucose, glucose-6-phosphate, fructose-6-phosphate, fructose-1,6-biphosphate, dihydroxyacetone phosphate, glyceraldehyde-3-phosphate, 1,3-bisphosphoglycerate, 3-phosphoglycerate, 2-phosphoglycerate, phosphoenolpyruvate and pyruvate. The first (preparatory) step of glycolysis requires energy (2 ATP + nicotinamide adenine dinucleotide (NAD-)), but more high-energy molecules are thereafter produced during the second (pay-off) phase (4 ATP + 2 reduced NAD). This process occurs in the cytoplasm and does not require O_2. It allows a net production of 2 ATP per glucose molecule or 3 ATP per glycogen molecule. In the absence of O_2, pyruvate can be transformed into lactate (whilst regenerating oxidised NAD), which can be utilised by various organs, including the brain and myocardium or muscle cells (e.g. type I), or converted into glucose via gluconeogenesis in the liver via the Cori cycle (Figure 3.1). In the presence of O_2, pyruvate and reduced NAD will further generate ATP in the mitochondria.

Citric Acid Cycle

Once in the mitochondria, pyruvate will lose a carbon dioxide group to form an acetyl-coA, which will enter the citric acid cycle (also called Krebs cycle or tricarboxylic acid (TCA) cycle) (Figure 3.1). The citric acid cycle can be briefly summarised as a series of eight enzyme-catalysed chemical reactions, representing the main part of the aerobic respiration. It is initiated with the formation of citrate from the combination of the acetyl-coA with oxaloacetate, followed by the successive production of isocitrate, alpha-ketoglutarate, succinyl coA, succinate, fumarate, malate and oxaloacetate. Oxaloacetate will then combine with a new molecule of acetyl-coA for another cycle. For every cycle, one ATP and three NADHs are produced. As a glucose molecule produces two pyruvate molecules, it will generate two ATPs and six reduced NADs through the citric acid cycle. Notably, both the transformation of pyruvate into acetyl-coA and the citric acid cycle release CO_2.

Electron Transport Chain and Oxidative Phosphorylation

The reduced NADs produced during glycolysis and the citric acid cycle are coenzymes containing electrons with a high transfer potential. These electrons can be transferred to O_2 in the mitochondrial membrane through a series of steps, ultimately producing a molecule of water (electrode transport chain). These redox reactions release energy at each step and can be used to pump hydrogen protons (H^+) through the inner

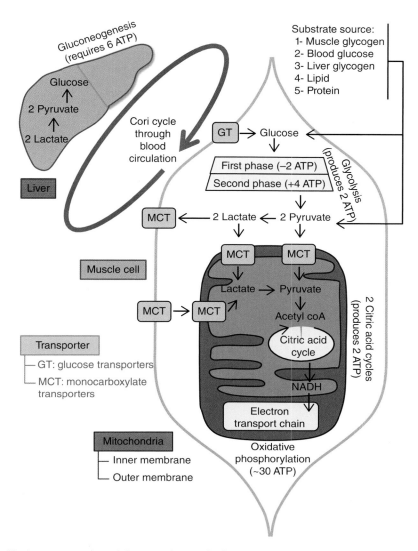

Figure 3.1 Simplified representation of the muscle metabolism

membrane towards the intermembrane space (Figure 3.1). This creates a pH gradient across the inner membrane. This electrical potential is used in a second phase (ATP synthase) to attach inorganic phosphate (Pi) to ADP in order to generate ATP.

In summary, the oxidation of one molecule of glucose through glycolysis, the citric acid cycle and oxidative phosphorylation could ideally produce 38 ATPs. However, reduced NAD transport from cytoplasm to mitochondria requires 2 ATPs, decreasing net ATP synthesis to 36. Moreover, leakage of protons and other inefficiencies may decrease the actual production of ATP in vivo to approximately 30 per molecule of glucose.

Interacting Energy Systems During Exercise

ATP provision relies on two anaerobic (phosphagen and glycolysis) and one aerobic pathway. Muscle phosphagens (i.e. ATP and PCr) represent a pool of immediately available energy for the onset of exercise, acute intensity changes and very high-intensity actions. There is, however, a limited pool of phosphagen. Phosphagen can be rapidly resynthesised by anaerobic glycolysis, allowing for repeated high-intensity exercise (sometimes referred to as the 'lactic anaerobic' pathway). According to the glycogen-shunt hypothesis, this rapid ATP/PCr resynthesis (Figure 3.2) may originate more from glycogen metabolism

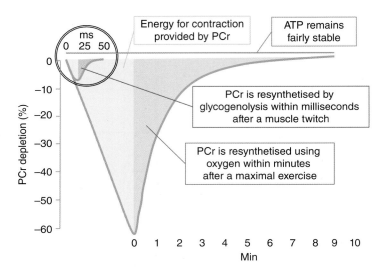

Figure 3.2 PCr depletion and resynthesis

(glycogenolysis) than from glucose metabolism (glycolysis) [2]. However, muscle acidosis resulting from the anaerobic glycolysis/glycogenolysis byproducts leads to muscle fatigue. Sustaining exercise relies therefore on oxidative phosphorylation (generally referred as the 'aerobic pathway'), and larger PCr resynthesis cannot be maintained without oxygen [3].

Phosphocreatine (PCr) and Glycolysis During Sprint(s)

The ATP requirement for muscle contraction can be instantaneously matched by PCr (Figure 3.2). Muscular PCr allows for fast and immediate ATP resynthesis, and represents 45–50% of the energy source for maximal sprinting (Figure 3.3). However, PCr stores can be reduced by 50% within seconds of sprint activity, and require more than 5 minutes to be fully restored (Figure 3.2). PCr availability is therefore likely to represent the main limiting factor during repeated sprints with recovery durations below 60 seconds. This mainly affects type IIx or IIb fibres that rely on PCr (more so than type I fibres). The remaining energy during a maximal sprint is derived from glycolysis. When sprinting activity is repeated, the contribution of glycolysis decreases dramatically [4], to be progressively replaced by aerobic pathways [5]. The high glycolytic activity during such high-intensity exercises leads to the accumulation of lactate, hydrogen ions and other byproducts.

Lactate Kinetics During High-Intensity Exercise

Lactate is constantly produced from pyruvate via the enzyme lactate dehydrogenase, with resting blood concentration approximately 0.5–2.0 mmol.L^{-1}. Used by various organs and cells, it is the primary energy source for neurons in the brain. During very intense exercise, however, lactate production during glycolysis will be higher than lactate flux and utilisation, and thus blood concentrations can reach over 20 mmol.L^{-1}. Consequently, it was believed during most of the 19th and 20th centuries that when lactate production exceeded buffering capacity, it caused a decrease in cellular pH (called lactate acidosis) and, in turn, muscle fatigue. However, acidosis is caused by reactions other than lactate production; lactate is simply an indirect marker of these coinciding reactions [6]. Following the seminal work of Prof. George Brooks, several studies have shown that lactate should be considered a substrate that can travel (Figure 3.1) and can be used intracellularly and intercellularly, rather than an end product [7]. Moreover, lactate production actually delays but does not cause acidosis, and if muscle did not produce lactate, acidosis and muscle fatigue would occur more quickly [6]. The muscle acidosis resulting from the anaerobic glycolysis byproducts generates muscle fatigue, and sustaining exercise relies therefore on oxidative phosphorylation.

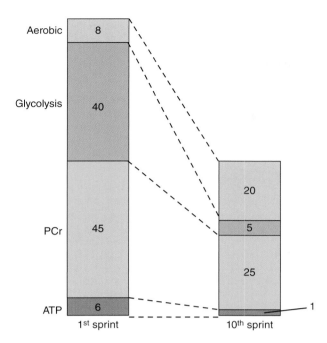

Figure 3.3 Example of energy contribution (arbitrary units) during sprints of less than 10 seconds, repeated with less than 30 seconds of rest (*Source*: Adapted from Gaitanos et al. [4] and Girard et al. [5])

$\dot{V}O_2$ Kinetics Responses to Submaximal Exercise

Oxidative phosphorylation requires the delivery of O_2 and the clearance of carbon dioxide (CO_2) through ventilatory, cardiovascular and muscular adaptations (Figure 3.4). Whilst pulmonary (p) and muscle (m) oxygen uptake ($\dot{V}O_2$) may closely match ATP requirement during steady-state moderate exercise, these adaptations are not immediate. At the onset of exercise, $m\dot{V}O_2$ requires ~2–3 minutes to reach steady state, during which the ATP supply is provided by muscle PCr, followed by anaerobic glycolysis. This nonoxidative contribution until steady state is termed 'O_2 deficit'.

Modelling the $p\dot{V}O_2$ response at the onset of exercise provides a valuable indicator of the underlying $m\dot{V}O_2$ profile (within 10%) and the magnitude of the incurred O_2 deficit, thus providing a physiological profile of the interaction between oxidative and nonoxidative metabolism during exercise [8]. After a short delay, representing the muscle-to-lung blood transit time, $p\dot{V}O_2$ rises along a time course that can be assessed by a single-exponential function. An exponential profile is effective for ensuring a rapid response, because it means that the highest rate of change will occur when the difference between what is required (ATP demand) and what is available is the greatest. Thus, besides the maximal $\dot{V}O_2$ ($\dot{V}O_{2max}$), the exponential rise in $p\dot{V}O_2$ as determined by the time constant (τ^1) in the transition to exercise intensity should also be considered a factor of aerobic exercise performance.

$\dot{V}O_2$ Responses Depend on Exercise Intensity

$p\dot{V}O_2$ kinetics during the early transition phase, and whether it reaches steady state or not, depends on exercise intensity. To provide a frame of reference for investigating $p\dot{V}O_2$ kinetics during exercise, four discrete exercise intensities can be proposed: moderate, heavy, severe and extreme (Figure 3.5). 'Moderate' is defined as all exercise intensities that fall below the blood lactate threshold (LT; the highest exercise $\dot{V}O_2$ achieved without a sustained increase in blood and muscle lactate concentration) or its noninvasive equivalent, the ventilatory threshold. Within this domain, $p\dot{V}O_2$ rises with single-exponential kinetics, following an initial short phase, and attains steady state within approximately 2–3 minutes (τ ~30 seconds), with an O_2 cost of exercise of ~10 mL.min^{-1}.W^{-1} [9].

$^1\tau$ is a measure of the time required for $\dot{V}O_2$ to reach 63% of the final amplitude.

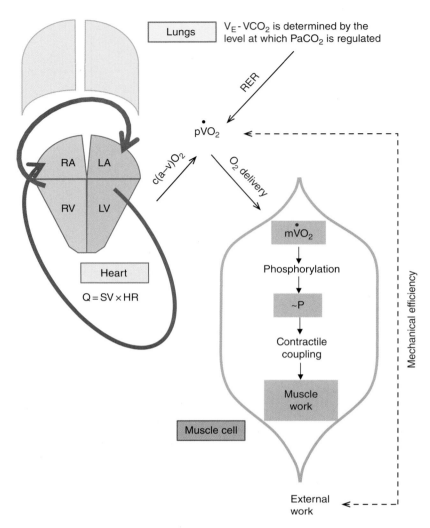

Figure 3.4 Interplay between respiratory, cardiovascular and muscular system. Gross mechanical efficiency can be estimated as the ratio of external work to the metabolic energy expenditure (pVO2). $PaCO_2$, arterial partial pressure of carbon dioxide; $c(a-v)O_2$, difference in O_2 content between systemic arterial and mixed venous blood; VE, minute ventilation; RER, respiratory exchange ratio; Q, cardiac output; SV, stroke volume; HR, heart rate; RQ, respiratory quotient

The upper boundary of the 'heavy' intensity is defined by the maximal lactate steady state (the highest power output at which a balance between the entry and removal of lactate within the blood is achieved) and/or the critical power (CP) (the asymptote of the hyperbolic relationship between power output and time to exhaustion) [10]. At this intensity, there is a nonlinear increase in the power output–$\dot{V}O_2$ relationship and the O_2 cost of exercise increases to 12–13 mL.min^{-1}.W^{-1}. p$\dot{V}O_2$ either reaches a delayed steady state above that predicted from lower power outputs or continues to increase until the end of exercise. This increased O_2 cost is termed the 'p$\dot{V}O_2$ slow component' [9]. Interestingly, the onset and amplitude of the p$\dot{V}O_2$ slow component are similar to the onset and amplitude of a slow-component phase in the fall of intramuscular PCr, as determined using phosphorus-31 magnetic resonance spectroscopy (^{31}P-MRS) in Layec et al. [11]. This suggests that the 'origin' of the p$\dot{V}O_2$ slow component in healthy participants resides within the contracting muscle, and to a lesser extent the O_2 cost of ventilation or cardiac work. The recruitment of higher-order type II muscle fibres and their associated metabolic properties, such as a low capacity for oxidative ATP synthesis and a higher O_2 and PCr cost for muscle contraction, has been proposed as the main causative factor for the slow-component phenomenon [10].

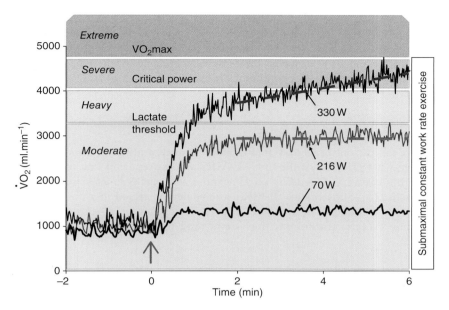

Figure 3.5 Illustration of the four exercise-intensity domains, with actual VO_2 response to moderate- (steady-state achievement) and severe- (slow component) intensity exercise in a representative trained subject. The vertical arrow delineates the onset of exercise

For severe-intensity exercises (i.e. above CP but below $\dot{V}O_{2max}$), following the exponential phase, the $p\dot{V}O_2$ slow component rises rapidly with time and attains $\dot{V}O_{2max}$. The higher the projected exercise intensity above CP, the lower the magnitude of the $p\dot{V}O_2$ slow component, such that at power outputs close to $\dot{V}O_{2max}$, the $p\dot{V}O_2$ response follows a single-exponential function that is truncated within minutes at $\dot{V}O_{2max}$ (Figure 3.5). During extreme-intensity exercise (i.e. beyond $\dot{V}O_{2max}$), the tolerable duration of exercise is usually <140 seconds (i.e. around four times a τ of ~30 s), with $\dot{V}O_{2max}$ normally achieved. No $p\dot{V}O_2$ slow component can be discerned here.

Measurement of Energy Sources

Power Output as a Surrogate for Anaerobic Metabolism

'Alactic' and 'lactic' anaerobic pathways are generally wrongly interpreted as physical tests to measure power output (e.g. from jump or sprint test), rather than metabolism per se. In the 1980s and 1990s, anaerobic performance was commonly classified as 'anaerobic power' and 'anaerobic capacity', estimated on cycle ergometer by the force–velocity test (repetitive short maximal sprints against increasing braking force) or the Wingate test (30 seconds' all-out sprint), respectively. Since the 2000s, the flywheel inertia has been integrated into power calculations, allowing maximal 'anaerobic' power testing to occur on a single sprint. This has since allowed for testing of repeat power, or 'repeated-sprint ability' (RSA). RSA is generally evaluated by calculating a decrement score across 5–10 maximal sprints, interspersed with short recovery periods (usually 24–30 seconds) [5]. However, all physical tests rely on the three energetic pathways.

Biochemical Method

The anaerobic pathway is sometimes indirectly assessed via the measure of certain metabolites, such as lactate or pyruvate. However, such measures depend on diffusion and elimination processes. It is therefore preferable to measure muscle rather than systemic concentrations. By comparing muscle biopsies taken prior to and after the first and last of 10 repeated sprints, Gaitanos et al. [4] showed a decrement in PCr concentration, an increase in metabolic byproducts (i.e. lactate and Pi) and a lowered pH. This technique has also been transferred from the laboratory to the sporting field, showing that glycogen depletion may persist for several days after sporting activities such as a football game [12]. Notably, this technique allows for the characterisation of different muscle fibre types, including: type I (predominantly oxidative, slow twitch characteristics), type IIa (both oxidative and glycolytic, moderately fast), type IIb (predominantly glycolytic, very fast) and type IIx (mixed myosin heavy chain from IIa and IIb). However, the temporal specificity of the biopsy technique is limited, and noninvasive techniques are preferred for continuous recording.

Nuclear Magnetic Resonance

^{31}P-MRS allows for noninvasive estimations of ATP, ADP, PCr and Pi concentrations (continuously, both at rest and during exercise), along with pH. One of the first ^{31}P-MRS studies reported that intracellular pH may drop to 6.0 or below, with a recovery depending on H^+ export, whereas post-exercise PCr recovery depends on oxidative metabolism [13]. Subsequent ^{31}P-MRS studies demonstrated that the kinetics of the muscle phosphates, specifically the breakdown of muscle PCr, holds a close temporal relationship with the exponential rise in $p\dot{V}O_2$ during exercise transitions, thus supporting the notion that two variables are mechanistically coupled [8].

Excess Post-Exercise Oxygen Consumption

Energy demands during transition phases have to be matched by PCr and glycolysis, but also by venous O_2 stores and possibly myoglobin desaturation. This 'oxygen debt' is compensated by an increased rate of O_2 intake following intense exercise, called 'excess post-exercise oxygen consumption' (EPOC). EPOC was originally linked to the clearance of lactic acid, but direct and indirect calorimeter experiments have shown that the kinetics of post-exercise $p\dot{V}O_2$ and lactate clearance are dissociated [14]. EPOC is thus linked to a range of factors that increase O_2 consumption, among which an elevated temperature may have a primary role [14]. These factors include recovery of hormone balancing, replenishment of fuel stores (including PCr), cellular repair and oxidation of lactate into pyruvate.

Oxygen Uptake

Human skeletal muscle is highly dependent upon oxidative metabolism. Resting $\dot{V}O_2$ is ~0.3 l.min^{-1} and can reach maximal values ($\dot{V}O_{2max}$) of ~5 L.min^{-1}. The measurement of whole-body $\dot{V}O_2$ by means of measuring pulmonary gas exchange has become an established method for studying energy expenditure in the field of both sports science and medicine. The maximum rate of energy supplied by aerobic metabolism is much less than that of the anaerobic system and is limited by the maximum rate of oxidative metabolism (expressed as $\dot{V}O_{2max}$). The assessment of changes in $p\dot{V}O_2$ (τ) is the most commonly used technique for measuring $p\dot{V}O_2$ kinetics, because it is noninvasive, relatively accessible and permits measurement of $p\dot{V}O_2$ kinetics whilst performing different exercise modalities (i.e. incremental, constant work rate, impulse or random sequence). Another feature commonly used to describe the $p\dot{V}O_2$ on-kinetics response is the $p\dot{V}O_2$ functional gain ($\Delta p\dot{V}O_2/\Delta WR$), which describes the efficiency (or its inverse) of a given exercise-intensity transition.

Muscle Oxygenation

Recent advances in near-infrared spectroscopy (NIRS; a noninvasive optical method which penetrates tissue several centimetres deep) provide the temporal resolution necessary to dynamically examine muscle micro-vascular haemoglobin concentration and oxygenation during exercise. Using multiple wavelengths in the near-infrared range (700–900 nm), the concentration of tissue constituents such as oxy-haemoglobin (HbO$_2$), deoxy-haemoglobin (HHb) and cytochrome c-oxidase can be quantified. Due to their identical spectral characteristics, haemoglobin and myoglobin are not separated in the near-infrared region. Whilst the NIRS signals obtained are considered to reflect the balance between O_2 delivery and utilisation, local $m\dot{V}O_2$ can be estimated by the use of an arterial or venous occlusion approach [15]. Furthermore, by normalising both the HHb and $p\dot{V}O_2$ signals, the time courses of adjustment for O_2 utilisation and O_2 extraction can be directly compared. Importantly, Grassi et al. [16] point out the 'striking similarities' between increases in [HHb] and decreases in the microvascular partial pressure of O_2 during the exercise on-transient. Nevertheless, because the precise contributions of arterial and venous circulations within the microvasculature cannot be known, NIRS does not provide a quantitative estimate of arteriovenous O_2 content difference. To summarise, NIRS offers the opportunity to evaluate the contribution of specific muscles to whole-body exercise, evaluate muscle oxygenation kinetics during and after exercise and gain insight into training-related changes. For a better understanding of the control of energy production during exercise in humans (i.e., inertia of O_2 delivery and O_2 utilisation mechanisms and alterations in muscle energy cost), it would be best to combine NIRS, ^{31}P-MRS and pulmonary gas exchange measurements [11].

Training Effect

Depending on the volume, intensity and frequency of exercise sessions, training leads to numerous adaptations, including cardiovascular, cardiorespiratory and metabolic adaptations, that will influence energy production and utilisation. In endurance-trained persons, these adaptations are commonly measurable via improvements in $\dot{V}O_{2max}$, efficiency or exercise economy, CP, $p\dot{V}O_2$ kinetics, LT and performance.

Anaerobic Energy Production

Performance increases from the first week of high-intensity (e.g. sprints) or resistance training, through an increase in muscle activation or an improved intermuscular coordination (e.g. agonist/antagonist ratio). Enzymatic, histological and structural muscle adaptations will only occur after ~4 weeks. Training can increase the muscle storage of high-energy phosphate (PCr) and other energy molecules (e.g. fats and carbohydrates). Training increases glycolytic enzymatic activity [17] and may enhance the rate of PCr resynthesis [18]. Training does not seem to clearly modify lactate production but does improve lactate clearance, suggesting an upregulation of the monocarboxilate transporter (MCT; Figure 3.1) [7]. Finally, training can promote an increase in fibre area (i.e. hypertrophy) and a change in fibre type. However, the change from an oxidative to a glycolytic type may be slower than the reverse.

Oxidative Phosphorylation

Prolonged periods of endurance training enhance mitochondrial oxidative enzyme activity and increase mitochondrial volume density in skeletal muscle. Such mitochondrial biogenesis adaptations, combined with the increase in capillaries and muscle blood flow in the trained muscles, improve the oxidative capacity of the endurance-trained muscle. Endurance training also increases the capacity of skeletal muscle to store glycogen and to use more fat as an energy source, leading to a glycogen storage economy. The increased capacity to use fat following endurance training results from an enhanced ability to mobilise free fatty acids from fat depots and an improved capacity to oxidise fat consequent to the increase in the muscle enzymes responsible for fat oxidation.

Following a 6-month endurance-training period, increases in $\dot{V}O_{2max}$ generally range from 15 to 20%. As indicated before, slower $p\dot{V}O_2$ kinetics is associated with a greater depletion of [PCr], greater accumulation of blood [lactate] and H^+ and a greater O_2 deficit. Cross-sectional studies examined by Jones and Koppo [19] have shown a faster $p\dot{V}O_2$ response (i.e. smaller τ, faster steady-state attainment) in trained than in untrained subjects. Notably, $\dot{V}O_{2max}$ is related to $p\dot{V}O_2$ kinetics in athletes with similar training programmes, and athletes with higher $\dot{V}O_{2max}$ values show faster τ values. In the same vein, longitudinal studies have shown training-induced reductions in τ during both moderate- and heavy-intensity exercise [19]. In the early stages of training, an intensification of 'parallel activation' of oxidative phosphorylation (i.e. all oxidative phosphorylation complexes, complex I, III and IV, ATP synthase, ATP/ADP and Pi carrier, are directly activated, probably by some $Ca2^+$-related mechanism) could account for the shortening of $p\dot{V}O_2$ response, preceding the enhanced mitochondrial biogenesis or capillarisation in the trained muscles.

Endurance or High-Intensity Intermittent Training?

Interestingly, repeated bouts of high-intensity exercise or high-intensity intermittent training (HIIT) have been shown to be better than endurance training (submaximal intensities) at inducing fat loss. HIIT corresponds to repeated short high-intensity exercise bouts (>80% $\dot{V}O_{2max}$ or >90% max. heart rate) lasting between 6 and 120 seconds, followed by a rest period consisting of between 12 seconds and 4 minutes; the total duration of exercise can last from 2.5 to 60.0 minutes. To date, there are some indications of changes in whole-body carbohydrate (decreased) and lipid oxidation (increased) after HIIT training; the latter may also improve glycaemic control and insulin sensitivity (explained in part by an increased glucose transporter type 4 in the muscles). HIIT may also improve aerobic adaptations, with some studies suggesting improved muscle oxidative potential (reflected by changes in the expression of a key metabolic regulator, peroxisome proliferator-activated receptor gamma coactivator 1-alpha (PGC-1 α)) after sprint-type training, and proposing that an increase in mitochondrial density and oxidative enzyme (citrate synthase) activity occurs with a lower weekly training volume. Thus, HIIT exercise may enhance mitochondrial metabolic capacity and/or oxygen supply at an early stage of a training period, which may speed up the p$\dot{V}O_2$ response at the onset of exercise. HIIT exercise involves all three energy systems, with the initial maximal-effort high-intensity bout using the ATP-PCr system to meet energy demands and glycolysis contributing to energy supply thereafter. The recovery period following HIIT exercise may play a large role in inducing an energy deficit, due to recovery processes associated with EPOC, including purine nucleotide metabolism.

Conclusion

Muscle contraction relies on ATP breakdown. Human can use various substrates to resynthesise ATP, some of which are instantaneously available within the muscle (e.g. PCr), others of which require multiple transformations (e.g. complex lipid). Acute ATP requirement at the onset of exercise or during transition-phase or high-intensity exercises will be covered by PCr. PCr stores are limited but can be rapidly resynthesised by anaerobic glycolysis. However, anaerobic glycolysis byproducts create muscle acidosis, and prolonged exercises therefore rely on oxidative phosphorylation. Oxidative phosphorylation requires cardiorespiratory adaptations for O_2 delivery and CO_2 clearance. These adaptations are not immediate but are trainable. The magnitude and rate of adaptation of oxygen uptake is a key factor in performance. Oxidative phosphorylation, glycolysis and PCr all work in conjunction, but their predominance in energy production depends first on exercise intensity and second on exercise duration.

References

1 Johnstone, A.M., Murison, S.D, Duncan, J.S. et al. Factors influencing variation in basal metabolic rate include fat-free mass, fat mass, age, and circulating thyroxine but not sex, circulating leptin, or triiodothyronine. *Am J Clin Nutr* 2005; **82**: 941–8.

2 Shulman, R.G. Glycogen turnover forms lactate during exercise. *Exerc Sport Sci Rev* 2005; **33**: 157–62.

3 Harris, R.C., Edwards, R.H., Hultman, E. et al. The time course of phosphorylcreatine resynthesis during recovery of the quadriceps muscle in man. *Pflugers Arch* 1976; **367**: 137–42.

4 Gaitanos, G.C., Williams, C., Boobis, L.H. and Brooks, S. Human muscle metabolism during intermittent maximal exercise. *J Appl Physiol* 1993; **75**: 712–19.

5 Girard, O., Mendez-Villanueva A. and Bishop, D. Repeated-sprint ability – Part I: Factors contributing to fatigue. *Sports Med* 2011; **41**: 673–94.

6 Roberds, R.A., Ghiasvand, F. and Parker, D. Biochemistry of exercise-induced metabolic acidosis. *Am J Physiol* 2004; **287**: R502–16.

7 Brooks, G.A. Cell–cell and intracellular lactate shuttles. *J Physiol* 2009; **587**: 5591–600.

8 Grassi, B. Oxygen uptake kinetics: old and recent lessons from experiments on isolated muscle in situ. *Eur J Appl Physiol* 2003; **90**: 242–9.

9 Perrey, S., Betik, A., Candau, R. et al. Comparison of oxygen uptake kinetics during concentric and eccentric cycle exercise. *J Appl Physiol* 2001; **91**: 2135–42.

10 Jones, A.M., Wilkerson, D.P., DiMenna, F. et al. Muscle metabolic responses to exercise above and below the 'critical power' assessed using 31P-MRS. *Am J Physiol* 2008; **294**: R585–93.

11 Layec, G., Bringard, A., Le Fur, Y. et al. Effects of a prior high-intensity knee-extension exercise on muscle recruitment and energy cost: a combined local and global investigation in humans. *Exp Physiol* 2009; **94**: 704–19.

12 Nybo, L., Girard, O., Mohr, M. et al. Markers of muscle damage and performance recovery after exercise in the heat. *Med Sci Sports Exerc* 2003; **45**: 860–8.

13 Taylor, D.J., Bore, P.J., Styles, P. et al. Bioenergetics of intact human muscle. A 31P nuclear magnetic resonance study. *Mol Biol Med* 1983; **1**: 77–94.

14 Gaesser, G.A. and Brooks, G.A. Metabolic bases of excess post-exercise oxygen consumption: a review. *Med Sci Sports Exerc* 1984; **16**: 29–43.

15 van Beekvelt, M.C., Shoemaker, J.K., Tschakovsky, M.E. et al. Blood flow and muscle oxygen uptake at the onset and end of moderate and heavy dynamic forearm exercise. *Am J Physiol* 2001; **280**: R1741–7.

16 Grassi, B., Pogliaghi, S., Rampichini, S. et al. Muscle oxygenation and pulmonary gas exchange kinetics during cycling exercise on-transitions in humans. *J Appl Physiol* 2003; 95: 149–58.

17 Costill, D.L., Coyle, E.F., Fink, W.F. et al. Adaptations in skeletal muscle following strength training. *J Appl Physiol* 1979; 46: 96–9.

18 McCully, K.K., Kakihira, H., Vandenborne, K. and Kent-Braun, J. Noninvasive measurements of activity-induced changes in muscle metabolism. *J Biomech* 1991; 21: 153–61.

19 Jones, A.M. and Koppo, K. Effect of training on VO2 kinetics and performance. In: A.M. Jones and D.C. Poole (eds) *Oxygen Uptake Kinetics in Sport, Exercise and Medicine.* New York: Routledge, 2005; pp. 373–99.

4 Cardiovascular Responses to Exercise

Julien D. Périard

Athlete Health and Performance Research Centre, ASPETAR, Qatar Orthopaedic and Sports Medicine Hospital, Doha, Qatar

Introduction

The cardiovascular system supplies oxygen (O_2) and nutrients to various tissues (e.g. muscle and brain) and removes carbon dioxide and waste products from the systemic circulation, both at rest and during exercise. However, the demands placed on the cardiovascular system during exercise are markedly intensified by the O_2 requirements of active skeletal and coronary muscle tissue. To ensure adequate perfusion, blood pressure rises and cardiac output ($\dot{Q}$) is enhanced as heart rate and stroke volume increase. Concomitantly, blood flow to inactive muscles and less active regions (e.g. splanchnic and renal) is reduced and redirected towards peripheral vascular beds (i.e. skin) to allow for metabolic heat dissipation. During exercise, the magnitude of adjustment in the cardiovascular response is primarily based on the relative intensity of effort, duration and muscle mass recruited. This chapter will examine the cardiovascular responses of healthy individuals performing acute and chronic exercise, focusing primarily upon the four components of maximal aerobic capacity ($\dot{V}O_{2max}$): heart rate, stroke volume, $\dot{Q}$ and O_2 extraction. Attention will be given not only to the cardiovascular responses to exercise in males and females but also to the ageing older (i.e. veteran) athlete.

Cardiovascular Responses to Aerobic Exercise

The Cardiovascular Response to Exercise Onset

The onset of dynamic exercise is characterised by an increase in heart rate and stroke volume, along with adjustments in $\dot{Q}$, arterial blood pressure, peripheral resistance and myocardial function. These adjustments are initiated by autonomic nervous system responses and by the need for O_2 delivery to active muscles. Typically, heart rate at rest varies between 60 and 90 beats.min^{-1}, but it can decrease to 30 beats.min^{-1} in endurance athletes (Table 4.1). The initial increase in heart rate stems from a withdrawal of parasympathetic activity and an increase in sympathetic stimulation (*neural control of exercise onset*). Stroke volume also increases in response to sympathetic stimulation or as a result of greater contractility. The increase in stroke volume, however, is mainly attributable to an enhanced venous return, due to the action of the muscle pump, which increases left ventricular end-diastolic volume (EDV). The increased volume and pressure (i.e. preload) cause the myocardium to stretch and contract more forcefully (i.e. the Frank–Starling mechanism), reducing left ventricular end-systolic volume (ESV) (Equation 4.1). During exercise at lower work rates (i.e. exercise intensities), changes in preload contribute more significantly to increases in stroke volume, whereas myocardial contractility has a larger influence on stroke volume when work rate intensifies. At rest in the upright position, stroke volume is between 50 and 60 ml.beat^{-1} in healthy individuals and 70 and 90 ml.beat^{-1} in aerobically trained athletes.

$$Stroke\,volume = EDV - ESV \qquad \text{(Equation 4.1)}$$

IOC Manual of Sports Cardiology, First Edition. Edited by Mathew G. Wilson, Jonathan A. Drezner and Sanjay Sharma.
© 2017 International Olympic Committee. Published 2017 by John Wiley & Sons, Ltd.

Cardiovascular parameter	Resting value	Range of values
Heart rate (beats.min⁻¹)	70	30–90
Stroke volume (ml)	75	50–90
End-diastolic volume (EDV) (ml)	125	65–240
End-systolic volume (ESV) (ml)	50	15–150
Cardiac output (l.min⁻¹)	5.25	4.0–8.0
Mean arterial blood pressure (mmHg)	93	70–115
Systolic blood pressure (SBP) (mmHg)	120	90–140
Diastolic blood pressure (DBP) (mmHg)	80	60–100

Table 4.1 Typical cardiovascular responses at rest for healthy individuals, along with the range of values observed in trained and sedentary individuals

As a consequence of the increase in heart rate and stroke volume, $\dot{Q}$ rises to meet the metabolic requirements associated with performing a given exercise task (Equation 4.2). Whilst the increase in heart rate is the primary factor mediating the rise in $\dot{Q}$, cardiac performance is also modulated by preload (the extent to which end-diastolic pressure stretches the ventricles), afterload (the resistance against which the heart must pump blood) and contractility (the intrinsic ability of the myocardium to shorten/contract).

$$\dot{Q} = heart\,rate \times stroke\,volume \qquad \text{(Equation 4.2)}$$

At the start of exercise, systolic blood pressure (SBP) increases in response to the initial increase in $\dot{Q}$. It typically increases from ~120 mmHg at rest in young (20–30 years) healthy individuals, following a similar pattern to that of heart rate. In contrast, diastolic blood pressure (DBP) remains relatively constant from rest (~80 mmHg) to exercise, decreasing occasionally, but by no more than 10 mmHg. As a result, mean arterial pressure (MAP) rises (Equation 4.3).

$$MAP = \frac{1}{3} \times \left(SBP - DBP \right) + DBP \qquad \text{(Equation 4.3)}$$

The redistribution of blood flow towards active muscle tissue during exercise is attributable to increased regional vasodilation. This occurs in response to variations in intramuscular pressure and the presence of vasoactive compounds (e.g. potassium ions, adenosine, acetylcholine and nitric oxide) [1]. The increased perfusion is also associated with sympathetic vasoconstriction in less active tissue (e.g. splanchnic organs) and nonactive muscles. These vasomotor responses decrease total peripheral resistance (TPR), which ultimately allows for muscle O_2 availability and MAP to increase (Equation 4.4).

$$TPR = \frac{MAP}{\dot{Q}} \qquad \text{(Equation 4.4)}$$

The initiation of exercise also increases the work of the heart, which must pump additional blood in response to the rise in $\dot{Q}$ towards not only the working muscles, but also the skin, for the purposes of heat dissipation. This results in an increase in myocardial O_2 uptake, which is represented by the rate pressure product (RPP) (Equation 4.5). The RPP, or double product, reflects the haemodynamic response and myocardial stress associated with the number of times the heart is required to beat per minute and the arterial blood pressure against which it is pumping.

$$RPP = heart\,rate \times SBP \qquad \text{(Equation 4.5)}$$

Neural Control of Exercise Onset

Cardiac function and blood pressure increase at the onset of exercise as a result of autonomic nervous system adjustments, which are characterised by parasympathetic withdrawal and sympathetic activation. The magnitude of these responses is proportional to exercise intensity and the muscle mass recruited.

Parasympathetic withdrawal causes an increase in heart rate, whilst sympathetic activation modulates a host of factors through the interaction of three distinct neural pathways: central command, the exercise pressor reflex and the arterial baroreflex. Briefly, central command activates motor and cardiovascular control centres within the brain to establish a pattern of autonomic activity based on the intensity of effort. The exercise pressor reflex in turn modulates sympathetic tone in relation to mechanical and metabolic signals originating from the contracting muscles (i.e. group III and IV muscle afferents). The sympathetic activity stemming from central command and the exercise pressor reflex modulates an increase in heart rate, myocardial contractility and venoconstriction (i.e. venous return), which increases stroke volume and, ultimately, $\dot{Q}$. The arterial baroreflex, activated via increases in blood pressure of between 60 and 180 mmHg sensed in the aorta and carotid arteries, modulates an inhibitory effect on sympathetic stimulation to ensure that excessive blood pressure variations are avoided. This is achieved through a progressive resetting of the baroreflex function curve (i.e. operating point, threshold and saturation pressures), allowing blood pressure regulation from rest to maximal exercise in an intensity-dependent manner. Recently, it has been proposed that arterial chemoreceptors also help maintain tonic levels of sympathetic activation during exercise [2].

The Cardiovascular Response to Prolonged Aerobic Exercise

The magnitude of adjustment in the cardiovascular response to prolonged dynamic exercise is determined by several factors, including exercise intensity, muscle mass, environmental conditions, training status and genetics. Further, a plateau in cardiovascular function occurs within 2–3 minutes of the beginning of light-to moderate-intensity exercise (40–75% $\dot{V}O_{2max}$), which is indicative of a metabolic steady state (Figure 4.1). This signifies the achievement of a balance between the energy required by working muscles and the rate of O_2 delivery for aerobic adenosine triphosphate (ATP) production.

Depending on exercise intensity, steady state may continue for between 10 and 30 minutes. Thereafter, a time-dependent change or 'drift' occurs in certain cardiovascular responses (Figure 4.1). This *cardiovascular drift* is characterised by a progressive increase in heart rate and decreases in stroke volume and MAP, whilst $\dot{Q}$ remains relatively stable [3]. Historically, cardiovascular drift was attributed to a peripheral redistribution of blood flow, which progressively reduced central venous and arterial pressure, along with stroke volume [4]. A more contemporary hypothesis suggests that the reduction in stroke volume is primarily due to an increase in intrinsic heart rate, mediated by the direct effect of temperature on the sinoatrial node and baroreflex modulation of sympathetic/parasympathetic activity, which decreases ventricular filling time and concomitantly EDV [5]. Although cardiovascular drift is observed during prolonged exercise regardless of environmental conditions, a greater drift develops under heat stress, which markedly impairs endurance exercise performance [4,6]. Similarly, the extent of cardiovascular drift is exacerbated by progressive dehydration [7], especially during exercise in the heat, as it increases heat storage and reduces the ability to tolerate exercise heat strain. This most likely occurs because of an inability to maintain $\dot{Q}$ and a reduction in skeletal muscle blood flow.

During prolonged submaximal exercise, the increase in MAP is critical, as it allows the blood flow requirements of various tissues (e.g. brain, heart, skin, skeletal muscles) to be met. The increase in MAP is mediated almost entirely by a rise in SBP, as changes in DBP are almost negligible. Given the large vasodilation occurring in active skeletal muscles and cutaneous vascular beds, TPR significantly decreases. However, MAP increases because the rise in $\dot{Q}$ is greater than the fall in TPR. In order to supply O_2 to working skeletal muscles, the myocardium also increases its O_2 demand and uptake. The increased work of the heart is reflected in the RPP.

Blood Flow Distribution During Aerobic Exercise

Exercise causes a redistribution of $\dot{Q}$, and hence blood flow, away from so-called inactive regions, towards active muscles. This redistribution results in a relative shift in the fraction of $\dot{Q}$ each region receives. Skeletal muscles receive a particularly large fraction, based on the increasing demand for O_2. From receiving a modest 18–20% of $\dot{Q}$ at rest, which is directed towards the entire musculature, active skeletal muscles receive upwards of 85% at $\dot{V}O_{2max}$. Interestingly, during exercise, active skeletal muscles rarely make up more than half of the entire muscle mass, even during maximal exercise. Nonetheless, the increase in skeletal muscle blood flow from rest to maximal exercise is substantial: from 750–1000 ml.min^{-1} (2–5 ml.100 g

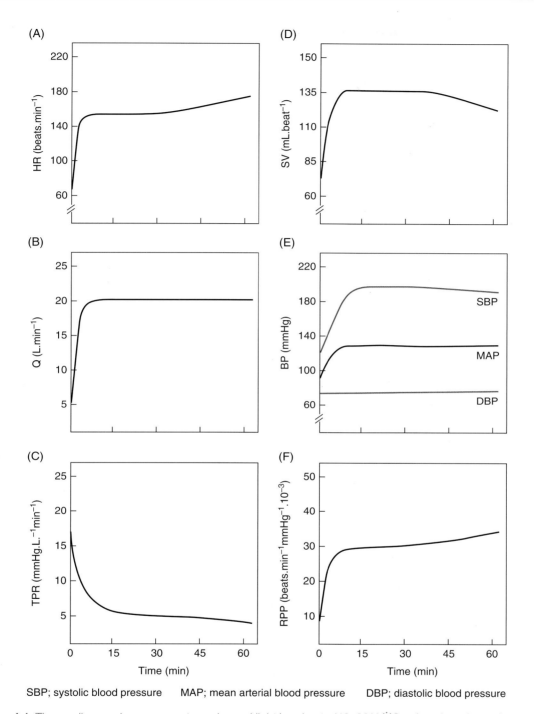

SBP; systolic blood pressure   MAP; mean arterial blood pressure   DBP; diastolic blood pressure

Figure 4.1 The cardiovascular response to prolonged light/moderate (40–60% $\dot{V}O_{2max}$) and moderate/intense (60–85% $\dot{V}O_{2max}$) dynamic exercise. During the first 10–30 minutes of exercise, a steady state occurs, whereby the cardiovascular system is able to meet whole-body metabolic requirements. As exercise persists, a drift occurs in cardiovascular function, despite the maintenance of a given absolute workload

muscle^{-1}.min^{-1}) to nearly 22 000 ml.min^{-1} in a healthy young individual with a maximal $\dot{Q}$ of 25 l.min^{-1} [8]. This represents an increase in skeletal muscle O_2 uptake from ~60 ml.min^{-1} to almost 4000 ml.min^{-1}. Notably, the increase in muscle blood flow during maximal exercise is limited by the requirement to maintain blood pressure, such that active muscles vasoconstrict if blood pressure cannot be maintained.

Whilst skeletal muscles receive a large fraction of the blood delivered to active muscles during exercise, coronary and respiratory muscle blood flow also increases. Coronary blood flow supplies the heart, a muscle that is always active. At rest in the supine position, coronary blood flow is ~250 ml.min^{-1}, or 5% of $\dot{Q}$. As exercise intensity increases, coronary blood flow can reach as much as 1000 ml.min^{-1} in a heart weighing 300 g. Given that blood flow to the heart is intimately linked with myocardial O_2 uptake, the RPP can be calculated in order to evaluate internal work. On the other hand, respiratory muscle blood flow during exercise is related to the increased work of breathing, which at $\dot{V}O_{2max}$ can account for 10–15% of total O_2 uptake. This fraction of O_2 uptake is observed at elevated ventilation rates (100–140 l.min^{-1}). At a ventilation of ~125 l.min^{-1}, for example, intercostal muscle blood flow is ~50 ml.100 ml^{-1}.min^{-1}.

The skin is the largest organ of the body, typically accounting for 6–10% of body mass in healthy individuals with a body surface area of 1.8–2.0 m^2. At rest in temperate conditions, skin blood flow is estimated to be 200–500 ml.min^{-1} (100–300 ml.m^{-2}.min^{-1}). During whole-body passive heating, however, maximal skin blood flow can reach 7000–8000 ml.min^{-1} (3500–4000 ml.m^{-2}.min^{-1}). Accordingly, the capacity of the cutaneous vasculature to vasodilate and receive high blood flows is secondary only to that of muscle. Hence, during exercise in the heat, competition for $\dot{Q}$ can develop between the skin and active skeletal muscle. Interestingly however, skin blood flow during exercise heat stress reaches only ~50% of maximal capacity, and even lower levels in temperate environments. Indeed, skin blood flow increases up to ~2 l.min^{-1} during submaximal exercise and decreases towards resting values or even lower during maximal exercise in cool conditions.

The cerebral circulation receives between 12 and 15% of $\dot{Q}$ at rest, or a blood flow of ~750 ml.min^{-1} (50–60 ml.100 g^{-1}.min^{-1}). Historically, it was thought that cerebral blood flow was unaffected or did not considerably vary during exercise because cerebral autoregulation maintained blood flow to the brain within a relatively narrow range in MAP (i.e. between 60 and 150 mmHg). However, it is now understood that cerebral blood flow increases with exercise intensity up to ~60% $\dot{V}O_{2max}$, after which it decreases towards baseline values [9,10]. This hyperventilation-induced cerebral vasoconstriction occurs mainly in response to a decrease in the partial pressure of arterial carbon dioxide.

The splanchnic organs include the liver, gastrointestinal tract (GIT), pancreas and spleen. At rest in the supine position, blood flow to this region is ~1500 ml.min^{-1} (~100 ml.100 g^{-1}.min^{-1} in the liver), which is ~25% of $\dot{Q}$. As exercise intensity increases, blood flow to the splanchnic organs decreases such that at $\dot{V}O_{2max}$, it is reduced to ~350 ml.min^{-1}. However, O_2 uptake remains relatively stable (50–60 ml.min^{-1}) in this region, owing to an increase in O_2 extraction from 4 ml.100 ml^{-1} at rest to 17 ml.100 ml^{-1} at $\dot{V}O_{2max}$ [8]. Similarly, the kidneys receive ~1200 ml.min^{-1} (~400 ml.100 g^{-1}.min^{-1}) at rest, making renal blood flow the second largest resting regional circulation, with ~20% of $\dot{Q}$. During exercise, renal blood flow decreases with the rise in work rate. However, given that the kidneys are overperfused, O_2 uptake only falls by ~3% from rest to $\dot{V}O_{2max}$, as O_2 extraction increases from 1.2 to 3.6 ml.100 ml^{-1}.

The Cardiovascular Response to Maximal Exercise

The cardiovascular response to prolonged dynamic exercise can be objectively quantified in relation to a maximal functional capacity (i.e. $\dot{V}O_{2max}$). The upper limit of this capacity reflects the ability of the cardiovascular systems to supply the working muscles with O_2 during intense exercise. The maximal volume of O_2 an individual can consume is typically measured during exercise performed at progressively increasing work rates until volitional fatigue (i.e. exhaustion), but it can also be quantified during supramaximal exercise (i.e. exercise performed at a workload 10–30% greater than required to achieve $\dot{V}O_{2max}$). The classical concept of $\dot{V}O_{2max}$ requires a plateau in O_2 uptake (Figure 4.2), despite further increases in workload [11]. Whilst this concept has been challenged due to inconsistencies in identifying a clear plateau during standard incremental tests, it has nonetheless been shown to be a true reproducible parametric measure of cardiorespiratory capacity during comparative continuous supramaximal exercise testing [12]. Accordingly, $\dot{V}O_{2max}$ has a day-to-day variability of 2–4% in individuals with sufficient motivation and anaerobic capacity. The calculation of $\dot{V}O_{2max}$ is based on the Fick principle (Equation 4.6). Accordingly, the magnitude by which maximal $\dot{Q}$ and a-vO_2 diff (the difference in O_2 concentration between arterial and mixed venous blood, or arteriovenous O_2 difference) can increase determines the upper limit to whole-body O_2 uptake. At rest, systemic a-vO_2 diff is usually ~4.5 ml.100 ml^{-1}, but it

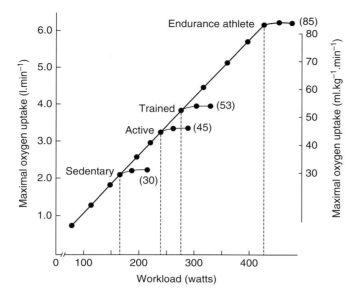

Figure 4.2 Maximal oxygen uptake in sedentary, active and trained individuals and elite endurance athletes (*Source*: Rowell [6]. Reproduced with permission of Wiley & Sons)

increases up to $16\,\mathrm{ml.100\,ml^{-1}}$ during maximal exercise. Interestingly, it can reach $18\,\mathrm{ml.100\,ml^{-1}}$ (90% extraction) in skeletal muscles at $\dot{V}O_{2max}$ [8].

$$\dot{V}O_{2max} = \dot{Q}_{max} \times a - vO_2\,diff_{max} \qquad \text{(Equation 4.6)}$$

As demonstrated in Figure 4.2, during dynamic upright exercise $\dot{V}O_{2max}$ increases as a function of workload from $\sim30\,\mathrm{ml.kg^{-1}.min^{-1}}$ in a population of young healthy, but sedentary males to $\sim85\,\mathrm{ml.kg^{-1}.min^{-1}}$ in highly trained endurance athletes [13]. The rise in heart rate during incremental exercise parallels that of O_2 uptake, reaching a plateau and maximum at around 195 beats.$\mathrm{min^{-1}}$, depending on age, gender and fitness level (Figure 4.3). In highly stressful conditions, such as hyperthermia or dehydration, heart rate can reach slightly higher values. Interestingly, myocardial cells possess the capacity to contract at more than 300 beats. $\mathrm{min^{-1}}$; however, heart rate seldom exceeds 210 beats.$\mathrm{min^{-1}}$, as ventricular filling time would be far too short above this.

The magnitude and nature of changes in stroke volume during exercise remain somewhat contentious. Previously, it was accepted that stroke volume increased with exercise intensity, but that a plateau occurred upon reaching 40–50% $\dot{V}O_{2max}$ [14]. Recently, however, progressive increases in stroke volume have been reported in both trained and untrained individuals during incremental exercise up to $\dot{V}O_{2max}$ [15]. The proposed pathway for the continued increase in stroke volume in trained individuals resides within an increased diastolic filling, enhanced contractility, larger blood volume and decreased cardiac afterload. In untrained individuals, stroke volume is suggested to continue increasing during exercise at intensities beyond 50% $\dot{V}O_{2max}$, due to a naturally occurring high blood volume. Other factors influencing stroke volume during intense or incremental exercise include age and gender. Further research is required to substantiate the level and intensity to which stroke volume can increase, however, as a comprehensive body of literature supports the notion that stroke volume decreases during intense exercise, especially at maximal effort (Figure 4.3). Correspondingly, the increase in $\dot{Q}$ during incremental exercise reflects changes in heart rate and stroke volume, and is nearly linear to that of O_2 uptake, with a slope of $6\,\mathrm{l.min^{-1}}$ per $1\,\mathrm{l.min^{-1}}$ increase in O_2 uptake. However, given that stroke volume generally decreases prior to the attainment of $\dot{V}O_{2max}$, the rise in $\dot{Q}$ at greater exercise intensities is achieved solely via increases in heart rate.

As with submaximal exercise, changes in blood pressure during maximal incremental exercise stem from adjustments in SBP. Indeed, SBP increases linearly with heart rate and O_2 uptake, plateauing at around 180–200 mmHg at $\dot{V}O_{2max}$. The rise in $\dot{Q}$ is responsible for increasing SBP, as it compensates for the decline

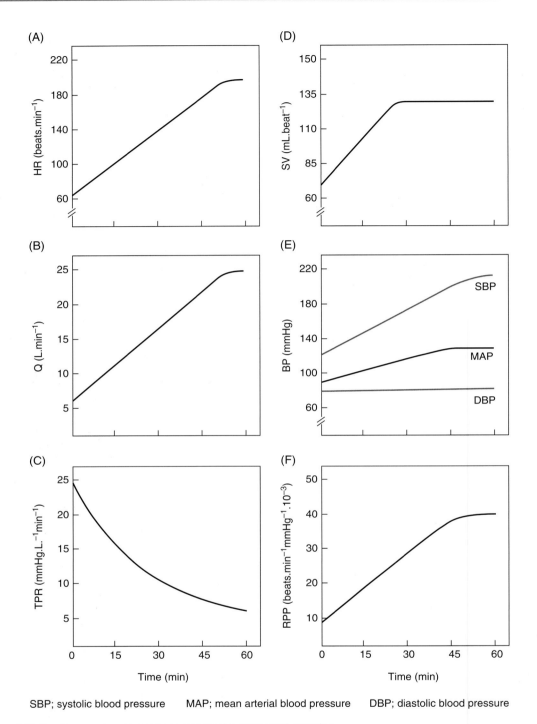

SBP; systolic blood pressure   MAP; mean arterial blood pressure   DBP; diastolic blood pressure

Figure 4.3 Cardiovascular response to maximal incremental exercise

in peripheral resistance. Moreover, the increase in SBP is relatively stable due to the vasomotor response occurring in active muscles (vasodilation) and inactive tissue (vasoconstriction). Conversely, DBP typically remains constant as exercise intensity increases, sometimes decreasing upon approaching $\dot{V}O_{2max}$. However, DBP is susceptible to decreasing during exercise performed under heat stress, where cutaneous vascular beds are more dilated and peripheral resistance is decreased. The decline in TPR during incremental exercise is curvilinear, reaching its nadir at $\dot{V}O_{2max}$. Despite the decrease in TPR, MAP does not decline during maximal exercise, since the increase in $\dot{Q}$ is quite large (Figure 4.3). Note that a fall in SBP towards the end of an incremental exercise test is particularly dangerous and warrants further investigation.

Gender Differences in the Cardiovascular Response to Aerobic Exercise

Males have a naturally higher percentage of lean muscle mass than females, along with a larger heart (size and volume). Males also possess greater O_2 carrying capacity than females, with a larger amount of red blood cells (~6%) and haemoglobin (10–15%). Despite these differences, the pattern of response in cardiovascular function during aerobic exercise is similar between genders, although the magnitude of response in certain parameters may vary. For example, heart rate is higher in females when performing submaximal exercise at a given absolute workload (e.g. 200W), whereas stroke volume is lower. The lower stroke volume is compensated for by a higher heart rate, which results in a similar or greater $\dot{Q}$ to that of males. This signifies that females exercise at a higher relative intensity (i.e. $\%\dot{V}O_{2max}$) than males when performing the same amount of absolute work. When matched for exercise intensity (e.g. 40 or 75% of peak workload), females demonstrate a lower $\dot{Q}$ in response to an elevated heart rate and reduced stroke volume compared with males, even when expressed in relation to body mass or body surface area [16]. However, O_2 extraction is increased in females, which emphasises the greater cardiac work required to exercise at the same relative intensity. Consequently, males rely on preload and enhanced use of the Frank–Starling mechanism to increase $\dot{Q}$, whilst in females it is supported by heart rate. It is suggested that part of the limitation associated with increasing stroke volume in females may stem from a blunted sympathetic response and higher basal vasodilator tone.

The increased relative intensity noted in females during submaximal exercise stems from males having an absolute $\dot{V}O_{2max}$ (i.e. $l.min^{-1}$) 40–60% greater than females. The disparity in $\dot{V}O_{2max}$ is mostly due to differences in lean muscle mass and heart size, because when expressed relative to body mass (i.e. $ml.kg^{-1}.min^{-1}$) the difference is reduced to 20–30%. It is further reduced to less than 15% when expressed as a function of lean body mass (i.e. $ml.kg$ lean body $mass^{-1}.min^{-1}$) [17]. Whilst expressing $\dot{V}O_{2max}$ in relation to lean body mass highlights the significance of muscle mass and adipose tissue in determining $\dot{V}O_{2max}$, it also highlights that excess fat is not the only factor influencing the difference in $\dot{V}O_{2max}$ between men and women. Indeed, both genders share the same innate ability to improve $\dot{V}O_{2max}$, and in similarly trained males and females there is no difference in maximal heart rate. However, because males have larger hearts, maximal stroke volume is higher, which leads to a maximal $\dot{Q}$ that is typically 30% higher than in females. Despite the difference in heart morphology, the mechanisms mediating the increase in stroke volume remain similar. As such, differences in stroke volume appear to be the primary cause of gender differences in increasing $\dot{Q}$ during submaximal and maximal aerobic exercise.

Males and females also display a similar pattern of response in blood pressure, peripheral resistance and myocardial O_2 demand during submaximal and maximal aerobic exercise. Whilst the DBP response to exercise is comparable between genders, SBP is higher in males during exercise at a given relative intensity. Consequently, MAP is greater in males at similar submaximal relative work rates, but also at the completion of maximal exercise. Given that males have a greater $\dot{Q}$ during submaximal exercise, TPR is usually lower than in females. TPR is similar during maximal exercise, however, owing to its marked decrease. Males tend to have a higher RPP at the completion of maximal exercise because of the exacerbated rise in SBP.

The Cardiovascular Response to Ageing

Ageing is associated with a decline in the ability to respond to physiological stress, partly as a result of age, but also due to the adoption of a sedentary lifestyle. The characteristic adjustments in cardiovascular function associated with the ageing process are reduced maximal heart rate, stroke volume, $\dot{Q}$ and O_2 uptake (Table 4.2). It is purported that $\dot{V}O_{2max}$ declines at a rate of ~10% per decade after the age of 30 in sedentary individuals. The primary pathway by which $\dot{V}O_{2max}$ is reduced lies in a decrease in stroke volume, along with lowered heart rate and O_2 extraction [18]. The decrease in stroke volume is related to a gradual decline in myocardial contractility and stiffening of the heart wall, which delays ventricular filling. Factors such as a slower relaxation of the ventricular wall, poor peripheral venous tone and decreased total blood volume (including plasma and red cell volume) also influence EDV and stroke volume. The reduction in maximal heart rate stems in part from a loss in muscle mass resulting from detraining, but also from diminished β-adrenergic responsiveness. The lower levels of O_2 extraction observed in aged individuals are associated with reductions in total haemoglobin, fibre/capillary ratio and muscle respiratory capacity, along with decreased mitochondrial mass and oxidative enzymes.

Cardiovascular parameter	Males				Females			
	Sedentary		Trained		Sedentary		Trained	
	Young	Old	Young	Old	Young	Old	Young	Old
Heart rate (beats.min⁻¹)	195	160	192	160	192	160	190	160
Stroke volume (ml)	120	100	150	120	85	80	110	90
Cardiac output (l.min⁻¹)	22	16	27	22	16	12	20	15
Mean arterial blood pressure (mmHg)	117	128	115	125	113	125	111	120
Systolic blood pressure (SBP) (mmHg)	195	205	195	205	175	195	180	190
Diastolic blood pressure (DBP) (mmHg)	78	90	75	85	82	90	77	85
Maximal oxygen uptake (ml.kg⁻¹.min⁻¹)	40	25	60	45	35	22	50	35

Table 4.2 Cardiovascular responses to maximal exercise in males and females in relation to training status (sedentary versus untrained) and age (young versus old)

During submaximal aerobic exercise at a given absolute workload, heart rate is similar or slightly higher in older individuals, whereas stroke volume and $\dot{Q}$ are lower. As a result, $\dot{V}O_{2max}$ during incremental exercise is achieved earlier. The pattern of response in blood pressure is similar in young and old individuals; however, older individuals have higher resting SBP and DBP. This upward shift is maintained during exercise, such that older individuals sustain a higher MAP for any given workload. The elevated blood pressure response stems from greater peripheral resistance, resulting from a loss of elasticity of the connective tissue in the vasculature. During maximal exercise, SBP may be 20–50 mmHg higher in older individuals, and DBP may be 15–20 mmHg higher. Given the higher heart rate and SBP responses experienced by the elderly, myocardial O_2 uptake is also higher during submaximal exercise. Whilst TPR decreases in older individuals during maximal exercise, the extent of this decrement is not as pronounced as in the young. Notably, because older individuals experience a greater decrease in maximal heart rate than they do an increase in SBP relative to younger individuals, the RPP at $\dot{V}O_{2max}$ is lower.

Importantly, regular exercise markedly attenuates the rate of loss in cardiovascular function and aerobic capacity (Table 4.2) [19]. Endurance training induces similar benefits in the elderly as it does in the young, with improvements in $\dot{V}O_{2max}$ of ~20% following 6 months of regular training. Moreover, trained older individuals often have a similar or greater $\dot{V}O_{2max}$ than untrained/sedentary younger individuals. Regular aerobic exercise reduces heart rate at submaximal workloads, along with resting and exercising SBP. Maximal stroke volume is increased with training, allowing for improvements in $\dot{Q}$ of over 3 l.min⁻¹. The changes mostly stem from peripheral adaptations, which facilitate the return of venous blood to the heart and enhance EDV. Hence, despite age-related reductions in cardiovascular performance, regular exercise induces adaptations that attenuate some of these reductions, improving SBP, stroke volume, $\dot{Q}$ and, ultimately, $\dot{V}O_{2max}$.

Cardiovascular Responses to Static Exercise

Exercise performed statically, or isometrically, involves the contraction of muscles in a fixed or stationary position (i.e. without movement). Several daily activities incorporate a static component, as do many sports (e.g. rowing, cycling, weightlifting, wrestling). The foremost difference in the cardiovascular response to static compared with dynamic exercise resides in its effect on active muscle blood flow. During an isometric contraction, muscle blood flow decreases in response to a swelling and stiffening of active muscle fibres, which increases intramuscular pressure and causes a mechanical constriction of the vessels. Although a similar constriction occurs during dynamic exercise, the rhythmic alternation between contraction and relaxation, such as in running, encourages blood flow through the muscle pump. As such, the hallmark of isometric exercise is a failure to ensure adequate blood flow to the contracting musculature when force production exceeds 10–30% of a maximal voluntary contraction (MVC). For example, blood flow to the quadriceps is greater during a sustained (30 minutes) contraction performed at 5% MVC than in one maintained for 8 minutes at 15% MVC or for 4 minutes at 25% (Figure 4.4) [20]. Indeed, despite the greater metabolic requirement of sustaining a contraction at 15 or 25% MVC, muscle blood flow remains much lower, indicating the significant impedance to blood flow. The level of impedance varies with muscle groups, as forearm (i.e. handgrip exercise) muscle blood flow

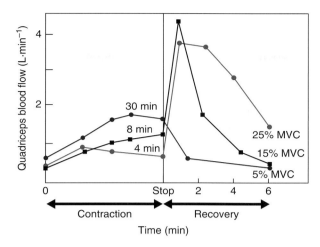

Figure 4.4 Blood flow to quadriceps muscle during contraction at 5 and 25% MVC and during a recovery period (*Source*: Sjøgaard et al. [20]. Reproduced with permission of Springer)

increases to 30–40% of MVC [21]. Whilst blood flow is impeded when contraction intensity exceeds a given level, the response during recovery compensates for the reduced flow noted during contraction (Figure 4.4).

The heart rate response to static exercise is caused by parasympathetic (i.e. vagal) withdrawal and sympathetic activation, with the magnitude of increase related to contraction intensity. In contrast, stroke volume remains relatively stable at lower contraction intensities (e.g. 10% MVC), whereas it decreases during high-intensity efforts. The decrease in stroke volume is purported to stem from a decrease in preload and increase in afterload. Nonetheless, $\dot{Q}$ increases during static exercise in response to the rise in heart rate. Interestingly, the increase in $\dot{Q}$ serves mostly to overperfuse regions not requiring an increase in blood flow (e.g. skin and inactive muscles), with systemic a-vO$_2$ often decreasing during static exercise.

The elevation in $\dot{Q}$ contributes to an increase in arterial blood pressure, as the decrease in peripheral resistance is minimal, especially in relation to the extent occurring during dynamic exercise. Moreover, the increase in arterial blood pressure – *the pressor response* – is disproportionate to the amount of work performed when compared with dynamic exercise. For example, submaximal dynamic exercise induces a large elevation in heart rate but a modest increase in SBP, imposing a volume load on the heart. In contrast, static/ isometric exercise causes a modest rise in heart rate but a marked increase in SBP, imposing a pressure load on the heart. Differences between males and females during static exercise are negligible, with heart rate, stroke volume and $\dot{Q}$ responding similarly, and MAP increasing slightly more in males. Like dynamic exercise, ageing results in lower heart rate, stroke volume and $\dot{Q}$ during static exercise, but a higher blood pressure response. For further discussion of the chronic effects of sustained and intensive physical activity upon the heart, see Chapter 5.

Conclusion

The magnitude and pattern of adjustment in the cardiovascular response to exercise are determined by several factors, including the nature of the task (e.g. dynamic versus static), work rate (i.e. relative exercise intensity), muscle mass involved, environmental conditions (e.g. heat and altitude), training status and genetics. Nonetheless, exercise is typically characterised by increases in heart rate and stroke volume, which lead to adjustments in $\dot{Q}$, arterial blood pressure, peripheral resistance and myocardial function. Part of these adjustments is a redistribution of $\dot{Q}$ (i.e. blood flow), which reflects the ability of the cardiovascular systems to supply the working muscles with O$_2$ during exercise. With chronic/regular training, this ability can be improved, leading to increased $\dot{V}O_{2max}$. Although the magnitude of response in certain cardiovascular parameters, such as $\dot{V}O_{2max}$, may vary between males and females during exercise, the pattern of response remains comparable. Similarly, whilst ageing reduces cardiovascular performance, regular exercise induces adaptations that attenuate some of these reductions, leading to improvements in blood pressure and aerobic performance that are equivalent to those seen in younger individuals.

References

1 Saltin, B., Radegran, G., Koskolou, M.D. and Roach, R.C. Skeletal muscle blood flow in humans and its regulation during exercise. *Acta Physiol Scand* 1998; **162**: 421–36.

2 Dempsey, J.A. New perspectives concerning feedback influences on cardiorespiratory control during rhythmic exercise and on exercise performance. *J Physiol* 2012; **590**: 4129–44.

3 Ekelund, L.G. Circulatory and respiratory adaptation during prolonged exercise of moderate intensity in the sitting position. *Acta Physiol Scand* 1967; **69**: 327–40.

4 Rowell, L.B. Human cardiovascular adjustments to exercise and thermal stress. *Physiol Rev* 1974; **54**: 75–159.

5 Coyle, E.F. and Gonzalez-Alonso, J. Cardiovascular drift during prolonged exercise: new perspectives. *Exerc Sport Sci Rev* 2001; **29**: 88–92.

6 Rowell, L.B. *Human Circulation: Regulation during Physical Stress*. New York: Oxford University Press, 1986.

7 Hamilton, M.T., Gonzalez-Alonso, J., Montain, S.J. and Coyle, E.F. Fluid replacement and glucose infusion during exercise prevent cardiovascular drift. *J Appl Physiol* 1991; **71**: 871–7.

8 Rowell, L.B. *Human Cardiovascular Control*. New York: Oxford University Press, 1993.

9 Moraine, J.J., Lamotte, M., Berre, J. et al. Relationship of middle cerebral artery blood flow velocity to intensity during dynamic exercise in normal subjects. *Eur J Appl Physiol Occup Physiol* 1993; **67**: 35–8.

10 Hellstrom, G., Fischer-Colbrie, W., Wahlgren, N.G. and Jogestrand, T. Carotid artery blood flow and middle cerebral artery blood flow velocity during physical exercise. *J Appl Physiol* 1996; **81**: 413–18.

11 Hill, A.V. and Lupton, H. Muscular exercise, lactic acid, and the supply and utilization of oxygen. *Quart J Med* 1923; **16**: 135–71.

12 Hawkins, M.N., Raven, P.B., Snell, P.G. et al. Maximal oxygen uptake as a parametric measure of cardiorespiratory capacity. *Med Sci Sports Exerc* 2007; **39**: 103–7.

13 Saltin, B. and Astrand, P.O. Maximal oxygen uptake in athletes. *J Appl Physiol* 1967; **23**: 353–8.

14 Åstrand, P.-O., Cuddy, T.E., Saltin, B. and Stenberg, J. Cardiac output during submaximal and maximal work. *J Appl Physiol* 1964; **19**: 268–74.

15 Vella, C.A. and Roberds, R.A. A review of the stroke volume response to upright exercise in healthy subjects. *Br J Sports Med* 2005; **39**: 190–5.

16 Wheatley, C.M., Snyder, E.M., Johnson, B.D. and Olson, T.P. Sex differences in cardiovascular function during submaximal exercise in humans. *SpringerPlus* 2014; **3**: 445.

17 Sparling, P.B. A meta-analysis of studies comparing maximal oxygen uptake in men and women. *Res Q Exerc Spor* 1980; **51**: 542–52.

18 Ogawa, T., Spina, R.J., Martin, W.H. et al. Effects of aging, sex, and physical training on cardiovascular responses to exercise. *Circulation* 1992; **86**: 494–503.

19 Stratton, J.R., Levy, W.C., Cerqueira, M.D. and Schwartz, R.S. Cardiovascular responses to exercise. Effects of aging and exercise training in healthy men. *Circulation* 1994; **89**: 1648–55.

20 Sjøgaard, G., Savard, G. and Juel, C. Muscle blood flow during isometric activity and its relation to muscle fatigue. *Eur J Appl Physiol Occup Physiol* 1988; **57**: 327–35.

21 Lind, A.R. and McNicol, G.W. Local and central circulatory responses to sustained contractions and the effect of free or restricted arterial inflow on post-exercise hyperaemia. *J Physiol* 1967; **192**: 575–93.

5 The Athlete's Heart: Impact of Age, Sex, Ethnicity and Sporting Discipline

Tracey Keteepe-Arachi and Nabeel Sheikh

St George's University of London, London, UK

Introduction

Participation in regular systematic intensive exercise is associated with a constellation of structural and functional cardiac adaptations comprising the 'athlete's heart'. The five- to sixfold increase in cardiac output ($\dot{Q}$) required for intense exercise results in chamber dilatation, ventricular hypertrophy, enhanced diastolic filling and changes in autonomic function, the consequences of which are frequently demonstrated on the resting 12-lead electrocardiogram (ECG). Manifestations of the athlete's heart are usually modest and fall well within defined limits of normality. Occasionally, however, a small proportion of athletes may demonstrate striking electrical and structural modifications, which overlap with those observed in cardiac diseases implicated in exercise-related sudden cardiac death (SCD). Differentiating physiology from cardiac pathology in such cases can prove challenging for the evaluating physician. The nature and extent of cardiac remodelling in response to exercise is determined by several important demographic factors, including the age, sex, ethnicity and the athlete's sporting discipline. The influence of these variables upon the athlete's heart is the focus of this chapter. Only athlete cohorts between 14 and 35 years old will be discussed.

Electrical Remodelling in the Athlete's Heart

Data based on observational studies from large athletic cardiovascular screening programmes have identified several common physiological ECG changes in athletes, which generally reflect increased vagal tone and chamber enlargement [1]. These include sinus bradycardia, first-degree and Mobitz type 1 second-degree atrioventricular block, isolated increases in QRS voltage, partial right-bundle branch block and the early repolarisation pattern [2].

A minority of athletes, however, may exhibit ECG changes frequently found in several cardiac conditions implicated in exercise-related SCD, making it difficult to distinguish between athlete's heart and cardiac pathology. To facilitate the differentiation of benign versus pathological ECG patterns in athletes, see Chapters 10–12.

Structural Remodelling in the Athlete's Heart

An increase in stroke volume is the predominant mechanism by which athletes are able to generate and maintain sizeable cardiac outputs for prolonged periods of time. Augmentation of stroke volume occurs through a combination of an increase in left ventricular (LV) end-diastolic volume (EDV), a decrease in LV end-systolic volume (ESV) and enhanced LV filling. Early studies based on M-mode echocardiography demonstrated that on average, athletes develop a 10% increase in end-diastolic diameter and a 15–20% increase in left ventricular wall thickness (LVWT) compared to the upper limits of normal for sedentary individuals [3].

IOC Manual of Sports Cardiology, First Edition. Edited by Mathew G. Wilson, Jonathan A. Drezner and Sanjay Sharma.
© 2017 International Olympic Committee. Published 2017 by John Wiley & Sons, Ltd.

Subsequent cross-sectional studies based on 2D echocardiography in large cohorts of elite athletes further quantified the structural cardiac changes of the athlete's heart. Pelliccia et al. [4] demonstrated an LV cavity size of >55 mm in almost 50% of 1309 adult Caucasian (white) predominately male Olympian athletes, with 14% revealing an extreme LV cavity dilatation of >60 mm. Based on these data, the upper limit of normal for LV cavity dimensions in white adult male athletes is currently regarded as ≤64 mm, although a minority of athletes participating in extreme endurance sports such as the Tour de France have been reported to demonstrate an LV cavity of ≥70 mm. A further study by the same group in 947 white Olympian athletes revealed LVWTs ranging between ≤7 and 16 mm; however, only 16 individuals (1.7%) demonstrated values ≥13 mm, in keeping with the range compatible with morphologically mild hypertrophic cardiomyopathy (HCM). Therefore, a value of ≤12 mm in white adult male athletes is currently regarded as the upper limit of normal for LVWT.

Although relatively neglected, new data from echocardiographic and cardiac magnetic resonance imaging (CMRI) studies have demonstrated that the right ventricle (RV) undergoes similar changes in mass, volume and function to the left, with cardiac remodelling occurring in a 'balanced' fashion [5–9]. Echocardiographic limits of normality with respect to RV chamber size have recently been proposed for adult athletes, although data are currently lacking in several cohorts [5–7].

The Influence of Age on the Athlete's Heart

The majority of the structural and electrical changes just described are derived from studies in white, adult (>18 years of age) cohorts. Exercise, however, also induces cardiac remodelling in younger athletes, who frequently start intense training regimes at increasingly younger ages in the pursuit of sporting excellence. This is of importance, given that adolescent and young-adult athletes appear to be particularly susceptible to SCD, making correct interpretation of structural and electrical data crucial in this cohort [10]. In general, younger athletes develop changes qualitatively similar to but quantitatively smaller in magnitude than those observed in adults.

Electrical Remodelling in Adolescent Athletes

Interpretation of a young athlete's ECG may prove particularly challenging due to the high prevalence of repolarisation anomalies, specifically morphological T-wave alterations, normally observed in individuals ≤16 years of age. These repolarisation changes compose the 'juvenile' ECG pattern, which is characterised by T-wave inversion in leads V1–V4 (Figure 5.1). The juvenile ECG pattern reflects RV dominance and a posteriorly directed repolarisation polarity in young children. With increasing age, the dominance transfers from RV to LV, with a resultant reversal of repolarisation polarity, which may be observed on the ECG progressing from left to right precordial leads. Eventually, after puberty, the adult ECG pattern is observed, with T-wave inversion limited to V1.

Persistence of the juvenile ECG pattern is recognised in post-pubertal adolescents and may overlap with the phenotype of cardiomyopathies and ion-channel disorders, leading to diagnostic difficulties. Papadakis et al. [11] compared ECG patterns in 1710 predominately white, male, adolescent athletes (mean age 16.0 ± 1.7 years) and 400 sedentary adolescent controls, finding no difference in the overall prevalence of T-wave inversion between the two groups (4 versus 3%, p = 0.46). T-wave inversion in the anterior leads was largely confined to V1–V2 and was almost always observed in athletes and controls aged <16 years. Only 0.8% of athletes and 0.5% of controls exhibited anterior T-wave inversion beyond V2. Detailed investigation of the majority of individuals with anterior T-wave inversion failed to identify sinister cardiac pathology, leading the authors to conclude that this pattern likely reflects the juvenile pattern in adolescent athletes. In contrast, T-wave inversion involving the inferior and/or lateral leads was not observed in controls and was observed infrequently in athletes (1.5%), in whom it was associated with left ventricular hypertrophy (LVH) or congenital cardiac abnormalities. This finding suggests that T-wave inversion in the inferior and/or lateral leads should prompt further investigation and long-term surveillance for an underlying cardiac disorder irrespective of the athlete's age.

Migliore et al. [12] performed a study of 2765 children aged between 8 and 18 years undergoing pre-participation cardiovascular evaluation, observing T-wave inversion in 5.7%. The majority of the T-wave inversion (4.7%) was localised to the right precordial leads, consistent with a juvenile pattern. The prevalence of right

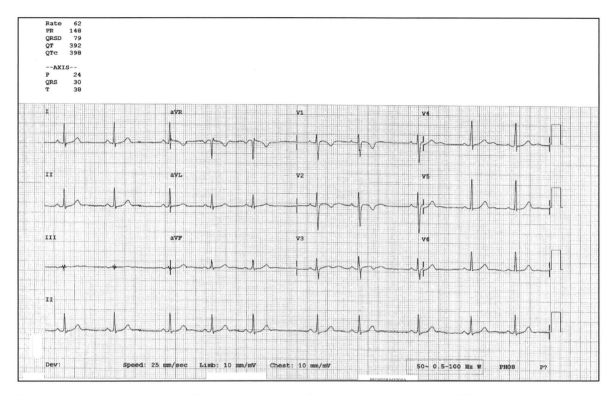

Figure 5.1 Example of a juvenile ECG pattern. Note the T-wave inversion in leads V1–V3

precordial T-wave inversion decreased significantly with increasing age and pubertal development, being found in 8.4% of children <14 years of age but only in 1.7% ≥14 years (p < 0.001). As in the study by Papadakis et al. [11], T-wave inversion in the lateral and inferior leads was rare (0.1 and 0.9%, respectively). Of the children with T-wave inversion, 2.4% were diagnosed with a cardiomyopathy (three with arrhythmogenic right ventricular cardiomyopathy (ARVC) and one with HCM). Of the three children with ARVC, all showed complete pubertal development and were ≥14 years of age. The individual diagnosed with HCM exhibited lateral T-wave inversion. The findings from this study reinforce the notion that T-wave inversion in the inferior and/or lateral leads in a young athlete or the persistence of anterior T-wave inversion beyond puberty warrants comprehensive evaluation and long-term follow-up.

Structural Remodelling

Makan et al. [13] examined LV cavity dimensions in 900 elite, predominately white male adolescent athletes with a mean age of 15.7 years. Compared with 250 healthy age- and sex-matched sedentary controls, the athletes exhibited a larger LV cavity (50.8 versus 47.9 mm), with a dimension of >54 mm being found in 18%, compared to none of the controls. An LV cavity exceeding predicted upper limits of normal was found in 13% of the athletes, and the range of cavity dimensions in these individuals was 52–60 mm. No adolescent athlete exhibited an LV cavity dimension >60 mm. Thus, the upper limit of normal for LV cavity dimensions in white male adolescent athletes may be regarded as ≤58 mm.

A study of 720 elite adolescent white athletes (mean age 15.7 ± 1.4 years) by Sharma et al. [14] compared LVWTs and LV cavity dimensions on echocardiography to 250 age-, gender- and body surface area-matched sedentary controls. On average, the athletes exhibited a 13% larger LVWT and 6% larger LV cavity dimension compared to controls. Although the LVWT exceeded the upper limits of normal in 38 athletes (5%), only 0.4% had an LVWT >12 mm (all male), and all demonstrated concomitant LV cavity dilatation. None of the controls exhibited an LVWT >11 mm. These data suggest that the upper limit of normal for LVWT may be regarded as ≤12 mm in male adolescent white athletes.

The Influence of Sex on the Athlete's Heart

Gender influences the athlete's heart independent of sporting discipline, age and body habitus. In general, changes occur to a greater extent in male than in female athletes. Although the exact mechanisms behind these sex differences are unclear, one possibility is variations in the amount of circulating androgens and in the density of androgen receptors.

Electrical Remodelling in Female Athletes

In a large study of 32 652 unselected athletes undergoing pre-participation cardiovascular evaluation, Pelliccia et al. [1] observed a higher prevalence of ECG abnormalities in males compared to females (12.4 versus 9.6%; $p = 0.001$). The same group documented significant differences between males and females in a study of 1005 consecutive athletes [15]: a significantly larger proportion of male athletes had either distinctly abnormal (17 versus 8%; $p < 0.001$) or mildly abnormal (28 versus 14%; $p < 0.001$) ECGs compared to female athletes. The majority of female athletes had normal ECGs (78 versus 55%; $p < 0.001$). These differences may be explained by the more subtle morphological adaptations to exercise demonstrated by females (see later), as well as a lower uptake in sports associated with more extensive electrical changes, such as rowing.

Structural Differences Between Male and Female Athletes

In a study of 1309 white adult Olympian athletes by Pelliccia et al. [4], although 12% of females had an enlarged LV cavity, none exhibited dimensions exceeding 55 mm. A further study by the same group compared cardiac dimensions in 600 female adult athletes, 738 elite male adult athletes and 65 sedentary female controls [16]. Compared to controls, both LV end-diastolic dimensions and LVWTs were greater in female athletes, by 6 and 14%, respectively. LV cavity dimensions exceeded normal limits (>54 mm) in 8% of female athletes, and were ≥60 mm in 1%. In contrast, none of the 600 female athletes' LVWTs exceeded >12 mm, compared to 2% of the males. Based on these data, the upper limits of normal for LV cavity dimensions and LVWTs in adult white female athletes are currently regarded as ≤57 and ≤11 mm, respectively.

Cardiac remodelling has also been observed in adolescent female athletes, but to a far lesser extent than in their male counterparts. In the study by Makan et al. [13], only 22% of adolescent athletes with LV cavity dilatation were females, and no female athlete exhibited an LV cavity >55 mm. Similarly, in the study by Sharma et al. [14], all female athletes had LVWTs of ≤11 mm. Thus, the upper limits of normal for LV cavity dimensions and LVWTs in adolescent white female athletes may be regarded as ≤54 and ≤11 mm, respectively.

The Influence of Ethnicity on the Athlete's Heart

The majority of the data presented so far have been derived from white cohorts, competing predominately in Europe and the US. Over the past 2 decades, however, ethnicity has emerged as an important determinant of cardiac adaptation to exercise. Increasing globalisation has provided athletes in all parts of the world with the opportunity to compete like never before, and data from pre-participation cardiovascular evaluation of these individuals has informed our understanding of the influence of ethnicity on the athlete's heart. From this perspective, the group most intensely studied has been athletes of African/Afro-Caribbean ethnicity (black athletes), whose participation rates in many sports are often disproportionately higher in Western countries than their prevalence in the general population.

Electrical Remodelling in Athletes of African/Afro-Caribbean Ethnicity

As with their white counterparts, black athletes reveal a high prevalence of training-related ECG changes, in particular ST-segment elevation, early repolarisation (ER) pattern and voltage criteria for LVH [17]. However, perhaps the most striking feature of cardiac remodelling in black athletes is the extent to which they develop electrical changes traditionally regarded as training-unrelated, in particular repolarisation abnormalities.

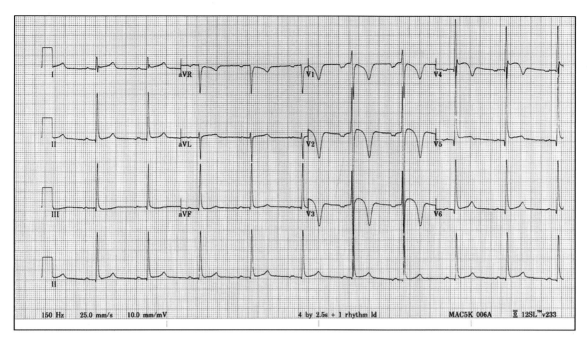

Figure 5.2 ECG from a black athlete demonstrating deep T-wave inversion in leads V1–V4. Note preceding convex ST-segment elevation and Sokolow–Lyon voltage criteria for LVH

Repolarisation Changes and T-Wave Inversion in Adult Male Black Athletes Black athletes have a higher prevalence of ER changes and T-wave inversion compared with white athletes. Magalski et al. [18] analysed the ECGs of 1959 elite adult male American football players and reported that electrical abnormalities were observed twice as commonly in black as in white athletes. T-wave inversion was 13 times more frequent. Papadakis et al. [17] compared the ECGs of 904 predominantly adult male black athletes with those from 1819 white adult male athletes, 119 black sedentary individuals and 52 black HCM patients. T-wave inversion was more than six times more prevalent in black compared to white athletes (22.8 versus 3.7%; p < 0.001), and was predominately confined to anterior leads V1–V4 (12.7%). When isolated to the anterior leads, T-wave inversion was usually associated with convex ST-segment elevation (in 64.3% of cases; Figure 5.2). Deep T-wave inversion (−0.2 mV or above) was also more common in black athletes compared to both white athletes and black controls (12.1 versus 1.0 and 1.7%, respectively; p < 0.001). T-wave inversion was far less common in the inferior and lateral leads in black athletes (6 and 4.1%, respectively). In contrast, almost all black HCM patients exhibited T-wave inversion (87.2%), the majority of which was in the lateral leads (76.9%). T-wave inversion isolated to V1–V4 and the inferior leads was much less common in black HCM patients (3.8 and 1.9%, respectively). ST-segment depression was frequently observed in black HCM patients, but was virtually absent in black athletes and controls (50.0 versus 0.4 and 0.0%, respectively; p < 0.001).

Comprehensive evaluation of athletes with T-wave inversion in this study failed to identify an underlying cardiomyopathy. However, during long-term follow-up, two black athletes and one white athlete were diagnosed with HCM. In keeping with a previous study in white athletes [19], all three individuals exhibited T-wave inversion in the inferior and/or lateral ECG leads. Importantly, none of the black athletes with T-wave inversion confined to V1–V4 were diagnosed with a cardiomyopathy. Based on these observations, T-wave inversion preceded by convex ST-segment elevation confined to V1–V4 in black athletes is considered an ethnic variant of physiological adaptation to exercise. However, T-wave inversion extending into the lateral leads should be considered abnormal regardless of ethnicity and investigated comprehensively to exclude an underlying cardiomyopathy, with long-term follow-up thereafter. At present, the precise significance of T-wave inversion confined to the inferior leads remains unknown; until further data are published, this pattern should be investigated with a minimum of echocardiography.

T-Wave Inversion in Adult Female Black Athletes T-wave inversion is also described in adult female black athletes, but to a far lesser extent. Rawlins et al. [20] compared the ECGs of 240 adult black female athletes to 200 adult white female athletes. As with males, black female athletes demonstrated a higher prevalence of repolarisation changes, including ST-segment elevation (11 versus 1%; $p < 0.001$), T-wave inversion (14 versus 2%; $p < 0.001$) and deep T-wave inversion (2 versus 0%; $p < 0.001$). All T-wave inversion in female black athletes was confined to V1–V3, with none revealing phenotypic features of a cardiomyopathy after further evaluation. Therefore, as with male athletes, T-wave inversion in the anterior leads is likely to represent an ethnically mediated variant in black female athletes. In contrast, the absence of T-wave inversion in the inferior or lateral leads suggests that these patterns should trigger comprehensive evaluation and follow-up.

T-Wave Inversion in Adolescent Black Athletes Striking ECG changes have also been described in younger black athletes. As with adults, voltage criteria for LVH and repolarisation abnormalities are more common in black athletes (ST-segment elevation 91 versus 56%, $p < 0.001$; deep T-wave inversion 14 versus 3%, $p < 0.05$) [21]. Sheikh et al. [22] studied both male and female black adolescent athletes and reported the prevalence of T-wave inversion to be fivefold greater in adolescent black compared to adolescent white athletes (22.8 versus 4.5%; $p < 0.001$), and almost twofold greater in adolescent black athletes than in sedentary adolescent black controls (22.8 versus 13.4%). As with adult black athletes, T-wave inversion in adolescent black athletes was predominantly confined to anterior leads V1–V4 (14.3%). The prevalence of T-wave inversion was higher in adolescent black male athletes compared to adolescent black female athletes (24.5 versus 16.7%; $p = 0.17$). Importantly, compared to 9% of adolescent black male athletes, none of the females exhibited deep T-wave inversion. This suggests that deep T-wave inversion in adolescent black female athletes should be viewed with caution and requires further investigation. Inferior and/or lateral T-wave inversion was observed with the same frequency in black adolescent athletes as in black adult athletes; although comprehensive evaluation of all athletes with T-wave inversion failed to reveal a cardiomyopathy in this study, the lower frequency of inferior and/or lateral T-wave inversion in this group and their association with cardiomyopathies warrant comprehensive evaluation and follow-up.

Structural Remodelling in Athletes of African/Afro-Caribbean Ethnicity

LV Chamber Dimensions in Black Athletes Most studies have revealed that black athletes demonstrate similar quantitative changes in LV cavity dimensions to white athletes. Therefore, the upper limits of normal for LV chamber dimensions in white athletes are also applicable to the black athletic population.

LVH in Black Athletes and the Influence of Age and Sex In contrast to LV cavity dimensions, several studies have demonstrated significantly greater mean LVWTs in black compared to white athletes. A UK study comparing cardiac dimensions in 300 male adult black and 300 male adult white athletes revealed significantly greater mean LVWTs in the former (11.3 ± 1.6 mm versus 10 ± 1.5 mm; $p < 0.001$). Importantly, 18% of black athletes exhibited an LVWT >12 mm in the range compatible with morphologically mild HCM, compared with just 4% of white athletes (Figure 5.3). Furthermore, 3% of black athletes demonstrated extreme degrees of LVH (≥ 15 mm), whereas the LVWT never exceeded 14 mm in white athletes [23]. The pattern of LVH in all athletes was homogenous and was associated with an LV cavity dilatation of between 55 and 66 mm. Furthermore, comprehensive evaluation of athletes with LVH failed to reveal the broader phenotypic features of HCM. A further collaborative study between the UK and France of 904 black and 1819 white athletes corroborated these findings, demonstrating LVWTs of >12 mm in 12.4% of black compared to just 1.6% of white athletes [17]. Irrespective of ethnicity, none of the athletes exhibited an LVWT of >16 mm.

Cardiac remodelling has also been studied in female black athletes. The aforementioned study by Rawlins et al. [20] showed that black female athletes demonstrated greater LVWTs compared to white female athletes (9.2 ± 1.2 versus 8.6 ± 1.2 mm; $p < 0.001$). However, the magnitude of LVWTs was significantly smaller: 3% of black female athletes revealed an LVWT of >11 mm, and none exhibited an LVWT of >13 mm. In comparison, none of the white female athletes revealed an LVWT of >11 mm.

Adolescent black athletes are also capable of developing significant LVH. Di Paolo et al. [21] reported a 5% larger mean LVWT in black compared to white adolescent athletes. LVH (LVWT ≥ 13 mm) was

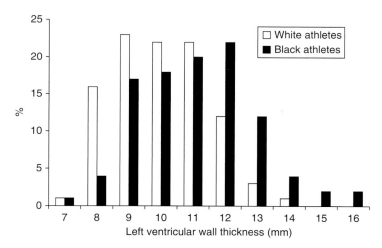

Figure 5.3 Distribution of maximal LVWTs in black and white athletes. Note the greater magnitude of LVH (maximal LVWT >12mm) in black athletes, with substantial LVH (maximal LVWT ≥15mm) in 3% (*Source*: Basavarajaiah et al. [23]. Reproduced with permission of Elsevier)

present in 2.6% black athletes compared to 0% of white athletes. In a larger study by Sheikh et al. [22], comprising 245 male and 84 female black adolescent athletes, 7% exhibited an LVH of >12mm, compared to just 0.6% of 903 white adolescent athletes and 0% of 134 sedentary adolescent black controls. Importantly, although none of the female adolescent athletes exhibited a wall thickness of >13mm, male adolescent black athletes were capable of developing significant LVH, up to and including 15mm. Furthermore, even in the very young (<16years), 5.5% of black athletes exhibited LVH, compared to 0% of white athletes. During further evaluation and follow-up of athletes with LVH, none exhibited features of HCM.

These studies suggest that the upper limit of normal for LVWTs should be regarded as ≤15mm in adult male black athletes and ≤12mm in adult female black athletes, and as ≤14mm in adolescent male black athletes and ≤11mm in adolescent female black athletes.

The RV in Black Athletes Recently, the nature of RV remodelling in black athletes has been examined. The issue is of pertinence given the high prevalence of T-wave inversion in RV leads V1–V4 in the black athletic population, which invariably raises the suspicion of ARVC. Zaidi et al. [7] examined RV dimensions in 300 elite black athletes, 375 elite white athletes and 153 sedentary controls (n = 69 black; all groups predominately male). Consistent with observations in white athletes, black athletes exhibited significantly greater RV and right ventricular outflow tract (RVOT) dimensions compared to controls, although they were marginally smaller than in white athletes. Although RVOT dilatation compatible with current diagnostic criteria for ARVC was frequently observed in both black and white athletes, nine (3%) black athletes exhibited concomitant anterior T-wave inversion, heightening the suspicion. Comprehensive evaluation of these nine individuals, including CMRI, failed to reveal features of ARVC, emphasising the limitations of applying diagnostic criteria derived from predominantly white, sedentary cohorts to black athletes.

Athletes of Other Ethnicities

Data on cardiac remodelling with exercise is also emerging for athletes of other ethnicities, including Arabic (Middle Eastern), South Asian and East Asian athletes. The data indicates that electrical and structural remodelling in these ethnicities is similar to that observed in white athletic cohorts, making ECG and echocardiographic interpretation criteria derived from white athletes applicable to these ethnic groups. However, more data are required in many ethnicities, particularly South and East Asian athletes.

Influence of Sporting Discipline on the Athlete's Heart

It is clear from the descriptions in this chapter that there is a direct relationship between exercise training and development of the athlete's heart. However, the extent and nature of both structural and electrical cardiac remodelling are also influenced by the type of exercise being performed.

Electrical Remodelling in Relation to Sporting Discipline

Exercise stimulates a resting bradycardia through changes in autonomic balance, which result in increased vagal tone and changes to the sinoatrial node. Additionally, the effects of chamber enlargement are directly manifest on the surface ECG. The prevalence of these electrical alterations in any athletic population is dependent upon the sporting discipline in question. Heart rate is generally lower in athletes engaged in dynamic exercise (also referred to as 'isotonic exercise' or 'endurance training'), such as running or cycling, than in those engaged in static exercise (also termed 'isometric exercise', 'strength training' or 'resistance training'), such as weightlifting or wrestling. Indeed, athletes engaged in dynamic exercise may exhibit marked sinus bradycardia of less than 30 beats.min^{-1}, asymptomatic pauses >2 seconds and junctional escape rhythms, all of which are overcome by exercise, suggesting a vagal origin [2]. Athletes performing dynamic exercise also reveal a higher prevalence of physiological electrical changes, reflecting chamber enlargement, including partial right-bundle branch block and voltage criteria for LVH [2, 15]. Pelliccia et al. [15] reported distinctly abnormal ECG patterns to be higher in those performing dynamic exercise, however. Cardiac pathology was demonstrated in only a minority of these athletes, the remainder revealing absolute increases in cardiac dimensions, including LV end-diastolic dimension and LVWT, suggesting a physiological basis.

Structural Remodelling in Relation to Sporting Discipline

The notion that sporting discipline has an influence on structural cardiac remodelling was first proposed by Moganroth et al. [24] in 1975, using echocardiography. The so-called 'Morganroth hypothesis' postulated that dynamic exercise, which involves sustained propulsion of the athlete through space rather than the generation of muscular force, places a predominant volume load on the heart. This results in 'eccentric hypertrophy', characterised by an increase in LV mass and wall thickness, with a proportional increase in LV EDV. In contrast, static exercise, which involves the generation of force but little movement of the athlete through space, places a pressure load on the heart and results in 'concentric hypertrophy', characterised by an increase in LV mass and wall thickness, but with normal LV EDV.

Although several studies have been consistent with the Morganroth hypothesis, particularly the concept of eccentric hypertrophy and large chamber dimensions with dynamic exercise, data from others suggest it is far from absolute and dichotomous. This likely reflects the fact that training regimes for most sports feature both dynamic and static aspects [25]. In keeping with LV adaptations, there is now considerable evidence derived from CMRI studies of eccentric RV remodelling in endurance athletes [8, 9]. More recent echocardiographic studies have confirmed these findings, reporting significantly larger right heart measurements (both chamber and outflow tract) in athletes performing dynamic as opposed to static exercise [5, 6].

Conclusion

Age, sex, ethnicity and sporting discipline have a significant impact on the nature and extent of cardiac remodelling in response to exercise. In general, adult male athletes, those of black ethnicity and those performing dynamic exercise tend to exhibit the largest cardiac dimensions and the most profound electrical alterations (Figure 5.4). Table 5.1 illustrates the current upper limits of normality for LV and RV chamber sizes and wall thicknesses in athletes of different ages, sexes and ethnicities, based on our current knowledge and the data presented in this chapter. Recognition and complete understanding of the influence of these demographic factors on the athlete's heart is crucial for the correct interpretation of an athlete's ECG and echocardiographic data during pre-participation cardiovascular evaluation.

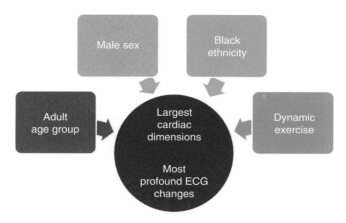

Figure 5.4 Impact of age, sex, ethnicity and sporting discipline on the athlete's heart

Athlete group	Gender	LV cavity dimension (mm)	LVWT (mm)	RV dimensions (mm)						
				RVOTP	RVOT1	RVOT2	RVD1	RVD2	RVD3	RVWT
Adult white	Male	≤64	≤12	≤40	≤43	≤32	≤55	≤47	≤109	≤6
	Female	≤57	≤11	≤37	≤40	≤29	≤49	≤43	≤100	≤5
Adolescent white	Male	≤58	≤12	–	–	–	–	–	–	–
	Female	≤54	≤11	–	–	–	–	–	–	–
Adult black	Male	≤62	≤15	≤40	≤43	≤32	≤55	≤47	≤109	≤6
	Female	≤56	≤12	≤37	≤40	≤29	≤49	≤43	≤100	≤5
Adolescent black	Male	≤62	≤14	–	–	–	–	–	–	–
	Female	≤57	≤11	–	–	–	–	–	–	–

Table 5.1 Upper limits of normal for LV and RV end-diastolic cavity dimensions and wall thicknesses, based on age, sex and ethnicity. RVOTP, right ventricular outflow tract dimension (parasternal); RVOT1, proximal right ventricular outflow tract dimension; RVOT2, distal right ventricular outflow tract dimension; RVD1, right ventricular basal dimension; RVD2, right ventricular mid-ventricular dimension; RVD3, right ventricular longitudinal dimension; RVWT, right ventricular free wall thickness.

– denotes data not available

References

1 Pelliccia, A., Culasso, F., Di Paolo, F.M. et al. Prevalence of abnormal electrocardiograms in a large, unselected population undergoing pre-participation cardiovascular screening. *Eur Heart J* 2007; **28**(16): 2006–10.
2 Corrado, D., Pelliccia, A., Heidbuchel, H. et al. Recommendations for interpretation of 12-lead electrocardiogram in the athlete. *Eur Heart J* 2010; **31**(2): 243–59.
3 Maron, B.J. Structural features of the athlete heart as defined by echocardiography. *J Am Coll Cardiol* 1986; **7**(1): 190–203.
4 Pelliccia, A., Culasso, F., Di Paolo, F.M. and Maron, B.J. Physiologic left ventricular cavity dilatation in elite athletes. *Ann Intern Med* 1999; **130**(1): 23–31.
5 Oxborough, D., Sharma, S., Shave, R. et al. The right ventricle of the endurance athlete: the relationship between morphology and deformation. *J Am Soc Echocardiogr* 2012; **25**(3): 263–71.
6 D'Andrea, A., Riegler, L., Golia, E. et al. Range of right heart measurements in top-level athletes: the training impact. *Int J Cardiol* 2013; **164**(1): 48–57.
7 Zaidi, A., Ghani, S., Sharma, R. et al. Physiological right ventricular adaptation in elite athletes of African and Afro-Caribbean origin. *Circulation* 2013; **127**(17): 1783–92.
8 Prakken, N.H., Velthuis, B.K., Teske, A.J. et al. Cardiac MRI reference values for athletes and nonathletes corrected for body surface area, training hours/week and sex. *Eur J Cardiovasc Prev Rehabil* 2010; **17**(2): 198–203.
9 Scharhag, J., Schneider, G., Urhausen, A. et al. Athlete's heart: right and left ventricular mass and function in male endurance athletes and untrained individuals determined by magnetic resonance imaging. *J Am Coll Cardiol* 2002; **40**(10): 1856–63.

10 Maron, B.J., Doerer, J.J., Haas, T.S. et al. Sudden deaths in young competitive athletes: analysis of 1866 deaths in the United States, 1980–2006. *Circulation* 2009; **119**(8): 1085–92.

11 Papadakis, M., Basavarajaiah, S., Rawlins, J. et al. Prevalence and significance of T-wave inversions in predominantly Caucasian adolescent athletes. *Eur Heart J* 2009; **30**(14): 1728–35.

12 Migliore, F., Zorzi, A., Michieli, P. et al. Prevalence of cardiomyopathy in Italian asymptomatic children with electrocardiographic T-wave inversion at pre-participation screening. *Circulation* 2012; **125**(3): 528–38.

13 Makan, J., Sharma, S., Firoozi, S. et al. Physiological upper limits of ventricular cavity size in highly trained adolescent athletes. *Heart* 2005; **91**(4): 495–9.

14 Sharma, S., Maron, B.J., Whyte, G. et al. Physiologic limits of left ventricular hypertrophy in elite junior athletes: relevance to differential diagnosis of athlete's heart and hypertrophic cardiomyopathy. *J Am Coll Cardiol* 2002; **40**(8): 1431–6.

15 Pelliccia, A., Maron, B.J., Culasso, F. et al. Clinical significance of abnormal electrocardiographic patterns in trained athletes. *Circulation* 2000; **102**(3): 278–84.

16 Pelliccia, A., Maron, B.J., Culasso, F. et al. Athlete's heart in women. Echocardiographic characterization of highly trained elite female athletes. *JAMA* 1996; **276**(3): 211–15.

17 Papadakis, M., Carre, F., Kervio, G. et al. The prevalence, distribution, and clinical outcomes of electrocardiographic repolarization patterns in male athletes of African/Afro-Caribbean origin. *Eur Heart Jour* 2011; **32**(18): 2304–13.

18 Magalski, A., Maron, B.J., Main, M.L. et al. Relation of race to electro-cardiographic patterns in elite American football players. *J Am Coll Cardiol* 2008; **51**(23): 2250–5.

19 Pelliccia, A., Di Paolo, F.M., Quattrini, F.M. et al. Outcomes in athletes with marked ECG repolarization abnormalities. *New Engl J Med* 2008; **358**(2): 152–61.

20 Rawlins, J., Carre, F., Kervio, G. et al. Ethnic differences in physiological cardiac adaptation to intense physical exercise in highly trained female athletes. *Circulation* 2010; **121**(9): 1078–85.

21 Di Paolo, F.M., Schmied, C., Zerguini, Y.A. et al. The athlete's heart in adolescent Africans: an electrocardiographic and echocardiographic study. *J Am Coll Cardiol* 2012; **59**(11): 1029–36.

22 Sheikh, N., Papadakis, M., Carre, F. et al. Cardiac adaptation to exercise in adolescent athletes of African ethnicity: an emergent elite athletic population. *Br J Sports Med* 2013; **49**(9): 585–92.

23 Basavarajaiah, S., Boraita, A., Whyte, G. et al. Ethnic differences in left ventricular remodeling in highly-trained athletes relevance to differentiating physiologic left ventricular hypertrophy from hypertrophic cardiomyopathy. *J Am Coll Cardiol* 2008; **51**(23): 2256–62.

24 Morganroth, J., Maron, B.J., Henry, W.L. and Epstein, S.E. Comparative left ventricular dimensions in trained athletes. *AnnI Intern Med* 1975; **82**(4): 521–4.

25 Spence, A.L., Naylor, L.H., Carter, H.H. et al. A prospective randomised longitudinal MRI study of left ventricular adaptation to endurance and resistance exercise training in humans. *J Physiol* 2011; **589**(Pt. 22): 5443–52.

6 Physical Activity in the Prevention and Management of Atherosclerotic Disease

John P. Buckley

Institute of Medicine, University Centre Shrewsbury and University of Chester, Chester, UK

Introduction

Led by the efforts of the World Health Organization (WHO), total physical activity per week in any form – and in addition to sport and intentional exercise – is increasingly being promoted globally as important to health and cardiovascular disease (CVD). The underpinning links between physical (in)activity and CVD discussed in this chapter highlight the importance of recognising the amount of activity undertaken within occupational settings and spontaneous play in children as significant influences on cardiovascular health. Much of the evidence has traditionally been related to moderate-to-vigorous cardiorespiratory endurance training. There is, however, increasing evidence on the benefits of focused muscular strength/endurance exercise and more frequent lower-intensity activity throughout one's waking hours, which affects metabolic risk factors (e.g. glucose, insulin and total daily energy expenditure).

Definitions Encompassing Physical Activity

'Physical activity' is an overarching term that encompasses all forms of human activity, as described in the following definitions. *Physical activity* is any human movement that is created by the contraction of skeletal muscle. *Exercise or exercise training* is also considered physical activity, but is performed in an organised structured manner, with an aim or a goal (e.g. fitness, health, performance, rehabilitation). Participation in *sport* is also included under the umbrella of 'physical activity'. *Physical fitness* is the ability or set of attributes required to perform any given physical activity/task and is reliant upon a combination of factors, including: aerobic capacity and endurance; muscular strength and endurance; joint mobility/flexibility and balance; coordination and skill; and metabolic function. *Sedentary behaviour* is a more recent area of investigation, with much attention focused on the ills of prolonged bouts of sitting. Independent of physical activity, the time one spends sitting is now accepted as a significant risk factor for cardiometabolic diseases.

Preventing CVD: The Continuum of Human Activity from Sedentary Behaviour to Moderate- to Vigorous-Intensity Physical Activity

The WHO has corroborated evidence and guidelines from around the world to define a healthy level of physical activity as at least 150 minutes of moderate-intensity or 75 minutes of vigorous-intensity activity per week. Rising concerns about daily sedentary behaviour, especially in the developed world, have however

IOC Manual of Sports Cardiology, First Edition. Edited by Mathew G. Wilson, Jonathan A. Drezner and Sanjay Sharma.
© 2017 International Olympic Committee. Published 2017 by John Wiley & Sons, Ltd.

Improved CVD risk factors	Improved arterial endothelial and myocardial integrity
• Blood lipids • Blood pressure • Blood glucose and insulin • Energy expenditure, adipose and visceral fat • Lean body mass • Psychological well being	• Nitric oxide vasodilatory responsiveness • Atheromatous plaque stability • Reduced inflammatory agents • Reduced myocardial irritability and arrhythmogenic potential

Figure 6.1 CVD risk factors and myocardial function elements affected by physical activity and exercise training (*Data sources*: Wienbergen and Hambrecht [5] and Gielen et al. [6])

highlighted that 150 minutes represents <2.5% of a person's waking hours. Many apparently active people meeting the 150-minute-per-week target are still at risk because many of their remaining waking hours (>60%) are spent sitting [1].

When delivering activity interventions, changes to both total daily energy expenditure (physical activity) and exercise capacity should be measured as independent outcomes across the prevention spectrum [2,3]. As summarised in Figure 6.1, prolonged periods of low- to moderate-level activity and spending more time on one's feet have now been linked to many cardiometabolic risk factors, while moderate to vigorous activity which increases cardiorespiratory capacity has direct effects on vascular, endothelial and myocardial function. Over the past 5 decades, the loss of energy expenditure in occupational and domestic life (200–300 kcal.day^{-1}) has continued to far outweigh what many people feel they are gaining by participating in sport, exercise and other intentional active leisure pursuits [4]. The greatest shift in physical activity patterns has therefore been from 'light' activity towards more sedentary behaviours, while the number of people engaged in moderate to vigorous activity is actually unchanged and in some cases has increased in the past 15 years. In response to this, the WHO's most recent target is to reduce physical inactivity by 10%. Globally, physical inactivity prevails on average in 40% of individuals with CVD; more alarming is that in developed countries, this figure rises to as much as 70% [2]. Many of the data have been collected from 'self-report', but where more objective accelerometer data have been collected, figures from the US and UK have shown 95% of the population being classified as inactive [1].

The scientific link between physical activity and cardiovascular health was first studied and then reported in the 1950s and 1960s by epidemiological and public health pioneers Jeremy Morris (UK) and Ralph Paffenbarger (US). This is not to disrespect that in 1772, Dr William Heberden (the physician who defined the term 'angina pectoris') reported to the Royal College of Physicians in London that a patient's angina symptoms were resolved by sawing wood for 30 minutes per day. It is of particular note that this is occupational activity, and not exercise or sport. All too often, exercise and sport can tend to become a focus of social health promotion schemes. The important fact to recognise is that the loss of activity in occupational settings, and not a lack of leisure-time sport or exercise, is the key agent underlying ill health. People who sit for most of their day at work have a 15% greater risk of premature mortality, compared with those who have a job which requires standing most of the day. It is interesting to note that Hippocrates also recognised the value of health-related activity coming from both 'natural exercise' (that which occurs in daily life) and 'artificial exercise' (sport and recreation). Examples from Brazil have highlighted the importance to health of changing the built environment, the workplace and leisure-time habits at home, as opposed to leisure, exercise and sports facilities/programmes [3].

In addition to avoiding prolonged periods of sitting, if people do engage in moderate to vigorous levels of activity, which lead to improved cardiorespiratory fitness, then all-cause and cardiovascular mortality are reduced by up to 50% [2]. It has been shown that the strength of this evidence is greatly improved when fitness is measured from an exercise test as opposed to self-reported physical activity in leisure time. Self-report physical-activity measures in large population cohorts have up until recently not been able to capture very well the non-exercise-activity component of daily movement (occupational and domestic) [1]. Even when an individual has other risk factors, such as high lipids, high blood pressure, diabetes, obesity, chronic lung disease, family history or smoking, exercise leads to a reduced CVD morbidity and mortality of between 20 and 50% [7]. The WHO and chief medical officers around the world have recently changed their advice regarding children and older or frail adults, cautioning against simply sitting too much. The recommended doses of aerobic activity (e.g. 150 minutes' moderate- or 75 minutes' vigorous-intensity per week) can be performed in multiple bouts of at least 10 minutes. With regard to strength training, it has beneficial effects on CVD risk factors, including blood glucose, insulin control and resting metabolic rate, as well as providing better functionality and quality of life for older, frailer individuals [6]. In terms of a specific structured exercise dose (frequency, duration and intensity) to improve cardiorespiratory fitness and muscular strength/ endurance, the guidelines for the prevention and rehabilitation of CVD are quite similar (see later).

Physical Activity within Rehabilitation and Secondary Prevention

One of the strengths of the exercise evidence base in CVD rehabilitation and secondary prevention is that it is mainly drawn from interventional randomised controlled trials (RCTs) [8]. For primary prevention, on the other hand, much of the evidence continues to be observational or epidemiological. This is not to say there are not practical confounders in the cardiac rehabilitation evidence. With respect to the lower-than-ideal uptake of cardiac rehabilitation globally [9], this may indicate a selection bias among patients entered into research trials: usually, they are Caucasian males between 45 and 65 years of age who are educated about and motivated to engage in participation. Education and socioeconomic status are strong key risk factors for CVD [8]. One of the challenges that most front-line cardiac rehabilitation professionals face is to offer a service that reflects the research trials; in many ways, the research trials are tightly controlled, with a high ratio of staff supervision, and they often exclude the types of participant (e.g. older, lower sociodemographic status, with many comorbidities) who are most in need of rehabilitation and secondary prevention guidance [8]. Furthermore, the modes of exercise used in these trials are often limited to just cycle ergometer and treadmill. Encouragingly, an increasing number of trials and guidelines recommend combining aerobic and strength training, which leads to better outcomes compared to aerobic exercise alone [6]. Rehabilitation programmes must always aim to be as full as possible, however, and must make the best use of the evidence base in order to support the case for an appropriately 'dosed' exercise component. The exercise dose is noted in Box 6.1 in terms of frequency, duration and intensity; it would seem frequency is a likely main culprit for people not attaining the correct 'dose'. There is little or no evidence on the effects of sedentary behaviour within secondary prevention, but it would seem sensible that the evidence from primary prevention of its links with cardiometabolic risk factors would apply.

Box 6.1   Exercise Training Recommendations for Enhancing Cardiorespiratory Fitness

- A *frequency* of 3–5 sessions per week
- An accumulated *duration* of sessions of 20–60 minutes, performed either continuously or with intervals of active recovery
- An *intensity* of moderate to vigorous effort (ranging from 40 to 75% of VO_{2max} or, for more precision, near to or at the ventilatory or lactate threshold); associated target heart rates and ratings of perceived exertion (RPEs) are typically used in practical settings to represent these ranges or thresholds of intensity (40–75% of heart rate reserve, Borg RPE score of 11–14 or Borg CR10 score of 2–5)
- Inclusion of *resistance/strength training* for 8 to 10 major muscle groups, performing 10 to 15 repetitions at an intensity up to 70% of a one-repetition maximum

(*Data sources*: AACVP [10], BACPR [11], Mezzani et al. [12], Conraads et al. [13])

The Cochrane Reviews of RCTs have clearly defined a relationship between aerobic training and cardiac mortality in patients with established coronary heart disease (CHD) [8]. The typical doses of activity they report have led to the recommendations summarised in Box 6.1, on the basis of which most guideline recommendations are made. From reviews of key evidence, it has been difficult to define a 'minimum' beneficial threshold of intensity in cardiac patients, due to a number of other competing factors at baseline (e.g. baseline fitness and previous activity levels), but there is confidence in outcomes when the exercise intensity exceeds 40% of VO_{2max}. In promoting a more flexible model for the provision of exercise (especially in lower-income or developing countries), which must be adapted to the psychological, sociological and geographical (clinic, community or home-based) needs of the patient, this intensity range also encompasses the effective lower-supervision, lower-intensity and lower-risk Australian model pioneered by Goble and

Worcester in the 1980s [14]. This model was designed to achieve the widest possible delivery of safe and beneficial rehabilitation in the disparate, low-population-density make-up of Australia.

The combined outcomes from the evidence for exercise-based rehabilitation have shown all-cause and cardiac mortality being reduced by 13 and 26%, respectively [8]. Furthermore, rehabilitation programmes that include regular aerobic training have shown a reduced incidence of recurrent myocardial infarction (MI) and unplanned hospital readmissions and an improved functional capacity and self-perceived quality of life [8]. In addition to the traditionally recommended exercise training goals, cardiovascular health and rehabilitation specialists need to place equal value on patients being as active as possible throughout their day, even if this includes lighter-intensity activity and avoiding prolonged periods of sitting [14,15].

The causal relationship between physical activity and the reduction of CVD has been attributed to multiple biological, psychological and social changes, which favourably alter a number of established atherogenic risk factors, including the integrity of both the coronary and systemic arterial endothelia and factors affecting or improving myocardial function [7]. Risk factors benefitting from physical activity include high blood pressure, dyslipidaemia and insulin resistance [15]. Whilst it can be argued that many of these risk factors can be managed medically, exercise has proven to have its own independent benefits on cardiovascular health in both primary and secondary prevention, including arterial endothelial integrity, as influenced by an enhanced vasodilatory responsiveness to exertion/stress, a reduction in the potential of atheromatous plaques to rupture and reduced inflammatory markers associated with the development of atheroma [5]. In one trial of stable angina patients, exercise proved more medically effective than angioplasty after 12 months, with a 12% event rate in the exercise group versus 30% in the angioplasty group.

Within a comprehensive model of cardiac rehabilitation, it has been estimated that half of the benefit comes from exercise training and the other half from reductions in the major risk factors (medical, psychological and lifestyle interventions), especially smoking [16]. However, the value of exercise in the longer term is an area that needs more attention. Programmes delivered for 12 weeks have reported maintenance of exercise capacity for up to 1.5 years [17], but few studies have provided data for periods longer than this. One of the only long-term studies, which followed patients up for 14 years [18], reported that those who attended more sessions within a 4-month rehabilitation period had greater survival at 14 years, but much of the influence was affected by smoking status. Questions arise around how long-term sustainability of physical activity and exercise capacity can be achieved when most programmes last for just 12 weeks, or 26 weeks at best. Efforts related to developing patients' self-management skills, behaviour and long-term maintenance of physical activity are thus a vital component of rehabilitation [19].

Early Commencement of Exercise Rehabilitation

The earliest possible commencement of exercise following a coronary event or intervention has now been demonstrated to be an important factor in preventing subsequent negative myocardial remodelling, and thus is included in recent recommendations [20]. Further benefits include a number of psychological factors (stress, anxiety and depression) [21]. The outpatient physical activity plan should be commenced following risk stratification and an assessment of functional capacity, which also becomes part of the risk stratification. Maximal exercise capacities <5 metabolic equivalents (METs) ($VO_{2max} \leq 17$ ml.kg^{-1}.min^{-1}) are associated with higher-risk patients and >7 METs with lower-risk. The evidence for early commencement and related strategies for increasing patient uptake of rehabilitation is robust, but more evidence is required on the most effective ways to influence adherence [19]. With the advancement of new 'personalised' and electronic technologies for monitoring, communicating, managing and measuring daily activity and exercise [22], it will be of interest for future investigators to evaluate their role in long-term adherence as part of or following a programme of rehabilitation.

There may be concern around early commencement of exercise for some patient groups, especially those who have recently undergone coronary artery bypass surgery (CABG), had a diagnosis of congestive heart failure, suffered an MI, received a heart transplant or received therapy and/or implantation of a device for controlling arrhythmias. Establishing a physical activity plan and exercise programme for some of these groups should be thought of as no different to prescribing beta-blocker medication to patients with heart failure, however. If the full recommended dose were to be given at the outset, it might put the patient at risk, but if the prescription and administration of the dose are titrated over weeks up to an optimised level, which works in concert with the expected adaptation/healing processes, the body will have time to adapt and adjust in a safe and effective way. For physical activity, this managed up-titration model should also be seen as a psychological and social process [11].

Reducing Risk of Exertion-Related Events

Whatever cardiovascular condition(s) a patient has, reducing the risk of provoking an exertion-related event is in part related to how the exercise programme is structured. This is of particular importance when starting rehabilitation early, which coincides with periods of healing and physiological stabilisation following an acute event, treatment and/or surgery. There are three factors that need to be considered when aiming to reduce the risk of an exertion-related event:

- assessment and risk stratification (see [10] for details);
- pre-activity screening and monitoring of patient status or of contraindications to physical activity;
- monitoring intensity and related levels of supervision.

Many guidelines and standards are written with the assumption of risk stratification and that contraindications will be set for individuals undergoing a maximal exercise test or moderate to vigorous supervised activity. Educating and training patients to self-monitor and self-manage their conditions is important if they are to feel confident to continue participating in the longer term. The level of exertion-related risk is dependent on a variety of parameters and on the context in which physical activity is being performed, including:

- exercise tests and assessments (submaximal or maximal);
- light- to moderate-intensity activity that is part of normal daily functioning at home, at work or as part of transport;
- nonsupervised moderate to vigorous activity (structured sessions or as part of work, leisure pursuits or transport);
- supervised structured moderate to vigorous activity.

Warm-Up and Cool-Down

All moderate to vigorous exercise sessions should be preceded by a graduated warm-up (up to <40% VO_{2max} or <40% HRR or < RPE 11) and followed by a de-graduating cool-down. The aim is to gradually upregulate (warm-up) and downregulate (cool-down) the following processes: adrenaline release; vasodilation to the heart, skeletal muscles and skin; bronchodilation; time to shift oxygen transport from the viscera to the exercising tissues; and blood glucose and muscle metabolism. Collectively, these considerations are aimed at preventing ischaemia, arrhythmia, postural hypotension and breathlessness and at reducing reliance on anaerobic muscle metabolism [23]. As in athletes, a well-controlled warm-up also leads to improved exercise performance, which may provide patients with a greater sense of satisfaction and confidence.

In order to cover all the activities required for a safe and effective programme, a 15-minute warm-up and 10-minute cool-down are recommended to ensure the necessary physiological processes have occurred to best prevent any adverse events of ischaemia, dyspnea, syncope or arrhythmia [10–12,23].

Medication Considerations

Key CHD medications, such as angiotensin-converting enzyme (ACE) inhibitors, beta-blockers, statins and nitrates, may interact with the physiological processes of exertion, especially when starting or ending with rest. These include augmenting the chances of exercise-related postural hypotension and muscle aches and fatigue, and downregulating fat metabolism but preventing heightened catecholamines related to arrhythmia [24]. However, the creation of postural hypotension as a result of moving from a seated or floor exercise to a standing one in the middle of a session could provoke acute reductions in venous return and thus reduce myocardial perfusion, leading to ischaemia.

For exercise testing and the prescription of beta-blockers or ivabradine, a reduction in maximum heart rate of 20–30 beats.min^{-1} should be expected [25].

Post-surgery and Early Rehabilitation

For all groups of CHD patients, uptake of exercise-based rehabilitation is usually greatest in those following CABG [26]. This is likely to be a result of the pathway of treatment and care for CABG being very predictable, timed and structured. Along with the overt visual reminder to the patient of the seriousness of their disease and of the surgical procedure, these facts seem to conspire towards patients more easily adopting and achieving the goals of rehabilitation (compared to other groups). This structure includes designated pre-surgery preparations and education, an in-patient phase of 5–7 days in hospital and up to 6 weeks' required convalescence [10].

It is recommended that structured moderate to more vigorous aerobic exercise training commence no earlier than 2 weeks post-hospital discharge, and more ideally at 4 weeks [27].

Post-surgery, Early Aerobic Activity and Strength Training

Commencing post-CABG rehabilitation early (~10 days post-discharge) should involve light-intensity aerobic activity, upper-body mobility and lower-limb strength training. There is now good evidence, which includes older people (>75 years), that it is safe and effective to commence normal resistance-strength training of the lower limbs (e.g. 10 to 15 repetitions at 60% per repetition maximum) at 2 weeks post-CABG discharge [28]. It has even been demonstrated that performing upper-body exercise with moderate weights soon after CABG surgery puts far less stress on the sternum than a forceful sneeze [29]. As a precaution, sternal stress can be greatly reduced if arm exercises are performed with the humerus held in adduction (elbows kept near to the thorax).

Note, however, that the key assumptions of all these elements is that the patient has recovered without complication and is feeling well, and that the surgical wounds in both the chest and the leg are healing well, without infection.

Typical Post-surgical Complications

Transient atrial fibrillation may be found in 25–30% of patients in the early postoperative period, or up to 60% following more complex surgery (e.g. addition of valve surgery). Atrial fibrillation is usually self-limited, and the vast majority of cases will revert to sinus rhythm within 24 hours. However, in a smaller proportion of patients, it can persist up to many weeks before spontaneously resolving [30]. Reviews reveal that predisposing factors to atrial fibrillation normally include advancing age, presence of heart failure, peripheral vascular disease (PVD), pulmonary disease and preoperative tachyarrhythmias or pericarditis. Pre-exercise risk stratification, screening, medical management and programme adaptation should therefore include all of these factors, and heart rate/symptom reporting should be routinely documented on a regular basis during the whole period of rehabilitation. It is important to ensure that participants with atrial fibrillation can use ratings of perceived exertion effectively, and to document the METs at which they are observably comfortable or struggling (either during an exercise assessment or during activities in which METs can be best and most accurately estimated, e.g. cycle ergometer, treadmill walking, stepping height and rate) [11].

Pre-surgery Exercise

The evaluation of pre-surgical cardiorespiratory fitness and exercise training is increasingly becoming common practice in many conditions, aimed at reducing surgical and post-surgical complications and at improving post-surgical health outcomes [31]. Survival rates at 12 years' follow-up have been reported as significantly favourable for those who received pre-CABG surgery exercise training [32]. Pre-surgery anxiety and depression are predictors of increased mortality, so psychological aspects of rehabilitation and the potential contributions that exercise may have alongside psychological interventions have been highlighted as important [33]. Furthermore, pre-surgery exercise influences post-surgery uptake and the outcomes of rehabilitation [33]. Inspiratory muscle training has also received some attention pre- and post-surgery, but larger trials or data sets are required to increase confidence in their validity.

Post-Angioplasty and Post-Myocardial Infarction

Compared to the >70% uptake in CABG groups, exercise-based rehabilitation uptakes in post-angioplasty and post-MI patients are much lower (<30 and <50%, respectively) [26]. Following treatment for MI and ischaemic heart disease, the earliest possible contact and commencement of rehabilitation have been shown to have some favourable influences on uptake of exercise [19,34].

Unlike CABG, hospital stays for those with coronary angioplasty (percutaneous coronary intervention, PCI) following either elective treatment or MI are now very short. This reduces the time available for inpatient rehabilitation and secondary prevention preparations. Furthermore, many patients are likely to return to normal aspects of their social and work life within a few weeks. Such achievements in medicine seem impressive, but this does reduce the amount of time available in which to engage with patients and encourage and support them to participate in exercise sessions and to provide advice on becoming more physically active in daily life. From this perspective alone, the value of commencing rehabilitation as soon as possible and of offering patients choices as to where and when (time of day) they can participate can be seen [19]. It is interesting to note that in the UK and Australia, neither an early return to work nor available transport to rehabilitation have been found to be significant reasons for not taking up rehabilitation [26,35].

Early exercise rehabilitation in stable patients following MI, which begins within 1 week of discharge and lasts for 12 weeks, prevents significant amounts of negative ventricular remodelling [20]. When exercise is delayed, there is a gradient effect, where with every 1-week delay in commencement, an extra 1 month of exercise training is required to achieve the same ventricular remodelling benefit. In all 12 studies (647 patients) included in Haykowsky et al. [20], the exercise intensity was >60% VO_2 peak, which is within the target intensity range recommended in many guidelines (see Box 6.1).

Post-Angioplasty Complications

An obvious cause for concern with early rehabilitation following angioplasty is that some patients may be in a vulnerable period for complications, which can lead to rehospitalisation within 30–60 days [36,37]. Between 10 and 20% of post-angioplasty patients will be readmitted to hospital within 30 days [38,39]. These patients tend to be either older, female or to have existing heart failure or chronic kidney disease [40]. Rehabilitation practitioners should therefore include these factors in their risk stratification and ensure symptom assessments are frequent, including encouraging patient self-monitoring.

Presenting symptoms of post-angioplasty complications include recurrent angina. Offering early exercise-based rehabilitation, which includes standardised preactivity screening by trained clinical staff, may actually enhance the chances of early detection of such complications and is known to reduce rehospitalisation rates by up to 58% (versus predicted rates) [8,19]. Compared with more sedentary individuals, patients who are regularly physically active (as part of a dedicated self-management programme) are likely to better detect and/or manage symptoms and recognise the onset of disease progression [21].

With the promotion of early rehabilitation, it will be interesting to see whether evidence emerges to show that exercise can contribute, like statins, to acute endothelial function and antithrombotic benefits. As noted earlier, exercise has shown some significant benefits for the longer-term effects of endothelial function and in the prevention of atheromatic events following rehabilitation, usually when commenced 4 weeks post-event. Recent evidence on the independent effect of exercise is less clear, however, because it is usually delivered as part of a lifestyle and risk-factor management package [6,19]. Future evaluation of the acute ameliorating effects of exercise commenced soon after angioplasty may help better highlight its independent benefits (singularly or collectively) in reducing endothelial dysfunction, thrombosis and restenosis.

Conclusion

For any individual, but especially those who are sedentary and inactive, the avoidance of sitting and regular performance of even light (but preferably moderate or vigorous) activity will at least reduce key CVD risk factors and at best act as an independent risk factor for reducing CVD morbidity and mortality in all groups (asymptomatic, symptomatic or post-medical intervention). Whilst this chapter has focused on the prevention and management of atherosclerotic disease, it is important to recognise that with advancements in medicine, emergency care and public education, survival rates from ischaemic heart disease have greatly improved. As a result, in conjunction with the rise in mean population ages in developed countries, the future of prevention and rehabilitation programmes will increasingly need to accommodate older people with heart failure, internal defibrillators, heart transplants and neurological and musculoskeletal comorbidities.

References

1 Maher, C., Olds, T., Mire, E. and Katzmarzyk, P.T. Reconsidering the sedentary behaviour paradigm. *PLoS One* 2014; **9**: e86403.

2 Hallal, P.C., Andersen, L.B., Bull, F.C. et al. Global physical activity levels: surveillance progress, pitfalls, and prospects. *Lancet* 2012; **380**: 247–57.

3 Mielke, G.I., Hallal, P.C., Malta, D.C. and Lee, I.M. Time trends of physical activity and television viewing time in Brazil: 2006–2012. *Int J Behav Nutr Phys Act* 2014; **11**: 101.

4 Church, T.S., Thomas, D.M., Tudor-Locke, C. et al. Trends over 5 decades in U.S. occupation-related physical activity and their associations with obesity. *PLoS One* 2011; **6**: e19657.

5 Wienbergen, H. and Hambrecht, R. Physical exercise and its effects on coronary artery disease. *Curr Opin Pharmacol* 2013; **13**: 218–25.

6 Gielen, S., Laughlin, M.H., O'Conner, C. and Duncker, D.J. Exercise training in patients with heart disease: review of beneficial effects and clinical recommendations. *Prog Cardiovasc Dis* 2015; **57**: 347–55.

7 Swift, D.L., Lavie, C.J., Johannsen, N.M. et al. Physical activity, cardiorespiratory fitness, and exercise training in primary and secondary coronary prevention. *Circ J* 2013; **77**: 281–92.

8 Heran, B.S., Chen, J.M., Ebrahim, S. et al. Exercise-based cardiac rehabilitation for coronary heart disease. *Cochrane Database Syst Rev* 2011;(7):CD001800.

9 Turk-Adawi, K., Sarrafzadegan, N. and Grace, S.L. Global availability of cardiac rehabilitation. *Nat Rev Cardiol* 2014; **11**: 586–96.

10 AACVPR. *Guidelines for Cardiac Rehabilitation and Secondary Prevention Programs 5th Edition With Web Resource.* Champaign, IL: Human Kinetics, 2013.

11 BACPR. *A Practical Approach to Exercise and Physical Activity in the Prevention and Management of Cardiovascular Disease.* London: British Association for Cardiovascular Prevention and Rehabilitation, 2014.

12 Mezzani, A., Hamm, L.F., Jones, A.M. et al. Aerobic exercise intensity assessment and prescription in cardiac rehabilitation: a joint position statement of the European Association for Cardiovascular Prevention and Rehabilitation, the American Association of Cardiovascular and Pulmonary Rehabilitation and the Canadian Association of Cardiac Rehabilitation. *Eur J Prev Cardiol* 2013; **20**: 442–67.

13 Conraads, V.M., Pattyn, N., De Maeyer, C. et al. Aerobic interval training and continuous training equally improve aerobic exercise capacity in patients with coronary artery disease: the SAINTEX-CAD study. *Int J Cardiol* 2015; **179**: 203–10.

14 ACRA. *Recommended Framework for Cardiac '04, National Heart Foundation of Australia and the Australian Cardiac Rehabilitation Association.* Canberra: Australian Cardiac Rehabilitation Association, 2004.

15 Deanfield, J. and Board, J. Joint British Societies' consensus recommendations for the prevention of cardiovascular disease (JBS3). *Heart* 2014; **100**: 1–67.

16 Taylor, R.S., Unal, B., Critchley, J.A. and Capewell, S. Mortality reductions in patients receiving exercise-based cardiac rehabilitation: how much can be attributed to cardiovascular risk factor improvements? *Eur J Cardiovasc Prev Rehabil* 2006; **13**: 369–74.

17 Blum, M.R., Schmid, J.P., Eser, P. and Saner, H. Long-term results of a 12-week comprehensive ambulatory cardiac rehabilitation program. *J Cardiopulm Rehabil Prev* 2013; **33**: 84–90.

18 Beauchamp, A., Worcester, M., Ng, A. et al. Attendance at cardiac rehabilitation is associated with lower all-cause mortality after 14 years of follow-up. *Heart* 2013; **99**: 620–5.

19 BACPR, Buckley, J.P., Furze, G. et al. BACPR scientific statement: British standards and core components for cardiovascular disease prevention and rehabilitation. *Heart* 2013; **99**: 1069–71.

20 Haykowsky, M., Scott, J., Esch, B. et al. A meta-analysis of the effects of exercise training on left ventricular remodeling following myocardial infarction: start early and go longer for greatest exercise benefits on remodeling. *Trials* 2011; **12**: 92.

21 McGillion, M., O'Keefe-Mccarthy, S., Carroll, S.L. et al. Impact of self-management interventions on stable angina symptoms and health-related quality of life: a meta-analysis. *BMC Cardiovasc Disord* 2014; **14**: 14.

22 Reid, R.D., Morrin, L.I., Beaton, L.J. et al. Randomized trial of an internet-based computer-tailored expert system for physical activity in patients with heart disease. *Eur J Prev Cardiol* 2012; **19**: 1357–64.

23 Williams, R.P., Manou-Stathopoulou, V., Redwood, S.R. and Marber, M.S. 'Warm-up angina': harnessing the benefits of exercise and myocardial ischaemia. *Heart* 2014; **100**: 106–14.

24 Carl, L., Gallo, J. and Johnson, P. *Practical Pharmacology in Rehabilitation.* Champaign, IL: Human Kinetics, 2014.

25 Joannides, R., Moore, N., Iacob, M. et al. Comparative effects of ivabradine, a selective heart rate-lowering agent, and propranolol on systemic and cardiac haemodynamics at rest and during exercise. *Br J Clin Pharmacol* 2006; **61**: 127–37.

26 NACR. National Audit for Cardiac Rehabilitation. York: British Heart Foundation, York University, 2014.

27 Hillis, L.D., Smith, P.K., Anderson, J.L. et al. 2011 ACCF/AHA guideline for coronary artery bypass graft surgery: a report of the American College of Cardiology Foundation/American Heart Association Task Force on Practice Guidelines. *Circulation*, 2011; **124**: e652–735.

28 Busch, J.C., Lillou, D., Wittig, G. et al. Resistance and balance training improves functional capacity in very old participants attending cardiac rehabilitation after coronary bypass surgery. *J Am Geriatr Soc* 2012; **60**: 2270–6.

29 Adams, J., Schmid, J., Parker, R.D. et al. Comparison of force exerted on the sternum during a sneeze versus during low-, moderate-, and high-intensity bench press resistance exercise with and without the valsalva maneuver in healthy volunteers. *Am J Cardiol* 2014; **113**: 1045–8.

30 Siribaddana, S. Cardiac dysfunction in the CABG patient. *Curr Opin Pharmacol* 2012; **12**: 166–71.

31 Santa Mina, D., Clarke, H., Ritvo, P. et al. Effect of total-body prehabilitation on postoperative outcomes: a systematic review and meta-analysis. *Physiotherapy* 2014; **100**: 196–207.

32 Rideout, A., Lindsay, G. and Godwin, J. Patient mortality in the 12 years following enrolment into a pre-surgical cardiac rehabilitation programme. *Clin Rehabil* 2012; **26**: 642–7.

33 Furze, G., Dumville, J.C., Miles, J.N. et al. 'Prehabilitation' prior to CABG surgery improves physical functioning and depression. *Int J Cardiol* 2009; **132**: 51–8.

34 Karmali, K.N., Davies, P., Taylor, F. et al. Promoting patient uptake and adherence in cardiac rehabilitation. *Cochrane Database Syst Rev* 2014;(**6**):CD007131.

35 Redfern, J., Ellis, E.R., Briffa, T. and Freedman, S.B. High risk-factor level and low risk-factor knowledge in patients not accessing cardiac rehabilitation after acute coronary syndrome. *Med J Aust* 2007; **186**: 21–5.

36 Khawaja, F.J., Shah, N.D., Lennon, R.J. et al. Factors associated with 30-day readmission rates after percutaneous coronary intervention. *Arch Intern Med* 2012; **172**: 112–17.

37 Moretti, C., D'Ascenzo, F., Omede, P. et al. Thirty-day readmission rates after PCI in a metropolitan center in Europe: incidence and impact on prognosis. *J Cardiovasc Med (Hagerstown)* 2015; **16**: 238–45.

38 Ludman, P.F. BCIS Audit Returns Adult Intervention Procedures. Available from: http://www.bcis.org.uk/resources/documents/BCIS%20Audit%202008%20for%20web%2016-10-09%20version%201.pdf (last accessed 24 May 2016).

39 Lam, G., Snow, R., Shaffer, L. et al. The effect of a comprehensive cardiac rehabilitation program on 60-day hospital readmissions after an acute myocardial infarction. *J Am Coll Cardiol* 2011; **57**: E597.

40 Wasfy, J.H., Rosenfield, K., Zelevinsky, K. et al. A prediction model to identify patients at high risk for 30-day readmission after percutaneous coronary intervention. *Circ Cardiovasc Qual Outcomes* 2013; **6**: 429–35.

Part 2
Preventing Sudden Cardiac Death in Athletes

7 Incidence and Aetiology of Sudden Cardiac Death in Athletes

Kimberly G. Harmon

University of Washington, Seattle, WA, USA

Introduction

The death of a seemingly healthy athlete is always shocking, and impacts not only the athlete but the surrounding community as well. The frequency of such an occurrence is the topic of much debate, with some stating the incidence is as high as 1 in 5000 in high-risk groups [1] and others likening it to death from a lightning strike [2]. The most common causes of sudden cardiac death (SCD) are also debated. In Europe and other parts of the world, autopsy-negative sudden unexplained death (AN-SUD) is the most common finding at autopsy after suspected SCD. In the US, hypertrophic cardiomyopathy (HCM) has long been viewed as the most common cause of SCD [3], although recent research challenges this assumption [1,4]. This chapter will examine the incidence of SCD in different age groups and populations, as well as the strengths of the methodologies used to arrive at these determinations. In addition, the causes of SCD in different ages, populations and parts of the world will be explored.

Developing a Numerator and Denominator

To develop an accurate estimate of the incidence of SCD, both a reliable numerator (cases identified) and an accurate denominator (population studied) are required. Uncertainty or variability in either the numerator or the denominator will result in imprecise estimates. Cases are identified in a number of ways, including mandatory reporting, voluntary registries and review of media reports, death certificates or insurance claims. Mandatory reporting of an athlete's death offers the most reliable method of case identification, but in most countries this is not required, and it may be difficult to determine whether SCD occurred in an athlete or in association with sporting activity. Registries are another way of collecting athlete deaths, but this method is subject to ascertainment bias, and typically the denominator is difficult to define.

Media Reports

Media reports are frequently used to identify cases of SCD, although the ability to accurately detect all deaths in a given population using this method is questionable. In one study in Denmark, where there is mandatory reporting of death, only 20% of identified athlete deaths were found by an extensive media search [5]. A follow-up study determined only 2% of overall sports-related SCD was identified through media searches (3% of this in noncompetitive athletes, 9% in competitive athletes) [6]. In another study tracking deaths primarily through media sources over 27 years, there was a steady increase in findings, which was attributed to improved media search strategies and the use of Internet search engines [3]. In a US study examining college athletes over 10 years, media reports identified 70% of athlete deaths, but significantly more were identified in higher-profile division I athletes (87%) than in lower-profile division II (61%) or division III (44%). SCDs identified by an internal database did not vary between divisions [1]. Studies using media reports to identify deaths in lower-profile populations, such as high-school or recreational athletes,

IOC Manual of Sports Cardiology, First Edition. Edited by Mathew G. Wilson, Jonathan A. Drezner and Sanjay Sharma.
© 2017 International Olympic Committee. Published 2017 by John Wiley & Sons, Ltd.

will likely miss a greater proportion of deaths. Although media reports are frequently the only option for case identification, this method clearly underestimates cases and leads to reduced assessments of the incidence of SCD.

Insurance Claims

Insurance claims have been used as a way to identify cases, but insurance for athletes typically only covers death occurring at a supervised team practice, game or activity, and thus encompasses only a fraction of an athlete's life. A study of Minnesota high-school athletes estimated the rate of SCD to be 1 in 917 000 athlete-years over the previous decade based on a review of insurance claims, which identified only one SCD during that time period [7]. However, a review of Minnesotan high-school athlete SCDs captured in a media database during the same time period demonstrated six SCDs [8]. Thus, although media reports identify only a fraction of total deaths, in this instance they detected six times as many SCDs as insurance claims. In a study of US college athletes, only 9% of deaths identified during a 10-year time period were indicated by insurance claims [1]. SCD rates based on insurance claims severely underestimate the incidence of SCD.

Activity at Time of Death

Initial studies of incidence in the US relied on data from the National Center for Catastrophic Injury Research (NCCSIR), whose mission is to conduct surveillance of catastrophic injuries and illnesses related to participation in organised sports. A death needs to have occurred within an hour of sporting activity in order for it to be included in the registry. At its inception, the purpose of the NCCSIR was to compare catastrophic injuries and deaths among sports in order to better inform rule and equipment changes, so death occurring outside of sport-related activity was not included in the registry. However, for cardiac-related morbidity, this distinction poses several problems. Many cardiac deaths which may be triggered or hastened by athletic participation occur outside of the heavy exertion of training. In fact, studies reporting activity at the time of SCD in both young populations and athletes demonstrate that 30–45% of deaths occurred during sleep or non-exertion [1,5,9–12]. In addition, the NCCSIR only represents 'organised sports'. Deaths that occurred whilst participating in club teams, intramurals, recreational teams, off-season practice, training or gym class are not included even if the athlete was also part of an 'organised' team. Therefore, although the NCCSIR served many of its stated objectives, cardiac risk in an athlete needs to be viewed from a broader perspective.

The NCCSIR has recently changed its surveillance practices regarding sudden cardiac arrest (SCA) and SCD to include cardiac events that occur in an athlete at any time.

Defining a Population

The incidence of SCD varies significantly with age. Therefore, when examining incidence rates, the age of the cohort needs to be clearly understood. From birth to 2 years, there is a high rate of SCD due to congenital heart disease (CHD); this then drops, and remains low until about the age of 14 [9,11,13]. There is not currently good evidence to suggest whether high-school (14–18) or college-age (19–24) athletes are at equal or disproportionate risk. It is evident, however, that after the age of 25, the risk of SCD goes up considerably, and that the majority of this increased risk is due to coronary artery disease (CAD) [9,11,13,14]. Data must be interpreted carefully in studies that include athletes both under 14 and over 25, as their incidence rates differ.

What about the Denominator?

Whilst it may be argued whether the incidence of SCD is 1 in 1 000 000 athlete-years or 1 in 50 000, it is still a rare enough occurrence to require large populations for study. There are few defined groups that are large enough to generate the number of deaths required to adequately study incidence and yet still track sufficiently for SCD occurrence. In the general population, population statistics can be used as a denominator, but it is more difficult to use them when determining the underlying percentage of athletes and their level of competition, creating significant room for error. In some countries, such as Italy, there is mandatory registration of athletes, which can be used as a denominator; this is also the case in the US military [15–18]. There are also well-defined athlete groups in the US, such as the National Collegiate Athletic Association (NCAA), although this covers a limited age group. When evaluating any study, the accuracy of the denominator needs to be clearly understood.

The Incidence of SCD

The reported incidence of SCD varies widely and is dependent on the population studied and the study methodology. Currently, 15 studies report on the incidence of SCD in athletes, of which six report on general athlete populations with broad age ranges (8–44), four report on college-age athletes (~18–24) and six examine high–school athletes (14–18) (Tables 7.1–7.3). The studies investigating the general population can be divided into two distinct groups, based on the classification of SCD as exertional or as occurring at any time. The three studies which include only exertional SCDs find incidence rates ranging from 1 in 300 000 to 1 in 82 645 athlete-years [5,13,19]. In one, by Van Camp et al. [19], cases were identified by media report prior to the advent of the Internet and the denominator was estimated based on participants in a variety of athletic associations. The other two studies are both from Denmark. They encompass two distinct time periods and identify cases from death certificates, with autopsies and medical records available for most. It is unlikely that many deaths were missed in these studies [5,6]. However, the presence of SCD could only be discerned from a review of the available records, and only if the athletes were exercising at the time of death [5,6]. The denominators were estimated from population surveys regarding athletic activity and then extrapolated to years in the study period. In addition, one of the studies included only a small number of cases – just three athlete SCDs per year over the 3-year study period – creating wide confidence intervals for incidence estimates (Table 7.1) [6].

There were three incidence studies examining SCD occurring at any time in athletes with broad age ranges, with incidence estimates ranging from 1 in 37 593 athlete-years to 1 in 163 934 [3,15,20]. In an Italian study which prospectively followed athletes over 20 years, the rate was 1 : 43 478 [15]. Similar incidence rates were found in an Israeli study, but this was a retrospective review of deaths noted in two newspapers from 1985 to 2009, with an estimated athlete denominator. This cohort included athletes up to 44 years of age, including a relatively large proportion of those who died from CAD, so rates may be higher than in studies with a lower age cut-off [20]. Studies utilising prospective identification of cases and including death in athletes occurring at any time demonstrate higher athlete SCD incidence numbers.

Four studies examine SCD in US college athletes, all of which provide similar estimates, ranging from 1 in 43 770 to 1 in 67 000 [1,12,21,22]. These studies include athletes with SCD on or off the court or field of play. Given the similarity of the estimates, this is likely an accurate representation of the incidence of SCD in college athletes, although there appear to be subgroups at substantially higher risk. Studies in US high-school athletes are more difficult to compare, due to methodological differences and difficulty with case identification. Two studies using insurance claims for case identification include only SCDs occurring with exertion whilst participating in an officially sponsored activity; these estimate the incidence of SCD to be 1 : 217 000–917 000 athlete years [7,23]. These rate are low, given that insurance claims represent a small fraction of total deaths [8]. Other studies look at both SCA and SCD, but only incidences that occur whilst physically on the high-school campus, again limiting the timeframe of surveillance [24,25]. One of these, which is survey-based, reports an SCD rate of 1 in 46 000 [24]. The other, which is prospective, reports 18 occurrences of SCA with an 89% survival rate, demonstrating the need to include SCA events with survival in calculations. The rate of SCA/SCD in this latter study is 1 in 87 719 athlete-years overall, and 1 in 57 000 in males [25]. The wide range of SCD estimates for high-school athletes reflects the need for better reporting and collection strategies.

There appear to be subgroups of athletes at higher risk for SCD. These include males, African/Afro-Caribbean athletes and basketball players [1,12,22]. In most studies, males represent 80–100% of those with SCD [1,3,5,7,19,22]. Some have suggested that this is because greater numbers of males participate in sport, but the difference is not large enough to account for the extremely high incidence of SCD [1,15]. In a prospective study of Italian athletes, males were 2.4 times more likely than females to have an SCD event [15], whilst in a study of college athletes, males had a 3.2 times higher risk [1]. A prospective study of high-school athletes

Author	Year	Country	Study design	Numerator	Denominator	Exertional or all deaths?	Years	Incidence of SCD	No. of years	Age range	Number of cardiac deaths
Van Camp	1996	US	Retrospective cohort	Registry/media search	Estimated	Exertional	1983–93	1 : 300 000	10	17–24	100
Holst	2010	Denmark	Retrospective cohort	Review of death certificates	Denmark population statistics Number of athletes estimated from survey	Exertional	2000–06	1 : 82 645 SrSCD (95% CI 1 : 50 000–147 089)	7	12 –35	15
Risgaard	2014	Denmark	Retrospective cohort	Review of death certificates	Denmark population statistics Number of athletes estimated from survey	Exertional	2007–09	Competetive athletes: 1 : 232 558 (95% CI 1 : 106 383–256 410) Noncompetetive athletes: 1 : 212 766 (95% CI 1 : 87 719–1 000 000)	3	12–35	Competetive: 3 Noncompetetive: 6
Corrado	2003	Italy	Prospective cohort study	Mandatory death reporting	Registered Italian athletes	All	1979–99	1 : 43 478	20	12–35	55
Maron	2009	US	Retrospective cohort	Registry/media search	Estimated	All	1980–2006	1 : 163 934	27	8–39	690

Table 7.1 Incidence of SCD in general populations of athletes

Author	Year	Country	Study design	Numerator	Denominator	Exertional or all deaths?	Years studied	Incidence	No. of years	Age range	Number of cardiac deaths
Drezner	2005	US	Retrospective survey	Survey	Athletes at surveyed schools	All		1 : 67 000	3.3		5
Harmon	2011	US	Retrospective cohort	Media database, internal NCAA list, insurance claims	Participation data from NCAA	All	2004–08	1 : 43 770	5	18–26	37
Maron	2014	US	Retrospective cohort	USRSDA Internal NCAA list for cardiac cases	Participation data from NCAA	All	2002–11	1 : 62 500	10	17–26	64
Harmon	2015	US	Retrospective cohort	Media database, internal NCAA list, insurance claims	Participation data from NCAA	All	2003–13	1 : 53 703	10	17–26	79

Table 7.2 Incidence of SCD in college athletes

Author	Year	Study design	Numerator	Denominator	Exertional or all deaths?	SCD or SCA/SCD	Years studied	Incidence	No. of years	Age range	Cardiac deaths
Maron	1998	Retrospective cohort	Insurance claims	Minnesota State High School League	Exertional during school-sponsored sport	SCD	1985–97	1 : 217 000 overall 1 : 129 000 male 0 female SCDs	12	16–17	3
Roberts	2013	Retrospective cohort	Insurance claims	Minnesota State High School League	Exertional during school-sponsored sport	SCD	1993–2012	1993–2012: 1 : 416 666 2002–12: 1 : 917 000	19	12–19	4
Drezner	2009	Cross-sectional survey	Survey	Number of student athletes reported by schools	All SCA/SCD occurring on-campus	SCA/SCD	2006–07	1 : 23 000 SCA/SCD 1 : 46 000 SCD	Within 6 months of survey	14–17	14
Maron	2012	Retrospective cohort	Registry/media search	Minnesota State High School League	Exertional	SCD	1986–2011	1 : 150 000	26	12–18	13
Toresdahl	2014	Prospective observational	Number of cases reported	Number of student athletes reported by schools	All SCA/SCD occurring on-campus	SCA/SCD	2009–11	1 : 87 719 SCA/SCD 1 : 57 000 male SCA/SCD	2	14–18	18 SCA/SCD 2 SCD
Drezner	2014	Restrospective cohort	Media reports	National Federation of State High School Associations	All SCA/SCD	SCA/SCD	2003–13	1 : 71 428 SCA/SCD 1 : 153 846 SCD	10	14–18	6 SCD 7 SCA

Table 7.3 Incidence of SCD in high-school athletes

demonstrated male athletes were 5.65 times more likely to have an SCA or SCD [25]. In studies that identify cases using media reports, this difference might be accounted for by the fact that the death of a male athlete is often higher-profile and therefore more likely to be reported on, but the same difference occurs in prospective studies and in studies using other methods of case identification.

African/Afro-Caribbean athletes also appear to be at higher risk. In studies of US college athletes, SCD is reported to occur three to five times more frequently in African/Afro-Caribbean athletes compared to Caucasian athletes. Many studies on the incidence of SCD do not report on the rate of SCD but note that African/Afro-Caribbean athletes appear to have a disproportionate number of deaths [3,18]. It has been noted that African/Afro-Caribbean athletes have a higher rate of abnormal electrocardiogram (ECG) patterns, although it is not clear whether these are false positives or early signs of pathology.

It also appears that male basketball players have an unusually high risk of SCD. In a study examining US college athletes, the risk of SCD was 1 in 9000 athlete-years, or 1 in 5000 for those in the upper divisions [1]. Higher rates of SCD in male basketball players compared to other athletes have also been noted in high school [8]. It is unclear why basketball players are at higher risk. Basketball is a highly dynamic sport and tends to select out a certain body habitus. More study is needed to better understand this finding.

Are Athletes at Greater Risk of SCD than Non-athletes?

Five studies compare the risk of SCD in athletes to that of the general population. Most suggest that SCD is more common in athletes. A prospective Italian study determined that athletes had a relative risk of SCD of 2.5 compared to non-athletes [15]. Another prospective study in France followed reporting of SCD by emergency-service responders and found that sports-related sudden death had a 4.5 times higher incidence than SCD in the general population [26]. Finally, a prospective study examining SCA/SCD in US high schools reported a 3.65 greater risk in athletes compared to non-athletes [25].

Two studies from Denmark suggest that SCD is 3.3–6.7 times more common in the general population than in athletes, but these compare exertional death in athletes with death occurring at any time in the general population, perhaps accounting for some of the disparity [5,6]. These are both retrospective reviews of death certificates and, in most cases, autopsy reports, and some cases may not have been correctly identified as athletes. It would appear that the preponderance of evidence supports athletes as being at higher risk for SCD.

Relative Frequency of SCD

The incidence of SCD has been compared to the risk of dying from a lightning strike [2], but this appears to be more metaphorical than factual. Over the last 9 years, there has been an average of 32 deaths per year from lightning strikes in the US [27]. With a population of approximately 320 000 000, that equates to a risk of death from lightning strike of 1 in 10 000 000 person-years. This is considerably different than even the most conservative estimate of SCD.

There has also been concern that car accidents, suicide and homicide are significantly more common than SCD in athletes [2], but true comparisons of rates require similar methods or populations. In a review of US college athlete deaths over a decade, the risk of death in an automobile accident was 1 in 27 000 athlete-years, or approximately twice the risk of an athlete SCD. However, athletes at higher risk, such as male basketball players, were three times more likely to have an SCD compared to death in a car accident [1]. In this same cohort, SCD occurred twice as frequently as both suicide and homicide. Comparative risks for younger athletes or for athletes in other countries are not available.

Aetiology of SCD

The most common finding at death in athletes with presumed SCD is a pathologically normal heart or AN-SUD [1,4,5,28]. In Italy, it appears that arrhythmogenic right ventricular cardiomyopathy (ARVC) is more common [15], and in the UK, left ventricular hypertrophy/possible HCM [29]. In both studies, autopsy of the heart was done at a specialised centre, which may have discovered findings that would have been missed at places with less expertise – this might account for some of the discrepancy. Genetic variation between regions of the world may also account for some differences in the causes of SCD in different countries. In the US, it has long been suggested that HCM is the most common cause of SCD, accounting for over a third of all cases; however, this information originates from the US Registry for Sudden Death in Athletes (USRSDA), which is based out of an HCM centre, likely creating ascertainment bias [3]. Studies of aetiology in the US are primarily autopsy-based, but there are significant differences in the training of those performing the autopsies and in the tests and methods used. Recent information from the US suggests HCM may be less common and AN-SUD more common than was previously appreciated [1,4]. Moving towards a standardised autopsy at specialised centres and molecular autopsy will improve our understanding of the aetiology of SCD.

Conclusion

The incidence of SCD in athletes varies with age, sex and sports played, with males, African/Afro-Caribbean athletes and basketball players at increased risk compared to other athletes. A wide range of incidences is reported in the literature, but much of the variability in similar populations can be attributed to differences in study methodology. Prospective studies of large, defined populations with mandatory reporting of death and specialised cardiac and molecular autopsies are optimal, but few exist. The incidence of SCD in athletes aged 18–24 years is about 1 in 50 000. After the age of 25–30, incidence increases drastically secondary to CAD. Worldwide, AN-SUD appears to be the most common finding after SCD. There is evidence that this is also true in the US, where HCM was previously determined to be the chief cause of SCD. SCD is the leading medical cause of death and the leading cause of exertional death, and is a comparable public health risk to automobile accidents, suicide and homicide in populations where direct comparisons have been made. As we move forward, systems with mandatory reporting and prospective identification of cases should improve estimates of the incidence of SCD. A good understanding of the incidence of SCD is critical to a correct appreciation of effective primary and secondary prevention measures.

References

1 Harmon, K. Incidence, etiology and comparitive frequency of sudden cardiac death in NCAA athletes: a decade in review. *Circulation* 2015; doi: 10.1161/CIRCULATIONAHA.115.015431.

2 Maron, B.J., Friedman, R.A., Kligfield, P. et al. Assessment of the 12-lead ECG as a screening test for detection of cardiovascular disease in healthy general populations of young people (12–25 years of age): a scientific statement from the American Heart Association and the American College of Cardiology. *Circulation* 2014; **130**: 1303–34.

3 Maron, B.J., Doerer, J.J., Haas, T.S. et al. Sudden deaths in young competitive athletes. Analysis of 1866 deaths in the United States, 1980–2006. *Circulation* 2009; **119**: 1085–92.

4 Harmon, K.G., Drezner, J.A., Maleszewski, J.J. et al. Pathogeneses of sudden cardiac death in national collegiate athletic association athletes. *Circ Arrhythm Electrophysiol* 2014; **7**: 198–204.

5 Holst, A.G., Winkel, B.G., Theilade, J. et al. Incidence and etiology of sports-related sudden cardiac death in Denmark – implications for preparticipation screening. *Heart Rhythm* 2010; **7**: 1365–71.

6 Risgaard, B., Winkel, B.G., Jabbari, R. et al. Sports-related sudden cardiac death in a competitive and a noncompetitive athlete population aged 12 to 49 years: data from an unselected nationwide study in Denmark. *Heart Rhythm* 2014; **11**: 1673–81.

7 Roberts, W.O. and Stovitz, S.D. Incidence of sudden cardiac death in Minnesota high school athletes 1993–2012 screened with a standardized pre-participation evaluation. *J Am Coll Cardiol* 2013; **62**: 1298–301.

8 Drezner, J.A., Harmon, K.G. and Marek, J.C. Incidence of sudden cardiac arrest in Minnesota high school student athletes: the limitations of catastrophic insurance claims. *J Am Coll Cardiol* 2014; **63**: 1455–6.

9 Pilmer, C.M., Kirsh, J.A., Hildebrandt, D. et al. Sudden cardiac death in children and adolescents between 1 and 19 years of age. *Heart Rhythm* 2014; **11**: 239–45.

10 Margey, R., Roy, A., Tobin, S. et al. Sudden cardiac death in 14- to 35-year olds in Ireland from 2005 to 2007: a retrospective registry. *Europace* 2011; **13**: 1411–18.

11 Winkel, B.G., Risgaard, B., Sadjadieh, G. et al. Sudden cardiac death in children (1–18 years): symptoms and causes of death in a nationwide setting. *Eur Heart J* 2014; **35**: 868–75.

12 Harmon, K.G., Asif, I.M., Klossner, D. and Drezner, J.A. Incidence of sudden cardiac death in national collegiate athletic association athletes. *Circulation* 2011; **123**: 1594–600.

13 Risgaard, B., Winkel, B.G., Jabbari, R. et al. Burden of sudden cardiac death in persons aged 1 to 49 years: nationwide study in Denmark. *Circ Arrhythm Electrophysiol* 2014; **7**: 205–11.

14 Meyer, L., Stubbs, B., Fahrenbruch, C. et al. Incidence, causes, and survival trends from cardiovascular-related sudden cardiac arrest in children and young adults 0 to 35 years of age: a 30-year review. *Circulation* 2012; **126**: 1363–72.

15 Corrado, D., Basso, C., Rizzoli, G. et al. Does sports activity enhance the risk of sudden death in adolescents and young adults? *J Am Coll Cardiol* 2003; **42**: 1959–63.

16 Corrado, D., Basso, C., Pavei, A. et al. Trends in sudden cardiovascular death in young competitive athletes after implementation of a preparticipation screening program. *JAMA* 2006; **296**: 1593–601.

17 Eckart, R.E., Scoville, S.L., Campbell, C.L. et al. Sudden death in young adults: a 25-year review of autopsies in military recruits. *Ann Intern Med* 2004; **141**: 829–34.

18 Eckart, R.E., Shry, E.A., Burke, A.P. et al. Sudden death in young adults: an autopsy-based series of a population undergoing active surveillance. *J Am Coll Cardiol* 2011; **58**: 1254–61.

19 Van Camp, S.P., Bloor, C.M., Mueller, F.O. et al. Nontraumatic sports death in high school and college athletes. *Med Sci Sports Exerc* 1995; **27**: 641–7.

20 Steinvil, A., Chundadze, T., Zeltser, D. et al. Mandatory electrocardiographic screening of athletes to reduce their risk for sudden death proven fact or wishful thinking? *J Am Coll Cardiol* 2011; **57**: 1291–6.

21 Drezner, J.A., Rogers, K.J., Zimmer, R.R. and Sennett, B.J. Use of automated external defibrillators at NCAA Division I universities. *Med Sci Sports Exerc* 2005; **37**: 1487–92.

22 Maron, B.J., Haas, T.S., Murphy, C.J. et al. Incidence and causes of sudden death in US college athletes. *J Am Coll Cardiol* 2014; **63**: 1636–43.

23 Maron, B.J., Gohman, T.E. and Aeppli, D. Prevalence of sudden cardiac death during competitive sports activities in Minnesota high school athletes. *J Am Coll Cardiol* 1998; **32**: 1881–4.

24 Drezner, J.A., Rao, A.L., Heistand, J. et al. Effectiveness of emergency response planning for sudden cardiac arrest in United States high schools with automated external defibrillators. *Circulation* 2009; **120**: 518–25.

25 Toresdahl, B.G., Rao, A.L., Harmon, K.G. and Drezner, J.A. Incidence of sudden cardiac arrest in high school student athletes on school campus. *Heart Rhythm* 2014; **11**: 1190–4.

26 Marijon, E., Tafflet, M., Celermajer, D.S. et al. Sports-related sudden death in the general population. *Circulation* 2011; **124**: 672–81.

27 Jensenius, J.S. A Detailed Analysis of Lightning Deaths in the United States from 2006 through 2014. Available from: http://www.lightningsafety.noaa.gov/fatalities/analysis06-14.pdf (last accessed 24 May 2016).

28 Suarez-Mier, M.P., Aguilera, B., Mosquera, R.M. and Sanchez-De-Leon, M.S. Pathology of sudden death during recreational sports in Spain. *Forensic Sci Int* 2013; **226**: 188–96.

29 de Noronha, S.V., Sharma, S., Papadakis, M. et al. Aetiology of sudden cardiac death in athletes in the United Kingdom: a pathological study. *Heart* 2009; **95**: 1409–14.

8 Cardiovascular Screening for the Prevention of Sudden Cardiac Death in Athletes

Antonio Pelliccia[1] and Domenico Corrado[2]

[1]Institute of Sport Medicine and Science, Rome, Italy
[2]Department of Cardiac, Thoracic and Vascular Sciences, University of Padua Medical School, Padua, Italy

Introduction

The sudden death of a young athlete from a cardiac disorder is particularly emotive and is often associated with considerable media coverage, drawing attention to the youth, their athletic prowess and the number of life years lost due to a cardiac disorder that could have been detected during life. The beneficial effects of regular and intensive exercise for the prevention of cardiovascular disease (CVD) are well known [1]. Paradoxically, however, individuals who harbour a serious cardiovascular abnormality may be susceptible to an increased risk of 'exercise-related' sudden cardiac death (SCD) [2]. Accordingly, pre-participation evaluation (PPE) is now advised as a strategy to screen for potentially life-threatening disorders [3], which if identified in a timely fashion can be appropriately managed through lifestyle modifications, pharmacotherapy and/or implantable cardioverter-defibrillators (ICDs), minimising the chance of an athlete suffering an adverse cardiac event.

The Risk of Sudden Death in Athletes

Cardiovascular pathology leading to SCD is the most common medical cause of death in athletes, with participation in competitive sport associated with a 2.8 times increased risk of SCD compared to sedentary individuals [4]. Competitive sport is not per se the cause for SCD, but rather the combination of intensive physical exercise with an underlying CVD can trigger a serious ventricular arrhythmia, ultimately leading to cardiac arrest. Furthermore, the type of pathologic substrate also has a significant effect upon event rates, with hypertrophic cardiomyopathy (HCM), arrhythmogenic right ventricular cardiomyopathy (ARVC) and congenital coronary arteries anomalies [9] appearing to be the prime culprits in most cases of SCD.

The exact incidence of SCD in athletes remains controversial. Variability in incidence rates is largely caused by differences in reporting methodology, the reliability of case identification and the accuracy of population denominators. Most published studies are based on media reports or catastrophic insurance claims as their primary method for case identification, often grossly underestimating SCD rates in athletes [2,5]. Recent data suggest that the incidence is significantly higher than previously reported [6,7], with an overall incidence of 1 : 50 000 in young athletes now considered a reasonable estimate. Furthermore, it is now known that male athletes are at consistently greater risk of SCD than females, with male African-descent athletes at a disproportionately greater risk than other ethnicities [6]. Within the Veneto region in Italy, we observed an annual incidence of SCD in young (<35 years) competitive athletes of approximately 3 : 100 000 [8]. This figure is derived from a prospective central registry covering the well-defined geographic area of Veneto, with accurate data on the classification of responsible cardiac conditions (the numerator), alongside robust athlete population figures calculated from sport federation registries (the denominator).

Rationale for Screening Competitive Athletes

There is universal agreement that exercise is a trigger for sudden cardiac arrest in individuals with underlying pathologic cardiac disorders. In addition, early detection of at-risk disorders and the mitigation of risk through activity restrictions and medical interventions are the very premises of PPE. Both the American Heart Association (AHA) and the European Society of Cardiology (ESC) agree 'that compelling justification exists for cardiovascular pre-participation screening on medical, ethical and legal grounds' [9,10]. This opinion has now been endorsed by several sporting organisations, including the International Olympic Committee (IOC) [11], Fédération Internationale de Football Association (FIFA) and Union Cycliste Internationale (UCI).

The Screening Programmes Implemented in Italy

The athlete population in Italy (including all ages and both genders) is estimated to be 6 million, ultimately representing the target for a national systematic PPE programme. As directed by the Italian government, dedicated sport medicine clinics are distributed across Italy, with one or more in most major towns. These clinics are run by specialists in sport medicine who, by law, are able to undertake PPE and provide medical clearance for athletes to engage in competition.

The PPE protocol set is governed by legislation, with only minor differences according to type of sport and level of participation. Accordingly, all individuals engaged in competitive sport are required to pass a medical examination that includes a personal and family history, physical examination and 12-lead electrocardiogram (ECG), plus additional testing if it is deemed necessary by the examining physician (Figure 8.1). In adult (over-40) competitive athletes, exercise ECG stress testing may also be undertaken in specific cases in accordance with recommendations set by the Italian Society of Sport Cardiology [12].

The screening protocol for elite competitors (i.e. Italian Olympic and Paralympic athletes) is broader than that dictated by the legislation for the general athlete population, and, with regard to the cardiovascular system, includes exercise ECG testing and echocardiography (Figure 8.1). These examinations are undertaken under the direction of the National Olympic Committee at the Institute of Sport Medicine and Science in Rome. Certain professional athletes (such as football players participating in the first and second national league) are examined by their team physician, in cooperation with selected consultants, within a medical programme organised by the Football Teams and the Italian Football Federation.

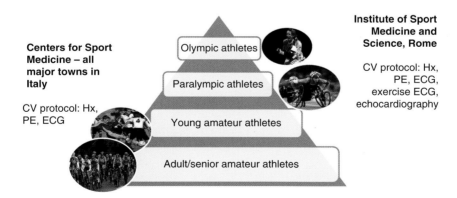

Figure 8.1 Pyramid of national screening programmes for athlete populations implemented in Italy. Young and adult/senior amateur athletes are examined at sport medicine clinics, found in all major towns across the country, by qualified sport medicine specialists, according to a protocol dictated by legislation (i.e. history-taking (Hx), physical examination (PE) and ECG). Elite athletes, selected for participation in the Olympic or Paralympic Games, are examined at the Institute of Sport Medicine and Science in Rome by qualified specialists in sport medicine and cardiologists, according to a protocol implemented by the Italian Olympic Committee (i.e. Hx, PE, ECG, exercise ECG and echocardiography)

Rationale for Including a 12-Lead ECG in the PPE

The available scientific evidence demonstrates that cardiac screening with personal history and physical examination alone has a very low sensitivity. Cardiovascular symptoms are often diffuse, possibly vague (e.g. palpitations, lightheadedness, fatigue) and frequent in adolescents and young adults. The sensitivity of cardiac screening is improved with the addition of ECG, as the vast majority of athletes with underlying cardiac abnormalities will have an abnormal ECG. It is now widely accepted that the 12-lead ECG, in addition to history and physical examination, substantially improves the diagnostic power of the screening. The ECG is abnormal in >90% of patients with HCM and in >60% of those with ARVC. Furthermore, the ECG is able to capture electrical cardiac conditions such as Wolff–Parkinson–White (WPW) syndrome, long and short QT syndromes, Brugada syndrome and Lènegre disease [3,8,13] Overall, these conditions account for two-thirds of the causes of SCDs in young athletes (Figure 8.2).

A recent systematic review/meta-analysis of evidence comparing screening strategies suggests that the ECG is five times more sensitive than history and 10 times more sensitive than physical exam, and that it has a higher positive likelihood ratio, lower negative likelihood ratio and lower false-positive rate than either. Specifically, Harmon et al. [14] reported that among 15 studies examining a total of 47 137 athletes, the sensitivity and specificity of ECG were 94/93%, history 20/94% and physical examination 9/97%, respectively. The overall false-positive rate of ECG (6%) was less than that of history (8%) or physical exam (10%). Positive likelihood ratios were 14.8 for ECG, 3.22 for history and 2.93 for physical examination. Negative likelihood ratios were 0.055 for ECG, 0.85 for history and 0.93 for physical exam. There were a total of 160 potentially lethal cardiovascular conditions detected, at a rate of 0.3%, or 1 in 294. The most common pathology was WPW (n = 67, 42%), followed by long QT syndrome (n = 18, 11%), HCM (n = 18, 11%), dilated cardiomyopathy (n = 11, 7%), coronary artery disease (CAD) or myocardial ischaemia (n = 9, 6%) and ARVC (n = 4, 3%). The authors concluded that the most effective strategy for screening for CVD in athletes is an ECG.

Efficacy of Screening to Identify Cardiac Disease Risk

A cardiac screening programme should be capable of identifying (or at least, raising suspicion for) the risk of SCD. Of 33 735 individuals screened at the Centre for Sport Medicine in Padua, Italy, 22 (0.07%) were identified as having HCM. Of these, 18 presented with an abnormal ECG (82%). If ECG was excluded from the PPE, only 5 (23%) athletes would have been identified, based upon a positive family history, symptoms and/or abnormal physical findings [15].

PPE is also able to identify a spectrum of cardiac abnormalities, including rhythm and conduction anomalies, valvular disease, systemic hypertension, congenital heart disease (CHD), vascular disease and myopericarditis. Of 42 386 athletes examined at the same sports medicine centre in Padua, 3914 (9%) demonstrated an abnormal personal and family history, physical examination and/or ECG, of whom 879 (2%) were ultimately considered to harbour a pathologic condition requiring sport restriction (Figure 8.3).

	ECG	Hx + PE
• HCM	≤90%	<10%
• ARVC	60–80%	<10%
• Dilated cardiomyopathy	30–60%	<10%
• Myocarditis	30–60%	<10%
• Marfan's syndrome	<10%	>90%
• Valvular disease	<10%	>90%
• Long- and short-QT syndrome	>80%	zero
• Brugada syndrome	>90%	zero
• Pre-excitation syndrome (WPW)	>90%	zero
• Congenital coronary artery anomalies	<10%	<10%

Figure 8.2 Estimated probability of identification of major CVDs, by history-taking (Hx), physical examination (PE) and 12-lead ECG in the context of a mass screening programme

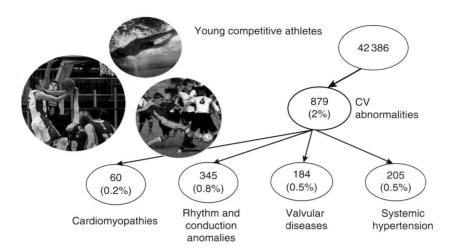

Figure 8.3 Spectrum of cardiovascular abnormalities detected at PPE by a combination of history-taking (Hx), physical examination (PE) and 12-lead ECG

Although these experiences suggest that ECG screening is efficient in identifying asymptomatic HCM athletes, a measure of caution is appropriate, in that 5–10% of young HCM patients may present with a normal ECG. In such instances, the use of echocardiography has been advised as a regular part of cardiac screening (as proposed by FIFA and the Union of European Football Associations (UEFA)). Whilst it is expected that echocardiography will increase sensitivity, it does come at a significant cost (economically and logistically), and is usually reserved for elite athletic settings with good economic resources.

Recently, we revised the results of the screening programme in place for Olympic athletes over the latest 10-year period. Of a population of 2300 athletes, a substantial subset of 6% was identified with cardiovascular abnormalities, either structural or electrical. Specifically, echocardiography was responsible for identifying (or confirming) the presence of several pathologic conditions, including arrhythmogenic cardiomyopathies and congenital cardiac and valvular disease, that would not have been identified by the ECG screening programme alone.

Similar results emerged from a selected population of 267 elite Paralympic athletes examined in the period 2004–12. The prevalence of cardiovascular abnormalities in this population was even larger, at 12%. Specifically, 9% of Paralympic athletes were identified with structural cardiac disease, such as hypertrophic and dilated cardiomyopathies, as well as idiopathic aortic root dilation, other than congenital or acquired valvular disease. In addition, 3% of the athletes presented major supraventricular or ventricular tachyarrhythmias in the absence of structural cardiac disease, selectively requiring radiofrequency (RF) ablation.

In conclusion, our data demonstrate that elite athletes may harbour cardiac abnormalities in an unsuspectedly large proportion, including at-risk pathologic conditions, without any appreciable limitation in their performance. This suggests that elite competitors may be exposed to an unacceptable risk in association with sport participation and that they deserve more comprehensive medical surveillance than commonly believed.

Impact of the Screening Programme on Cardiac Mortality

The only robust evidence to show that PPE is lifesaving is based on the Italian experience. Mortality data derived from a time-trend analysis of the incidence of deaths in a 26-year period (1979–2004) [8] after the introduction of PPE demonstrate that the annual incidence of sudden death in athletes decreased by 89%, from 3.6 per 100 000 person-years in the pre-screening period to 0.4 per 100 000 person-years in the post-screening period. By comparison, the incidence of death in an unscreened nonathletic population of the same age did not significantly change over the same time. Death by the cardiomyopathies was greatly reduced, with the proportion of athletes identified and disqualified due to HCM and ARVC doubling from the early to the late screening period. Consequently, this study was the first to substantiate that a systematic national screening programme can significantly decrease mortality via effective identification and disqualification of athletes with an underlying and unsuspected cardiomyopathy.

To date, the results of the Italian experience have not been reproduced by any other research groups. The major criticism of our registry mortality data is based on the Israel experience, as reported by Steinvil et al. [16], who claim that the yearly incidence of athletic field deaths in Israel did not change between 1985–96 (2.54 per 100 000 persons) and 1997–2009 (2.66 per 100 000 persons) despite the introduction of a cardiac screening programme using 12-lead ECG. Ultimately, their data suggest that efforts to prevent SCD in young athletes through ECG-based screening strategies are likely worthless. We believe, however, that major methodological limitations largely diminish Steinvil et al.'s conclusion. First, the number of athlete SCDs was derived from searching just two newspapers (i.e. not from a systematic SCD registry). This method of data capture is known to largely underreport cardiac events [6]. Second, the size of the population of competitive athletes was not known, but estimated. In conclusion, the Steinvil et al. [16]. study is fatally flawed as the incidence of SCD was calculated from an uncertain number of events in an uncertain number of athletes.

Maron et al. [17] compared death rates in young Italian athletes (from Veneto) screened with ECG and in American athletes from Minnesota (a demographically similar population) who had been screened by history and physical examination only (i.e. without ECG). Maron et al. found that over a comparable 11-year period (1993–2004), 12 deaths were reported in Veneto and 11 in Minnesota. When analysed as deaths per 100 000 person-years, Veneto exceeded Minnesota for all years combined (1.87 for 1979–2004 vs 1.06 for 1985–2007, respectively; $p = 0.006$), although the two regions did not differ significantly for 1993–2004 (0.87 vs 0.93, respectively; $p = 0.88$). The study concluded that SCDs in young competitive athletes occurred at a low rate in both Veneto and Minnesota, despite different screening strategies. Consequently, Maron et al. questioned the inclusion of an ECG in screening programmes, as it had little effect on decreasing athlete SCD. However, yet again, caution in drawing this conclusion is needed, as, like in Israel, the numerator used to calculate incidence of SCDs in the American athletes was derived from insurance claims and media reports – methods consistently considered invalid [6].

Costs of Systematic Screening across Italy

National Screening Programme

Implementation of the national screening programme in Italy has been feasible thanks to the limited costs involved in setting up a mass programme and the modest governmental support. The history, physical examination and ECG performed by qualified physicians (sport medicine specialists) costs around €50–60 per athlete. This cost is paid by the athlete or their athletic team, except for athletes younger than 18 years, for whom the expense is covered by the National Health System. If additional testing is required (usually echocardiography), it is covered by the athletic team or in small part by the National Health System, at an average cost of €120. The proportion of athletes requiring additional testing is approximately 9%, generating a modest additional impact on the overall cost of screening [15].

If undertaking a cost-effectiveness analysis, it is worth considering that young athletes/patients with a genetic cardiomyopathy or electrical disease may survive for many decades if identified in a timely manner and have a normal or near-normal life expectancy thanks to appropriate management. Moreover, the benefit of the screening goes beyond the identification of index athletes, because it may result in the identification of other affected family members, potentially saving additional lives. However, the large number of life-years saved is rarely considered when calculating the cost-effectiveness ratio of a cardiac screening programme.

Several analyses have attempted to quantify the cost of the Italian screening protocol when applied to countries – namely, the US – reporting conflicting results. Wheeler et al. [18] estimated that adding ECG to history and physical examination when screening young athletes would save 2.06 life-years per 1000 athletes screened, at a cost of USD42 000 per life-year saved. The addition of ECG remained cost-effective in a broad range of sensitivity analyses. However, different results were reported by Halkin et al. [19], who computed the costs of diagnostic testing for the estimated 8.5 million US athlete population over a 20-year period, based on Medicare lists, and concluded that the cost per life-year saved would be largely in excess of USD500 000, which is clearly prohibitive.

Based upon the Italian experience, we believe that the costs of cardiac screening should be computed as a package, whereby PPE (i) is considered as preventive medicine that targets healthy individuals in the vast majority of cases and (ii) is performed by sports medicine physicians and not cardiologists. We acknowledge that reimbursement of any preventive medicine programme does not currently exist in Medicare.

The legitimacy of reimbursement would require a change in cultural attitudes and in medical policy in the US, where cardiac screening is unlikely to be federally supported. Therefore, we believe that most of the purported obstacles to the implementation of 12-lead ECG screening reflect cultural, philosophical and social differences between our societies, more than economic reasons.

Screening Olympic and Paralympic Athletes

Italy has a bespoke screening programme for its Olympic and Paralympic athletes, at an average cost of €300–500 per athlete. However, it should be noted that the true cost is lower if it is considered that the medical personnel who undertake the screening are employed to do so by various sporting federations, with all medical equipment and facilities owned by the Italian Olympic Committee.

When assessing the cost/efficiency of the screening programmes in Olympic and Paralympic athletes, some considerations should not be missed. The screening represents just a small part of the routine expenses of elite athletes, which include medical treatments and insurance coverage, as well as a variety of costs related to training, coaching, technical equipment, travel and lodging. When compared with revenues, the costs (particularly for screening) become modest, or even negligible.

Limitations of Screening Programmes

Most of the criticism of the implementation of cardiovascular screening in other countries is based on practical considerations, including a lack of adequate economic resources, the absence of appropriately trained physicians and the potential for a high rate of false-positives, leading to unnecessary additional investigations, which obviously increase the cost of any screening programme.

Addressing the False-Positive ECG Conundrum

In 2010, the ESC produced 'revised' recommendations for the interpretation of athlete ECGs [20]. This was in response to an increasing number of sporting governing bodies undertaking pre-participation cardiovascular screening and producing an unacceptably high yield of false-positive reports, arising from the misinterpretation of physiological ECG changes commonly observed in athletes. To demonstrate improved specificity, the authors reanalysed the ECGs of 1005 highly trained athletes reported a decade earlier [21]. Originally, 402 athletes (40%) presented an abnormal ECG (so called 'group 2' changes). This was lowered to 11% using the 2010 ESC recommendations. As an example, in a large, unselected population of 32 652 young and adolescent individuals entering the screening programme, the ECG pattern was judged abnormal in 3853 (or 11.8%); however, most of these abnormalities (7%) were either prolonged PR intervals, incomplete RBBBs or early repolarisation patterns, commonly believed to be innocent expression of the exercise training. Other ECG changes, which required additional testing (as potential expressions of cardiac disease), were present in just 4.8% of the athlete population [22].

However, it has since been demonstrated that certain black ethnic populations, such as African, Afro-Caribbean and black Latin-American, continue to demonstrate a high prevalence of abnormal ECGs (~20–40%) when using the 2010 ESC recommendations [23]. To address this issue, in 2012, an international team of experts produced the 'Seattle Criteria' [24]: a revision of ECG interpretation guidelines for athletes, aimed at providing greater accuracy in identifying those with cardiac pathology, whilst also attempting to reduce the false-positive rate. The Seattle Criteria have demonstrated favourable results over the ESC recommendations, reducing the number of ECGs previously considered abnormal (17 to 4%) in a population of high-level athletes, whilst still identifying all athletes with cardiac pathology.

Recently, additional 'Refined Criteria' for the interpretation of athletes' ECGs have been proposed [25]. Riding et al. [26] observed that the Refined Criteria reduced the prevalence of an abnormal ECG from 11.6% when using the Seattle Criteria and from 22.3% when using the 2010 ESC recommendations to just 5.3% ($p < 0.0001$). Further, specificity was significantly improved to 94% across all athlete ethnicities (Arabic, black African and Caucasian; $p < 0.0001$) compared with the Seattle Criteria (specificity 87.5%) and ESC recommendations (specificity 76.6%). Importantly, 100% sensitivity for serious cardiac pathologies was maintained. It is therefore likely that the Refined Criteria will be adopted for widespread use in the interpretation of athletes' ECGs in coming years.

Legal Considerations

For over 30 years, Italy has had legislation that enforces cardiac screening and the use of a sports medicine physician to undertake and interpret screening results. Understandably, there is concern in other countries with different cultural and social backgrounds over 'systematic' or 'mandatory' cardiac screening and the autonomous rights of the individual athlete. This legal debate is heightened if one considers the possible misdiagnosis of cardiac pathology in an athlete or the clearance for competitive sport of an athlete harbouring a serious cardiac pathology. Both situations would have a devastating effect (personally, professionally and financially) upon the athlete and their immediate family, whilst for the physician in question, it would trigger legal complaints and civil charges that would have to be resolved in the public and medical courts. Concern over legal consequences represents one of the major reasons of resistance to widespread diffusion of the ECG screening in countries that do not have national screening programmes.

CAD and Other Undetected Abnormalities

One of the major limitations of the 12-lead ECG is the inability to detect, or even raise suspicion of, the presence of congenital coronary artery anomalies or premature atherosclerotic coronary disease. Only a modest subset of young athletes with congenital coronary artery anomalies present with symptoms, such as syncope or chest pain. Even if an exercise-ECG stress test is included, it rarely induces ischaemia, and therefore, most athletes remain undetected. In adult and senior athletes, the identification of silent ischaemic coronary disease is hampered by the low sensibility of exercise-ECG stress testing. Whilst computed tomography (CT) angiography has the potential to identify and characterise the coronary lesions, it is logistically and financially unfeasible to include this test in the routine work-up of a systematic screening programme.

Finally, sudden death may also be caused by a number of other less common diseases that remain undetectable on ECG, either because of a nonarrhythmic mechanism (spontaneous aortic rupture or bicuspid aortic valve) or because they are not related to the heart (bronchial asthma or ruptured cerebral aneurysm). Blunt, nonpenetrating and often innocent-appearing blows to the precordium may trigger ventricular fibrillation without structural injury to the ribs, sternum or heart (commotio cordis).

Conclusion

There is consensus agreement from both the American College of Cardiology (ACC)/AHA and the ESC that compelling justification exists for cardiovascular pre-participation screening on medical, ethical and legal grounds. Whilst agreement on the implementation of screening may exist, there remains a difference in opinion regarding the methods employed to assess cardiovascular risk. For over 30 years, Italy's systematic cardiac screening programme has demonstrated that a significantly greater number of athletes' lives can be saved with the inclusion of a 12-lead ECG than by history and physical examination alone. At present, the ECG screening protocol is recognised as the best medical practice for screening purposes, and it is currently supported by the ESC Sport Cardiology, IOC and international federations including FIFA and UCI.

In conclusion, athlete screening should be seen as 'preventative medicine' aimed at protecting the lives of young individuals, in the same vein as other benevolent health care strategies, including the prevention of obesity, diabetes mellitus, hypertension and CAD. Indeed, the prospect of identifying a sinister cardiac disorder in a young person is associated with disproportionately better outcome at a much lower cost than any of these other conditions.

References

1 Perk, J., De Backer, G., Gohlke, H. et al. European Guidelines on cardiovascular disease prevention in clinical practice (version 2012). *Eur Heart J* 2012; **33**: 1635–701.

2 Maron, B.J., Doerer, J.J., Haas, T.S. et al. Sudden deaths in young competitive athletes. Analysis of 1866 deaths in the United States, 1980–2006. *Circulation* 2009; **119**: 1085–92.

3 Corrado, D., Basso, C., Schiavon, M. et al. Pre-participation screening of young competitive athletes for prevention of sudden cardiac death. *J Am Coll Cardiol* 2008; **52**: 1981–9.

4 Corrado, D., Basso, C., Rizzoli, G. et al. Does sports activity enhance the risk of sudden death in adolescents and young adults ? *J Am Coll Cardiol* 2003; **42**: 1959–63.

5 Maron, B.J., Haas, T.S., Murphy, C.J. et al. Incidence and causes of sudden death in US college athletes. *J Am Coll Cardiol* 2014; **63**: 1636–43.

6 Harmon, K.G., Asif, I.M., Klossner, D. et al. Incidence of sudden cardiac death in national collegiate athletic association athletes. *Circulation* 2011; **123**: 1594–600.

7 Harmon, K.J., Drezner, J.A., Wilson, M.G. and Sharma, S. Incidence of sudden cardiac death in athletes: a state-of-the-art review. *Br J Sports Med* 2014; **48**: 1185–92.

8 Corrado, D., Basso, C., Pavei, A. et al. Trends in sudden cardiovascular death in young competitive athletes after implementation of a preparticipation screening program. *JAMA* 2006; **296**: 1593–601.

9 Maron, B.J., Thompson, P.D., Ackerman, M.J. et al. Recommendations and considerations related to preparticipation screening for cardiovascular abnormalities in competitive athletes: 2007 update: a scientific statement from the American Heart Association Council on Nutrition, Physical Activity, and Metabolism: endorsed by the American College of Cardiology Foundation. *Circulation* 2007; **115**: 1643–55.

10 Corrado, D., Pelliccia, A., Bjornstad, H.H. et al. Cardiovascular pre-participation screening of young competitive athletes for prevention of sudden death: proposal for a common European protocol. *Eur Heart J* 2005; **26**: 516–24.

11 Ljungqvist, A., Jenoure, P., Engebretsen, L. et al. The International Olympic Committee (IOC) Consensus Statement on periodic health evaluation of elite athletes March 2009. *Br J Sports Med* 2009; **43**: 631–43.

12 Biffi, A., Delise, P., Zeppilli, P. et al. Italian cardiological guidelines for sports eligibility in athletes with heart disease. *J Cardiovasc Med (Hagerstown)* 2013; **14**(7): 477–99.

13 Sharma, S., Merghani, A. and Gati, S. Cardiac screening of young athletes prior to participation in sports. Difficulties in detecting the fatally flawed among the fabulously fit. *JAMA Intern Med* 2015; **175**(1): 125–7.

14 Harmon, K.G., Zigman, M. and Drezner, J.A. The effectiveness of screening history, physical exam, and ECG to detect potentially lethal cardiac disorders in athletes: a systematic review/meta-analysis. *J Electrocardiol* 2015; **48**(3): 329–38.

15 Corrado, D., Basso, C., Schiavon, M. and Thiene, G. Screening for hypertrophic cardiomyopathy in young athletes. *New Engl J Med* 1998; **339**: 364–9.

16 Steinvil, A., Chundadze, T., Zeltser, D. et al. Mandatory electrocardiographic screening of athletes to reduce their risk for sudden death proven fact or wishful thinking? *J Am Coll Cardiol* 2011; **57**: 1291–6.

17 Maron, B.J., Haas, T.S., Doerer, J.J. et al. Comparison of U.S. and Italian experiences with sudden cardiac deaths in young competitive athletes and implications for preparticipation screening strategies. *Am J Cardiol* 2009; **104**: 276–80.

18 Wheeler, M.T., Heidenreich, P.A., Froelicher, V.F. et al. Cost-effectiveness of preparticipation screening for prevention of sudden cardiac death in young athletes. *Ann Intern Med* 2010; **152**: 276–86.

19 Halkin, A., Steinvil, A., Rosso, R. and Viskin, S. Preventing sudden death of athletes with electrocardiographic screening: what is the absolute benefit and how much will it cost? *J Am Coll Cardiol* 2012; **60**(22): 2271–6.

20 Corrado, D., Pelliccia, A., Heidbuchel, H. et al. Recommendations for interpretation of 12-lead electrocardiogram in the athlete. *Eur Heart J* 2010; **31**(2): 243–59.

21 Pelliccia, A., Maron, B.J., Culasso, F. et al. Clinical significance of abnormal electrocardiographic patterns in trained athletes. *Circulation* 2000; **102**: 278–84.

22 Pelliccia, A., Culasso, F., Di Paolo, F. et al. Prevalence of abnormal electrocardiograms in a large, unselected population undergoing preparticipation cardiovascular screening. *Eur Heart J* 2007; **28**: 2006–10.

23 Papadakis, M., Carre, F., Kervio, G. et al. The prevalence, distribution, and clinical outcomes of electrocardiographic repolarization patterns in male athletes of African/Afro-Caribbean origin. *Eur Heart J* 2011; **32**(18): 2304–13.

24 Drezner, J.A., Ackerman, M.J., Anderson, J. et al. Electrocardiographic interpretation in athletes: the 'Seattle Criteria'. *Br J Sports Med* 2013; **47**(3): 122–4.

25 Sheikh, N. and Sharma, S. Refining electrocardiography interpretation criteria in elite athletes: redefining the limits of normal. *Eur Heart J* 2014; **35**(44): 3078–80.

26 Riding, N.R., Sheikh, N., Adamuz, C. et al. Comparison of three current sets of electrocardiographic interpretation criteria for use in screening athletes. *Heart* 2014; **101**(5): 384–90.

9 Comparison of Pre-participation Evaluations for Assessing Cardiovascular Risk in Athletes

Ramy S. Abdelfattah[1] and Mathew G. Wilson[2–4]

[1]Stanford Cardiology Sports Medicine Clinic, Stanford University, Stanford, CA, USA
[2]Department of Sports Medicine, ASPETAR, Qatar Orthopaedic and Sports Medicine Hospital, Doha, Qatar
[3]Research Institute of Sport and Exercise Sciences, Liverpool John Moores University, Liverpool, UK
[4]Research Institute of Sport and Exercise Sciences, University of Canberra, Canberra, ACT, Australia

Introduction

When an organisation, school, institution or health care provider considers performing or is involved in the pre-participation cardiovascular screening of athletes, questions arise: Which guidelines provide the best evidence-based approach to screening? Which protocol best permits early identification of athletes at risk of sudden cardiac death (SCD)? Whilst the medicolegal and ethical responsibility of any clinician dealing with an athlete is to provide the best medical care available, many medical and cardiology societies and sporting organisations have created their own pre-participation evaluations (PPEs) to assess cardiovascular risk in athletes. Thus, for clinicians clearing young athletes for participation, there is a lack of consistency and consensus over which protocol to follow [1].

Over the past 20 years, the major controversy in sports cardiology has been whether or not the 12-lead electrocardiogram (ECG) should be included in pre-participation screening. Increased attention arose after the publication of the 2005 European Society of Cardiology (ESC) guidelines endorsing a 12-lead ECG protocol [2]. Unfortunately, validation and improvement of the non-ECG elements has been disappointedly neglected. Consequently, this chapter will compare the five most common PPE protocols: the American Heart Association (AHA) 12 elements (and their recent 14-element update); the Pre-participation Physical Evaluation Monograph, including its 4th edition (4th Monograph); the ESC protocol; the International Olympic Committee (IOC) protocol; and the Pre-Competition Medical Assessment (PCMA) of the Fédération Internationale de Football Association (FIFA).

American Heart Association (AHA)

In 1996, the AHA proposed 12 elements for the pre-participation cardiovascular screening of athletes in the AHA Scientific Statement [3]. These elements were unaltered in a 2007 update [4], which was a reaction to the movement to include the ECG as part of the PPE. This update contended that incorporating a 12-lead ECG in pre-participation screening in the US was impractical and would require considerable resources. Although it stated that such a screening programme would detect greater numbers of athletes with heart disease, many difficulties would prevent such a national programme, including the effects of a false-positive, cost-efficiency

IOC Manual of Sports Cardiology, First Edition. Edited by Mathew G. Wilson, Jonathan A. Drezner and Sanjay Sharma.
© 2017 International Olympic Committee. Published 2017 by John Wiley & Sons, Ltd.

Personal history[a]
1. Chest pain/discomfort/tightness/pressure related to exertion
2. Unexplained syncope/near-syncope[b]
3. Excessive and unexplained dyspnoea/fatigue or palpitations, associated with exercise
4. Prior recognition of a heart murmur
5. Elevated systemic blood pressure
6. Prior restriction from participation in sports
7. Prior testing for the heart, ordered by a physician

Family history[a]
8. Premature death (sudden and unexpected or otherwise) before 50 years of age attributable to heart disease in one or more relatives
9. Disability from heart disease in a close relative <50 years of age
10. Hypertrophic or dilated cardiomyopathy, long QT syndrome or other ion channelopathies, Marfan syndrome or clinically significant arrhythmias; specific knowledge of genetic cardiac conditions in family members

Physical examination
11. Heart murmur[c]
12. Femoral pulses to exclude aortic coarctation
13. Physical stigmata of Marfan syndrome
14. Brachial artery blood pressure (sitting position)[d]

Table 9.1 The 14-element AHA recommendations for pre-participation cardiovascular screening of competitive athletes

[a] Parental verification is recommended for high-school and middle-school athletes

[b] Judged not to be of neurocardiogenic (vasovagal) origin; of particular concern when occurring during or after physical exertion

[c] Refers to heart murmurs judged likely to be organic and unlikely to be innocent; auscultation should be performed with the patient in both the supine and standing positions (or with Valsalva maneuver), specifically to identify murmurs of dynamic left ventricular outflow tract obstruction

[d] Preferably taken in both arms

considerations and practical difficulties. The AHA stated that false-positive screening diagnoses would generate unnecessary life consequences, with emotional, financial and medical burdens for the athlete, their family, their team and their institution, including unnecessary additional tests and procedures, anxiety, uncertainty and the possibility of disqualification without justification. To date, these claims have not been substantiated by scientific study. The AHA recommended that cardiovascular athletic screening with history and physical examination be performed only by physicians. When impractical, it suggested that nurse practitioners or physician-assistants perform the screening – if they have the correct training, medical skills and background.

In 2014, the AHA updated the number of elements from 12 to 14 (10 for personal and family history and 4 for physical examination) (Table 9.1) [5]. The 14 elements added palpitations and chest tightness or pressure associated with exercise to the chest pain element, as well as two new elements concerning any prior restriction from participation in sports or any prior cardiac testing ordered by a physician. A positive response or finding in 1 or more of the 14 items may be judged sufficient for further cardiovascular evaluation. The AHA recommends parental verification of the responses to the history questions obtained from minors.

The differences between the AHA 12 and 14 elements are relatively minor and are based on consensus opinion rather than evidence. The accuracy of screening questionnaires in identifying athletes with conditions associated with SCD has been called into question [6,7], and simply expanding a screening tool from 12 to 14 elements may not have the desired effect when the deficiency is in the tool itself. Unfortunately, the AHA document focused on the opinion that the ECG is impractical as part of a screening protocol rather than considering advances made in the ECG screening of young athletes.

Pre-participation Physical Evaluation Monograph 4th Edition (4th Monograph)

In 1992, five organisations (American Academy of Family Medicine, American Academy of Pediatrics, American Medical Society for Sports Medicine, American Orthopedic Society for Sports Medicine and American Osteopathic Academy of Sports Medicine) developed the Pre-Participation Physical Evaluation

Personal history
- Has a doctor ever denied or restricted your participation in sports for any reason?
- Have you ever passed out or nearly passed out DURING or AFTER exercise?
- Have you ever had discomfort, pain, tightness or pressure in your chest during exercise?
- Does your heart ever race or skip beats (irregular beats) during exercise?
- Has a doctor ever told you that you have any heart problems? If so, check all that apply: ☐ High blood pressure ☐ Heart murmur ☐ High cholesterol ☐ Heart infection ☐ Kawasaki disease ☐ Other:
- Has a doctor ever ordered a test for your heart (e.g. ECG, echocardiogram)?
- Do you get lightheaded or feel more short of breath than expected during exercise?
- Have you ever had an unexplained seizure?
- Do you get tired or short of breath more quickly than your friends during exercise?

Family history
- Has any family member or relative died of heart problems or had any unexpected or unexplained sudden death before the age of 50 (including drowning, unexplained car accident or SIDS)?
- Does anyone in your family have: hypertrophic cardiomyopathy, Marfan syndrome, arrhythmogenic right ventricular cardiomyopathy, long or short QT syndrome, Brugada syndrome or catecholaminergic polymorphic ventricular tachycardia?
- Does anyone in your family have a heart problem, pacemaker or implanted defibrillator?
- Has anyone in your family had unexplained fainting, seizures or near drowning?

Physical examination
- Murmurs (auscultation, standing, supine ± Valsalva)
- Location of point of maximal impulse (PMI)
- Simultaneous femoral and radial pulses
- Marfan stigmata (kyphoscoliosis, high-arched palate, pectus excavatum, arachnodactyly, arm span > height, hyperlaxity, myopia, mitral valve prolapse, aortic insufficiency)

Table 9.2 The 4th PPE Monograph history and physical examination elements

Monograph to guide physicians through the PPE process for young athletes from middle school through college. The American College of Sports Medicine joined the effort for the development of the 3rd edition in 2005, and the AHA collaborated with development of the 4th edition 2010 [8].

The 4th Monograph made important changes to the SCD screening questions by including unexplained or undiagnosed seizure activity, drowning, unexplained car accidents and sudden infant death syndrome (SIDS) in the personal and family history questionnaires (Table 9.2). Additionally, the Monograph recommends that syncope issues be addressed in routine preventive health discussions with athletes and their guardians, because of their importance in identifying any child at risk of sudden death. Whilst the 4th Monograph does not recommend the ECG, it includes ECG criteria for physicians applying it as part of screening. The 4th-edition personal and family history questions were shown in one study of adolescent athletes to have a high false-positive response rate (31.3%) whilst detecting conditions posing risk for SCD [6].

European Society of Cardiology (ESC)

In 2005, the consensus statement of the Study Group on Sports Cardiology of the Working Group on Cardiac Rehabilitation and Exercise Physiology of the ESC published a proposal for a European protocol for cardiovascular pre-participation screening of young competitive athletes (Table 9.3) [2]. The consensus document recommended the ECG, assuming its efficacy as a screening tool based on the 25-year Italian experience [9].

The ESC recommends that the PPE screening should start at the beginning of competitive athletic activity, age 12–14 years for most sports, and be repeated on a regular basis at least every 2 years. It also recommends that the PPE be performed by a physician with the specific training, skills, knowledge and cultural background required to identify those cardiovascular diseases (CVDs) responsible for exercise-related sudden death. The ESC suggests providing postgraduate residency training programmes in sports medicine (and sports cardiology) full-time for 4 years, as in Italy.

Personal history
- Exertional chest pain or discomfort
- Syncope or near-syncope
- Irregular heartbeat or palpitations
- Shortness of breath or fatigue out of proportion to the degree of exertion

Family history
- A close relative(s) who has experienced a premature heart attack or sudden death (aged <55 in males and <65 in females)
- Family history of cardiomyopathy, Marfan syndrome, long QT syndrome, Brugada syndrome, severe arrhythmias, coronary artery disease or other disabling CVDs

Physical examination
- Marfan features (musculoskeletal/ocular)
- Diminished and delayed femoral artery pulses
- Mid- or end-systolic clicks, a second heart sound (single or widely split and fixed with respiration), marked heart murmurs (any diastolic and systolic grade ≥2/6)
- Irregular heart rhythm
- Brachial blood pressure >140/90 mmHg (on >1 reading)

Table 9.3 The ESC questionnaire and physical examination components for pre-participation cardiovascular screening of competitive athletes

International Olympic Committee (IOC)

In 2004, the IOC created its own PPE for national Olympic committee physicians to use before sending athletes to the Olympic Games (Table 9.4). It is worth placing the IOC PPE in the context of the international population for which it was designed. Combining the athlete participation figures from the Beijing and London Olympics, there were 22 156 athletes competing for 205 countries. Excluding European and North American countries, there were 32 African, 32 Asia-Pacific, 32 Latin American, 14 Middle Eastern and 8 South Asian nations [10].

In 2009, the IOC published consensus recommendations on periodic health evaluation in elite athletes [11]. The IOC statement reiterated that the main purpose of the evaluation was to screen for injuries or medical conditions that might place an athlete at risk and endorsed the inclusion of an ECG in the cardiovascular screening of athletes. Whilst the PPE protocol was not made obligatory prior to competition, the IOC highlighted the importance of balancing the ethical and legal aspects to help protect the rights and responsibilities of athletes, physicians and sporting organisations. It recommended that the PPE should be performed in the primary interest of the athlete under the responsibility of a physician trained in sports medicine. Whilst the IOC recommended that the physician strongly discourage the athlete from continuing training when evidence from the PPE identifies serious risk – until the necessary medical measures have been taken – it also stated that it remains the responsibility of the athlete to decide whether to continue training or not [11].

Fédération Internationale de Football Association (FIFA)

FIFA, through its medical committee, FIFA Medical Assessment and Research Centre (F-MARC), developed a standardised PCMA and implemented it at the Men's 2006 FIFA World Cup and the 2007 FIFA Women's World Cup [12]. After undertaking an assessment of the feasibility of and compliance with performing a comprehensive PCMA in participating teams at the FIFA U-17 and U-20 Women's World Cups 2010, FIFA decided to make the PCMA a compulsory requirement for all FIFA competitions.

The PCMA was designed not only to investigate conditions that predispose an individual to SCD but also to identify the risk of future injuries or other health issues that would be detrimental to successful participation. The cardiovascular section of the FIFA PCMA is an extensive 55-step document (Table 9.5); it also includes an ECG and echocardiogram.

Comparison of the Five Protocols

All basic components of the five PPEs are comparable: physical exam, medical history and family history; however, use of more advanced screening tools such as ECG varies. Optimally, PPEs should be simple to administer, ensure good sensitivity and specificity and provide the clinician with sufficient guidance when

For all participants	Potentially detectable cardiovascular conditions
Personal history Questionnaire by examining physician: 1. Have you ever fainted or passed out when exercising? 2. Do you ever have chest tightness? 3. Does running ever cause chest tightness? 4. Have you ever had chest tightness, cough or wheezing which made it difficult for you to perform in sports? 5. Have you ever been treated/hospitalised for asthma? 6. Have you ever had a seizure? 7. Have you ever been told that you have epilepsy? 8. Have you ever been told to give up sports because of health problems? 9. Have you ever been told you have high blood pressure? 10. Have you ever been told you have high cholesterol? 11. Do you have trouble breathing or do you cough during or after activity? 12. Have you ever been dizzy during or after exercise? 13. Have you ever had chest pain during or after exercise? 14. Do you have or have you ever had racing of your heart or skipped heartbeats? 15. Do you get tired more quickly than your friends during exercise? 16. Have you ever been told you have a heart murmur? 17. Have you ever been told you have a heart arrhythmia? 18. Do you have any other history of heart problems? 19. Have you had a severe viral infection (e.g. myocarditis or mononucleosis) within the past month? 20. Have you ever been told you had rheumatic fever? 21. Do you have any allergies? 22. Are you taking any medications at the present time? 23. Have you routinely taken any medication in the past 2 years?	Any cardiovascular condition
Family history *Questionnaire by examining physician* 24. Has anyone in your family less than 50 years old: • Died suddenly and unexpectedly? • Been treated for recurrent fainting? • Had unexplained seizure problems? • Had unexplained drowning when swimming? • Had an unexplained car accident? • Had a heart transplantation? • Had a pacemaker or defibrillator implanted? • Been treated for irregular heart beat? • Had heart surgery? 25. Has anyone in your family experienced sudden infant death (cot death)? 26. Has anyone in your family been told they have Marfan syndrome?	Inherited cardiomyopathy (hypertrophic, arrhythmogenic, dilated) Inherited heart rhythm problem/cardiac ion channel diseases (long and short QT syndrome, Brugada syndrome, Lenegre disease, catecholaminergic polymorphic ventricular tachycardia) Connective-tissue disorders
General 27. Peripheral pulses 28. Marfan stigmata 29. Cardiac auscultation: rate/rhythm 30. Murmur: systolic/diastolic obstruction and systolic click 31. Blood pressure	Coarctation of the aorta, aortic dilatation, mitral valve prolapse (MVP), ventricular ectopic beats, structural heart disease, outflow tract obstruction, aortic valve (AV) disease Hypertension

Table 9.4 Lausanne recommendations: sudden cardiovascular death in sport under the umbrella of the IOC medical commission

A. Heart and lung personal symptoms		Date of last cardiovascular exam	
	Never	Within the last 4 weeks	Before the last 4 weeks
Chest pain or tightness			
Shortness of breath			
Asthma			
Cough			
Bronchitis			
Palpitations/arrhythmias			
Other heart problems			
Dizziness			
Syncope			
Chest pain after exercise			
Hypertension			
Heart murmur			
Abnormal lipid profile			
Seizures			
Advised to give up sport			
More quickly tired than teammates			
Diarrhoea illness			
	No	Yes	
Smokes			
Consumes alcohol			
Wears contact lenses or glasses			

B. Family history (male relatives <55 years, female relatives <65 years)					
	None	Father	Mother	Sibling	Other
Sudden cardiac death (SCD)					
Sudden infant death					
Coronary heart disease					
Cardiomyopathy					
Hypertension					
Recurrent syncope					
Arrhythmias					
Heart transplant					
Heart surgery					
Pacemaker/defibrillator					
Marfan syndrome					
Unexplained drowning					
Unexplained car accident					
Stroke					
Diabetes					
Cancer					
Other (arthritis etc.)					

Table 9.5 FIFA Pre-Competition Medical Assessment (PCMA). Only relevant sections related to cardiovascular screening are presented

(Continued)

C. General physical exam

Thyroid gland	☐ normal	☐ abnormal
Lymph nodes/spleen	☐ normal	☐ abnormal
Lungs		
• Percussion	☐ normal	☐ abnormal
• Breath sounds	☐ normal	☐ abnormal
Abdomen		
• Palpation	☐ normal	☐ abnormal
Marfan criteria	☐ no	☐ yes, please specify: • chest deformities • long arms and legs • flat footedness • scoliosis • lens dislocation • other:_____

D. Cardiovascular system examination

Rhythm	☐ normal	☐ arrhythmic
Heart sounds	☐ normal	☐ abnormal, please specify: • split • paradoxically split • 3rd heart sound • 4th heart sound
Heart murmurs	☐ no	☐ yes, please specify: • systollic intensity:____/6 • diastollic intensity:____/6 • clicks • changes during valsalva manoeuver • changes on abruptly standing up
Peripheral oedema	☐ no	☐ yes
Jugular veins (45° position)	☐ normal	☐ abnormal
Hepatojugular reflux	☐ no	☐ yes
Blood vessels		
• Peripheral pulses	☐ palpable	☐ not palpable
• Delay in femoral pulses	☐ no	☐ yes
• Vascular bruits	☐ no	☐ yes
• Varicose veins	☐ no	☐ yes
Heart rate (after 5 minutes' rest)	_____/min	
Blood pressure (in supine position after 5 minutes' rest)		
• Right arm	____/____mmHg	
• Left arm	____/____mmHg	
• Ankle	____/____mmHg	

Table 9.5 *(cont'd)*

obtaining positive responses. Their goal is to enable clinicians to make an informed decision as to whether an athlete requires further cardiovascular work-up beyond basic screening.

Personal History

The major problem with all five of the protocols is that none is evidence-based. None of the questions or recommended elements were validated prior to publication and all are based on consensus opinion. Since publication, many studies have demonstrated a low sensitivity and a high response rate for the screening heart health questions.

The five protocols agree on questioning about history of chest pain, fatigue, shortness of breath, chest tightness/discomfort, palpitations and/or syncope (Table 9.6). However, they differ in the way they ask about the symptom and its relation to exercise. For example, in evaluating syncope, the ESC and FIFA protocols enquire about syncope and pre-syncope but the AHA, IOC and 4th Monograph ask about syncope or fainting specifically during or after exercise. The 4th Monograph asks about lightheadedness during or after exercise in a separate question. The IOC and FIFA protocols uniquely include history of dizziness (but do not specify whether this refers to vertigo or lightheadedness). Also, the FIFA protocol asks twice about any history of chest pain (related and not related to exercise) and includes a question on shortness of breath – but not in relation to exercise, unlike the four other protocols.

Item	AHA	ESC	IOC	FIFA	4th Monograph
Chest pain (during or after exercising)	Y	Y	Y	Y	Y
More quickly tired/fatigued than teammates	Y	Y	Y	Y	Y
Heart murmur	Y	Y	Y	Y	Y
High blood pressure	Y	Y	Y	Y	Y
Shortness of breath (during or after exercising)	Y	Y	Y	Y	Y
Chest tightness/discomfort	Y	Y	Y	Y	Y
Palpitations/racing of the heart/skipped heartbeats (during or after exercising)	Y	Y	Y	Y	Y
(Near) syncope/(near) loss of conscious/fainted/passed out (during or after exercising)	Y	Y	Y	Y	Y
Advised to give up sport/restriction on participation	Y		Y	Y	Y
Dizziness/lightheadedness (during or after exercise)			Y	Y	Y
Abnormal lipid profile			Y	Y	Y
Other heart problem			Y	Y	Y
Seizures			Y	Y	Y
Cough/asthma			Y	Y	
Heart arrhythmia			Y	Y	
Previous cardiac investigation (ECG, echocardiogram etc.)	Y				Y
Rheumatic fever/allergies			Y		
Bronchitis/diarrhoea				Y	
Epilepsy			Y		
Alcohol/smoking				Y	
Medications at the present time or during the past 2 years			Y		
Contact lenses/glasses				Y	
Severe viral infection within the past month			Y		

Table 9.6 Comparison of the personal history sections of the five protocols

Item	AHA	ESC	IOC	FIFA	4th Monograph
Sudden death	Y	Y	Y	Y	Y
Arrhythmia	Y	Y	Y	Y	Y
Marfan syndrome	Y	Y	Y	Y	Y
Cardiomyopathy	Y	Y		Y	Y
Heart surgery	Y		Y	Y	
Pacemaker/implanted defibrillator			Y	Y	Y
Unexplained fainting/drowning			Y	Y	Y
Unexplained car accident/sudden infant death			Y	Y	Y
Disabled from heart disease	Y	Y			
Heart transplant			Y	Y	
Unexplained seizures			Y		Y
Coronary heart disease		Y		Y	
Cardiac treatment	Y				
Hypertension/stroke/cancer/diabetes/arthritis				Y	

Table 9.7 Comparison of the family history sections of the five protocols

Many of the questions asked within the cardiovascular sections of the IOC and FIFA protocols are of little value when looking for cardiac conditions that may predispose to SCD. Some of these questions may be pertinent for a team physician from a general health perspective when managing athletes participating at the Olympic Games or the World Cup but are of less importance when attempting to identify an athlete with an inherited, congenital or acquired cardiac disease. It is also unclear why the FIFA protocol differentiates personal cardiac symptoms before and during the prior 4 weeks. For example, an athlete who experienced syncope with palpitations 2 months ago would receive the same cardiac work-up if they presented with these symptoms within the last 2 weeks.

Family History

The five protocols recommend questioning about any history of premature heart attack or SCD (Table 9.7). The age at which an SCD occurs is important. Whilst most sudden deaths over the age of 35 are due to coronary artery atheromas, we would be significantly concerned about the health of a young athlete with a family history of SCD in a first-degree relative who died unexpectedly at between 5 and 35 years of age. Yet, age ranges and gender distinction are different between the protocols, for unknown reasons. Whilst the ESC and FIFA protocols recommend a specific age range according to gender (≤55 years in males and ≤65 years in females), the AHA, IOC and 4th Monograph recommend a different age range without any gender distinction (<50 years). Although the five protocols enquire about a family history of arrhythmia, the AHA protocol specifically asks about inherited arrhythmias. The ESC protocol gives examples of what to look for (long QT syndrome, Brugada syndrome and severe arrhythmias), whilst the 4th Monograph gives a lengthy list of conditions to consider.

Physical Examination

As part of the physical examination, all five protocols recommend measuring blood pressure, listening for heart murmurs during auscultation and checking for features suggestive of Marfan stigmata (Table 9.8). The ESC protocol guides clinicians to look for skeletal and ocular features of Marfan. The FIFA protocol provides more stigmata details, including chest deformities, long arms and legs, flat footedness, scoliosis and lens dislocation. The 4th Monograph provides further details: kyphoscoliosis, high-arched palate, pectus excavatum, arachnodactyly, arm span > height, hyperlaxity, myopia, mitral valve prolapse (MVP) and aortic insufficiency. Importantly, no protocol provides specific methods for the elements of the physical exam, and all assume that these are standardised.

Item	AHA	ESC	IOC	FIFA	4th Monograph
Marfan stigmata	Y	Y	Y	Y	Y
Murmur	Y	Y	Y	Y	Y
Delay/weakness in femoral pulse	Y	Y		Y	Y
Blood pressure	Y	Y	Y	Y	Y
Peripheral pulse	Y		Y	Y	Y
Rhythm		Y	Y	Y	
Heart sounds		Y	Y	Y	
Heart rate			Y	Y	
Clicks		Y	Y		
Point of maximal impulse (PMI) location					Y
Varicose veins/vascular bruits				Y	
Peripheral oedema/jugular venous pressure (JVP)/hepatojugular reflux				Y	
Cuff pressure between two arms	Y				

Table 9.8 Comparison of the physical examination sections of the five protocols

ECG and Ancillary Tests

The ESC, IOC and FIFA protocols incorporate a resting ECG, but only FIFA requires an echocardiogram. Evidence for including an echocardiogram is not provided. The recommendation of ECG (or not) is the singular major difference between the US and other guidelines, with growing evidence supporting inclusion of the ECG. The value of the ancillary tests is covered in Chapters 14–17 and will not be discussed further here.

Considerations

Personal and Family History Considerations

There are many problems with the use of any of the five cardiovascular screening questionnaires. We have consistently shown that personal symptoms are poor predictors of cardiovascular abnormalities [13]. High rates of positive responses create a medicolegal dilemma when gathered by health care providers without adequate training or experience in the symptoms or conditions of concern in young athletes. Since the reaction to a positive response is not standardised, this may lead to variation in practice, along with expensive and unnecessary testing and delay. At Stanford, the AHA 12-element screening questions produce a positive response in up to 25% of athletes: even more than the ECG when either the Stanford or the Seattle ECG criteria are applied (under 6%) [14]. In a study of US high-school athletes, 31% required additional evaluation because of medical or family history responses and 8% because of physical examination findings [6]. This is matched by data from Qatar, where 22% of athletes had at least one finding on history and physical examination that warranted additional cardiovascular examination. This false-positive rate is important, as no athlete was identified with an inherited cardiac disease on the basis of history and physical examination alone [15]. Thus, it is clear that more evidence-based questioning is required to increase sensitivity and specificity and so reduce the unnecessarily high level of false-positive responses.

A challenge to developing accurate questions about cardiovascular warning symptoms is that many of the symptoms overlap with the expected physiological responses to intense physical exertion, including shortness of breath, fatigue and even chest tightness or lightheadedness. How an athlete interprets these symptoms as a normal response to training or an abnormal response of concern for a cardiopulmonary limitation also varies and lacks uniformity. In a perfect world, a physician would use an open-ended enquiry in assessing the risk posed by a sport, with prompting questions regarding high-risk symptoms. These could include:

• Have you ever lost consciousness and fallen to the ground during or immediately after exercise?
• Have you been bothered by racing or skipping of your heart beat during or immediately after exercise?

- Have you ever had chest pain or pressure at maximal exercise that was not related to breathing, lasted minutes and was other than sharp and stabbing?

Without appropriate follow-up questions to distinguish the clinically significant from the extraneous, all positives might result in unnecessary testing, delay and cost. Using this approach may reduce the high false-positive rate inherent to questionnaires. Whatever approach is taken, the critical issue is that the follow-up questions should enable the physician to make a reasonable decision regarding the potential cardiovascular risk of the positive response [16].

Perhaps the question, 'Is there a family history of SCD in a first-degree relative under 35 years of age?' is the most important. In a study which examined 470 SCD victims aged 1–35 years and followed up their first- and second-degree relatives for 11 years, Ranthe et al. [17] concluded that 'cardiovascular diseases co-aggregated significantly with SCD in families, with young first-degree relatives at greatest risk. Results clearly indicate that family members of young SCD victims should be offered comprehensive and systematic screening, with focus on the youngest relatives.' In a retrospective review of 112 paediatric patients with a family history of sudden arrhythmic death syndrome, Wong et al. [18] concluded 'the yield of screening pediatric relatives is significant and higher when focused on 1st degree relatives and on inherited cardiac conditions such as LQTS [long QT syndrome]'. Accordingly, we suggest that all five PPEs have set an age limit that is far too high, and that lowering the age for familial cardiac disease to less than 40 would be more appropriate.

Physical Exam Considerations

Marfan's syndrome is a relatively rare condition, and reminders of the physical stigmata of Marfan's syndrome are potentially helpful for physicians with less experience. However, stigmata are rare and not particularly sensitive (see Chapter 22). It is unlikely that many young athletes over 6 feet tall with long arms will have Marfan's without other markers being present. Any elevation of blood pressure over 140/90 should lead to serial exams to see if this is a consistent finding, and any athlete with consistent elevations should undergo further evaluation and treatment.

Subtle physical exam findings are unlikely to be detected except by the most skilled examiners. Fixed splitting of the second heart sound is normal in the supine position and only abnormal when sitting or standing. Each cardiologist seems to have their own method of doing a Valsalva manoeuvre, and only one-quarter of athletes with hypertrophic cardiomyopathy (HCM) will have an obstructive component at rest. The value of squatting to detect MVP is uncertain, as severe MVP is usually accompanied by a murmur heard in any position. Diastolic murmurs are the most difficult to hear, yet are nearly always associated with pathology. Auscultation for aortic insufficiency, the most common cause of diastolic murmurs, should be performed in the sitting position, with the athlete leaning forward during expiration – a recommendation not made in any of the five protocols. In the mass PPE environment, any diastolic murmur and/or loud systolic murmur should lead to a more thorough exam in a physician's office or by an echocardiogram.

General PPE Considerations

In an attempt to determine the effectiveness of different components of the PPE screening in order to detect potentially lethal cardiac disorders in athletes, Harmon et al. [19] recently undertook a systematic review/meta-analysis of over 47 000 participants who underwent cardiovascular screening. Their meta-analysis demonstrated that the sensitivity and specificity of history questions were 20/94%, those of physical exam were 9/97% and those of ECG were 94/93%. The overall false-positive rate of history was 8%, that of physical exam was 10% and that of ECG was 6%. Harmon et al. [19] concluded: 'the most effective strategy for screening for cardiovascular disease in athletes is the ECG, and the use of history and physical exam alone as a screening tool should be reevaluated'.

To lessen false-positive rates and increase sensitivity, we suggest including elements of the 4th Monograph (seizures, other findings suggestive of inherited arrhythmic diseases), lowering the age for family history questions to 40 (to avoid coronary artery disease (CAD)-associated events) and focusing on symptoms during or after exercise. We also suggest providing specific accompanying questions to the questioning physician, to help reduce unnecessary further cardiovascular examinations. This is imperative, since not all physicians have the clinical experience or training to evaluate athletes. In this way, the family physician or mass-screening physician can serve as a gate keeper to expensive and unnecessary evaluations.

Conclusion

In conclusion, no PPE will identify all cardiac conditions, and some athletes with normal evaluations may have a cardiac event, due either to undetected cardiac conditions or to conditions that develop later. It is clear, however, that the cardiac risk elements in the five protocols discussed in this chapter result in more false-positives than do current athlete-specific ECG criteria. More research is needed to improve the accuracy of screening medical and family history questions. The use of follow-up questions to assess responses and guide the reaction of health care providers to their final interpretation must be specified. Mandating the currently available screening questionnaires creates more problems than does judiciously adding ECG to PPEs.

Acknowledgements

We acknowledge the scientific contribution and advice of Prof. Victor Froelicher, Dr Nathan Riding and Prof. Sanjay Sharma in the production of this chapter.

References

1 Asplund, C.A. and Asif, I.M. Cardiovascular preparticipation screening practices of college team physicians. *Clin J Sport Med* 2014; **24**: 275–9.

2 Corrado, D., Pelliccia, A., Bjornstad, H.H. et al. Cardiovascular pre-participation screening of young competitive athletes for prevention of sudden death: proposal for a common European protocol. Consensus Statement of the Study Group of Sport Cardiology of the Working Group of Cardiac Rehabilitation and Exercise Physiology and the Working Group of Myocardial and Pericardial Diseases of the European Society of Cardiology. *Eur Heart J* 2005; **26**: 516–24.

3 Maron, B.J., Thompson, P.D., Puffer, J.C. et al. Cardiovascular preparticipation screening of competitive athletes. A statement for health professionals from the Sudden Death Committee (clinical cardiology) and Congenital Cardiac Defects Committee (cardiovascular disease in the young), American Heart Association. *Circulation* 1996; **94**: 850–6.

4 Maron, B.J., Thompson, P.D., Ackerman, M.J. et al. Recommendations and considerations related to preparticipation screening for cardiovascular abnormalities in competitive athletes: 2007 update: a scientific statement from the American Heart Association Council on Nutrition, Physical Activity, and Metabolism: endorsed by the American College of Cardiology Foundation. *Circulation* 2007; **115**: 1643–55.

5 Maron, B.J., Friedman, R.A., Kligfield, P. et al. Assessment of the 12-lead ECG as a screening test for detection of cardiovascular disease in healthy general populations of young people (12–25 years of age): a scientific statement from the American Heart Association and the American College of Cardiology. *Circulation* 2014; **130**: 1303–34.

6 Fudge, J., Harmon, K.G., Owens, D.S. et al. Cardiovascular screening in adolescents and young adults: a prospective study comparing the Pre-Participation Physical Evaluation Monograph 4th Edition and ECG. *Br J Sports Med* 2014; **48**: 1172–8.

7 Price, D.E., McWilliams, A., Asif, I.M. Electrocardiography-inclusive screening strategies for detection of cardiovascular abnormalities in high school athletes. *Heart Rhythm* 2014; **11**: 442–9.

8 American Academy of Family Physicians, American Academy of Pediatrics, American College of Sports Medicine et al. *Preparticipation Physical Evaluation*, 4th edn. Elk Grove Village, IL: American Academy of Pediatrics, 2010.

9 Corrado, D., Basso, C., Pavei, A. et al. Trends in sudden cardiovascular death in young competitive athletes after implementation of a preparticipation screening program. *JAMA* 2006; **296**: 1593–601.

10 Bille, K., Figueiras, D., Schamasch, P. et al. Sudden cardiac death in athletes: the Lausanne Recommendations. *Eur J Cardiovasc Prev Rehabil* 2006; **13**: 859–75.

11 Ljungqvist, A., Jenoure, P., Engebretsen, L. et al. The International Olympic Committee (IOC) Consensus Statement on periodic health evaluation of elite athletes March 2009. *Br J Sports Med* 2009; **43**: 631–43.

12 Dvorak, J., Grimm, K., Schmied, C. and Junge, A. Development and implementation of a standardized precompetition medical assessment of international elite football players – 2006 FIFA World Cup Germany. *Clin J Sport Med* 2009; **19**: 316–21.

13 Wilson, M.G., Basavarajaiah, S., Whyte, G.P. et al. Efficacy of personal symptom and family history questionnaires when screening for inherited cardiac pathologies: the role of electrocardiography. *Br J Sports Med* 2008; **42**: 207–11.

14 Pickham, D., Zarafshar, S., Sani, D. et al. Comparison of three ECG criteria for athlete pre-participation screening. *J Electrocardiol* 2014; **47**: 769–74.

15 Wilson, M.G., Chatard, J.C., Carre, F. et al. Prevalence of electrocardiographic abnormalities in West-Asian and African male athletes. *Br J Sports Med* 2012; **46**: 341–7.

16 Asif, I.M., Yim, E.S., Hoffman, J.M. and Froelicher, V. Update: Causes and symptoms of sudden cardiac death in young athletes. *Phys Sportsmed* 2015; **43**: 44–53.

17 Ranthe, M.F., Winkel, B.G., Andersen, E.W. et al. Risk of cardiovascular disease in family members of young sudden cardiac death victims. *Eur Heart J* 2013; **34**: 503–11.

18 Wong, L.C., Roses-Noguer, F., Till, J.A. and Behr, E.R. Cardiac evaluation of pediatric relatives in sudden arrhythmic death syndrome: a 2-center experience. *Circ Arrhythm Electrophysiol* 2014; **7**: 800–6.

19 Harmon, K.G., Zigman, M. and Drezner, J.A. The effectiveness of screening history, physical exam, and ECG to detect potentially lethal cardiac disorders in athletes: a systematic review/meta-analysis. *J Electrocardiol* 2015; **48**: 329–38.

10 Normal Electrocardiographic Findings in Athletes

Mathew G. Wilson[1–3] and Victoria Watt[1]

[1]Department of Sports Medicine, ASPETAR, Qatar Orthopaedic and Sports Medicine Hospital, Doha, Qatar
[2]Research Institute of Sport and Exercise Sciences, Liverpool John Moores University, Liverpool, UK
[3]Research Institute of Sport and Exercise Sciences, University of Canberra, Canberra, ACT, Australia

Introduction

The purpose of pre-participation screening is to identify pre-existing cardiovascular abnormalities, and thereby reduce the potential for adverse cardiac events and loss of life. Many pre-participation screening programmes include a resting 12-lead electrocardiogram (ECG). The concerns for physicians when interpreting an athlete's ECG include both missing a dangerous cardiac condition and generating false-positive interpretations, causing unnecessary investigations and potential restriction of sporting activity. This chapter focuses on the physiological ECG adaptations commonly found in athletes to help guide physicians when distinguishing between normal ECG adaptations and abnormal ECG findings associated with pathological cardiac conditions.

Normal ECG Findings in Athletes

Sustained, regular and intensive exercise (≥ 6 hours per week) is associated with a number of ECG changes that reflect increased vagal tone and enlarged cardiac chamber size. These ECG findings in athletes are considered to reflect physiological adaptations to regular exercise and do not require further evaluation (Table 10.1).

Sinus Bradycardia

Three criteria must be met to diagnose sinus rhythm: (i) there must be a P-wave before every QRS complex; (ii) there must be a QRS complex after every P-wave; and (iii) the P-wave must have a normal axis in the frontal plane (0–90°). In normal sinus rhythm, the heart rate is determined by the balance between the sympathetic and parasympathetic nervous systems. In healthy adults, sinus rhythm ≤ 60 beats.min^{-1} is considered 'sinus bradycardia'. In athletes, resting sinus bradycardia is a common finding due to increased vagal tone; it is particularly prevalent in endurance athletes. In the absence of symptoms such as fatigue, dizziness or syncope, a heart rate ≥ 30 beats.min^{-1} should be considered normal in a well-trained athlete. Sinus bradycardia should disappear with the onset of physical activity.

Sinus Arrhythmia

Heart rate usually increases slightly during inspiration and decreases slightly during expiration. This normal, physiological fluctuation in heart rate, termed 'sinus arrhythmia', can be exaggerated in athletes, resulting in an irregular heart rate. This is considered a normal finding and should not be confused with sinus node dysfunction ('sick sinus syndrome'). Differentiating features that suggest sinus node dysfunction include

IOC Manual of Sports Cardiology, First Edition. Edited by Mathew G. Wilson, Jonathan A. Drezner and Sanjay Sharma.
© 2017 International Olympic Committee. Published 2017 by John Wiley & Sons, Ltd.

1 Sinus bradycardia (≥30 beats.min⁻¹)

2 Sinus arrhythmia

3 Ectopic atrial rhythm

4 Junctional escape rhythm

5 First-degree AV block (PR interval >200 ms)

6 Mobitz type I (Wenckebach) second-degree AV block

7 Incomplete RBBB

8 QRS voltage criteria for LVH and RVH

9 Early repolarisation (ST elevation, J-point elevation, J-waves or terminal QRS slurring)

10 Convex ('domed') ST segment elevation combined with T-wave inversion in leads V1–V4 in black/African athletes

11 T-wave inversion in V1–V3 in young adolescent athletes (<16 years old)

Table 10.1 Normal ECG findings in athletes

AV, atrioventricular; RBBB, right bundle branch block; LVH, left ventricular hypertrophy; RVH, right ventricular hypertrophy

lack of rhythmic changes in the heart rate, abrupt sustained rate increases and decreases, prolonged pauses or periods of sinus arrest, inappropriate rate responses to exercise (including slowed acceleration and an inappropriately rapid deceleration) and any association with clinical symptoms such as exercise intolerance, pre-syncope or syncope. In sinus arrhythmia, the P-wave axis remains normal in the frontal plane and the fluctuation in heart rate should resolve with the onset of exercise.

Junctional Escape Rhythm

A junctional escape (or nodal) rhythm occurs when the QRS rate is faster than the resting P-wave or sinus rate, which is typically slower in athletes due to increased vagal tone (Figure 10.1). The QRS rate for junctional rhythms is usually less than 100 beats.min⁻¹, and the QRS complex is narrow (<120 ms) unless the baseline QRS has a bundle branch block. Sinus rhythm should resume with the onset of physical activity.

Ectopic Atrial Rhythm

In an ectopic atrial rhythm, P-waves are present but have a different morphology to the sinus P-wave, typically with a rate ≤100 beats.min⁻¹. Ectopic P-waves are most easily seen when they are negative in the inferior leads (II, III and aVF). Occasionally, two different P-wave morphologies may be seen; this is known as a 'wandering atrial pacemaker'. Ectopic atrial rhythms occur due to a slowed resting sinus rate caused by increased vagal tone in athletes. Sinus rhythm should resume with the onset of physical activity.

First-Degree Atrioventricular Block

In first-degree atrioventricular (AV) block, the PR interval is prolonged (>200 ms) but each P-wave is followed by a QRS complex and the R–R interval is regular (Figure 10.2). This represents a delay in AV nodal conduction in athletes, due to increased vagal activity or intrinsic AV node changes, and typically resolves with the onset of exercise.

Second-Degree Atrioventricular Block (Mobitz Type I/ Wenckebach Phenomenon)

In Mobitz type I second-degree AV block, the PR interval progressively lengthens from beat to beat until there is a nonconducted P-wave with no QRS complex (Figure 10.3). The first PR interval after the dropped beat is shorter than the last conducted PR interval *before* the dropped beat. This represents a greater disturbance of AV nodal conduction than first-degree AV block, but is usually a normal finding in asymptomatic, well-trained athletes. One-to-one conduction should return with the onset of exercise.

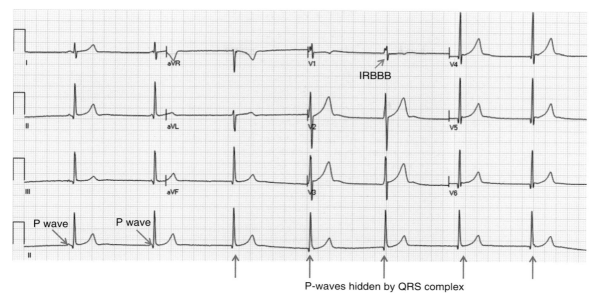

Figure 10.1 A 28-year-old asymptomatic Caucasian handball player demonstrating a junctional escape rhythm and incomplete right bundle branch block (IRBBB)

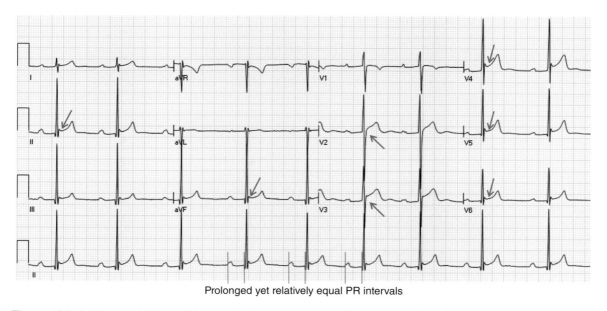

Prolonged yet relatively equal PR intervals

Figure 10.2 A 29-year-old black African football player demonstrating sinus bradycardia (57 beats.min⁻¹), marked first-degree AV block (309 ms) and early repolarisation (arrows) in leads II, aVF, V2–V6

Incomplete Right Bundle Branch Block

Incomplete right bundle branch block (IRBBB) presents with a QRS duration ≤120 ms with a right bundle branch block (RBBB) pattern: terminal R-wave in lead V1 (rsR′) and wide terminal S-wave in leads I and V6 (Figure 10.4A). This may be observed in up to 60% of athletes [1]. It has been suggested that the mildly delayed conduction is caused by right ventricular remodelling (with increased cavity size and resultant increased conduction time), rather than an intrinsic delay within the His–Purkinje system itself [2].

Isolated IRBBB in an asymptomatic athlete with a negative family history and normal physical examination does not require further evaluation. However, physicians should be aware of three key points.

97

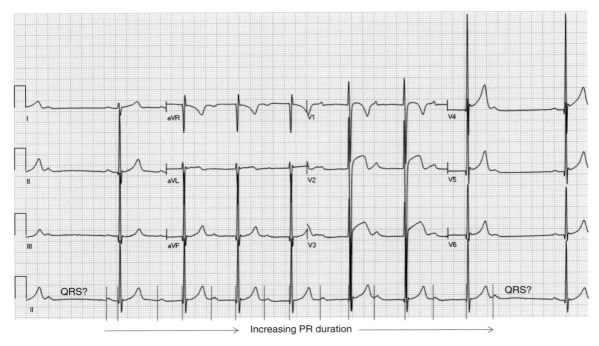

Increasing PR duration

Figure 10.3 A 17-year-old asymptomatic black African basketball player demonstrating Mobitz type I second-degree AV block, early repolarisation in V2–V5 and voltage criteria for left ventricular hypertrophy (LVH)

First, IRBBB can be associated with atrial septal defects (ASDs), and thus other ECG changes suggestive of ASDs should be excluded (such as right- or leftward axis, voltage criteria for right ventricular hypertrophy (RVH), right atrial hypertrophy, inverted P-waves in the inferior leads and first-degree AV block). Some of these ECG changes are common in well-trained athletes, so physical examination may provide further information. Whilst normal cardiac auscultation does not exclude a haemodynamically significant ASD, there are a number of clinical signs that may be apparent, including fixed splitting of the second heart sound, a systolic ejection murmur over the pulmonary valve and a right ventricular heave with a loud pulmonary component of the second heart sound, if there is concomitant pulmonary hypertension [3].

Second, IRBBB may be seen in patients with arrhythmogenic right ventricular cardiomyopathy (ARVC) [4]. However, in ARVC, other ECG abnormalities may be present, such as T-wave inversion involving the right precordial leads beyond V2 in individuals over 14 years old, low limb lead voltages, prolonged S-wave upstroke, localised prolongation of the QRS complex (>110 ms) in leads V1–V3, epsilon waves (reproducible low-amplitude signals at the end of the QRS complex) and premature ventricular beats with a left bundle branch block (LBBB) morphology (Figure 10.4B) [5].

Third, IRBBB should not be confused with Brugada syndrome (Figure 10.4C), which is characterised by marked J-point elevation (high take-off ≥2 mm), followed by a coved (type I Brugada) and downsloping ST segment with a negative T-wave in one or more leads in V1–V3 [6]. These ECG changes reflect the underlying repolarisation abnormalities found in Brugada syndrome, rather than delayed right ventricular activation, which manifests as isolated IRBBB.

Early Repolarisation

Early repolarisation is a common finding in trained athletes and is considered a benign ECG pattern in apparently healthy, asymptomatic individuals. Until recently, early repolarisation was simply referred to as 'ST elevation', but updated definitions include J-waves or terminal QRS slurring, with and without ST-segment elevation [7]. Early repolarisation is most common in the precordial leads but can be present in any lead, and is found in up to 88% of high-level athletes [8]. See Chapter 13 for an extensive review (and illustrative ECGs) of early repolarisation in athletes. To date, no data support the association between early repolarisation and sudden cardiac death (SCD) in athletes. Accordingly, all patterns of early repolarisation, including inferolateral subtypes, should be considered normal variants in athletes.

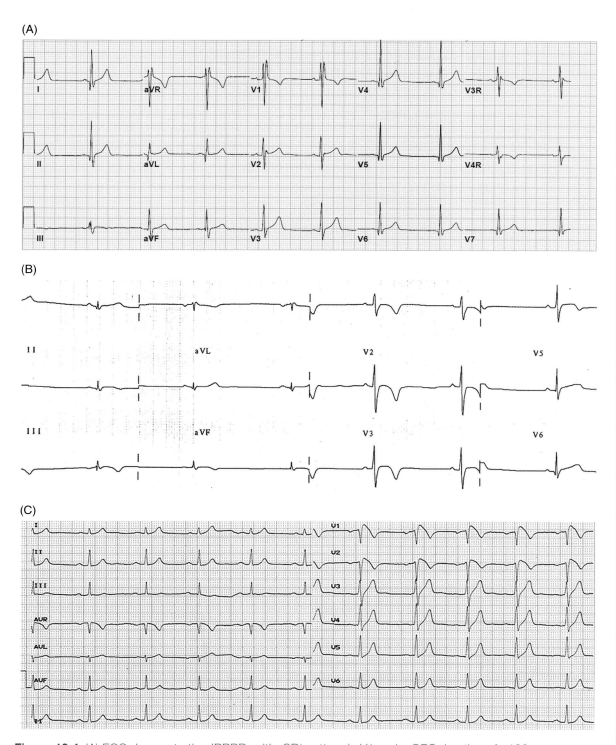

Figure 10.4 (A) ECG demonstrating IRBBB, with rSR′ pattern in V1 and a QRS duration of <120 ms. (B) ECG of a patient with arrhythmogenic right ventricular cardiomyopathy (ARVC) showing inverted T-waves in V1–V4, low limb lead voltages and delayed S-wave upstroke. (C) ECG demonstrating a typical type 1 Brugada pattern

QRS Voltage Criteria for Left Ventricular Hypertrophy

In athletes, intensive conditioning leads to cardiac remodelling, with increased cavity dimensions and wall thicknesses. These structural changes can be reflected on the ECG as an increase in QRS amplitude [9]. The most commonly used voltage criteria for left ventricular hypertrophy (LVH) is the Sokolow–Lyon index (S-V1 + R-V5 > 35 mm), but it is well known that QRS voltage is not a reliable predictor of LVH on echocardiography or cardiac magnetic resonance imaging [10], and >50% of well-trained athletes meet voltage criteria for LVH on ECG [8]. QRS voltage is influenced by a number of factors, including body habitus, age, left ventricular size and left ventricular mass. Males, athletes and black/African individuals typically have higher QRS voltage, while obesity, older age and pulmonary disease may be associated with lower QRS voltage [11].

In patients with hypertrophic cardiomyopathy (HCM), isolated increased QRS voltage is uncommon, being seen in around 2% of cases [12]. However, HCM and other causes of pathological LVH are often associated with a number of other ECG abnormalities, such as T-wave inversion, ST depression and pathological Q-waves. Accordingly, isolated increased QRS voltage in an asymptomatic athlete with a negative family history *in the absence of other ECG abnormalities* is not a reliable indicator of LVH or HCM and thus does not require further evaluation. See Chapters 11 and 19 for further information on the ECG abnormalities found in HCM.

Repolarisation Findings in Relation to Age and Ethnicity

An athlete's age and ethnicity have a significant impact upon their cardiovascular remodelling response to physical activity (see Chapter 5). It is now recognised that there are specific repolarisation patterns in young adolescents and, specifically, in black/African athletes that are normal variants and should be distinguished from abnormal findings suggestive of a pathologic cardiac disorder [13].

T-wave inversion is commonly observed in young adolescent athletes <16 years of age. These repolarisation changes are often called the 'juvenile' ECG pattern, which is characterised by T-wave inversion in leads V1–V3. This repolarisation pattern reflects right ventricular dominance and a posteriorly directed repolarisation polarity in young children. With increasing age, the dominance transfers from right to left, with a resultant reversal of repolarisation polarity, which may be observed on the ECG. Eventually, after puberty, the adult ECG pattern is observed, with T-wave inversion limited to V1. Accordingly, T-wave inversion in V1–V3 in an asymptomatic athlete <16 years of age without a family history of SCD does not require further testing.

As mentioned previously, early repolarisation is common in athletes and is usually characterised by an elevated ST segment with upward concavity, ending in a positive (upright 'peaked') T-wave. However, there is also a normal variant of early repolarisation observed in up to 23% of black/African athletes, characterised by an elevated ST segment with upward convexity ('dome–shaped'), followed by a negative T-wave confined to leads V1–V4 (Figure 10.5) [14]. The presence of either the common or the variant repolarisation pattern in asymptomatic black/African athletes with a negative family history does not require additional testing. It should be noted, however, that T-wave inversion in the lateral leads (V5–V6) is always considered abnormal and requires additional testing to rule out HCM or other cardiomyopathies [15].

Repolarisation variants in black/African athletes must also be distinguished from pathological repolarisation changes in the anterior precordial leads found in ARVC and Brugada-pattern ECGs. In ARVC, the ST segment is usually isoelectric prior to T-wave inversion (Figure 10.4B), in contrast to the 'domed' ST-segment elevation which is the hallmark feature of the normal repolarisation variant in black/African athletes (Figure 10.5). In Brugada-pattern ECGs, the marked J-point elevation and downsloping ST segment prior to T-wave inversion (Figure 10.4C) distinguishes this from the 'domed' ST segment elevation preceding the negative T-wave in black/African athletes. All pathological repolarisation changes in the anterior precordial leads suggesting either ARVC or possible Brugada syndrome require additional testing.

Criteria for Interpretation of the Athletes' ECGs

In 2010, the European Society of Cardiology (ESC) produced 'revised' recommendations for the interpretation of ECGs of athletes [16]. This was in response to an increasing number of sports governing bodies undertaking pre-participation cardiovascular screening and producing an unacceptably high yield of false-positive reports, arising from misinterpretation of physiological ECG changes commonly observed

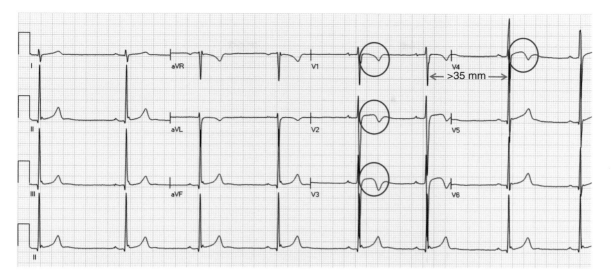

Figure 10.5 A 17-year-old asymptomatic black/African football player demonstrating 'domed' ST elevation followed by T-wave inversion in leads V1–V4 (circles) and voltage criteria for LVH

in athletes. To demonstrate improved specificity, the authors reanalysed the ECGs of 1005 highly trained athletes reported a decade earlier [17]. Originally, 40% (402) presented an abnormal ECG (so called 'group 2' changes). This was lowered to 11% using the 2010 ESC recommendations. However, it has since been demonstrated that certain black ethnic populations, such as African, Afro-Caribbean and black Latin American, continue to demonstrate a high prevalence of abnormal ECGs (~20–40%) when using the 2010 ESC recommendations [1,8,18].

To address this issue, in 2012, an international team of experts produced the 'Seattle Criteria' [19]: a revision of ECG interpretation guidelines for athletes, aimed at providing greater accuracy in identifying those with cardiac pathology, whilst also attempting to reduce the false-positive rate. The Seattle Criteria have demonstrated favourable results compared to the ESC recommendations, reducing the number of ECGs previously considered abnormal (from 17 to 4%) in a population of high-level athletes, whilst still identifying all athletes with cardiac pathology [20].

Recently, however, additional 'Refined Criteria' for the interpretation of athletes' ECGs have been published [21]. These Refined Criteria were produced following an analysis of data derived from an interpretation of the ECGs of over 5000 athletes utilising both the ESC recommendations and the Seattle Criteria. Sheikh et al. [21] demonstrated that the ECG patterns of isolated atrial enlargement (left and right), axis deviation (left and right) and RVH, found in both the ESC recommendations and the Seattle Criteria, provided an extremely low diagnostic yield for cardiac pathology. A unique feature of this investigation was a validation assessment in 103 young athletes with confirmed HCM, whereby the Refined Criteria identified 98.1% of HCM cases.

The Refined Criteria differ from the ESC recommendations and the Seattle Criteria in that asymptomatic athletes without a family history of SCD do not receive further cardiovascular evaluation when presenting with the following recognised training-related ECG changes *in isolation*: (i) left atrial enlargement (LAE); (ii) right atrial enlargement (RAE); (iii) left axis deviation (LAD); (iv) right axis deviation (RAD); and (v) Sokolow–Lyon voltage criteria for RVH. In line with the Seattle Criteria, a corrected QT interval (QTc, corrected by Bazett's formula) of ≤470 ms in male and ≤480 ms in female athletes is considered normal. In addition, T-wave inversion preceded by convex ST-segment elevation in leads V1–V4 *in asymptomatic black athletes only* does not require further investigation. However, importantly, the presence of *two or more* of ECG patterns (i)–(v) *does* warrant secondary investigation (Figure 10.6).

It is worth noting that the Refined Criteria are not an evolution of the 2012 Seattle Criteria, but use ECG parameters from both the 2010 ESC recommendations and the Seattle Criteria. To date, only one other group has utilised these new Refined Criteria. Riding et al. [22] observed that the Refined Criteria reduced the prevalence of an abnormal ECG to just 5.3% (p < 0.0001), from 11.6% when using the Seattle Criteria and from 22.3% when using the 2010 ESC recommendations. Further, specificity was significantly improved

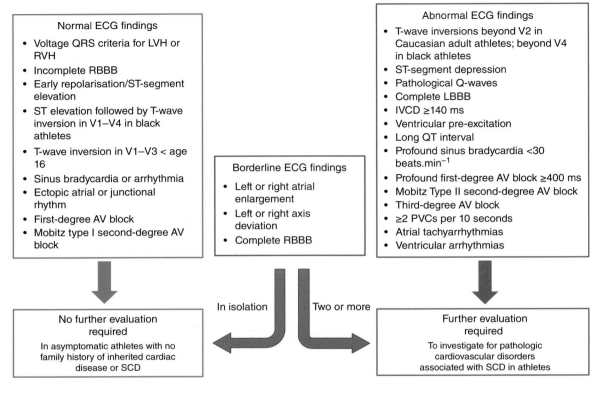

Figure 10.6 Definition of an abnormal ECG using the Refined Criteria. AV, atrioventricular; RBBB, right bundle branch block; LVH, left ventricular hypertrophy; LBBB, left bundle branch block; IVCD, intraventricular conduction delay; SCD, sudden cardiac death

to 94% across all athlete ethnicities (Arabic, black African and Caucasian; p < 0.0001) (compared to 87.5% with the Seattle Criteria and 76.6% with the ESC recommendations). Importantly, 100% sensitivity for serious cardiac pathologies was maintained. It is hoped that the Refined Criteria will be adopted for widespread use in the interpretation of athletes' ECGs in coming years.

Conclusion

An increasing number of sports governing bodies are adopting ECG screening as part of the pre-participation assessment of athletes, and ECG screening is recommended by the current ESC, Fédération Internationale de Football Association (FIFA) and International Olympic Committee (IOC) guidelines. A well-trained athlete will undergo structural cardiac remodelling, and this is apparent on the resting 12-lead ECG. It is thus essential that the ECG is interpreted correctly, in the context of the athlete's age, ethnicity and level of fitness. The ECG can provide valuable information when interpreted properly, accounting for the electrical and structural changes that are a common result of regular training. A false-positive report can be just as devastating to the athlete as confirmation of significant cardiac pathology, with both leading to further investigations and potential restriction of sporting activity – unnecessary in the former case, essential in the latter. Therefore, ECG findings related to athletic adaptation must be distinguished from changes suggestive of an underlying pathological disorder. This is critical in the evaluation of athletes, both to avoid a false-positive result and to identify athletes at risk of SCD.

References

1 Wilson, M.G., Chatard, J.C., Carre, F. et al. Prevalence of electrocardiographic abnormalities in West-Asian and African male athletes. *Br J Sports Med* 2012; **46**: 341–7.
2 Langdeau, J.B., Blier, L., Turcotte, H. et al. Electrocardiographic findings in athletes: the prevalence of left ventricular hypertrophy and conduction defects. *Can J Cardiol* 2001; **17**: 655–9.

3 Webb, G. and Gatzoulis, M.A. Atrial septal defects in the adult. Recent progress and overview. *Circulation* 2006; **114**: 1645–53.

4 Corrado, D., Basso, C. and Thiene, G. Arrhythmogenic right ventricular cardiomyopathy: diagnosis, prognosis, and treatment. *Heart* 2000; **83**: 588–95.

5 Marcus, F.I., McKenna, W.J., Sherrill, D. et al. Diagnosis of arrhythmogenic right ventricular cardiomyopathy/dysplasia. Proposed modification of the task force criteria. *Circulation* 2010; **121**: 1533–41.

6 Bayés de Luna, A., Brugada. J., Baranchuk, A. et al. Current electrocardiographic criteria for diagnosis of Brugada pattern: a consensus report. *J Electrocard* 2012; **45**: 433–42.

7 Perez, M.V., Friday, K. and Froelicher, V. Semantic confusion: the case of early repolarization and the J point. *Am J Med* 2012; **125**: 843–4.

8 Riding, N.R., Salah, O., Sharma, S. et al. ECG and morphologic adaptations in Arabic athletes: are the European Society of Cardiology's recommendations for the interpretation of the 12-lead ECG appropriate for this ethnicity? *Br J Sports Med* 2014; **48**: 1138–43.

9 Corrado, D., Biffi, A., Basso, C. et al. 12-lead ECG in the athlete: physiological versus pathological abnormalities. *Br J Sports Med* 2009; **43**: 669–76.

10 Sohaib, S.M., Payne, J.R., Shukla, R. et al. Electrocardiographic (ECG) criteria for determining left ventricular mass in young healthy men; data from the LARGE Heart study. *J Cardiovasc Magn Reson* 2009; **11**: 2.

11 Hancock, E.W., Deal, B.J., Mirvis, D.M. et al. AHA/ACCF/HRS recommendations for the standardization and interpretation of the electrocardiogram. Part V: Electrocardiogram changes associated with cardiac chamber hypertrophy: a scientific statement from the American Heart Association Electrocardiography and Arrhythmias Committee, Council on Clinical Cardiology; the American College of Cardiology Foundation; and the Heart Rhythm Society: endorsed by the International Society for Computerized Electrocardiology. *Circulation* 2009; **119**: e251–61.

12 Ryan, M.P., Cleland, J.G., French, J.A. et al. The standard electrocardiogram as a screening test for hypertrophic cardiomyopathy. *Am J Cardiol* 1995; **76**: 689–94.

13 Sheikh, N., Papadakis, M., Ghani, S. et al. Comparison of electrocardiographic criteria for the detection of cardiac abnormalities in elite black and white athletes. *Circulation* 2014; **129**: 1637–49.

14 Sheikh, N., Papadakis, M., Carre, F. et al. Cardiac adaptation to exercise in adolescent athletes of African ethnicity: an emergent elite athletic population. *Br J Sports Med* 2013; **47**: 585–92.

15 Schnell, F., Riding, N., O'Hanlon, R. et al. Recognition and significance of pathological T-wave inversions in athletes. *Circulation* 2015; **131**: 165–73.

16 Corrado, D., Pelliccia, A., Heidbuchel, H. et al. Recommendations for interpretation of 12-lead electrocardiogram in the athlete. *Eur Heart J* 2010; **31**: 243–59.

17 Pelliccia, A., Maron, B.J., Culasso, F. et al. Clinical significance of abnormal electrocardiographic patterns in trained athletes. *Circulation* 2000; **102**: 278–84.

18 Papadakis, M., Carre, F., Kervio, G. et al. The prevalence, distribution, and clinical outcomes of electrocardiographic repolarization patterns in male athletes of African/Afro-Caribbean origin. *Eur Heart J* 2011; **32**: 2304–13.

19 Drezner, J.A., Ackerman, M.J., Anderson, J. et al. Electrocardiographic interpretation in athletes: the 'Seattle Criteria'. *Br J Sports Med* 2013; **47**: 122–4.

20 Brosnan, M., La Gerche, A., Kalman, J. et al. The Seattle Criteria increase the specificity of preparticipation ECG screening among elite athletes. *Br J Sports Med* 2013; **48**: 1144–50.

21 Sheikh, N., Papadakis, M., Ghani, S. et al. Comparison of ECG criteria for the detection of cardiac abnormalities in elite black and white athletes. *Circulation* 2014; **129**: 1637–49.

22 Riding, N.R., Sheikh, N., Adamuz, C. et al. Comparison of three current sets of electrocardiographic interpretation criteria for use in screening athletes. *Heart* 2015; **101**: 384–90.

11 Abnormal Electrocardiographic Findings in Athletes: Recognising Changes Suggestive of Cardiomyopathy

Gherardo Finocchiaro and Michael Papadakis

Cardiovascular and Cell Sciences Research Centre, St George's University of London, London, UK

Introduction

Primary cardiomyopathies collectively account for the majority of sudden cardiac deaths (SCDs) in young athletes. They are often inherited, and sudden death during exercise may be the first manifestation of the disease. In an attempt to prevent such tragedies, many learned scientific and sporting organisations, including the International Olympic Committee (IOC), recommend pre-participation cardiovascular evaluation in athletes to detect quiescent myocardial disease. The screening modality of choice is the 12-lead electrocardiogram (ECG), as studies have demonstrated that the majority of individuals with cardiomyopathies, commonly implicated in SCD in young athletes, have an abnormal ECG. Up to 98% of patients with hypertrophic cardiomyopathy (HCM) and 80% of patients with arrhythmogenic right ventricular cardiomyopathy (ARVC) exhibit an abnormal ECG phenotype, which often predates the structural manifestations observed on imaging studies [1,2].

Fundamental to the interpretation of an athlete's ECG is a clear understanding of the ECG phenotypes that indicate an underlying cardiomyopathy and their differentiation from ECG changes related to cardiac adaptation due to regular exercise. In addition, ECG interpretation should be guided by the demographic characteristics of the athlete. It is well established that up to 40% of athletes of African/Afro-Caribbean (black) ethnicity exhibit ECG phenotypes that would be suggestive of cardiac disease in Caucasian (white) athletes [3,4]. Conversely, female athletes are less likely to exhibit ECG changes that overlap with cardiomyopathies compared to their male counterparts [5]. As such, ECG phenotypes that would be considered a normal variant in a male black athlete may be a cause of concern for female white athletes. In an attempt to aid physicians with the interpretation of an athlete's ECG, the European Society of Cardiology (ESC) and other learned groups have devised algorithms that attempt to differentiate benign (also referred to as type 1 or training-related) changes from those likely to indicate pathology (also referred to as type 2 or training-unrelated), which warrant comprehensive cardiac evaluation [6–8].

This chapter provides an up-to-date review of the ECG findings suggestive of cardiomyopathy in athletes, and where appropriate offers a comparison with current recommendations. In addition, it provides a practical algorithm for the investigation of ECG abnormalities (Figure 11.1).

IOC Manual of Sports Cardiology, First Edition. Edited by Mathew G. Wilson, Jonathan A. Drezner and Sanjay Sharma.
© 2017 International Olympic Committee. Published 2017 by John Wiley & Sons, Ltd.

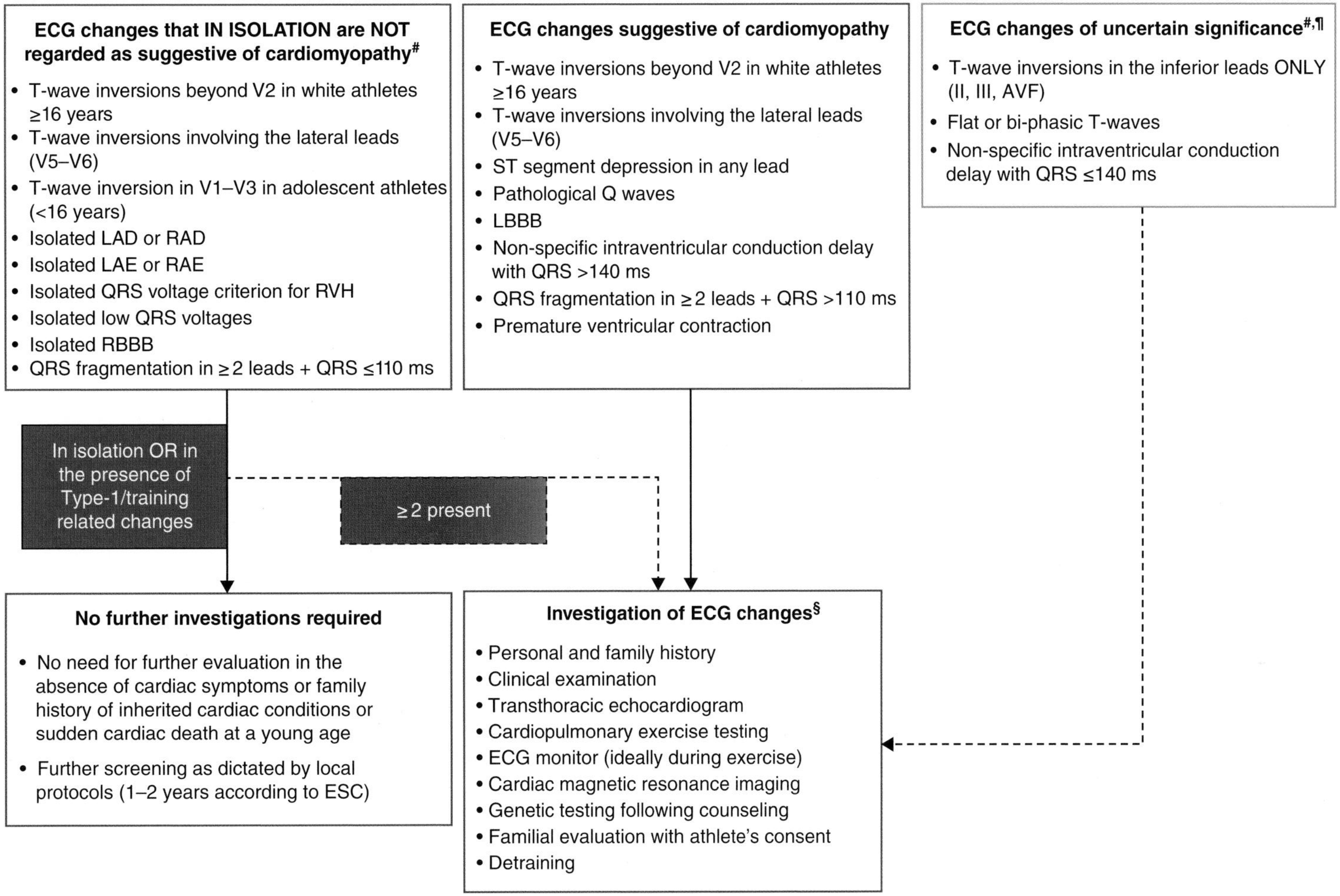

ECG changes that IN ISOLATION are NOT regarded as suggestive of cardiomyopathy[#]

- T-wave inversions beyond V2 in white athletes ≥16 years
- T-wave inversions involving the lateral leads (V5–V6)
- T-wave inversion in V1–V3 in adolescent athletes (<16 years)
- Isolated LAD or RAD
- Isolated LAE or RAE
- Isolated QRS voltage criterion for RVH
- Isolated low QRS voltages
- Isolated RBBB
- QRS fragmentation in ≥2 leads + QRS ≤110 ms

ECG changes suggestive of cardiomyopathy

- T-wave inversions beyond V2 in white athletes ≥16 years
- T-wave inversions involving the lateral leads (V5–V6)
- ST segment depression in any lead
- Pathological Q waves
- LBBB
- Non-specific intraventricular conduction delay with QRS >140 ms
- QRS fragmentation in ≥2 leads + QRS >110 ms
- Premature ventricular contraction

ECG changes of uncertain significance[#,¶]

- T-wave inversions in the inferior leads ONLY (II, III, AVF)
- Flat or bi-phasic T-waves
- Non-specific intraventricular conduction delay with QRS ≤140 ms

In isolation OR in the presence of Type-1/training related changes

≥2 present

No further investigations required

- No need for further evaluation in the absence of cardiac symptoms or family history of inherited cardiac conditions or sudden cardiac death at a young age
- Further screening as dictated by local protocols (1–2 years according to ESC)

Investigation of ECG changes[§]

- Personal and family history
- Clinical examination
- Transthoracic echocardiogram
- Cardiopulmonary exercise testing
- ECG monitor (ideally during exercise)
- Cardiac magnetic resonance imaging
- Genetic testing following counseling
- Familial evaluation with athlete's consent
- Detraining

Figure 11.1 Flow chart of ECG changes related to cardiomyopathy. *Preceded by J-point elevation and convex ST-segment elevation. [+]'Juvenile' ECG pattern. [§]The complement and order of investigations may differ depending on clinical suspicion, local expertise and availability. Most ECG phenotypes suggestive of cardiomyopathy will require further follow-up even if initial evaluation is negative. [¶]May warrant further investigation until further data become available. [#]In the absence of clinical or other ECG features suggestive of cardiomyopathy.

T-Wave Inversion

Not all T-wave inversion is pathological. All individuals, irrespective of athletic activity, are allowed T-wave inversion in leads III, AVR and V1. T-wave inversion, however, is the most common ECG feature of primary myocardial disease, with certain patterns being indicative of specific conditions. T-wave inversion is seen in 55–85% of patients with ARVC, commonly affecting the anterior leads, extending beyond V1 and up to V4 [2]. Similarly, up to 85% of patients with HCM demonstrate T-wave inversion on their ECG, but in contrast to ARVC, it is predominantly the inferolateral leads that are affected, with only a minority (4%) of patients exhibiting isolated T-wave inversion in the anterior leads [3].

Anterior T-Wave Inversion in Athletes

Anterior T-wave inversion is a normal variant in children. As the child goes through puberty, the anterior T-wave inversions gradually resolve and eventually disappear. The term 'juvenile ECG pattern' is widely used – in the absence of symptoms, signs or family history of cardiac disease – to denote T-wave inversion beyond lead V2 in adolescents who have not reached physical maturity. The juvenile pattern is present in 10–15% of white athletes aged 12 years, but only in 2.5% of white athletes aged 14–15 years (Figures 11.2A,B) [9,10]. Anterior T-wave inversion that extends beyond lead V2 is extremely rare (0.1%) in white athletes aged >15 years (or in younger athletes who have completed puberty, when formal assessment by a paediatrician is feasible) and should raise suspicion of ARVC [9,10]. T-wave inversion confined to V1–V2 may be present in up to 2% of adolescent white athletes and is only a minor diagnostic criterion for ARVC. The need for further evaluation of such athletes is a matter of some controversy, and the wider consensus in the scientific community is that in the absence of symptoms or a family history of concern, further evaluation is not required.

Anterior T-wave inversion may also be an ECG marker of physiological adaptation to exercise. T-wave inversion in leads V1–V4 preceded by J-point elevation and convex ST-segment elevation is considered part

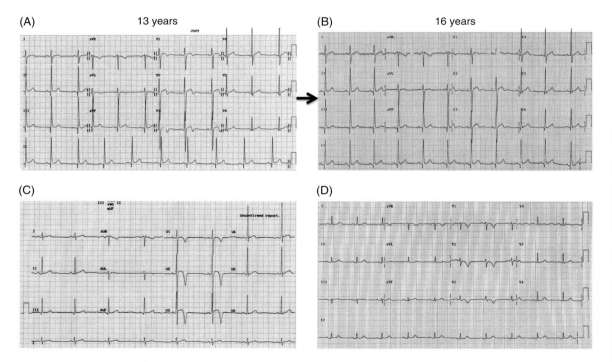

Figure 11.2 ECG examples of anterior T-wave inversion. (A) Adolescent athlete demonstrating the 'juvenile' ECG pattern, with anterior T-wave inversion up to V3. (B) Regression of T-wave inversion to V1 by the age of 16 years (post-puberty). (C) Anterior, deep T-wave inversion in a black marathon runner, preceded by J-point elevation and convex ST-segment elevation. (D) A patient with ARVC and anterior T-wave inversion. Note the absence of J-point elevation and the isolelectric/mildly depressed ST segment preceding the T-wave inversion

of the 'black athlete's heart' and should not result in further investigations, in the absence of other clinical or ECG features of cardiomyopathy (Figures 11.2C). Papadakis et al. [3] demonstrated that up to 13% of male black athletes exhibit isolated T-wave inversion in leads V1–V4, commonly preceded by convex ST-segment elevation. None of these athletes showed symptoms or signs of cardiomyopathy despite comprehensive evaluation and a 5-year follow-up period. Similar findings have been described in female and adolescent black athletes. Anterior T-wave inversion preceded by an isoelectric or depressed ST segment in athletes ≥16 years is abnormal and requires investigation for ARVC (Figure 11.2D).

Lateral T-Wave Inversion in Athletes

Irrespective of the demographics of the athlete, there are certain T-wave inversion patterns that should always raise suspicion of underlying cardiomyopathy and prompt comprehensive evaluation. Even if pathology is not identified in the first instance, subsequent surveillance is prudent, with repeat evaluation annually, or sooner should the athlete become symptomatic. Such patterns include T-wave inversions that affect two or more lateral leads (I, aVL, V5, V6). In cases of cardiomyopathy, lateral T-wave inversions may commonly extend to the inferior territory (II, III, aVF), are deep (≥2 mm) and are frequently associated with ST-segment depression (Figure 11.3). Minor T-wave inversion (<2 mm) should also be treated with suspicion, as there is no compelling evidence to suggest that athletes with minor T-wave inversion in the lateral or inferolateral leads are at lower risk of harbouring a cardiomyopathy.

In a study of 12 550 athletes referred for pre-participation screening, Pelliccia et al. [11] followed 81 athletes with widespread deep T-wave inversions and initial normal echocardiographic studies for a period of 9 years. All five (6%) athletes who developed morphologically detectable cardiomyopathy during surveillance evaluations exhibited lateral T-wave inversion (3 HCM, 1 ARVC, 1 dilated cardiomyopathy (DCM)). Similarly, in a study of almost 3000 athletes (33% black) by Papadakis et al. [3], only 3 out of 1243 (0.2%) were ultimately diagnosed with HCM. All three athletes had deep inferolateral T-wave inversion. In the same study, the authors reported on ECG findings in a small cohort of HCM patients (n = 52). Of the 43 (83%) with pathological T-waves, 93% demonstrated T-wave inversion in the lateral leads. Finally, in a recent study by Schnell et al. [12], the authors performed a comprehensive evaluation of 155 asymptomatic athletes who exhibited deep T-wave inversion in two or more leads. Of the 155 athletes, 137 (88%) exhibited deep T-wave inversion affecting the lateral leads, commonly (n = 100; 65%) present in the inferolateral territories (II, III, aVF, V5, V6). The high prevalence of lateral T-wave inversion was associated with a high diagnostic yield of

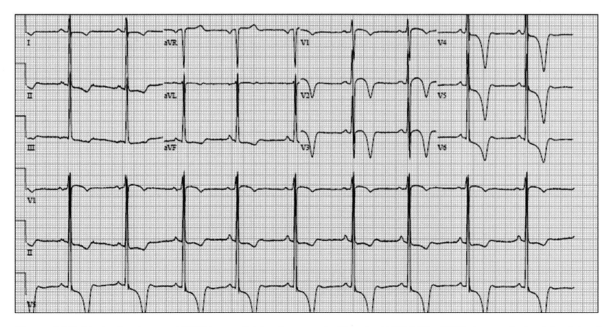

Figure 11.3 Markedly abnormal ECG in an athlete diagnosed with apical HCM. The ECG demonstrates inferolateral T-wave inversion with deep T-wave inversion and ST segment depression in V4–V6

cardiomyopathies (41%), with HCM being the predominant diagnosis. Cardiac magnetic resonance imaging (CMRI) emerged as the investigation of choice, as it identified almost 90% of athletes with myocardial disease and assigned a diagnosis in 24 athletes in whom the transthoracic echocardiogram was reported as 'suspicious' (n = 10) or normal (n = 14).

Inferior T-Wave Inversion in Athletes

The exact significance of inferior T-wave inversion, when present in isolation, remains uncertain. Inferior T-wave inversion has been reported in up to 6% of healthy black athletes and 2% of white athletes but is also occasionally observed in individuals with cardiomyopathy. It would be reasonable to consider this pattern abnormal until more data are available.

Flat or Biphasic T-Waves in Athletes

There are no data relating to the significance of flat or biphasic T-waves. As with T-wave inversion, most physicians would recommend further evaluation of biphasic T-waves where the negative portion is >1 mm in depth in two or more leads.

ST-Segment Depression

Assessment of the ST segment requires a good-quality ECG to accurately determine the isoelectric line. The isoelectric line, also known as the 'base line', is best determined by the line between the end of the T-wave and the beginning of the P-wave. ST-segment depression is a common finding in cardiomyopathies, especially HCM, and is present in up to 50% of patients [3]. Studies indicate that the presence of ST-segment depression on the resting ECG of HCM patients predicts exercise-induced subendocardial ischemia. In addition, when present in lateral leads I and AVL, ST-segment depression seems to confer increased risk of SCD [13]. On the other hand, ST-segment depression is extremely rare (<0.5%) in healthy athletes, and thus always warrants further investigation and follow-up.

Pathological Q-Waves

Q-waves are a normal component of the ECG. There is lack of consensus regarding the definition of a pathological Q-wave, and the existence of multiple diagnostic criteria is a source of confusion. This issue is important, since the presence of pathological Q-waves always warrants further evaluation and follow-up of the athlete to look for potential cardiomyopathy. Most existing criteria examine the depth and duration of the Q-waves and require their presence in two or more contiguous leads, excluding aVR. A Q-wave duration of ≥40 ms and an absolute depth of >3 mm are considered pathological criteria by some, whereas others recommend a Q-wave amplitude ≥25% of the ensuing R-wave. Utilising different combinations of these criteria, scientific panels have devised a number of definitions. The World Health Organization (WHO) defines pathological Q-waves as those with a duration ≥40 ms and an amplitude ≥25% of the ensuing R-wave in two contiguous leads. The Seattle Criteria define pathological Q-waves in athletes as those >40 ms in duration or >3 mm in depth in two or more leads, excluding leads III and aVR [7]. The Seattle criterion is supported by the results of a study by Konno et al. [14], who tested a number of different criteria in 148 HCM patients and reported the Seattle definition as having the highest sensitivity (69%) and specificity (90%). However, a recent study comparing athletes and patients with HCM demonstrated that a revised Q-wave definition of ≥40 ms or a Q/R ratio of ≥0.25 in two contiguous leads reduced the false-positive rate without compromising the sensitivity [4].

Voltage Criterion for Left Ventricular Hypertrophy

The ECG of trained athletes often exhibits the isolated voltage criterion for left ventricular hypertrophy (LVH) (e.g. the Sokolow–Lyon or the Cornell criterion). Although such a criterion is considered by convention to reflect physiological left ventricular remodelling, it correlates poorly with left ventricular mass in young athletes. Conversely, the presence of isolated QRS voltage criterion for LVH is unusual (1.9%) in

HCM patients, in whom pathological LVH is commonly associated with additional ECG features, including T-wave inversion, ST-segment depression, pathological Q-waves, left atrial enlargement (LAE), left axis deviation (LAD) and delayed intrinsicoid deflection [1]. As such, the presence of high QRS voltages in the absence of other ECG or clinical markers suggestive of pathology is considered part of the normal and training-related ECG changes in athletes and should not prompt referral for further evaluation [6,7].

Voltage Criterion for Right Ventricular Hypertrophy

As with the voltage criterion for LVH, the voltage criterion for right ventricular hypertrophy (RVH) is fairly common in athletes. A study by Zaidi et al. [15] identified the Sokolow–Lyon (R in [V1] + S in [V5 or V6] >1.05 mV) voltage criterion for RVH in 12% of young athletes but only 6% of a control sedentary population. The same study identified a poor correlation between the presence of ECG criteria for RVH and increased right ventricular wall thickness on echocardiography, with ECG criteria having a positive predictive value (PPV) between 0 and 11% for the detection of echocardiographic RVH. Most importantly, however, the authors reviewed the ECGs of 68 patients with ARVC and demonstrated that none exhibited QRS voltages for RVH in isolation [15]. Based on these considerations, it is reasonable to conclude that isolated QRS-voltage for RVH represents part of the normal spectrum of physiological cardiac adaptations to exercise, and that in the absence of other ECG or clinical markers of pathology it does not require referral of the athlete for further evaluation.

Intraventricular Conduction Abnormalities and QRS Fragmentation

Left Bundle Branch Block

The prevalence of left bundle branch block (LBBB) in apparently asymptomatic, predominantly middle-aged individuals ranges from 0.1 to 0.8%. It is even less common in young, healthy athletes. However, LBBB is commonly observed in cardiomyopathies, particularly DCM, and it has important prognostic implications. In a large series of 608 patients with DCM, LBBB was present in one-third of the cohort (31%) at baseline ECG. Another 11.2% of the same cohort developed LBBB during follow-up, and new-onset LBBB was a predictor of all-cause mortality [16]. Isolated LBBB is also occasionally (2%) observed in HCM [1]. Based on the results of existing literature, all individuals with LBBB should be investigated comprehensively, and even if no cardiovascular pathology is identified in the first instance, they should be followed up on a long-term basis. A recent study by Mahmod et al. [17] reinforced the value of CMRI in such patients. The authors reported on 54 asymptomatic patients with LBBB referred for CMRI. Of the 25 patients who had an abnormal echo, CMRI confirmed the diagnosis in 19 (76%) and provided clinically relevant additional information in 13 (52%), including the diagnosis of cardiac sarcoid. In the 29 patients with normal echocardiograms, CMRI detected subclinical cardiomyopathy in one-third, including DCM, LVH and one case of Ebstein anomaly.

Right Bundle Branch Block

The right bundle branch block (RBBB) morphology is characterised by an rSR′ pattern in lead V1 and a qRS pattern in lead V6. When the RBBB pattern is associated with a QRS duration of ≥120 ms, it is termed 'complete RBBB', whereas a QRS duration <120 ms is termed 'incomplete' or 'partial' RBBB. Incomplete RBBB is a fairly common ECG phenotype in both young athletes and sedentary individuals, and its presence, in isolation, does not correlate with cardiac pathology. Studies employ different definitions for incomplete RBBB, resulting in significant variation of its prevalence. Some studies define incomplete RBBB as any rSR′ pattern in lead V1, whilst others require evidence of QRS prolongation of between 100 and 120 ms. Utilising the first definition, the prevalence of incomplete RBBB in athletes ranges from 10 to 50%, compared to 5–10% in sedentary controls, depending on the demographics of the cohorts studied [3,9,18]. The latter definition leads to a reduction in the overall prevalence of incomplete RBBB to 5–10% in athletes and 2–5% in sedentary subjects [15].

Complete RBBB is present in up to 3% of athletic individuals, and its exact significance remains uncertain. In contrast to LBBB, the presence of RBBB in isolation does not appear to relate to cardiac pathology. Kim et al. [19] observed a positive correlation between increasing QRS duration in athletes with the RBBB pattern and increasing right ventricular size and left ventricular mass. Although long-term follow-up data are necessary, the authors concluded that both incomplete and complete RBBB may be ECG phenotypes of cardiac adaptation to exercise and that in the absence of other features suggestive of disease, they do not require further evaluation. Such features would include: cardiovascular symptoms; a family history of cardiac disease or SCD; fixed split of the second heart sound or murmur on auscultation, consistent with an ostium secundum atrial septal defect; anterior T-wave inversion extending beyond lead V2, LBBB morphology ventricular ectopy or epsilon waves suggestive of ARVC; and suspicion of the Brugada ECG phenotype.

Nonspecific Intraventricular Conduction Delay

Nonspecific intraventricular conduction delay is defined as a QRS duration of >110 ms without the specific patterns of LBBB or RBBB. Its exact significance is unknown, and it can be observed in both cardiomyopathies and healthy athletes. The ESC recommends further evaluation of all athletes with QRS prolongation, whilst the Seattle group places emphasis on athletes in whom the QRS duration is severely prolonged (>140 ms). Other specific features of note include localised prolongation of the QRS complex in the anterior leads, associated with epsilon waves and delayed S-wave upstroke, which can be a marker of ARVC [2].

QRS Fragmentation

Fragmentation of the QRS complex is defined as the presence of additional R-waves (R′) or the presence of notches in the R- or S-waves in two contiguous leads (Figure 11.4). The presence of a fragmented QRS is considered to represent distortion of signal conduction and of the depolarisation process within ventricles associated with myocardial scar and myocardial fibrosis. Peters et al. [20] analysed the ECGs of 360 ARVC patients and compared them to 52 controls. Fragmented QRS complexes were present in 85% of the patients, compared to only 4% of controls. The authors concluded that the presence of fragmented QRS complexes in the right precordial leads could be used as a screening tool for ECGs suspicious of ARVC. Other studies have associated the presence of fragmented QRS complexes with increased arrhythmic risk in patients with cardiomyopathies.

The prevalence and significance of isolated QRS fragmentation in athletes is unknown. In the presence of QRS prolongation (>110 ms), further evaluation is considered prudent. A narrow QRS complex in an asymptomatic athlete without relevant family history or cardiovascular risk factors is not deemed to warrant investigation.

Voltage Criteria for QRS-Axis Deviation and Atrial Enlargement

LAD and right axis deviation (RAD) are defined by convention as a QRS axis of $\leq -30°$ and $\geq +120°$, respectively. LAE is defined as a biphasic P-wave in lead V1 with a negative component of ≥ 40 ms duration and ≥ 0.1 mV (1 mm) depth, whilst right atrial enlargement (RAE) is defined as a P-wave amplitude ≥ 2.5 mm in leads II, III and aVF. Both the ESC and Seattle groups consider LAD and LAE to be ECG phenotypes that should prompt further evaluation of athletes [6,7]. These recommendations are based on the fact that both LAD and LAE are common findings in cardiomyopathies, being present in up to 12 and 44% of HCM patients, respectively. The recommendations are less clear about RAD and RAE. In contrast to LAD and LAE, both groups have removed isolated RAD or RAE from the list of ECG phenotypes suggestive of cardiac disease. At the same time, however, both discuss RAD and RAE within the context of underlying heart disease, suggesting that they should be evaluated further. RAD can be a feature of ARVC, RAE has been reported in up to 20% of HCM patients, and both may be present in pulmonary hypertension. Importantly, however, in the great majority of patients, voltage criteria for axis deviation or atrial enlargement are either present simultaneously or are associated with additional ECG anomalies suggestive of cardiomyopathy.

Axis deviation and atrial enlargement can also be common findings in healthy athletes. Sharma et al. [18] identified RAD in 16% of adolescent athletes, compared to 6% of healthy, age-matched controls. None of the adolescent athletes in this cohort exhibited LAD. In the same study, LAE and RAE were present in 14 and 16% of athletes, respectively. Studies in predominantly adult athletes in Italy and the UK reported RAD and LAD in a smaller proportion (~1% each) [3,21]. The same studies reported a variable prevalence of the voltage criterion for atrial enlargement, with ethnicity being an important determinant. In one study, by Papadakis et al. [3], the voltage criterion for LAE was present in almost 9% of black athletes, compared to

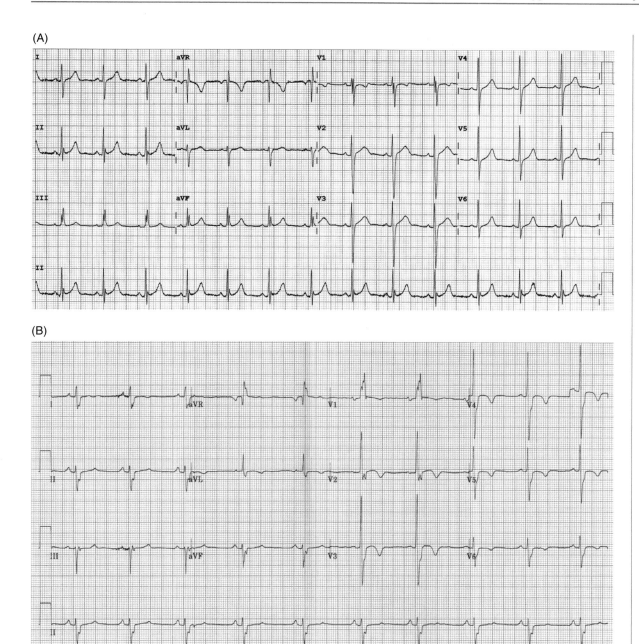

Figure 11.4 ECGs demonstrating QRS fragmentation. (A) Isolated QRS fragmentation of the inferior leads and lead V1 with a narrow QRS complex in a young individual. (B) QRS fragmentation affecting most leads with an associated broad QRS complex, RBBB pattern, anterolateral T-wave inversion and LAD in a patient with HCM

only 3% of white athletes, whilst the voltage criterion for RAE was present in 6% of black athletes and 0.3% of white. Further studies by Gati et al. [22] and Sheikh et al. [4] suggest that the presence of isolated voltage criteria for axis deviation or atrial enlargement on an athlete's ECG does not correlate with quiescent cardiomyopathy. Consequently, exclusion of these criteria from ECG phenotypes that warrant further investigations improves the specificity of ECG as a screening tool, without compromising its sensitivity. This notion is further supported by the study of Riding et al. [23] in a mixed population of white, black and Arabic athletes from the Gulf region of the Middle East. Based on the available evidence, the presence of the voltage criterion for LAD, RAD, LAE or RAE, in isolation, should not prompt further investigation of asymptomatic athletes with no family history of cardiac disease or SCD. The presence of 2 or more of these findings together still warrants consideration for more evaluation until additional information is available.

Premature Ventricular Contraction

Premature ventricular contractions (PVCs) are defined as QRS complexes >100 ms that are not preceded by a triggering P-wave. They can be a marker of pathology, but are also seen in healthy athletes as a result of increased vagal tone and resting bradycardia and can subside after detraining. In a study by Biffi et al. [24], of 70 athletes with ventricular arrhythmias, defined as ≥2000 PVCs and/or one or more burst of nonsustained ventricular tachycardia over 24 hours, who de-trained, 16 demonstrated complete reversibility with no PVCs on follow-up ECG monitor and 54 demonstrated only partial or no reversibility. None of the athletes with complete resolution demonstrated evidence of cardiovascular pathology on further investigation and follow-up. In contrast, 20 of the 54 athletes (37%) in whom arrhythmias persisted exhibited evidence of cardiac disease (cardiomyopathy in 10, mitral valve prolapse in 6 and myocarditis in 4). The morphology of the PVC may provide the clinician with clues relating to its aetiology. Extrasystoles originating from the right ventricle typically show an LBBB pattern, with a predominantly negative QRS complex in V1. LBBB morphology and an inferior axis (positive QRS complex in leads II, III and aVF) indicate a right ventricular outflow tract origin, consistent with idiopathic right ventricular outflow tract arrhythmia, which is a benign condition. Conversely, LBBB morphology and a superior axis (negative QRS complex in leads II, III and aVF) indicate a right ventricular free wall or apex origin and are more suggestive of ARVC. In addition, there is mounting evidence that genetically susceptible athletes competing at high-endurance events may be prone to right ventricular arrhythmias due to exercise-induced right ventricular dysfunction.

Comprehensive evaluation of the athlete is mandated in the presence of multiple and/or multifocal PVCs during an ECG strip, especially in the presence of symptoms or a family history of SCD or cardiomyopathy. Learned consensus panels do not recommend further evaluation of athletes with a single PVC on a 12-lead ECG strip in the absence of other features suggestive of cardiac disease. In the authors' experience of screening more than 20 000 athletes, PVCs are a rare finding, being present in 0.5% of ECGs. Moreover, it is impossible to assess the burden or significance of a PVC based on a snapshot of the rhythm strip. We would therefore recommend further evaluation of any athlete with a PVC on their ECG, with a transthoracic echocardiogram to exclude underlying structural heart disease and a 24-hour ECG monitor to assess the burden of ventricular ectopy. Further evaluation will depend on initial results.

Other ECG Phenotypes Associated with Cardiomyopathy

Low Voltages in the Limb Leads

Low voltage in limb leads is defined as a QRS amplitude ≤5 mm in each of the limb leads (I, II and III). Low voltages are frequently observed in athletes and the normal population, so in isolation should not prompt further evaluation for cardiac disease. Low limb-lead voltages, however, may also be a feature of ARVC and cardiac amyloidosis and should not be ignored in the context of clinical or other ECG features suggestive of cardiomyopathy [2].

Ventricular Pre-excitation

Ventricular pre-excitation manifests on the 12-lead ECG with a short PR interval and a delta (Δ) wave (slurred upstroke) at the origin of the QRS complex, commonly referred as the Wolff–Parkinson–White (WPW) pattern. Evidence of ECG pre-excitation may be present in 1 in 300 individuals in the general population. The risk of SCD relates to potential atrioventricular re-entry tachycardia, which in the context of atrial fibrillation may culminate in ventricular fibrillation. The majority of cases are congenital and are not associated with any structural cardiac abnormality. However, ventricular pre-excitation may be associated with structural heart disease, notably Ebstein anomaly and HCM. The association of LVH, often severe, and the presence of ventricular pre-excitation should raise suspicion of a glycogen-storage disease produced by LAMP2 or PRKAG2 mutations [25]. A diagnosis of an inherited glycogen storage disease has important implications relating to treatment and prognosis for both the individual and their family.

Conclusion

The interpretation of an athlete's ECG should be performed by individuals with experience in sports cardiology in order to minimise the burden of unnecessary investigations. It is clear that the overlap between physiological adaptation to exercise and cardiomyopathies remains substantial, and there are still a number of unanswered questions relating to the significance of certain ECG phenotypes. During the past decade, however, there have been a significant number of studies in large athletic populations of diverse demographic characteristics, which combined with a comparison to patients with known cardiomyopathy allow – for the first time – for the development of evidence-based, individualised recommendations to distinguish abnormalities on an athlete's ECG suggestive of cardiomyopathy.

References

1 Lakdawala, N.K., Thune, J.J., Maron, B.J. et al. Electrocardiographic features of sarcomere mutation carriers with and without clinically overt hypertrophic cardiomyopathy. *Am J Cardiol* 2011; **108**: 1606–13.

2 Jain, R., Dalal, D., Daly, A. et al. Electrocardiographic features of arrhythmogenic right ventricular dysplasia. *Circulation* 2009; **120**: 477–87.

3 Papadakis, M., Carrè, F., Kervio, G. et al. The prevalence, distribution, and clinical outcomes of electrocardiographic repolarization patterns in male athletes of African/Afro-Caribbean origin. *Eur Heart J* 2011; **32**: 2304–13.

4 Sheikh, N., Papadakis, M., Ghani, S. et al. Comparison of electrocardiographic criteria for the detection of cardiac abnormalities in elite black and white athletes. *Circulation* 2014; **129**: 1637–49.

5 Rawlins, J., Carre, F., Kervio, G. et al. Ethnic differences in physiological cardiac adaptation to intense physical exercise in highly trained female athletes. *Circulation* 2010; **121**: 1078–85.

6 Corrado, D., Pelliccia, A., Heidbuchel, H. et al. Recommendations for interpretation of 12-lead electrocardiogram in the athlete. *Eur Heart J* 2010; **31**: 243–59.

7 Drezner, J.A., Ackerman, M.J., Anderson, J. et al. Electrocardiographic interpretation in athletes: the 'Seattle criteria'. *Br J Sports Med* 2013; **47**: 122–4.

8 Drezner, J.A., Ashley, E., Baggish, A.L. et al. Abnormal electrocardiographic findings in athletes: recognising changes suggestive of cardiomyopathy. *Br J Sports Med* 2013; **47**: 137–52.

9 Papadakis, M., Basavarajaiah, S., Rawlins, J. et al. Prevalence and significance of T-wave inversions in predominantly Caucasian adolescent athletes. *Eur Heart J* 2009; **30**: 1728–35.

10 Migliore, F., Zorzi, A., Michieli, P. et al. Prevalence of cardiomyopathy in Italian asymptomatic children with electrocardiographic T-wave inversion at preparticipation screening. *Circulation* 2012; **125**: 529–38.

11 Pelliccia, A., Di Paolo, F.M., Quattrini, F.M. et al. Outcomes in athletes with marked ECG repolarization abnormalities. *N Engl J Med* 2008; **358**: 152–61.

12 Schnell, F., Riding, N., O'Hanlon, R. et al. Recognition and significance of pathological T-wave inversions in athletes. *Circulation* 2015; **131**: 165–73.

13 Haghjoo, M., Mohammadzadeh, S., Taherpour, M. et al. ST-segment depression as a risk factor in hypertrophic cardiomyopathy. *Europace* 2009; **11**: 643–9.

14 Konno, T., Shimizu, M., Ino, H. et al. Diagnostic value of abnormal Q waves for identification of preclinical carriers of hypertrophic cardiomyopathy based on a molecular genetic diagnosis. *Eur Heart J* 2004; **25**: 246–51.

15 Zaidi, A., Ghani, S., Sheikh, N. et al. Clinical significance of electrocardiographic right ventricular hypertrophy in athletes: comparison with arrhythmogenic right ventricular cardiomyopathy and pulmonary hypertension. *Eur Heart J* 2013; **34**: 3649–56.

16 Aleksova, A., Carriere, C., Zecchin, M. et al. New-onset left bundle branch block independently predicts long-term mortality in patients with idiopathic dilated cardiomyopathy: data from the Trieste Heart Muscle Disease Registry. *Europace* 2014; **16**: 1450–9.

17 Mahmod, M., Karamitsos, T.D., Suttie, J.J. et al. Prevalence of cardiomyopathy in asymptomatic patients with left bundle branch block referred for cardiovascular magnetic resonance imaging. *Int J Cardiovasc Imaging* 2012; **28**: 1133–40.

18 Sharma, S., Whyte, G., Elliott, P. et al. Electrocardiographic changes in 1000 highly trained junior elite athletes. *Br J Sports Med* 1999; **33**: 319–24.

19 Kim, J.H., Noseworthy, P.A., McCarty, D. et al. Significance of electrocardiographic right bundle branch block in trained athletes. *Am J Cardiol* 2011; **107**: 1083–9.

20 Peters, S., Trümmel, M. and Koehler, B. QRS fragmentation in standard ECG as a diagnostic marker of arrhythmogenic right ventricular dysplasia-cardiomyopathy. *Heart Rhythm* 2008; **5**: 1417–21.

21 Pelliccia, A., Maron, B.J., Culasso, F. et al. Clinical significance of abnormal electrocardiographic patterns in trained athletes. *Circulation* 2000; **102**: 278–84.

22 Gati, S., Sheikh, N., Ghani, S. et al. Should axis deviation or atrial enlargement be categorised as abnormal in young athletes? The athlete's electrocardiogram: time for re-appraisal of markers of pathology. *Eur Heart J* 2013; **34**: 3641–8.

23 Riding, N.R., Sheikh, N., Adamuz, C. et al. Comparison of three current sets of electrocardiographic interpretation criteria for use in screening athletes. *Heart* 2015; **101**: 384–90.

24 Biffi, A., Maron, B.J., Verdile, L. et al. Impact of physical deconditioning on ventricular tachyarrhythmias in trained athletes. *J Am Coll Cardiol* 2004; **44**: 1053–8.

25 Arad, M., Maron, B.J., Gorham, J.M. et al. Glycogen storage diseases presenting as hypertrophic cardiomyopathy. *N Engl J Med* 2005; **352**: 362–72.

12 Abnormal Electrocardiographic Findings in Athletes: Recognising Changes Suggestive of Primary Electrical Disease

Jordan Prutkin

Division of Cardiology, Section of Electrophysiology, Center for Sports Cardiology, University of Washington, Seattle, WA, USA

Introduction

The 12-lead electrocardiogram (ECG) has significant power to identify primary electrical diseases of the heart or to detect electrical abnormalities suggestive of an underlying cardiomyopathy that need further evaluation. These primary electrical diseases are typically ion channelopathies, which usually have no structural abnormalities manifest on imaging. Several specific ECG findings may be suggestive or diagnostic of a primary electrical abnormality of the heart. Recognition of these ECG findings is necessary to determine the risk of sudden cardiac arrest (SCA) in the athlete. This chapter will describe 12-lead ECG findings suggestive of electrical abnormalities of the heart and the evaluation that should be instituted when these are present (Table 12.1).

Long QT Interval

Long QT syndrome is demonstrated on an ECG as a prolonged QT interval. It is an inherited arrhythmia syndrome in which there is an increased risk of syncope, torsade de pointes, ventricular fibrillation and SCA. The underlying basis for long QT syndrome is a prolongation in the action potential duration due to delayed cellular repolarisation in the ventricles. Whilst at least 13 genes have been found to cause long QT syndrome, the three most common types (LQT1, LQT2 and LQT3) represent about 80% of cases [1]. These are caused by loss-of-function mutations in the two potassium channels KCNQ1 and KCNH2 in LQT1 and LQT2, respectively, and a gain-of-function mutation in SCN5A in LQT3. Long QT syndrome has a predominantly autosomal-dominant inheritance, known as the Romano–Ward syndrome, although Jervell and Lange-Nielsen syndrome is a rare autosomal-recessive form associated with sensorineural deafness, and 5–10% of cases are de novo mutations [1].

Evaluation of the QT interval on the ECG is the primary way of diagnosing long QT syndrome. However, several factors can influence the QT interval, the most important of which is heart rate. When the sinus rate is faster, the QT interval shortens, and when the sinus rate is slower, the QT interval lengthens. Therefore, several different correction formulas have been created to adjust the QT interval for the heart rate. The most common

---

IOC Manual of Sports Cardiology, First Edition. Edited by Mathew G. Wilson, Jonathan A. Drezner and Sanjay Sharma.
© 2017 International Olympic Committee. Published 2017 by John Wiley & Sons, Ltd.

ECG finding	Definition	Evaluation
Long QT interval	QTc ≥470 ms (male) QTc ≥480 ms (female) QTc ≥500 ms (marked QT prolongation)	Review medications and repeat ECG Consider exercise ECG test, electrolyte testing, family screening and genetic testing Consider direct referral to a heart rhythm specialist for a QTc ≥500 ms
Short QT interval	QTc ≤320 ms	Repeat ECG Consider referral to heart rhythm specialist, family screening and genetic testing
Type 1 Brugada pattern	ST elevation ≥2 mm (high take-off) with downsloping ST-segment elevation followed by a negative symmetric T-wave in one or more leads in V1–V3	Consider referral to heart rhythm specialist, family screening and genetic testing If the pattern is indeterminate, repeat ECG with leads V1–V2 in second intercostal space
Wolff–Parkinson–White (WPW) pattern	PR interval ≤120 ms, delta wave and QRS duration ≥120 ms	Exercise ECG test to determine whether there is abrupt loss of the bypass pathway Consider electrophysiology (EP) study in those without abrupt pathway loss or those performing moderate–high-intensity sports
Supraventricular tachycardia (SVT)	Narrow complex tachycardia with heart rate >100 beats.min⁻¹, atrial fibrillation or atrial flutter	Urgent treatment, if needed If stable, conduct 24-hour ECG monitoring, exercise ECG testing and echocardiogram Consider cardiac magnetic resonance imaging (MRI) or EP study as clinically indicated
Sinus tachycardia	Sinus rhythm >130 beats.min⁻¹	Repeat ECG Conduct laboratory testing, including electrolytes, complete blood count (CBC) and thyroid tests Review medications and performance enhancing drugs
Premature ventricular contractions (PVCs)	Two or more PVCs per 10-second tracing (consider one PVC in highly trained endurance athletes ≥25 years old or with other clinical suspicion of cardiac disease)	Conduct 24-hour ECG monitoring, exercise ECG testing and echocardiogram If there are ≥2000 PVCs or nonsustained ventricular tachycardia on 24-hour ECG monitor, consider cardiac MRI
Ventricular arrhythmias	Couplets, triples, nonsustained or sustained ventricular tachycardia	Conduct 24-hour ECG monitoring, exercise ECG testing, echocardiogram and cardiac MRI
Profound sinus bradycardia	≤30 beats.min⁻¹	Repeat ECG after mild exercise activity Consider exercise ECG or other testing based on clinical suspicion
Profound first atrioventricular (AV) block	PR interval ≥400 ms	Repeat ECG after mild exercise activity Consider exercise ECG or other testing based on clinical suspicion
Second-degree Mobitz type II AV block	Intermittently dropped QRS complexes with a fixed PR interval	Conduct 24-hour ECG monitoring, exercise ECG testing, echocardiogram and cardiac MRI, and refer to heart rhythm specialist
Third-degree (complete) AV block	AV dissociation with more P-waves than QRS complexes	Conduct 24-hour ECG monitoring, exercise ECG testing, echocardiogram and cardiac MRI, and refer to heart rhythm specialist

Table 12.1 Abnormal electrical findings on an athlete's ECG and possible evaluation

is Bazett's correction, which should be used for screening purposes as it is used in existing population-based studies to define normal QT intervals corrected (QTc) for heart rate. Using Bazett's formula, $QTc = QT/\sqrt{RR}$, where the RR interval is measured in seconds. The formula is most accurate for a heart rate of 60–90 beats.min^{-1}. It overestimates the QTc interval at fast heart rates and underestimates it at slower ones. Therefore, in those with a borderline or abnormal QTc with bradycardia of <50 beats.min^{-1}, it may be necessary to perform a small amount of aerobic activity in order to increase the heart rate, while in those with tachycardia >100 beats.min^{-1} a prolonged period of rest may be required.

Many athletes have sinus arrhythmia, which leads to a respiratory variation in heart rate and the RR interval. The best method by which to calculate the QTc in this setting is to average the QT intervals on all beats on the rhythm strip and divide by the average RR interval [2].

Whilst it is usually clear where to begin measurement of the QT interval (the beginning of the QRS complex), one of the most difficult aspects is determining the end of the T-wave. It is essential not to include the U-wave in the measurement, as this will falsely increase the QT interval and U-waves are frequently seen in athletes with bradycardia. It is best to examine leads II or V5, which are frequently present on the rhythm strip at the bottom of 12-lead ECGs. The 'teach the tangent' or 'avoid the tail' method can be used to define the end of the T-wave [3]. This involves drawing a straight line on the downslope of the T-wave to where it intersects with the baseline (Figure 12.1). This intersection is the end of the QT interval. Use of this method should exclude the U-wave as part of the measurement.

Certain T-wave morphologies can be suggestive of long QT syndrome genotypes, although this may not always be sensitive or specific. For instance, a notched T-wave in the lateral precordial leads, even in the presence of a normal QT interval, may suggest LQT2 [4].

Accurate measurement of the QT interval can be difficult even for experienced cardiologists and electrophysiologists [5]. The computer read of the raw QT interval is accurate about 90–95% of the time, and it is usually very accurate in measuring the RR interval [6]. Therefore, the easiest way of calculating the QTc is to manually measure the QT interval as just described and then compare the measured QT interval with the computer-derived measure. If the hand-measured QT is within 10 ms, then the computer-derived QTc measure is accurate. Otherwise, it is best to use the hand-measured QT interval but use the computer-measured RR interval, or heart rate, to determine the QTc (RR = 60/heart rate).

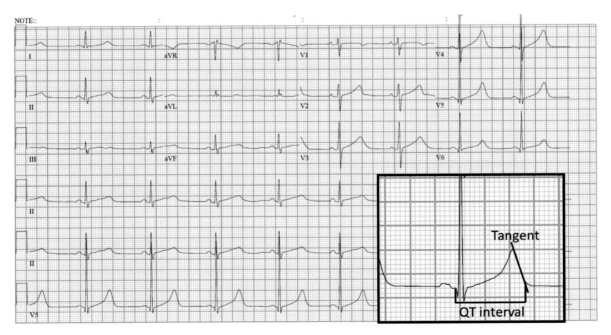

Figure 12.1 ECG of a patient with long QT syndrome. The inset shows a tangent line on the downslope of the T-wave. The QT interval is measured from the beginning of the QRS to where the tangent intersects the baseline. In this example, the QT interval measures 570 ms and the heart rate is 52 beats.min^{-1}, giving a QTc of 531 ms using Bazett's formula

There is no definite QTc value that equates to long QT syndrome, as there is a bell curve of QTc values in the general population, which overlaps somewhat with those who have genetically confirmed long QT syndrome. For screening purposes, it is imperative to choose a QTc interval that represents an appropriate balance of sensitivity and specificity in order to determine which QTc cutoff requires further evaluation in an asymptomatic athlete with no significant family history. A QTc cutoff of ≥470 ms in males and ≥480 ms in females is recommended [6] Even at values above these cutoffs, a diagnosis of long QT syndrome is not definitive. If the QTc is ≥500 ms, this is marked QT prolongation and more likely represents true long QT syndrome.

If a prolonged QT interval is found, a repeat ECG should be completed to confirm the finding, preferably on a different day. It is important to complete a thorough family history, looking for sudden death, syncope and unexplained drowning or motor vehicle accidents that may have been caused by polymorphic ventricular tachycardia or ventricular fibrillation. In addition, a personal history of syncope or seizures (which may actually be due to nonsustained ventricular arrhythmias) should be completed. The medication list should be examined for QT-prolonging medications. If possible, it is best to obtain ECGs of first-degree relatives to see whether there is a familial prolongation of the QT interval, which would be more concerning. Laboratory testing for electrolytes should be completed. An exercise treadmill test should be considered, to assess whether the QTc shortens to <480 ms at the 4th minute of recovery. If the QT interval is prolonged on two ECGs or if there is a personal or family history of syncope, seizures or sudden death, especially with QTc intervals ≥500 ms, expert consultation should be obtained.

Short QT Interval

Short QT syndrome is much less common than long QT syndrome, with fewer than 200 patients reported in the literature [7]. Like long QT syndrome, short QT syndrome is caused by mutations in ion-channel genes, although only a small proportion of genetic mutations have thus far been discovered. For screening purposes, because of the overlap between normal and short QT intervals and the rare incidence of this syndrome, a QTc interval of ≤320 ms should be considered abnormal, warranting further evaluation. Even at this value, short QT syndrome is not definitively diagnosed. Diagnostic criteria using a point-scoring system have been created, which include a short QTc, a J-point to T-peak interval <120 ms, a history of cardiac arrest or polymorphic ventricular tachycardia/ventricular fibrillation, a family history of short QT syndrome and genetic mutations [8].

Brugada Pattern

Brugada syndrome is defined by a characteristic ECG pattern in leads V1–V3, associated with ventricular fibrillation and sudden death. It is an autosomal-dominant disease with variable penetrance. The predominance of mutations have been found in sodium channels, with the most common being SCN5A. It typically presents with symptoms in middle-aged males, and is the second highest cause of death in young men from Thailand [9]. It is thought that the majority of cases of sudden unexplained death syndrome (SUDS), known as 'Bangungut' in the Phillipines, 'Pokkuri' in Japan and 'Lai Tai' in Thailand, are due to Brugada syndrome.

It can be difficult to correctly identify the ECG pattern, as it can sometimes be subtle, but also because the pattern may occur only intermittently on ECG. The type 1 Brugada pattern has been associated with SCA. This pattern demonstrates coved ST elevation in leads V1–V3, although it may sometimes be seen only in V1. The ST elevation is ≥2 mm, with a downsloping ST segment, which may be straight or concave, that continues into an inverted T-wave (Figure 12.2A). Typically, the QT interval is normal, although it may be slightly prolonged in V1–V3.

An elevated ST segment with T-wave inversions due to an early repolarisation pattern may often be seen in athletes, making the diagnosis of Brugada syndrome difficult. The ST_J/ST_{80} ratio can be helpful in differentiation (Figure 12.2B). This ratio looks at the height of the ST segment at the J-point versus the height 80 ms after the J-point. If the ratio is >1, it has high sensitivity and specificity for Brugada syndrome, whilst if it is <1, it is normal [10]. Stated another way, if the ST segment is downsloping in the first 80 ms, it is consistent with Brugada syndrome, but if it is upsloping, then it is normal. In addition, the high take-off is usually not peaked in Brugada syndrome, as might be seen in right bundle branch block (RBBB).

In patients in whom the ECG is ambiguous, a Brugada pattern may be more easily seen if ECG leads V1 and V2 are moved up to the second intercostal space.

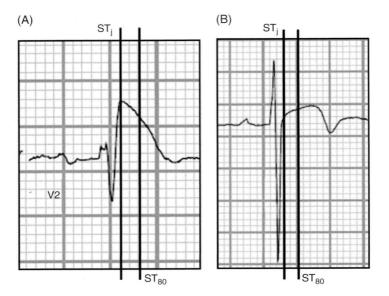

Figure 12.2 (A) Type 1 Brugada pattern in lead V2, which shows ≥2 mm ST elevation, downsloping ST segment, and T-wave inversion. The ST_j/ST_{80} ratio, which is the height of the ST segment at the J-point and 80 ms later, is >1. (B) Early repolarisation pattern in V2. The ST_j/ST_{80} ratio here is <1

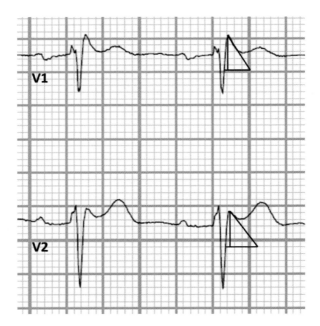

Figure 12.3 Type 2 Brugada pattern in leads V1–V2. A line is dropped 5 mm down from the r′ and a second line is drawn on the downslope of the ST segment. A third horizontal line is then drawn starting 5 mm below the r′ from the S wave and intersecting with the downslope of ST segment. If this third line is ≥4 mm (160 ms), then it is a type 2 pattern. In this example, the duration of the line is <4 mm in V1 but ≥4 mm in V2, making this a type 2 pattern

In the past, three Brugada patterns were described, but more recent criteria have combined two of them, as they were not felt to be significantly different [11]. The new type 2 Brugada pattern has a saddleback ST segment. There is a high take-off of the r′ portion of the QRS, followed by a positive T-wave in V2. In those with a type 2 pattern, sodium channel blockers such as ajmaline, flecainide, procainamide or pilsicainide will sometimes convert the pattern to type 1. The type 2 pattern can also be difficult to differentiate from a normal athlete's ECG. The best criterion to use in differentiating the two is the duration of the base of a triangle created at the r′ (Figure 12.3). A line is dropped 5 mm straight down from the r′ and a second line is drawn as a tangent along the downslope of the ST segment [12]. A third, horizontal line is then drawn from 5 mm below the r′ from the S wave to the intersection with the second line. If this line is ≥4 mm or 160 ms, it is more consistent with a type 2 pattern.

Phenocopies of Brugada syndrome have been reported, which are nongenetic causes that can induce the Brugada pattern. These include metabolic conditions, mechanical compression, myocardial ischaemia, myocardial or pericardial disease and inappropriate ECG filtering, amongst several other causes [13]. If one of these is found, and the ECG pattern resolves when the medical condition improves, then it is likely not Brugada syndrome.

If there is a Brugada pattern, expert consultation should be obtained. This might include family evaluation and genetic testing.

Wolff–Parkinson–White Pattern

The Wolff–Parkinson–White (WPW) pattern occurs in about 1–3 in 1000 people, with a slightly higher prevalence among first-degree family members [14]. About 65% of adolescents and 40% of those over age 30 years with the WPW pattern are asymptomatic [14].

The WPW pattern on ECG is characterised by a short PR interval ≤120 ms, prolonged QRS duration ≥120 ms and a slurred QRS upstroke/downstroke called a delta wave (Figure 12.4). The underlying aetiology is a bypass pathway, or accessory connection, between the atria and ventricles. The pathway location, which can be anywhere along the atrioventricular (AV) annuli, as well as the conduction speed of the pathway relative to the conduction speed of the AV node, will determine the delta-wave vector and QRS morphology. Therefore, there is no single ECG lead to use to decide whether WPW is present.

In some cases, the findings of WPW are subtle and the pattern difficult to confirm. A positive QRS in lead V1 in the absence of RBBB may raise suspicion for WPW, although there may be other causes for this, including right ventricular hypertrophy (RVH). In addition, left-sided bypass pathways, since they are far away from the sinus node, may not be obviously seen on an ECG, as the AV node will conduct sooner, and the QRS will not show the WPW pattern. Bypass pathways that are weakly conducting (with a low risk of SCA) may only intermittently be seen on ECG.

A short PR interval alone is not sufficient for a diagnosis of WPW. Since athletes often have a slow sinus rate, it is possible to see ectopic atrial rhythms, some of which may originate near the AV node, which can give a

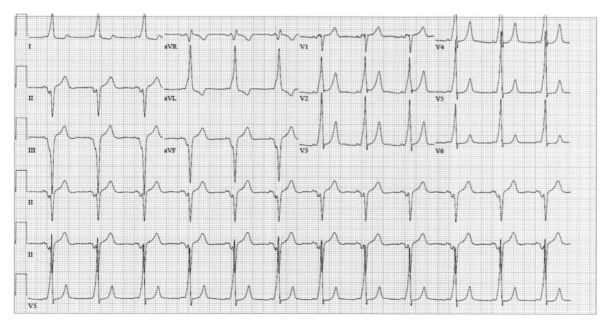

Figure 12.4 WPW pattern showing a PR interval ≤120 ms, QRS duration ≥120 ms and slurred QRS upstroke/downstroke (delta wave)

short PR interval, but the QRS is normal in duration and appearance. Another possibility is that the sinus rate is slow enough that there is a junctional escape rhythm which has a rate just a little faster than the atrial rate. In this situation, the PR interval may be short, leading to the appearance of a pseudo-delta wave, since it is the P-wave causing apparent QRS widening (Figure 12.5). There is usually respiratory variability in the P-wave and QRS rates, which can differentiate sinus bradycardia with a junctional escape rhythm. There are also some atypical intracardiac pathways, such as a fasciculoventricular pathway connecting the right bundle and ventricular tissue, which can give a WPW appearance on ECG but do not cause arrhythmias or SCA, although they can only be differentiated during an electrophysiology (EP) study. Finally, there are some patients with enhanced AV nodal conduction or Lown–Ganong–Levine syndrome who have a short PR interval but normal QRS appearance who do not develop arrhythmias or SCA (Figure 12.6).

The most common rhythm abnormality in those with WPW is atrioventricular reciprocating tachycardia (AVRT), a type of paroxysmal supraventricular tachycardia (SVT). In this arrhythmia, conduction occurs down the AV node and up the bypass pathway. Less commonly, conduction occurs down the bypass pathway and up the AV node. The conduction speed of the bypass pathway, in general, is unrelated to the possibility of developing AVRT. Symptoms include palpitations, chest pain, shortness of breath, dizziness and, rarely, syncope. It is very rarely a life-threatening rhythm.

Patients with WPW are also at increased risk of atrial fibrillation and atrial flutter, and the biggest concern is rapid conduction down the bypass pathway, leading to ventricular fibrillation and SCA. Most patients with WPW will have some symptoms prior to SCA, but for some patients (especially younger individuals) SCA may be the first presentation [14].

The incidence of SCA in those with WPW has been difficult to quantify in various studies due to methodological limitations, but it is approximately 1.1–4.5 per 1000 patient-years [14–16].

If a patient with a WPW pattern is found, a thorough evaluation for symptoms should be completed. If there are symptoms, the patient should be referred to a heart-rhythm specialist for EP study to assess the conduction properties of the bypass pathway and possible ablation to eliminate the pathway. The best predictor of a high-risk pathway that should be ablated is a shortest pre-excited RR interval in AF of ≤250 ms.

For the asymptomatic patient, the initial steps should be an echocardiogram (as there is a relationship between WPW and Ebstein anomaly and some types of cardiomyopathy) and an exercise treadmill test to look for *abrupt* loss of bypass pathway conduction (Figure 12.7). If the pathway slowly disappears or is continuously

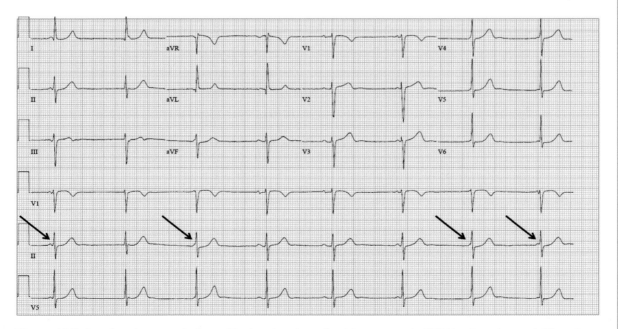

Figure 12.5 Junctional escape rhythm with sinus bradycardia giving a pseudo-WPW pattern (arrows). There is a respiratory sinus arrhythmia and the junctional beats cause near-simultaneous P-waves and QRS complexes (arrows), which have the appearance of a short PR and delta wave

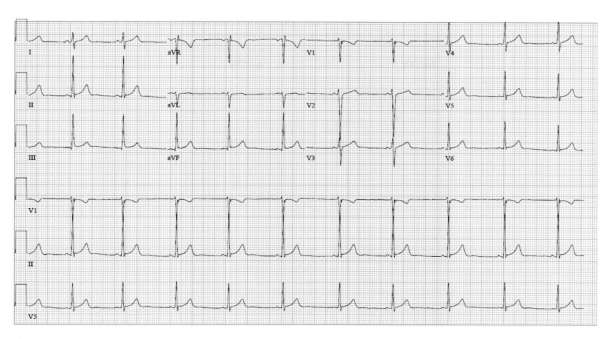

Figure 12.6 Lown–Ganong–Levine syndrome. The PR interval measures 100 ms, but the QRS is normal, with no delta wave

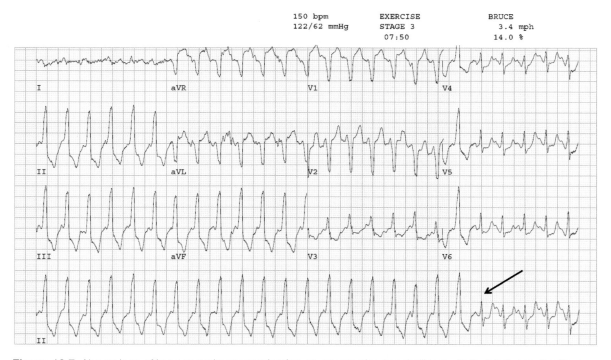

Figure 12.7 Abrupt loss of bypass pathway conduction on an exercise treadmill test. At 7 : 50 during the Bruce protocol, at a heart rate of 150 beats.min⁻¹, there is abrupt lengthening of the PR interval and narrowing of the QRS complex (arrow), suggesting the bypass pathway is low risk for SCA

present even at maximum heart rates during exercise testing, the patient should be referred to a heart-rhythm specialist for EP study. If the pathway abruptly disappears during exercise testing, then the risk of SCA is low due to slow conduction across the bypass pathway during higher heart rates, making it unlikely that rapid AF could degenerate into ventricular fibrillation. The athlete can be allowed to participate without restrictions.

An EP study can be considered in those who do not lose the pathway abruptly on exercise testing, especially those in moderate- to high-intensity sports, although some have argued that the risk of SCA approximates the risk of complications from an EP study and is not necessary for the asymptomatic patient [14]. If symptoms develop later, evaluation by a heart-rhythm specialist should be completed.

Supraventricular Tachycardias

Whilst rarely seen on screening ECGs (just 2 out of 32 561 young athletes in one study [17]), SVT can reflect pathology that needs further evaluation. AF and atrial flutter are atrial arrhythmias that can rapidly conduct through the AV node to the ventricles, especially in a young person. Whilst the rhythms themselves are only very rarely life-threatening, they can be associated with other disorders that can lead to SCA. These include WPW, long QT syndrome, short QT syndrome, Brugada syndrome and any type of cardiomyopathy. There is also an elevated rate of stroke and other thromboembolic events, although this risk is typically low in young people in the absence of cardiomyopathy, hypertension or diabetes. Patients with AF or atrial flutter need an echocardiogram, 24-hour Holter and exercise treadmill test. Depending on the clinical situation, cardiac magnetic resonance imaging (MRI), EP study, familial evaluation and/or genetic testing may be indicated. Use of performance-enhancing medications should also be questioned.

Paroxysmal SVT, which includes AV nodal re-entrant tachycardia, AVRT and atrial tachycardia, is exceedingly rare on a screening ECG, as it is usually accompanied by symptoms and typically includes urgent management to slow the heart rate. This can include the Valsalva manoeuvre, carotid sinus massage or facial dunking in ice water, which enhance vagal tone to the AV node and may terminate the arrhythmia. Ideally, these manoeuvres are completed whilst an ECG rhythm strip is obtained to document how the rhythm ends, which can help define the type of SVT. A repeat ECG should then be obtained whilst in normal sinus rhythm to determine whether there are other abnormalities, including a WPW pattern. Athletes with SVT should have an echocardiogram and should be referred to a heart-rhythm specialist to consider EP study and ablation.

Whilst sinus tachycardia is unlikely to be the only manifestation of cardiac disease, a resting heart rate >130 beats.min^{-1} in the screening setting will most commonly represent anxiety, but may also indicate anaemia, thyroid disease, dehydration, fever, medications or performance-enhancing drugs. An ECG should be repeated after a few minutes to see whether the heart rate is still elevated, and further evaluation should be considered for consistently elevated heart rates without explanation.

Premature Ventricular Contractions and Ventricular Arrhythmias

In those with cardiac disease, premature ventricular contractions (PVCs) and ventricular arrhythmias may be the first manifestation. The differential diagnosis is large, including idiopathic PVCs, arrhythmogenic right ventricular cardiomyopathy (ARVC), myocarditis, hypertrophic or dilated cardiomyopathies, myocardial infarction, left ventricular noncompaction, sarcoidosis and inherited arrhythmia syndromes, such as catecholaminergic polymorphic ventricular tachycardia (CPVT). If two PVCs are seen on a screening ECG, further evaluation should be completed.

One study divided 355 athletes into groups based on the number of PVCs found on a 24-hour Holter [18]. In those with <2000 PVCs, no significant myocardial disease was found. However, in those with ≥2000 PVCs, 10% had ARVC, 5.5% had myocarditis and 5.5% had dilated cardiomyopathy. Some studies have suggested de-training for 3–6 months and a repeat Holter monitor to count PVCs [19]. Whilst de-training led to a significant decrease in PVCs in one study, retraining afterwards led to a recurrence of PVCs, although not as many as at baseline [19]. Another study showed no effect of de-training [20]. This suggests that at least some element of a decrease in PVCs found on repeat Holter monitoring is due to regression to the mean, and that athletic training does not cause PVCs. De-training may be considered if there is a concern that myocarditis is the cause and time is needed for healing, but otherwise it does not seem to offer benefit.

The most common location for PVCs is from the right ventricular outflow tract (RVOT), the area just below the pulmonic valve. These PVCs have an ECG morphology with a left bundle branch block (LBBB)-like pattern and inferior axis (positive in leads II, III and aVF and negative in aVL) (Figure 12.8). They are normally benign, however, although they can also be seen in those with myocardial disease.

Compared to other ECG findings, PVCs are the most transitory, as they occur sporadically. Therefore, someone with frequent PVCs may have a normal ECG if the ECG is not done at the moment the PVCs are occurring.

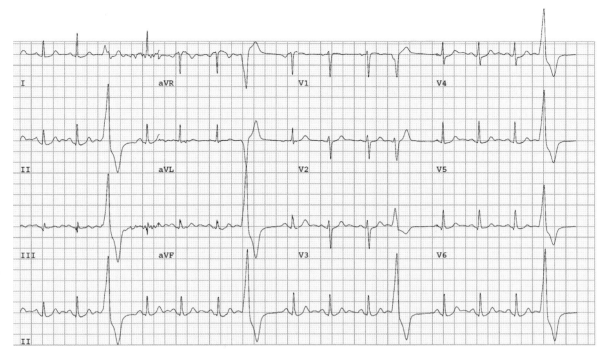

Figure 12.8 PVCs from the RVOT in a quadrigeminal pattern. They have an LBBB-like pattern and are positive in leads II, III and aVF (inferior axis). Notably, there are no T-wave inversions in leads V2–V3 and no epsilon wave, meaning they are less likely to be due to ARVC, although this does not rule out the diagnosis

If two PVCs are seen on the ECG, then an evaluation must be performed, as this suggests they have more frequent PVCs throughout the day. At a minimum, this should include a 24-hour ambulatory ECG, echocardiogram and exercise stress test. If the ambulatory ECG shows ≥2000 PVCs or nonsustained ventricular tachycardia, then there should be more intensive evaluation looking for cardiac disease, especially if the PVCs are not coming from the RVOT or if there are multiple PVC morphologies, couplets or nonsustained or sustained ventricular tachycardia. This may include a cardiac MRI, signal-averaged ECG, coronary artery disease (CAD) evaluation, longer-term ECG monitoring, EP study (including possible ablation) or cardiac biopsy. Such athletes should have serial evaluation in the future, as the PVCs may be the first sign of occult cardiac disease.

ARVC is one of the more concerning diseases on the differential. It can be difficult to diagnose due to its variable manifestations, and a scoring system with major and minor criteria has been developed to aid in its diagnosis [21]. A major criterion is nonsustained or sustained VT with an LBBB morphology and superior axis (negative in leads II, III, and aVF), suggesting a right ventricular origin not from the RVOT. Two of the minor diagnostic criteria for ARVC are >500 PVCs in 24 hours and nonsustained or sustained VT with an RVOT morphology. Classically, ARVC has been thought to be a genetic disease, although there is some emerging evidence that there may also be an exercise-induced form, where repeated induced stress of the right ventricle from ultra-endurance sport (e.g. triathlon, cycling) induces ARVC [22]. If there is a concern for either genetic or gene-elusive ARVC, there should be a lower threshold for considering the Holter study abnormal. In addition, if there is a clinical suspicion of myocardial disease for other reasons, then a single PVC may require further evaluation.

Sinus Bradycardia

Athletes commonly have slower sinus rates, with endurance athletes often having sinus bradycardia, defined as a heart rate <60 beats.min^{-1}, due to changes in autonomic tone and to downregulation of ionic currents in the heart. Frequently, they may have heart rates in the 30s or 40s, especially whilst sleeping. This is normal, physiologic and asymptomatic in most athletes, although there are data to suggest a higher need for pacemaker implants later in life [23].

A heart rate ≤30 beats.min^{-1} or a pause ≥3 seconds in an '*awake*' athlete may be abnormal. Frequently, this will be accompanied by a junctional escape rhythm. If the athlete is asymptomatic, a brief episode of exercise should be completed and a repeat ECG obtained. If the heart rate increases, then no further evaluation or therapy is needed. If the heart rate does not increase with this light exercise, a formal treadmill test should be completed. Athletes may commonly have bradycardia and long sinus pauses whilst sleeping due to high parasympathetic tone, but this is a normal finding and does not indicate that treatment is needed. If the athlete has symptoms of fatigue with exertion and cannot obtain a target heart rate with exercise, or has dizziness at rest associated with bradycardia, than appropriate evaluation and treatment may be needed, including a pacemaker.

Heart Block

First-degree heart block, defined as a PR interval ≥200 ms, is a normal finding in athletes due to high vagal tone and slowed conduction through the AV node (Figure 12.9). Even profound AV block can be seen out to 400 ms or longer at times, which may be accompanied by sinus bradycardia. This may reflect normal physiology, but in some situations may be pathologic. If the PR interval is ≥400 ms, the athlete should do quick exercises to briefly increase sympathetic and decrease parasympathetic tones, to see whether the PR interval shortens appropriately. If it shortens, the athlete is asymptomatic, the family history does not include a pacemaker or sudden death and there are no other ECG abnormalities, then it is reasonable to assume this is normal physiology. If not, then further evaluation with a formal exercise test or Holter monitor should be considered.

In some athletes at rest, there may be such high parasympathetic input that there is Mobitz I second-degree AV block, also known as Wenckebach (Figure 12.10). In this scenario, the ECG shows intermittently dropped QRS complexes, where there is a P-wave and no QRS. The key finding is that the PR interval progressively increases on each beat until the dropped QRS, and the first PR interval after the dropped beat is shorter than the last conducted PR interval before the dropped beat. This is a normal finding at rest in athletes. It may be helpful to have the athlete do a small amount of exercise, as in sinus bradycardia and first-degree AV block, to see whether there is normalisation of 1 : 1 AV-node conduction.

Mobitz II second-degree AV block is pathologic. This usually represents conduction system disease below the AV node in the His–Purkinje system. The ECG finding is dropped QRS complexes, but the PR interval is fixed, with no change pre and post dropped beats (Figure 12.11). It can sometimes be difficult to determine whether Mobitz I or II second-degree AV block is present; this requires close examination of the PR

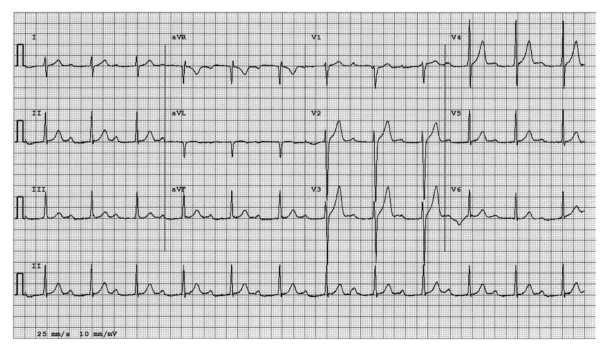

Figure 12.9 First-degree AV block with a PR interval measuring 386 ms. This is a normal finding in athletes

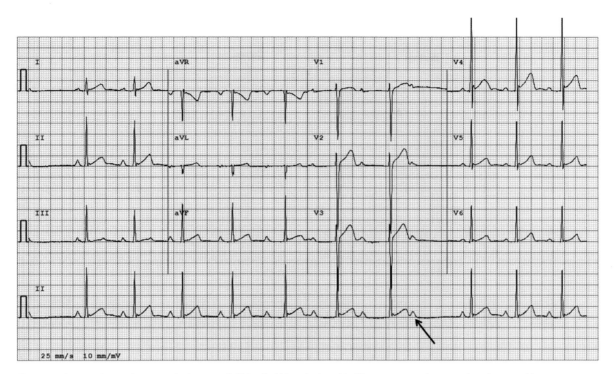

Figure 12.10 Mobitz I second-degree AV block (Wenckebach). The arrow points to the dropped beat. The PR interval on the conducted beat prior to the dropped beat is longer than the PR interval on the first return beat

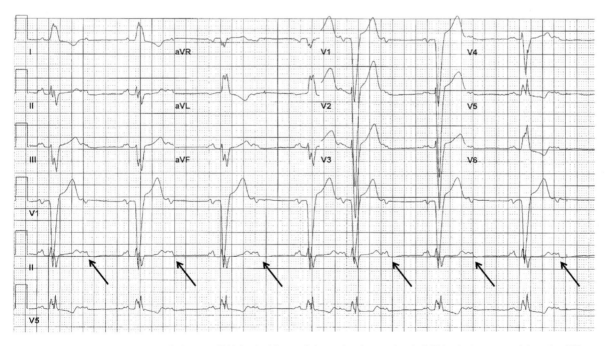

Figure 12.11 Mobitz II second-degree AV block. Most of the strip shows 2 : 1 AV block, but examining the PR intervals on the beats just before and after the dropped beat (arrows) shows the PR interval is fixed and indicates Mobitz II second-degree AV block. Note that the conducted beats have an LBBB pattern, suggesting there is conduction-system disease and possible cardiomyopathy

interval. Mobitz II is much less common than Mobitz I, unrelated to exercise training, and it can be a marker for myocardial disease such as sarcoidosis or myocarditis – or it may be a direct abnormality of the conduction system.

Complete AV block is also unusual in an awake athlete, although it may be seen whilst sleeping. With complete AV block, also known as 'third-degree AV block', there is AV dissociation, with more P-waves than QRS complexes. A junctional escape rhythm has a narrow QRS, whilst a ventricular escape rhythm has a wide QRS. Since many athletes have such slow sinus rates, they can have junctional or ventricular escape rhythms, which are not the same as complete AV block. The key finding with complete heart block is that there are more P-waves than QRS complexes and that the P-wave rate is regular.

If complete AV block is seen, it should be directly referred to a heart-rhythm specialist for evaluation. This can include an echocardiogram, cardiac MRI, treadmill test and/or 24-hour Holter monitor. Usually, a pacemaker should be implanted.

Sudden Death Syndromes with a Normal ECG

It is important to mention that there are electrical disorders of the heart which are not found on a screening ECG but can predispose to sudden death.

Catecholaminergic Polymorphic Ventricular Tachycardia

CPVT affects about 1 in 10 000 individuals and is one cause of SCA during exercise in those with normal hearts. It is a disorder of cardiac ion channels, predominantly the ryanodine receptor (RYR2). It typically affects children and adolescents, and will present with syncope or SCA with exercise or strong emotional events that trigger adrenergic release.

Since the resting ECG is normal in CPVT, an exercise ECG test should be considered in those with syncope during exertion. During the early portion of the exercise test, the ECG is normal, but as workload increases, PVCs start to appear. This is in contrast to benign normal heart PVCs, which typically decrease in response to exercise. Eventually, as exertion increases further, there is development of polymorphic PVCs and eventually polymorphic RR, typically in a bidirectional pattern, where the QRS axis rotates 180° every other beat. This is an unusual type of RR and is highly specific (although insensitive) for CPVT [24]. Other common findings on exercise testing in those with CPVT are ventricular bigeminy, couplets and nonsustained ventricular tachycardia.

Idiopathic Ventricular Fibrillation

Some patients with SCA of unexplained cause despite extensive evaluation have idiopathic ventricular fibrillation. These patients have a normal ECG, so will not be found on screening.

Conclusion

The ECG is a valuable resource for the detection of electrical abnormalities in many cardiac disorders, including inherited arrhythmia syndromes such as channelopathies, as well as for electrical manifestations of cardiomyopathies. Appropriate athlete-specific ECG interpretation can be used as a screening or diagnostic test to find disorders with an increased risk of SCA during sport. Referral to a cardiologist or heart-rhythm specialist is recommended when the diagnosis is unclear or expert evaluation is needed.

References

1 Ackerman, M.J., Priori, S.G., Willems, S. et al. HRS/EHRA expert consensus statement on the state of genetic testing for the channelopathies and cardiomyopathies. *Heart Rhythm* 2011; **8**: 1308–39.
2 Johnson, J.N. and Ackerman, M.J. The prevalence and diagnostic/prognostic utility of sinus arrhythmia in the evaluation of congenital long QT syndrome. *Heart Rhythm* 2010; 7: 1785–9.
3 Postema, P.G., De Jong, J.S., van der Bilt, I.A. and Wilde, A.A. Accurate electrocardiographic assessment of the QT interval: teach the tangent. *Heart Rhythm* 2008; 5: 1015–18.

4 Malfatto, G., Beria, G., Sala, S. et al. Quantitative-analysis of T-wave abnormalities and their prognostic implications in the idiopathic long QT-syndrome. *J Am Coll Cardiol* 1994; **23**: 296–301.

5 Viskin, S., Rosovski, U., Sands, A.J. et al. Inaccurate electrocardiographic interpretation of long QT: the majority of physicians cannot recognize a long QT when they see one. *Heart Rhythm* 2005; **2**: 569–74.

6 Drezner, J.A., Ackerman, M.J., Cannon, B.C. et al. Abnormal electrocardiographic findings in athletes: recognising changes suggestive of primary electrical disease. *Br J Sports Med* 2013; **47**: 153–67.

7 Mazzanti, A., Kanthan, A., Monteforte, N. et al. Novel insight into the natural history of short QT syndrome. *J Am Coll Cardiol* 2014; **63**: 1300–8.

8 Gollob, M.H., Redpath, C.J. and Roberts, J.D. The short QT syndrome: proposed diagnostic criteria. *J Am Coll Cardiol* 2011; **57**: 802–12.

9 Nademanee, K. Sudden unexplained death syndrome in Southeast Asia. *Am J Cardiol* 1997; **79**: 10–11.

10 Zorzi, A., Leoni, L., Di Paolo, F.M. et al. Differential diagnosis between early repolarization of athlete's heart and coved-type brugada electrocardiogram. *Am J Cardiol* 2015; **115**: 529–32.

11 Bayes De Luna, A., Brugada, J., Baranchuk, A. et al. Current electrocardiographic criteria for diagnosis of Brugada pattern: a consensus report. *J Electrocardiol* 2012; **45**: 433–42.

12 Serra, G., Baranchuk, A., Bayés-De-Luna, A. et al. New electrocardiographic criteria to differentiate the Type-2 Brugada pattern from electrocardiogram of healthy athletes with r'-wave in leads V1/V2. *Europace* 2014; **16**: 1639–45.

13 Anselm, D.D. and Baranchuk, A. Brugada phenocopy: redefinition and updated classification. *Am J Cardiol* 2013; **111**: 453.

14 Cohen, M.I., Triedman, J.K., Cannon, B.C. et al. PACES/HRS expert consensus statement on the management of the asymptomatic young patient with a Wolff-Parkinson-White (WPW, ventricular preexcitation) electrocardiographic pattern. *Heart Rhythm* 2012; **9**: 1006–24.

15 Cain, N., Irving, C., Webber, S. et al. Natural history of Wolff-Parkinson-White syndrome diagnosed in childhood. *Am J Cardiol* 2013; **112**: 961–5.

16 Pappone, C., Vicedomini, G., Manguso, F. et al. Wolff-Parkinson-White syndrome in the era of catheter ablation: insights from a registry study of 2169 patients. *Circulation* 2014; **130**: 811–19.

17 Marek, J., Bufalino, V., Davis, J. et al. Feasibility and findings of large-scale electrocardiographic screening in young adults: data from 32 561 subjects. *Heart Rhythm* 2011; **8**: 1555–9.

18 Biffi, A., Pelliccia, A., Verdile, L. et al. Long-term clinical significance of frequent and complex ventricular tachyarrhythmias in trained athletes. *J Am Coll Cardiol* 2012; **40**: 446–52.

19 Biffi, A., Maron, B.J., Culasso, F. et al. Patterns of ventricular tachyarrhythmias associated with training, deconditioning and retraining in elite athletes without cardiovascular abnormalities. *Am J Cardiol* 2011; **107**: 697–703.

20 Delise, P., Lanari, E., Sitta, N. et al. Influence of training on the number and complexity of frequent VPBs in healthy athletes. *J Cardiovasc Med* 2011; **12**: 157–61.

21 Marcus, F.I., Mckenna, W.J., Sherrill, D. et al. Diagnosis of arrhythmogenic right ventricular cardiomyopathy/dysplasia: proposed modification of the task force criteria. *Circulation* 2010; **121**: 1533–41.

22 Heidbüchel, H. and La Gerche, A. The right heart in athletes. Evidence for exercise-induced arrhythmogenic right ventricular cardiomyopathy. *Herzschrittmacherther Elektrophysiol* 2012; **23**: 82–6.

23 Baldesberger, S., Bauersfeld, U., Candinas, R. et al. Sinus node disease and arrhythmias in the long-term follow-up of former professional cyclists. *Eur Heart J* 2008; **29**: 71–8.

24 Horner, J.M. and Ackerman, M.J. Ventricular ectopy during treadmill exercise stress testing in the evaluation of long QT syndrome. *Heart Rhythm* 2008; **5**: 1690–4.

13 Effective Echocardiographic Assessment of the Athlete: Basic Examination to Advanced Imaging Techniques

David Oxborough

Research Institute for Sports and Exercise Sciences, Liverpool John Moores University, Liverpool, UK

Introduction

Echocardiography is a routine investigation that provides the operator with a 'window' into the structure and function of the heart. The role of echocardiography as a primary investigation in the pre-participation screening of the athlete is debatable, but its value within a secondary care setting is unequivocal (i.e. acting upon abnormal electrocardiographic (ECG) findings or in the assessment of an athlete with symptoms and/or family history of sudden cardiac death (SCD)). In the past, the grey zone between physiological adaptation and cardiac pathology was large and the sensitivity and specificity of echocardiography were poor. The advent of new echocardiographic technologies employed at rest and/or during exercise has improved the diagnostic capabilities of the discipline. In conjunction with a greater understanding of what is considered 'normal' for the athlete's heart, these newer technologies have helped to narrow the effective grey zone and provide renewed confidence in effective athlete management.

The aim of this chapter is to describe a practical and systematic process for undertaking an echocardiogram in an athlete in order to differentiate physiological adaptation from cardiac pathology. There are generally four stages to the examination: (i) reflection on pre-examination details obtained from the ECG, clinical questionnaires/examinations and specific athlete demographics: (ii) examination utilising conventional echocardiographic techniques at rest; (iii) application of novel techniques at rest; and (iv) consideration of the need to obtain functional data during a short exercise stimulus. In support of this process, diagnostic algorithms to aid in interpretation have been provided.

Stage 1: Pre-echocardiographic Information

As with any referral for echocardiography, adequate information should be provided to guide the operator towards the focus of the examination. An understanding of athlete demographics, including age, sex, body size, ethnicity and sporting discipline, will also enable a more accurate interpretation (see Table 13.1). It is

IOC Manual of Sports Cardiology, First Edition. Edited by Mathew G. Wilson, Jonathan A. Drezner and Sanjay Sharma.
© 2017 International Olympic Committee. Published 2017 by John Wiley & Sons, Ltd.

Sex	Cardiac chamber dimensions in female athletes rarely fall outside of the established 'normal range'. In particular, a left ventricular wall thickness >11mm warrants further investigation It is common for both female and male athletes to demonstrate a degree of eccentric remodelling of all cardiac chambers
Age	Highly trained junior athletes still develop cardiac remodelling in response to physiological conditioning, but this is often at a lower magnitude than in senior athletes That aside, where structural values fall outside the echocardiographic 'normal ranges', a functional assessment is key
Ethnicity	Left and right ventricular cavity sizes are similar between African/Afro-Carribean and White athletes, but wall thicknesses and left atrium size are often larger in the African/Afro-Carribean athlete There is a lack of data pertaining to the structure and function of Asian athletes, although there is no significant difference in ECG findings between West Asian and white athletes. The lack of available data on Asian ethnicity suggests that standard criteria as applied to white athletes should be utilised
Body surface area (BSA)	The relationship between body size and chamber dimensions is well established, and therefore *all* chamber dimensions should be indexed for BSA. That aside, cardiac adaptation to exercise involves eccentric hypertrophy beyond what may be attributable to body composition alone
Symptoms	A history of exertional chest pain, syncope or near-syncope, irregular heartbeat or palpitations, shortness of breath or fatigue out of proportion with the degree of exertion should direct the operator to closely assess for potential causes of sudden cardiac death (SCD). Symptoms are not specific, and therefore it is important to ensure all possible causes are excluded. That aside, it is important to be aware that exertional chest pain may direct further evaluation for coronary anomalies, whilst syncope may be related to outflow obstruction or an arrhythmogenic substrate, such as in arrhythmogenic right ventricular cardiomyopathy (ARVC) or hypertrophic cardiomyopathy (HCM)
ECG changes	The types of ECG change that present on an athlete's ECG will further guide the focus of the examination. For example, T-wave inversion in leads V1–V3 will direct a more focused assessment of the right heart. Lateral T-wave inversion is considered pathological and warrants further investigation
Training volume/level	Elite athletes are likely to demonstrate a greater degree of physiological cardiac adaptation than those who train at a much lower intensity
Sporting type	It is apparent that specific sporting disciplines create a specific stimulus that directs the degree of eccentric hypertrophy. Endurance athletes (cyclists, rowers, long-distance runners) are likely to have a greater degree of eccentric hypertrophy of all chambers than athletes who engage in sport of a combined stimulus (soccer, tennis, hockey) or strength (powerlifting, wrestling, judo)

Table 13.1 Demographic factors that require consideration prior to examination

outside the scope of this chapter to provide an in-depth assessment of all of these contributing factors, but see Chapter 5 and the following sources: Baggish and Wood [1], Riding et al. [2], Sheikh and Sharma [3], Whyte et al. [4] and Utomi et al. [5].

It is also important, a priori, to document, where possible, the normal ranges for data to be collected in any structured echocardiogram. Due to the multifactorial nature of the athlete's heart phenotype, it is challenging to provide a clear normal range. In view of this, this chapter recommends a common-sense approach that utilises standard nonathlete normative data as a starting point. Where values fall outside of the 'normal range' for a nonathlete, a functional assessment is key. At every stage, a consideration of athlete demographics should be integrated into the final interpretation, and algorithms to aid this process are presented at the relevant points within the chapter. In addition, data from key studies and meta-analyses for left ventricular size and function in female and male athletes [4–6] have been included (see Table 13.2). Table 13.2 also provides non-gender-specific cut-offs for right ventricular structure, obtained from three large studies [7–9]. It is important to acknowledge that body size directly influences cardiac size, and in the extremes of anthropometry, values above the proposed upper limits may be observed [2]. In view of this, the data in both the tables and the diagnostic algorithms should only be used to guide subsequent assessment, rather than to provide definitive diagnostic information.

Many of the echocardiographic indices of structure and function can be affected by volume load [10] and recent high-intensity training [11], and hence it is appropriate to ensure that the athlete is well hydrated and refrains from exercise for at least 6 hours prior to the examination. There are also data to suggest that the

Parameter	Male athlete	Female athlete
Left ventricular dimension diastole (mm)	59	56
Left ventricular interventricular septal thickness (mm)	12	11
Left ventricular posterior wall thickness (mm)	11	11
Left ventricular mass (g)	263	243
RVOT$_1$ (mm)	44	
RVOT$_2$ (mm)	41	
RVD$_1$ (mm)	49	
RVD$_2$ (mm)	44	
RVD$_3$ (mm)	92	

Table 13.2 Upper limits for left and right ventricular structures in elite athletes

RVOT, right ventricular outflow tract; RVD, right ventricular dimension.

magnitude of athletic cardiac adaptation increases in tandem with the progression of the competitive sporting season [12,13]. It is therefore important to give some consideration to seasonal variance, particularly when undertaking a serial assessment.

Stage 2: Standard Echocardiographic Examination

The athlete's echocardiogram should not be considered as basic or minimal, and therefore current echocardiographic guidelines for a complete examination should be followed [14]. According to the American Society of Echocardiography (ASE), the examination should utilise the range of acoustic windows available. In addition, two-dimensional (2D) Doppler, M-mode Doppler and tissue Doppler imaging (TDI) should all be integrated into the routine assessment. The examination should be undertaken using an ultrasound system that is capable of acquiring data from the specific modalities under the control of an experienced and accredited sonographer. The use of a quality-assurance programme will help to ensure standards are high and that parity is evidenced between operators [15].

The Left Ventricle

The structure of the athlete's left ventricle adapts in response to repeated exposure to an increased volume or pressure load during acute exercise. The extent and magnitude of phenotypical expression are dependent upon the athlete's demographic profile [1]. Although there is growing evidence to refute the existence of true physiological concentric hypertrophy (increase in wall thicknesses with normal left ventricular cavity size) [16], the presence of left ventricular eccentric hypertrophy (balanced increase in wall thicknesses and cavity size) is well established (see Figure 13.1) [6]. The presence of hypertrabeculation (more than three trabeculations) is common in highly trained athletes, and appears to be more prevalent in athletes of African/Afro-Caribbean ethnicity (see Figure 13.2) [17]. In view of this, it is important that the examination involves accurate and reproducible measurements, including cavity dimensions, wall thicknesses and left ventricular mass.

It is not uncommon to observe 'reduced' left ventricular systolic function, as determined by global ejection fraction [12] and/or systolic myocardial velocities, particularly in those athletes with large ventricles and slow heart rates. This is a consequence of the resting state, where the large ventricle is able to generate an adequate stroke volume with minimal contractility. In these athletes, it is important to exclude pathology, and an assessment following a short exercise stimulus may be warranted (see later). Chronic cardiac adaptation from exercise training does not cause any degradation in left ventricular diastolic function [18], and there is some evidence to suggest that early diastolic function in the athlete, even at rest, is superior to that in a sedentary individual [19,20], with early to late diastolic ratios (E/A) from both Doppler and TDI often being above 2. In mild phenotypes of conditions such as hypertrophic cardiomyopathy (HCM) and dilated cardiomyopathy (DCM), it is unlikely that significant diastolic dysfunction will exist, and hence a more subtle reduction in left ventricular relaxation may be apparent. This may manifest as a reduction in the E/A

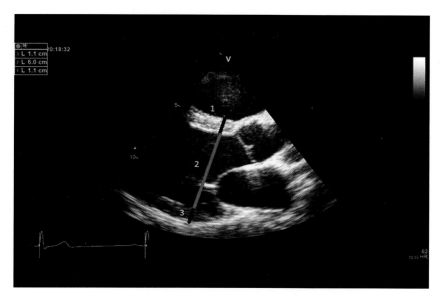

Figure 13.1 Parasternal long-axis orientation highlighting increased left ventricular cavity size in an elite athlete

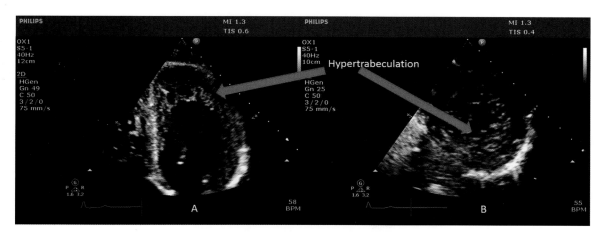

Figure 13.2 Left ventricular hypertrabeculation in an elite athlete

ratio (not necessarily reversed, but close to 1), in conjunction with absolute values of early diastolic myocardial velocities (E′) <9 cm.s^{-1}. These findings are by no means clear indicators of pathology, but should prompt the operator to request further investigations. Figure 13.3 highlights the transmitral E/A ratio and septal myocardial velocities in an athlete and a patient with a very mild phenotype of HCM.

Linear dimensions should be made from a parasternal long-axis orientation as per standard recommendations [14]. It is important to remember that values from M-mode and 2D echocardiography can vary, and therefore it is recommended that the same modality is used consistently. Due to the heterogeneous phenotype expression in pathological left ventricular hypertrophy, it is considered appropriate to provide a range of measurements of wall thickness from throughout the ventricle. This can be achieved by measuring the anteroseptum, the inferosetpum, the posterior wall and the lateral wall from the base and mid left ventricular levels using a parasternal short-axis orientation. In addition, two measurements at the apex can be used to exclude apical hypertrophy (see Figure 13.4).

Left ventricular geometry should be determined using a combination of left ventricular mass and relative wall thickness. Relative wall thickness is calculated by summating septal and posterior wall thickness in diastole and dividing into the left ventricular diastolic cavity dimension. Left ventricular geometry can be reported as 'normal', 'concentric remodelling' (increased relative wall thickness (>0.42) with normal

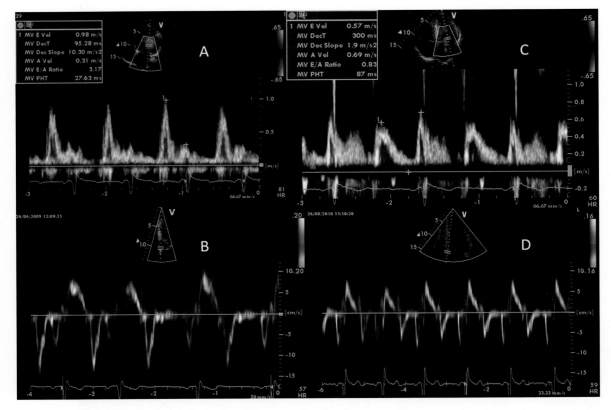

Figure 13.3 Transmitral Doppler and septal myocardial velocities from an elite athlete (A and B) and a patient with a mild phenotype of HCM (C and D)

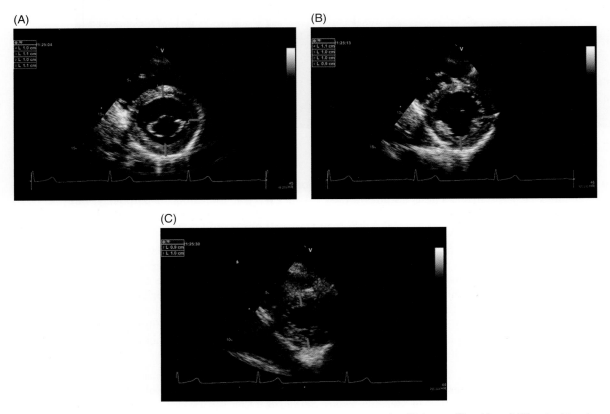

Figure 13.4 Location of left ventricular wall thickness measurements at the (A) base, (B) mid and (C) apical levels

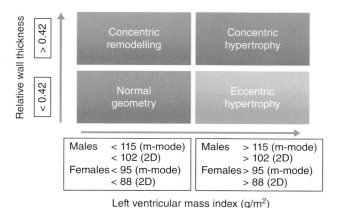

Figure 13.5 Schematic diagram demonstrating criteria for left ventricular geometry

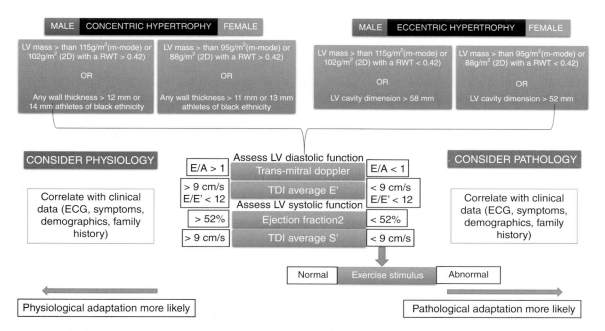

Figure 13.6 Diagnostic algorithm for the assessment of the left ventricle in the athlete

mass), 'concentric hypertrophy' (increased relative wall thickness (>0.42) and mass) or eccentric hypertrophy (normal relative wall thickness (<0.42) with increased mass) according to published criteria (see Figure 13.5) [14].

Left ventricular end-diastolic and systolic volumes should be calculated using a Simpsons biplane methodology, and a global ejection fraction can be derived. In order to assess left ventricular global diastolic function, standard transmitral Doppler should be utilised, providing peak velocities in early (E) and late (A) diastole and their ratio (E/A), early diastolic deceleration time and isovolumic relaxation time. Pulsed-wave TDI should be included in the standard examination and should be assessed at the septal and lateral mitral annulus as a minimum. An overall grading of left ventricular diastolic function should be offered, and additional measurements can be made where appropriate, in accordance with diastolic guidelines [21].

The diagnostic algorithm seen in Figure 13.6 provides a workflow guide for interpretation of the athlete's left ventricle. Left ventricular geometry should be the initial starting point, followed by a full functional assessment. Table 13.2 provides a guideline of upper limits, based on pooled data.

The Right Ventricle

During acute exercise, the right ventricle is subjected to a disproportionate wall stress [22], adapting in conjunction with an elevated preload. The primary manifestation is eccentric hypertrophy. There is no evidence to suggest that any athlete develops right ventricular concentric hypertrophy; if this is found then further investigations are warranted. Like the left ventricle, the right ventricle appears to adapt to a greater extent in athletes involved in highly dynamic sports, such as rowing, cycling and football; there is little evidence to support right ventricular adaptation in resistance-based athletes [8]. The location of the adaptation is important in view of the geometrically complex right ventricle. There is a greater degree of adaptation at the right ventricle inflow (sinus) than at the outflow (infundibulum), and this is a useful marker for athletic adaptation [7]. These data are supported elsewhere [9], and they highlight the extent of right ventricular adaptation in the athletic population. Figure 13.7 demonstrates marked right ventricular enlargement at the inflow, with an increased right to left ventricle ratio in an elite athlete.

The justification for the assessment of right ventricular structure in the pre-participation screening setting is primarily based on confirming or excluding arrhythmogenic right ventricular cardiomyopathy (ARVC). Conventional echocardiography has relatively poor sensitivity for ARVC, due to a variable phenotypic expression and disease progression [23]. In view of this, it is extremely important to provide accurate linear right ventricular dimensions in order to exclude the presence of major echocardiographic criteria for the disease [24]. The specificity of echocardiography for ARVC is lower in athletes than in the general population and is driven by physiological right ventricular enlargement. This is confounded by limited normative athletic right ventricular values and rather conservative normal ranges for the general population [25]. It is therefore important to provide a functional assessment of the right ventricle and to be aware that major criteria for ARVC require both structural and functional elements. Conventional and 2D imaging using fractional area change (FAC) and tricuspid plane systolic excursion (TAPSE) are very useful in such situations, in that measurements of longitudinal function and overall area change are usually normal in the athlete [8]. Furthermore, the often localised dysfunction observed in ARVC is unlikely to occur in the athlete's heart.

In order to fully assess right ventricular structure, a range of measurements are recommended. The outflow can be assessed based on parasternal long- and short-axis orientations to provide linear dimensions in end-diastole of the proximal outflow ($RVOT_{PLAX}$ and $RVOT_1$) and distal outflow ($RVOT_2$) (see Figure 13.8). Lateral movement of the transducer from an apical four-chamber orientation will allow for a modified image of the right ventricular sinus/inflow, and careful rotation will allow the ultrasound beam to interrogate the widest part of the right ventricle, whilst ensuring the aortic root is closed. A linear dimension of the widest point in the first third will give RVD_1, mid-level is defined at the level of the left ventricular papillary muscle as RVD_2, and the length measured from apex to tricuspid annulus is termed RVD_3 (see Figure 13.9). Right ventricular area should be traced in both diastole and systole, and a right ventricular fractional area charge

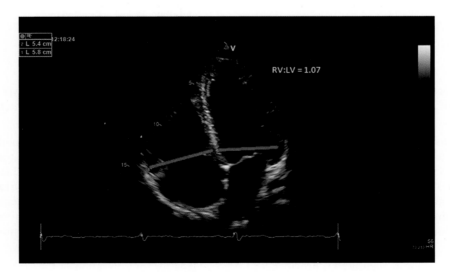

Figure 13.7 Apical four-chamber orientation demonstrating disproportionate enlargement of the right ventricular cavity in an elite athlete

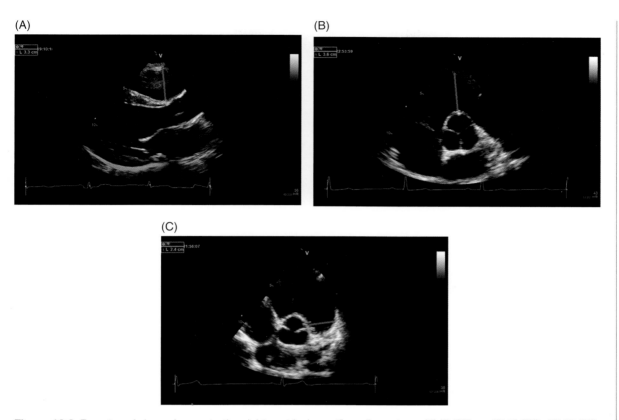

Figure 13.8 Parasternal views demonstrating right ventricular outflow dimensions: (A) $RVOT_{PLAX}$, (B) $RVOT_1$, (C) $RVOT_2$

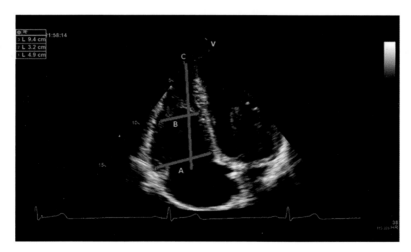

Figure 13.9 Modified apical four-chamber orientation demonstrating right ventricular inflow dimensions: (A) RVD_1, (B) RVD_2, (C) RVD_3

(RVFAC) can be calculated based on the area difference divided by the end-diastolic area. TAPSE can be achieved by moving the transducer medially and aligning longitudinal right ventricular lateral wall movement with the ultrasound beam. In addition, TDI should be acquired from the lateral tricuspid annulus and systolic and diastolic velocities should be reported. Although TDI-derived myocardial velocities are not part of the 'echocardiographic criteria' for ARVC, a reduced systolic velocity $<12\,cm.s^{-1}$ should raise suspicion (see Figure 13.10). It is also sensible to provide a measure of pulmonary artery systolic pressure as derived from the tricuspid regurgitant continuous-wave Doppler signal.

The diagnostic algorithm for interpretation of the right ventricular is presented in Figure 13.11.

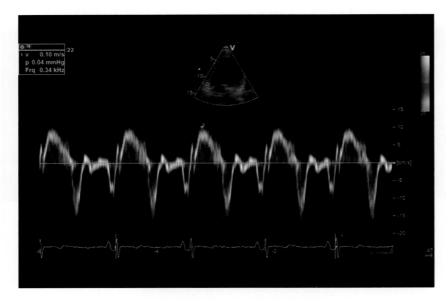

Figure 13.10 Pulsed-wave TDI of the right ventricular lateral wall demonstrating systolic myocardial velocity <12 cm.s^{-1}

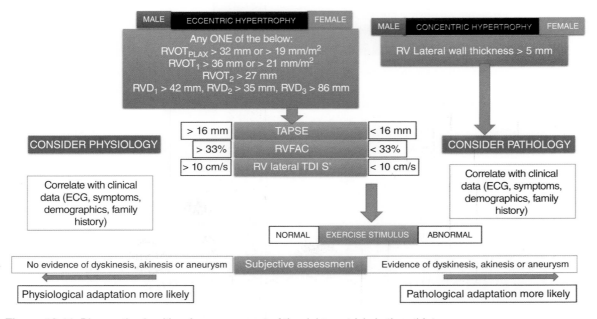

Figure 13.11 Diagnostic algorithm for assessment of the right ventricle in the athlete

The Left and Right Atria

In the myopathic heart, atrial enlargement occurs secondary to an elevation in ventricular filling pressures [26] or coexisting valve disease with or without the presence of ventricular systolic dysfunction [27]. This is a pertinent point, in that atrial dilatation appears to be a common morphological adaptation in the athlete's heart [28,29]. Like ventricular structure, atrial enlargement in the athlete appears to be more prevalent in those involved in highly dynamic sporting activities such as rowing, cycling, ice hockey and football [30]. Athletes involved in a low-dynamic sporting discipline (<50% oxygen consumption) do not appear to develop left or right atrial enlargement [31]. It is likely the stimulus for atrial dilatation is therefore related to an increase in preload during acute isotonic exercise. There are very few data related to the impact of

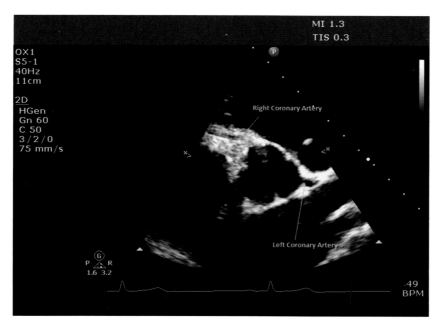

Figure 13.12 Parasternal short-axis orientation demonstrating left and right coronary ostia

other athlete demographics on atrial adaptation, but it is likely that ethnicity, gender and age will have a small but significant effect. In the pre-participation screening setting, the presence of atrial dilatation should not raise any concerns, as long as there is no evidence of delayed ventricular relaxation or elevation in filling pressures. That aside, it is sensible to make an accurate assessment of atrial volume using a biplane method for completeness and for serial assessment.

The incidence of atrial arrhythmias is more common in veteran endurance athletes [32], and although the mechanisms are not fully understood, there is evidence in the general population relating atrial size to arrhythmic burden [33]. In this population, echocardiography may play an important role in providing predictive criteria (elevated left atrial size) for the development of more frequent paroxysmal or even chronic atrial fibrillation.

The Coronary Ostia

It has been reported that coronary artery anomalies account for between 14 and 19% of SCD in young athletes [34–36]. Echocardiography can play an important role in excluding any abnormality by identifying the accurate location of the left and right coronary ostia, particularly in those athletes who are symptomatic. The ostia are located using a parasternal short-axis orientation at the level of the aortic valve, and careful tilting and rotation of the transducer is required to provide clear imaging of the vessels (see Figure 13.12). When the ostia cannot be visualised, further investigations are recommended.

Stage 3: Novel Echocardiographic Indices

Strain Imaging

The exponential development in ultrasound imaging technology over the past few decades has led to a significant improvement in the quality and availability of quantitative analysis tools for the assessment of cardiac mechanics. A 2013 professional body consensus statement from the American, European and Japanese Societies of Echocardiography [37] described the important *potential* role that strain imaging may have in a range of clinical conditions. It stated that based on a lack of consistency in vendor methodology and variable reproducibility, the techniques are still not ready for routine practice. The JUSTICE study [38] was aimed at establishing normative longitudinal strain from different vendors and patient ages, and although there is some vendor variance, this is less apparent between the ages of 20 and 40 (elite athlete age). When considering the role of strain imaging in differentiating physiology from pathology, it is important to draw from these papers and provide a common-sense approach to its application. There are a number of important points that require consideration prior to integrating the technique into the examination: (i) do not rely solely on strain imaging as a means to differentiate physiological from pathological cardiac adaptation; (ii) standardise the methodology, including optimisation of frame rates, depth, region of interest and equipment manufacturer; and (iii) consider the timing/profile of the waveforms, as well as peak values. This chapter focuses on the use of strain derived from a myocardial speckle-tracking technique (Lagangrian strain), which will provide different values to those obtained from a tissue-velocity (Eulerian) dataset [39]. Having raised these important issues, it is appropriate to highlight the corroborative value of the technique, which is achieved by supporting and building upon information generated from conventional 2D, Doppler and TDI modalities.

The Left Ventricle

Left ventricular mechanics are complex. During systole, myocardial shortening occurs in both longitudinal and circumferential planes. The outcome of reduced myocyte length and the law of conservation of mass is a displacement of the muscle mass into the left ventricular cavity in the form of radial thickening. In addition, the longitudinal fibres are arranged in a helical manner from base to apex, resulting in rotation/twist in opposite directions at the base and apex, leading in turn to torsion down the length of the ventricle. Collectively, these forces work to produce an optimal stroke volume. Resting cardiac mechanics in the athlete's heart have been described, albeit with some inconsistencies. A 90-day endurance-training programme in university rowers induced an increase in longitudinal and radial strain, but with regional changes in circumferential strain (increased free wall strain and decreased septal strain) [40]. The higher levels of strain observed in this study have also been observed in cross-sectional studies [41], with others demonstrating a higher magnitude of left ventricular twist in the athletic population [42]. The findings from other studies are in contrast to these data and highlight reduced systolic mechanics in athletes when compared to sedentary controls [43]. These heterogeneous findings are probably linked to the individual variability observed in structural adaptation and very likely related to left and, more importantly, right ventricular geometry. Figure 13.13 highlights the strain profiles resulting from a range of left ventricular mechanisms in an elite boxer prior to and following 3 months of intense resistance and endurance training (1 week prior to an international fight) [44]. Note the marked reduction in basal radial and septal circumferential strain and the increase in inferoposterior circumferential strain, probably secondary to right ventricular enlargement. It is also apparent that there is preserved global longitudinal strain and increased torsion at 3 months. Not all athletes develop right-sided enlargement as those with a resistance focus to their sporting discipline do. The strain profiles of the latter will be different to those of the athlete engaged in endurance training and more in keeping with those seen prior to the 3 months' intensive training shown in Figure 13.13.

In the HCM heart, longitudinal fibres (whose abundance is greater within the ventricular endocardium) may become fibrosed or ischaemic and therefore dysfunctional. In this setting, circumferential fibres will compensate and overall ejection fraction will be maintained. Global left ventricular longitudinal strain in patients with HCM, elite athletes with hypertrophy and sedentary controls has been studied [45], showing a lack of any difference in global strain between athletes and controls but a marked reduction in peak strain in the HCM patients. It is apparent that global longitudinal strain provides similar discriminatory power to standard conventional echocardiographic parameters. Other studies have demonstrated similar findings [41], but all show clear abnormal HCM phenotypes that are apparent from conventional imaging alone. The diagnostic challenge is, therefore, not in this patient group but in those athletes in the grey zone (i.e. possible mild phenotypes of HCM). A unique study provided data from HCM patients and athletes with similar wall thicknesses and applied longitudinal and circumferential strain analyses [46]. It demonstrated a lower endocardial longitudinal strain in HCM compared to professional football players, with no significant difference in circumferential strain. These peak values in isolation provided relatively poor sensitivity and specificity, but when used in ratio to relative wall thickness, specificity was as high as 95%. Furthermore, a small study in HCM patients and athletes shows that a global longitudinal strain value of less than −10% provides sensitivity and specificity of 80 and 95%, respectively, which can be further improved when incorporating standard TDI cut-offs [47]. Figure 13.14 highlights global longitudinal and circumferential strain in a patient with HCM. Note the variability in regional values, with basal longitudinal strain below −10% and peak deformation extending past aortic valve closure, as well as the compensation in circumferential function, required maintain stroke volume. Compare this to the elite athlete in Figure 13.13B,C.

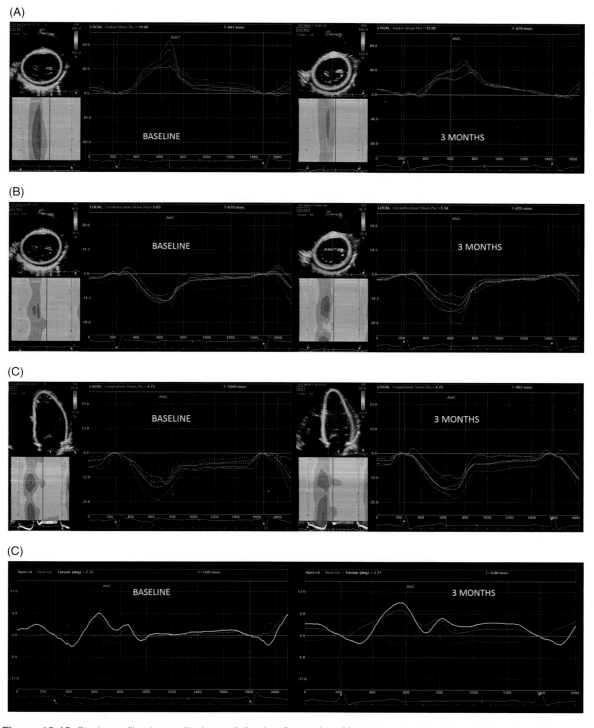

Figure 13.13 Strain profiles in an elite boxer following 3 months of intensive mixed training: (A) basal radial, (B) basal circumferential, (C) longitudinal, (D) twist/torsion

Other work has highlighted a marked reduction in left ventricular mechanics, including ventricular twist, in patients with overt phenotypes of HCM [48]. There is, however, a lack of data pertaining to comprehensive mechanics in those patients with a mild phenotype of the disease. It is clear that further work is required to fully profile the HCM heart from a mechanical perspective, and at this stage strain imaging provides only additional support to conventional data.

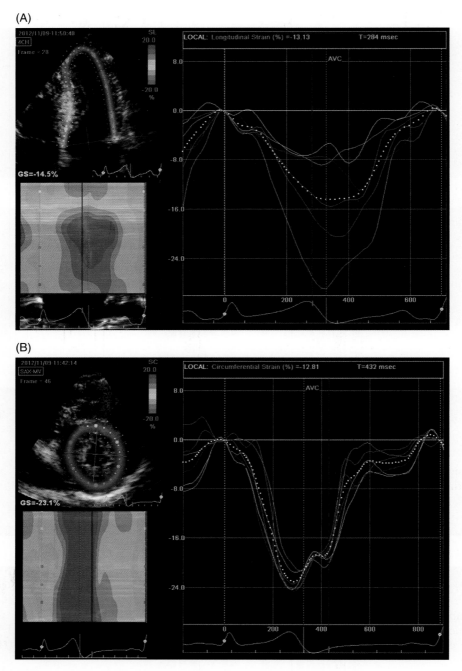

Figure 13.14 Longitudinal and circumferential strain profiles in nonobstructive HCM

As already discussed, the differentiation of DCM from athlete's heart can be challenging due to some athletes presenting with lower normal ejection fractions and systolic TDI myocardial velocities. Longitudinal strain has been highlighted as an early marker of left ventricular dysfunction in idiopathic and extrinsic DCM [49], and, therefore, may provide value in excluding early pathological progression in the athletic population. It is not possible to define an absolute cut-off, but serial assessment may be more insightful. Where values are borderline or mildly reduced, follow-up echocardiography can be used to determine whether there is a further reduction in strain. Data obtained from patients undergoing chemotherapy highlight a 10–15% decrease in global longitudinal strain, predicting a future reduction in left ventricular ejection fraction [50]. Figure 13.15 demonstrates global longitudinal strain in a patient with DCM and only

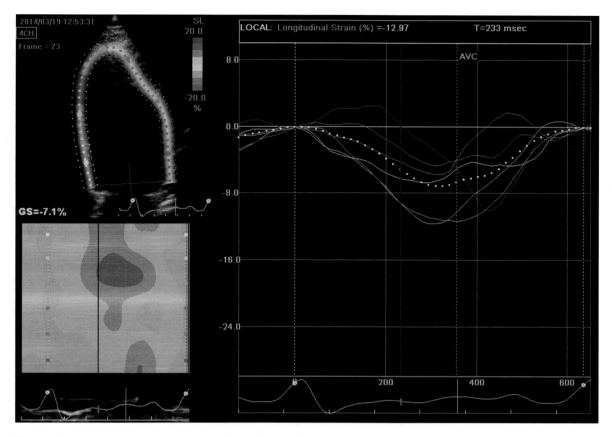

Figure 13.15 Longitudinal strain in a patient with DCM (mildly enlarged left ventricle)

a mildly dilated left ventricular cavity (61 mm). In addition, timing data for left ventricular twist may be helpful, with some evidence to suggest that left ventricular twist mechanics are prolonged in the early stages of DCM, resulting in a delayed untwist and mildly impaired relaxation [51].

The Right Ventricle

Cardiac mechanics within the right ventricle are very different to those of the left ventricle, and imaging is challenging due to the complex geometry. In view of this, right ventricular strain is predominantly constrained to longitudinal deformation [52], although some studies have attempted circumferential and multiplane assessment [53]. An important finding in the athlete's heart is what we consider to be a base-to-apex gradient, with higher strain values observed at the apex. This gradient has been shown to be higher in the athlete's heart than in healthy controls due to reduced basal strain in those athletes with enlarged cavities [54]. The mechanisms underpinning this are not fully understood, but it is likely that the change in right ventricular geometry and the need for a lower contractile state to generate an adequate stroke volume may play a part. Although it appears that there are regional variances in strain related to right ventricular geometry, global strain (as an average of the three myocardial segments: base, mid and apex) does not appear to be related to right ventricular size [7], and furthermore a cut-off value for differentiating physiology from pathology of less than −15% has been proposed.

There is currently a lack of data directly comparing cardiac mechanics in the athlete's heart to those in ARVC, although absolute peak values appeared to be significantly reduced in ARVC when compared to healthy controls in a study by Teske et al. [54]. It is important to note that overt functional abnormalities were apparent in most of the ARVC patients included in this study, and therefore strain imaging does not really provide additional value. In patients with mild phenotypes, absolute peak values may be nondiscriminatory, but the timing of peak contractility may be helpful. Figure 13.16 demonstrates longitudinal strain in an elite athlete and a 'negative phenotype'/'positive genotype' ARVC patient. Although there is a normal

(A)

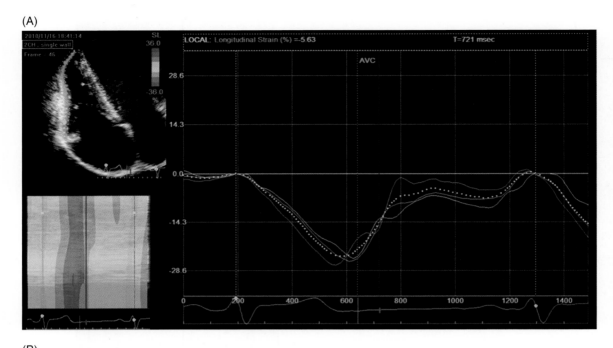

(B)

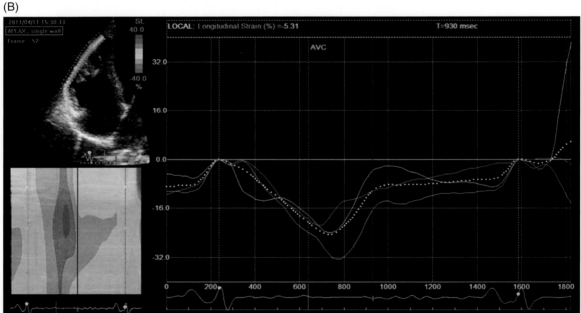

Figure 13.16 Right ventricular strain in (A) an elite athlete and (B) a 'negative-phenotype' ARVC patient

peak value (global right ventricular strain −25%), there is a delay in time to peak deformation after pulmonary valve closure in the patient with ARVC. This finding is anecdotal, and it is clear that further work is required to establish temporal strain profiles in a range of patients with ARVC.

3D Echocardiography

Three-dimensional (3D) ultrasound imaging is a relatively recent development, allowing for real-time assessment of cardiac chambers and function. The technique is now becoming useful in the clinical setting [14] and has been used to determine structure in the athlete's heart [55]. The few studies that have applied the technique

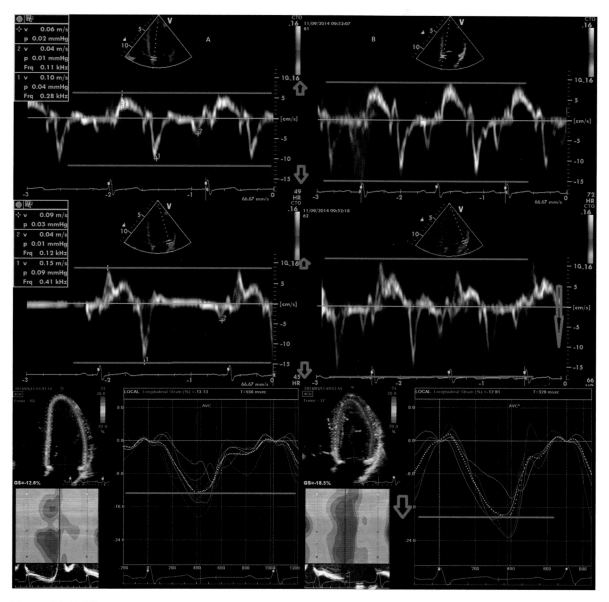

Figure 13.17 TDI and strain profiles (A) at rest and (B) following a short exercise stimulus in an elite athlete

to the left ventricle have not observed anything unique when compared to what we understand from 2D imaging (i.e. chamber enlargement as determined by volumes and cardiac mass). D'Andrea et al. [56] conducted a large study aimed at determining right ventricular volumes and right ventricular ejection fractions in endurance- and strength-trained athletes, and their findings confirm what has already been established using 2D techniques. Imaging the right ventricle and excluding localised areas of hypertrophy, dyskinesis or aneurysm in order to exclude HCM/ARVC may provide value over and above that obtained from standard echocardiography [57]. Further work is required to realise the potential of this technique. There has been an attempt to define 3D strain imaging in the athletic population [58], but based on current technology and still relatively low frame rates, it is difficult to provide adequate rationale for its inclusion in the assessment of the athlete's heart.

Stage 4: The Role of Exercise

This chapter has frequently alluded to the potential diagnostic role of exercise testing in the athlete who presents with borderline to reduced ventricular systolic and/or diastolic function. The physiological mechanisms for this presentation are based upon the enlarged chamber requiring minimal contractility in order to maintain an adequate stroke volume at rest. During exercise, the athlete's heart is able to generate a much greater reserve than is seen in the nonathlete, allowing for the increased stroke volumes that are required for optimal cardiac output and arteriovenous oxygen exchange. This is demonstrated by an increase in contractility, improved untwist and, ultimately, early diastolic filling, as determined by conventional and strain imaging. In patients with DCM, the diseased myocardium is unable to generate sufficient reserve and contractility in response to an exercise stimulus, and contractility and filling do not improve or even deteriorate. A similar finding can be seen in the right ventricle of the athlete, with work by La Gerche et al. [59] highlighting a normalisation of reduced basal right ventricular strain during incremental exercise [59]. Although there is no evidence highlighting the direct right ventricular response to exercise in ARVC, the lack of ability to increase stroke volumes in pulmonary hypertension and the negative chronic impact of exercise in ARVC patients do suggest right ventricular reserve would be lower than is seen in physiological adaptation.

The type of exercise stimulus required has not been clearly defined, but a short isometric exercise has been shown to differentiate types of DCM, and a supine cycle ergometer causing an increase in heart rate of 50% should be sufficient [49]. Figure 13.17 demonstrates normal changes in TDI and strain following a short cycling exercise in a healthy athlete with low resting values.

Conclusion

This chapter has highlighted the important role of echocardiography in the assessment of the athlete's heart. Conventional 2D Doppler and TDI are fundamental to the assessment, and a high-quality, all-encompassing examination is required. When interpreting the results, it is important to consider the athlete's demographic profile, clinical correlates and family history and to provide a safe and considered opinion on the echocardiographic findings. The diagnostic algorithms can be used as a guide, but it is important to remember the heterogeneous presentation of both the athlete's heart and cardiomyopathies, and, therefore, a common-sense approach is sensible. The additional use of strain imaging and an exercise stimulus may aid the diagnosis, and it is important to acknowledge that multimodality and corroborative investigations are central to the overall assessment of the athlete.

References

1 Baggish, A.L. and Wood, M.J. Athlete's heart and cardiovascular care of the athlete: scientific and clinical update. *Circulation* 2011; **123**: 2723–35.
2 Riding, N.R., Salah, O., Sharma, S. et al. Do big athletes have big hearts? Impact of extreme anthropometry upon cardiac hypertrophy in professional male athletes. *Br J Sports Med* 2012; **46**(Suppl. 1): i90–7.
3 Sheikh, N. and Sharma, S. Impact of ethnicity on cardiac adaptation to exercise. *Nature Rev Cardiol* 2014; **11**: 198–217.
4 Whyte, G.P., George, K., Nevill, A. et al. Left ventricular morphology and function in female athletes: a meta-analysis. *Int J Sports Med* 2004; **25**: 380–3.
5 Utomi, V., Oxborough, D., Whyte, G.P. et al. Systematic review and meta-analysis of training mode, imaging modality and body size influences on the morphology and function of the male athlete's heart. *Heart* 2013; **99**: 1727–33.
6 Pelliccia, A., Culasso, F., Di Paolo, F.M. and Maron, B.J. Physiologic left ventricular cavity dilatation in elite athletes. *Ann Intern Med* 1999; **130**: 23–31.
7 Oxborough, D., Sharma, S., Shave, R. et al. The right ventricle of the endurance athlete: the relationship between morphology and deformation. *J Am Soc Echocardiogr* 2012; **25**: 263–71.
8 D'Andrea, A., Riegler, L., Golia, E. et al. Range of right heart measurements in top-level athletes: the training impact. *Int J Cardiol* 2013; **164**: 48–57.
9 Zaidi, A., Ghani, S., Sharma, R. et al. Physiological right ventricular adaptation in elite athletes of African and Afro-Caribbean origin. *Circulation* 2013; **127**: 1783–92.
10 Burns, A.T., La Gerche, A., D'Hooge, J. et al. Left ventricular strain and strain rate: characterization of the effect of load in human subjects. *Eur J Echocardiogr* 2010; **11**: 283–9.
11 Banks, L., Sasson, Z., Busato, M. and Goodman, J.M. Impaired left and right ventricular function following prolonged exercise in young athletes: influence of exercise intensity and responses to dobutamine stress. *J Appl Physiol* 2010; **108**: 112–19.
12 Abergel, E., Chatellier, G., Hagege, A. et al. Serial left ventricular adaptations in world-class professional cyclists: implications for disease screening and follow-up. *J Am Coll Cardiol* 2004; **44**: 144–9.
13 D'Ascenzi, F., Pelliccia, A., Cameli, M. et al. Dynamic changes in left ventricular mass and in fat-free mass in top-level athletes during the competitive season. *Eur J Prev Cardiol* 2015; **22**: 127–34.
14 Lang, R.M., Badano, L.P., Mor-Avi, V. et al. Recommendations for cardiac chamber quantification by echocardiography in adults: an update from the American Society of Echocardiography and the European Association of Cardiovascular Imaging. *J Am Soc Echocardiogr* 2015; **28**: 1–39.e14.

15 Marwick, T.H. When is a number not a number? Quality control arrives in the imaging laboratory. *JACC CardiovascI Imaging* 2011; **4**: 830–2.

16 Utomi, V., Oxborough, D., Ashley, E. et al. Predominance of normal left ventricular geometry in the male 'athlete's heart'. *Heart* 2014; **100**: 1264–71.

17 Gati, S., Chandra, N., Bennett, R.L. et al. Increased left ventricular trabeculation in highly trained athletes: do we need more stringent criteria for the diagnosis of left ventricular non-compaction in athletes? *Heart* 2013; **99**: 401–8.

18 George, K.P., Naylor, L.H., Whyte, G.P. et al. Diastolic function in healthy humans: non-invasive assessment and the impact of acute and chronic exercise. *European J Appl Physiol* 2010; **108**: 1–14.

19 D'Ascenzi, F., Cameli, M., Zacà, V. et al. Supernormal diastolic function and role of left atrial myocardial deformation analysis by 2D speckle tracking echocardiography in elite soccer players. *Echocardiography* 2011; **28**: 320–6.

20 Kovacs, A., Apor, A., Nagy, A. et al. Left ventricular untwisting in athlete's heart: key role in early diastolic filling? *Int J Sports Med* 2014; **35**: 259–64.

21 Nagueh, S.F., Appleton, C.P., Gillebert, T.C. et al. Recommendations for the evaluation of left ventricular diastolic function by echocardiography. *J Am Soc Echocardiogr* 2009; **22**: 107–33.

22 La Gerche, A., Heidbüchel, H., Burns, A.T. et al. Disproportionate exercise load and remodeling of the athlete's right ventricle. *Med Sci Sports Exerc* 2011; **43**: 974–81.

23 Romero, J., Mejia-Lopez, E., Manrique, C. and Lucariello, R. Arrhythmogenic right ventricular cardiomyopathy (ARVC/D): a systematic literature review. *Clin Med Insights Cardiol* 2013; **7**: 97–114.

24 Marcus, F.I., McKenna, W.J., Sherrill, D. et al. Diagnosis of arrhythmogenic right ventricular cardiomyopathy/dysplasia: proposed modification of the task force criteria. *Circulation* 2010; **121**: 1533–41.

25 Rudski, L.G., Lai, W.W., Afilalo, J. et al. Guidelines for the echocardiographic assessment of the right heart in adults: a report from the American Society of Echocardiography endorsed by the European Association of Echocardiography, a registered branch of the European Society of Cardiology, and the Canadian Society of Echocardiography. *J Am Soc Echocardiogr* 2010; **23**: 685–713.

26 D'Andrea, A., De Corato, G., Scarafile, R. et al. Left atrial myocardial function in either physiological or pathological left ventricular hypertrophy: a two-dimensional speckle strain study. *Br J Sports Med* 2008; **42**: 696–702.

27 Roşca, M., Popescu, B., Beladan, C.C. et al. Left atrial dysfunction as a correlate of heart failure symptoms in hypertrophic cardiomyopathy. *J Am Soc Echocardiogr* 2010; **23**: 1090–8.

28 Pellicia, A., Maron, B., Di Paolo, F. et al. Prevelance and clinical significance of left atrial remodelling in competitive athletes. *J Am Coll Cardiol* 2005; **46**: 690–6.

29 Gabrielli, L., Bijnens, B.H., Butakoff, C. et al. Atrial functional and geometrical remodeling in highly trained male athletes: for better or worse? *European J Appl Physiol* 2014; **114**: 1143–52.

30 Wilhelm, M., Roten, L., Tanner, H. et al. Gender differences of atrial and ventricular remodeling and autonomic tone in nonelite athletes. *Am J Cardiol* 2011; **108**(10): 1489–95.

31 McClean, G., George, K., Lord, R. et al. Chronic adaptation of atrial structure and function in elite male athletes. *Eur Heart J Cardiovasc Imaging* 2014; **16**: 417–22.

32 Andersen, K., Farahmand, B., Ahlbom, A. et al. Risk of arrhythmias in 52 755 long-distance cross-country skiers: a cohort study. *Eur Heart J* 2013; **34**: 3624–31.

33 Cui, Q., Zhang, W., Wang, H. et al. Left and right atrial size and the occurrence predictors in patients with paroxysmal atrial fibrillation. *Int J Cardiol* 2008; **130**: 69–71.

34 Maron, B.J., Haas, T.S., Murphy, C.J. et al. Incidence and causes of sudden death in US college athletes. *J Am Coll Cardiol* 2014; **63**: 1636–43.

35 Harmon, K.G., Drezner, J., Wilson, M.G. and Sharma, S. Incidence of sudden cardiac death in athletes: a state-of-the-art review. *Br J Sports Med* 2014; **48**: 1185–92.

36 Sheppard, M.N. Aetiology of sudden cardiac death in sport: a histopathologist's perspective. *Br J Sports Med* 2012; **46**(Suppl. 1): i15–21.

37 Mor-Avi, V., Lang, R.M., Badano, L.P. et al. Current and evolving echocardiographic techniques for the quantitative evaluation of cardiac mechanics: ASE/EAE consensus statement on methodology and indications endorsed by the Japanese Society of Echocardiography. *J Am Soc Echocardiogr* 2011; **24**: 277–313.

38 Takigiku, K., Takeuchi, M., Izumi, C. et al. Normal range of left ventricular 2-dimensional strain. *Circ J* 2012; **76**: 2623–32.

39 Lord, R.N., George, K., Jones, H. et al. Reproducibility and feasibility of right ventricular strain and strain rate (SR) as determined by myocardial speckle tracking during high-intensity upright exercise: a comparison with tissue Doppler-derived strain and SR in healthy human hearts. *Echo Res Pract* 2014; **1**: 31–41.

40 Baggish, A.L., Yared, K., Wang, F. et al. The impact of endurance exercise training on left ventricular systolic mechanics. *Am J Physiol Heart Circ Physiol* 2008; **295**: H1109–16.

41 Richand, V., Lafitte, S., Reant, P. et al. An ultrasound speckle tracking (two-dimensional strain) analysis of myocardial deformation in professional soccer players compared with healthy subjects and hypertrophic cardiomyopathy. *Am J Cardiol* 2007; **100**: 128–32.

42 Weiner, R.B., Hutter, A.M., Wang, F. et al. The impact of endurance exercise training on left ventricular torsion. *JACC Cardiovasc Imaging* 2010; **3**: 1001–9.

43 Nottin, S., Doucende, G., Schuster-Beck, I. et al. Alteration in left ventricular normal and shear strains evaluated by 2D-strain echocardiography in the athlete's heart. *J Physiol* 2008; **586**: 4721–33.

44 Oxborough, D., George, K., Utomi, V. et al. Acute response and chronic stimulus for cardiac structural and functional adaptation in a professional boxer. *Oxf Med Case Rep* 2014; **1**: 65–8.

45 Afonso, L., Kondur, A., Simegn, M. et al. Two-dimensional strain profiles in patients with physiological and pathological hypertrophy and preserved left ventricular systolic function: a comparative analyses. *BMJ Open* 2012; **2**: 1–8.

46 Kansal, M.M., Lester, S.J., Surapaneni, P. et al. Usefulness of two-dimensional and speckle tracking echocardiography in 'gray zone' left ventricular hypertrophy to differentiate professional football player's heart from hypertrophic cardiomyopathy. *Am J Cardiol* 2011; **108**: 1322–6.

47 Butz, T., van Buuren, F., Mellwig, K. et al. Two-dimensional strain analysis of the global and regional myocardial function for the differentiation of pathologic and physiologic left ventricular hypertrophy: a study in athletes and in patients with hypertrophic cardiomyopathy. *Int J Cardiovasc Imaging* 2011; **27**(1): 91–100.

48 Zhang, H., Wang, H., Sun, T. et al. Assessment of left ventricular twist mechanics by speckle tracking echocardiography reveals association between LV twist and myocardial fibrosis in patients with hypertrophic cardiomyopathy. *Int J Cardiovasc Imaging* 2014; **30**(8): 1539–48.

49 Okada, M., Tanaka, H., Matsumoto, K. et al. Subclinical myocardial dysfunction in patients with reverse-remodeled dilated cardiomyopathy. *J Am Soc Echocardiogr* 2012; **25**: 726–32.

50 Plana, J.C., Galderisi, M., Barac, A. et al. Expert consensus for multimodality imaging evaluation of adult patients during and after cancer therapy: a report from the American Society of Echocardiography and the European Association of Cardiovascular Imaging. *J Am Soc Echocardiogr* 2014; **27**(9): 911–939.

51 Pacileo, G., Baldini, L., Limongelli, G. et al. Prolonged left ventricular twist in cardiomyopathies: a potential link between systolic and diastolic dysfunction. *Eur J Echocardiogr* 2011; **12**: 841–9.

52 Meris, A., Faletra, F., Conca, C. et al. Timing and magnitude of regional right ventricular function: a speckle tracking-derived strain study of normal subjects and patients with right ventricular dysfunction. *J Am Soc Echocardiogr* 2010; **23**: 823–31.

53 Forsha, D., Risum, N., Kropf, P.A. et al. Right ventricular mechanics using a novel comprehensive three-view echocardiographic strain analysis in a normal population. *J Am Soc Echocardiogr* 2014; **27**: 413–22.

54 Teske, A.J., Cox, M.G., De Boeck, B.W. et al. Echocardiographic tissue deformation imaging quantifies abnormal regional right ventricular function in arrhythmogenic right ventricular dysplasia/cardiomyopathy. *J Am Soc Echocardiogr* 2009; **22**: 920–7.

55 Schiros, C.G., Ahmed, M.I., Sanagala, T. et al. Importance of three-dimensional geometric analysis in the assessment of the athlete's heart. *Am J Cardiol* 2013; **111**: 1067–72.

56 D'Andrea, A., Riegler, L., Morra, S. et al. Right ventricular morphology and function in top-level athletes: a three-dimensional echocardiographic study. *J Am Soc Echocardiogr* 2012; **25**: 1268–76.

57 Atsumi, A., Ishizu, T., Kameda, Y. et al. Application of 3-dimensional speckle tracking imaging to the assessment of right ventricular regional deformation. *Circ J* 2013; **77**: 1760–8.

58 Vitarelli, A., Capotosto, L., Placanica, G. et al. Comprehensive assessment of biventricular function and aortic stiffness in athletes with different forms of training by three-dimensional echocardiography and strain imaging. *Eur Heart J Cardiovasc Imaging* 2013; **14**: 1010–20.

59 La Gerche, A., Burns, A.T., D'Hooge, J. et al. Exercise strain rate imaging demonstrates normal right ventricular contractile reserve and clarifies ambiguous resting measures in endurance athletes. *J Am Soc Echocardiogr* 2012; **25**: 253–62.e1.

14 Early Repolarisation in Athletes

Greg Mellor and Elijah R. Behr

Cardiac Research Centre, St George's University of London, London, UK

Introduction

The early repolarisation (ER) pattern was first described as an electrocardiographic (ECG) entity more than 50 years ago, and was shown to be more common in young adults, males, African/Afro-Caribbean (black) individuals and athletes [1]. Whilst originally thought to be entirely benign, recent evidence has demonstrated that ER is associated with an increased risk of sudden cardiac death (SCD).

Early Repolarisation Syndrome

In a landmark study, Haïssaguerre et al. [2] showed that ER, defined by J-point elevation ≥0.1 mV in the inferolateral leads, was more common in survivors of idiopathic ventricular fibrillation than in age- and sex-matched controls. The findings were replicated in other studies, leading to the recognition of early repolarisation syndrome (ERS) [3]. ERS is characterised by ventricular fibrillation in an individual (most often male) in the presence of ER on the ECG after exclusion of all other possible aetiologies. Characteristically, there is augmentation of the ER pattern at the time of the cardiac arrest, which usually occurs during sleep or at rest, when vagal tone is presumed to predominate.

Defining ER

Historical definitions of ER focused on the anterior and lateral precordial leads. An early report of 'the normal RS-T elevation variant' [1] describes 'elevated take-off of the ST-segment at the end of the QRS (the J junction) with downward concavity of the ST-segment and symmetrical T waves'. However, Haïssaguerre et al. [2] refined the diagnosis of ER, focusing on the inferior (II, III, aVF) and lateral (I, aVL, V4–V6) ECG leads. The right-sided precordial leads (V1–V3) were ignored to avoid confusion with Brugada syndrome and arrhythmogenic right ventricular cardiomyopathy (ARVC), both of which are associated with right ventricular depolarisation and repolarisation abnormalities. The defining feature of ER is elevation of the junction between the terminal QRS complex and the ST segment: the J-point. J-point elevation, the so-called 'J-wave', must be present in two consecutive leads and of >0.1 mV in amplitude to be considered positive (Figures 14.1–14.3). In addition to J-point amplitude, other features are significant. The J-point morphology may be described as notched, with a positive upstroke in the terminal portion of QRS, or slurred, with continuity between the QRS and ST segment (Figures 14.1–14.3). The contour of the associated ST segment is also important, and may differentiate between higher- and low-risk forms (see later). The ST segment is classified as rapidly ascending if there is ≥0.1 mV ST elevation within 100 ms of the J-point. Otherwise, it is classified as horizontal/descending (Figures 14.1–14.3). Indeed, the latter pattern is more common in cardiac arrest survivors [4].

IOC Manual of Sports Cardiology, First Edition. Edited by Mathew G. Wilson, Jonathan A. Drezner and Sanjay Sharma.

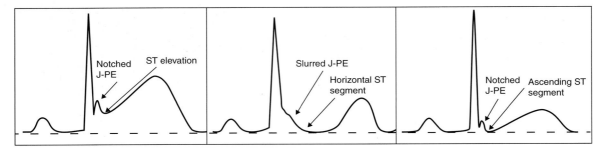

Figure 14.1 Schematic of varying ER morphologies. (A) High-amplitude J-point notching with ST elevation and a rapidly ascending ST segment. (B) Slurred J-point elevation with a horizontal ST segment (<0.1 mV ST elevation 100 ms after J-point). (C) Notched J-point elevation with a rapidly ascending ST segment (≥0.1 mV ST elevation 100 ms after J-point)

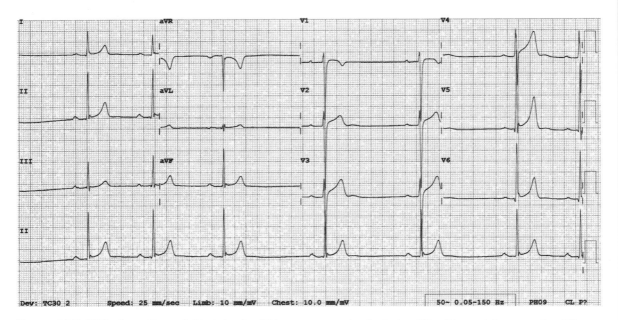

Figure 14.2 ECG of an elite cyclist training for 30 hours per week, displaying ER with a rapidly ascending ST segment typically seen in athletes. Note other ECG features of athletic training, including sinus bradycardia, first-degree heart block and isolated voltage criteria for LVH

ER in the General Population

Although idiopathic ventricular fibrillation and ERS are rare, interest in the ER pattern was fuelled by several large-cohort studies investigating the significance of the ER pattern in the general population. These demonstrated an increased risk of SCD associated with the ER pattern in middle age and beyond.

The largest study included 10 864 Finnish individuals with a mean age of 44 years at the time of enrolment [5]. ER was present in 5.8% of the cohort and individuals with ER in the inferior leads had an increased risk of death from arrhythmia (heart rate 1.43, 95%CI 1.06–1.94, p=0.03) over a 25-year follow-up period. This only became apparent, however, at least a decade after the initial ECG. High-amplitude (≥0.2 mV) J-point elevation in the inferior leads was associated with the highest risk (heart rate 2.92, 95%CI 1.45–5.89). The same investigators subsequently went on to identify high- and low-risk forms of ER by analysing the associated ST-segment morphology within the same population cohort (see previous definitions) [6]. Those with ER with a horizontal/descending ST segment had a higher risk of sudden arrhythmic death (age- and sex-adjusted heart rate 1.43, 95%CI 1.05–1.94) than those without ER, whereas individuals with ER and a

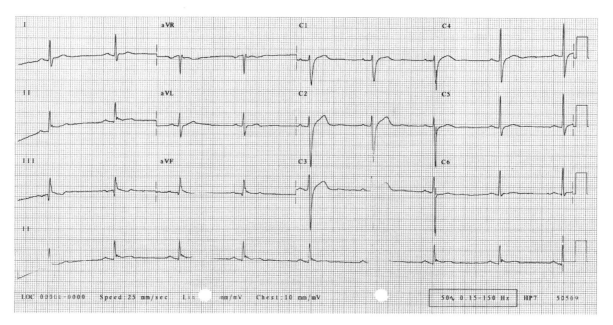

Figure 14.3 ECG of a cardiac arrest survivor diagnosed with ERS. The ECG shows high-amplitude inferior J-point notching with a horizontal/descending ST segment

rapidly ascending ST segment had no significantly increased risk (adjusted heart rate 0.89, 95%CI 0.52–1.55). In addition, ER has been shown to increase susceptibility to ventricular fibrillation in the context of other cardiac pathologies, including acute coronary syndrome, Brugada syndrome and long QT syndrome, and so is increasingly recognised as a risk modifier for ventricular arrhythmia [7–9]. The precise mechanism underlying the arrhythmogenesis of ER remains unclear. The prevailing view proposes enhanced and heterogeneous repolarising currents between the epi- and endocardium during phase 1 of the action potential, leading to a transmural voltage gradient and phase 2 re-entry [10]. Other investigators have suggested a subtle structural component in horizontal ER.

Prevalence of ER in Athletes

ER is more common in athletes than in the general population. Prevalence has been reported variably, depending on the definitions used and the population studied. Older reports show the prevalence to be as high as 58% in a cohort of marathon runners [11] using historical ER definitions. Reports from Italy's national pre-participation screening programme state 34% of adult elite athletes have the ER pattern, comprising 'upward ST-segment elevation in ≥2 peripheral or precordial leads, beginning from an elevated J-point and continuing with an upsloping shape into the T-wave' [12].

Care must be taken when comparing older studies that use historical definitions of ER to modern studies that refer to inferolateral J-point elevation. However, even when using modern definitions, ER remains common in athletes. In a study of 503 US college-level athletes, ER was present in 30% [13]. The presence of ER was associated with male gender and isolated voltage criteria for left ventricular hypertrophy (LVH). As in other studies, ER with a rapidly ascending ST segment was the predominant form in athletes, accounting for 85% of cases. ER was more commonly seen in the lateral than the inferior leads – another feature common to other athletic cohorts.

ER is a dynamic phenomenon that waxes and wanes as training levels vary. The relationship between ER and physical exercise was demonstrated in another cohort of US collegiate athletes who were studied before and after a 90-day period of athletic training [14]. Using modern definitions of ER, the prevalence in the initial cohort of 879 participants was 25.1%. A subgroup of 148 athletes was examined a second time after a 90-day training period. Athletes were either rowing crew (representing endurance athletes) or American football players (representing power athletes). In addition, these athletes had transthoracic echocardiography performed at baseline and after the training period. The prevalence of ER increased from 37.2 to 52.7% following the training period (p = 0.003). This increase was driven by changes seen in the endurance athletes (63.2 vs 39.7%, p = 0.03); the increase in the power athletes was not significant (44.9 vs 35.9%, p = 0.25). Both groups of athletes demonstrated features of structural athletic remodelling on echocardiography. There were, however, no significant associations between left ventricular parameters and the ER pattern, suggesting ER is a purely electrophysiological phenomenon. Increased vagal tone is thought to underlie the increase in ER seen with training, although there is little experimental evidence to confirm this.

Prognosis of ER in Athletes

There are no prospective studies of the prognosis of ER in athletes, and so its significance is not entirely known. Several studies have reported a benign prognosis in athletes with ER, but these are universally limited by small cohort sizes and/or short follow-up periods. In addition to the study of US college athletes, which reported no events in a total follow-up of around 1500 person-years, several other athlete cohorts have reported follow-up data. A Spanish study followed up 299 athletes, aged 20.1 ± 6.4 years at enrolment, for an average of 24 years (7176 person-years) [15]. ER was present in 31.4% of athletes (97.5% with a rapidly ascending ST segment). When assessed again after retirement from professional sport, ER remained in 54.3% of originally positive cases. Those in whom ER remained were more likely to have continued regular exercise for ≥5 hours per week (47.6 vs 28.5%, p = 0.004). There was no increased risk of cardiovascular events or mortality associated with ER. A study of 704 Italian Olympic-level athletes [16] reported that ER was present in 14%. There were no clinical events in the ER group after a mean follow-up period of 6 ± 4 years (4224 person-years). Whilst these results can be interpreted as reassuring, large prospective studies with long follow-up durations are required.

A single case–control study presented contrasting results, showing an association between inferolateral ER and SCD in athletes [17]. The ECGs of 21 athletes who had suffered a cardiac arrest were compared to those of 365 unmatched athletic controls taken during routine pre-participation screening. However, the definitions of ER were not in line with contemporary studies. The prevalence of J-waves and/or 'QRS slurring' was reported separately to the prevalence of 'ST elevation'. Furthermore, J-point elevation ≥0.05 mV was considered positive, rather than the accepted >0.1 mV cutoff. The authors concluded that QRS slurring in any inferolateral lead (28.6 vs 7.6%, p = 0.006) and 'a J-wave and/or QRS slurring without ST elevation in the inferior and lateral leads' were more prevalent in cardiac arrest victims (28.6 vs 7.9%, p = 0.007) than in athletic controls. Further limitations may also have contributed to this study's contradictory findings. The control group was not matched for age, sex or training volume, and consequently there was an unexpectedly low prevalence of ER. This was in stark contrast to other studies, which consistently show a high prevalence of ER in athletes. Notably, the example ECGs offered in the original paper show ER with a horizontal/descending ST segment in the cardiac arrest victim, compared to ER with a rapidly ascending ST segment in a healthy control. Whilst conclusions cannot be drawn from single examples, ER with a horizontal ST segment is not typical in athletes. It is possible to reanalyse the data from this study using the contemporary classification of ER. When presented in this way, the prevalence in healthy controls is much higher (51%). There is also no significant difference in ER prevalence between the two groups (57 vs 51%, p = 0.6). However, ER with a horizontal/descending ST segment does appear to be more common in the cardiac arrest group (38 vs 16%, p = 0.01). These 'reworked' results resemble other case–control studies of idiopathic ventricular fibrillation in nonathletes and are not suggestive of a higher risk associated with ER in athletes (Table 14.1).

It has been suggested that the most convincing evidence of the benign nature of ER in athletes is its high prevalence in this group [18]. Assuming an SCD rate in athletes of 1 : 100 000 per annum and a prevalence of ER of 25%, then even if every SCD victim had ER, the odds of SCD occurring in athletes with ER would be 1 : 25 000 per annum. Therefore, although the relative risk would be fourfold higher, the absolute increase in risk would only be 0.003%. The true incremental mortality risk would likely be even lower given that an alternative cause of death is found in the majority of athletic SCD.

Finally, it is worth reflecting upon the similarities between the historical descriptions of ER and modern descriptions of ER with a rapidly ascending ST segment. Both are associated with athletes and with a benign prognosis. J-point elevation in the inferior leads with a horizontal/descending ST segment appears to be associated with increased risk in the older general population. It is, however, uncommon in athletes, and not a feature of the 'athlete's ECG'. Its significance therefore remains unclear in this group.

	Case (n = 21)	Control (n = 365)	Relative risk	p
Any ER	12 (57)	187 (51)	1.1	0.6
Inferior	3 (14)	24 (7)	2.2	0.18
Lateral	3 (14)	107 (29)	0.5	0.14
Inferolateral	6 (29)	56 (15)	1.9	0.11
Ascending ER	4 (24)	149 (41)	0.5	0.08
Inferior	1 (5)	13 (4)	1.3	0.78
Lateral	2 (10)	79 (22)	0.4	0.18
Inferolateral	1 (5)	47 (13)	0.4	0.27
Horizontal ER	8 (38)	58 (16)	2.4	**0.01**
Inferior	2 (10)	11 (3)	3.2	0.11
Lateral	1 (5)	38 (10)	0.5	0.4
Inferolateral	5 (24)	9 (2)	9.7	**<0.001**

Table 14.1 Reworking of data produced by Cappato et al. [17] with more commonly used ER classifications. Cases with 'ST elevation' were included as having ER with a rapidly ascending ST segment, as per convention

Conclusion

ER is common in athletes. It is typically associated with a rapidly ascending ST segment and is more often seen in the lateral leads. The ECG pattern increases with endurance training and is expected to reduce following a period of de-training. Whilst there is a lack of evidence to fully confirm a benign prognosis of ER in athletes, there is also no evidence of clinically actionable increased risk. Therefore, the presence of ER with an ascending ST segment on an athlete's ECG should be considered a normal training-related phenomenon and should not prompt any further investigation [19]. Inferior ER associated with a horizontal/descending ST segment is not typical in athletes, and whilst it may be associated with a small increase in risk of SCD later in life, the lack of effective risk-stratification tools and the time lag between detection and increased risk preclude further investigation. As with any suspicious presentation, however, if there are sinister symptoms such as cardiac syncope or a family history of unexplained and/or premature SCD, then further investigation is warranted.

References

1 Wasserburger, R.H. and Alt, W.J. The normal RS-T segment elevation variant. *Am J Cardiol* 1961; **8**: 184–92.
2 Haïssaguerre, M., Derval, N., Sacher, F. et al. Sudden cardiac arrest associated with early repolarization. *New Engl J Med* 2008; **358**(19): 2016–23.
3 Priori, S.G., Wilde A.A., Horie, M. et al. Executive summary: HRS/EHRA/APHRS expert consensus statement on the diagnosis and management of patients with inherited primary arrhythmia syndromes. *Europace* 2013; **15**(10): 1389–406.
4 Rosso, R., Glikson, E., Belhassen, B. et al. Distinguishing 'benign' from 'malignant early repolarization': the value of the ST-segment morphology. *Heart Rhythm* 2012; **9**(2): 225–9.
5 Tikkanen, J.T., Anttonen, O., Junttila, M.J. et al. Long-term outcome associated with early repolarization on electrocardiography. *New Engl J Med* 2009; **361**(26): 2529–37.
6 Tikkanen, J.T., Junttila, M.J., Anttonen, O. et al. Early repolarization: electrocardiographic phenotypes associated with favorable long-term outcome. *Circulation* 2011; **123**(23): 2666–73.
7 Tikkanen, J.T., Wichmann, V., Junttila, M.J. et al. Association of early repolarization and sudden cardiac death during an acute coronary event. *Circ Arrhythm Electrophysiol* 2012; **5**(4): 714–18.
8 Kawata, H., Morita, H., Yamada, Y. et al. Prognostic significance of early repolarization in inferolateral leads in Brugada patients with documented ventricular fibrillation: a novel risk factor for Brugada syndrome with ventricular fibrillation. *Heart Rhythm* 2013; **10**(8): 1161–8.
9 Laksman, Z.W., Gula, L.J., Saklani, P. et al. Early repolarization is associated with symptoms in patients with type 1 and type 2 long QT syndrome. *Heart Rhythm* 2014; **11**(9): 1632–8.
10 Antzelevitch, C. and Yan, G.X. J-wave syndromes. From cell to bedside. *J Electrocardiol* 2011; **44**(6): 656–61.
11 Zoneraich, S., Rhee, J.J., Zoneraich, O. et al. Assessment of cardiac function in marathon runners by graphic noninvasive techniques. *Ann NY Acad Sci* 1977; **301**: 900–17.

12 Pelliccia, A., Culasso, F., Di Paolo, F.M. et al. Prevalence of abnormal electrocardiograms in a large, unselected population undergoing pre-participation cardiovascular screening. *Eur Heart J* 2007; **28**(16): 2006–10.

13 Junttila, M.J., Sager, S.J., Freiser, M. et al. Inferolateral early repolarization in athletes. *J Interv Card Electrophysiol* 2011; **31**(1): 33–8.

14 Noseworthy, P.A., Weiner, R., Kim, J. et al. Early repolarization pattern in competitive athletes: clinical correlates and the effects of exercise training. *Circ Arrhythm Electrophysiol* 2011; **4**(4): 432–40.

15 Serra-Grima, R., Doñate, M., Álvarez-García, J. et al. Long term follow-up of early repolarization pattern in elite athletes. *Am J Med* 2015; **128**(2): 192.e1–9.

16 Quattrini, F.M., Pelliccia, A., Assorgi, R. et al. Benign clinical significance of J-wave pattern (early repolarization) in highly trained athletes. *Heart Rhythm* 2014; **11**(11): 1974–82.

17 Cappato, R., Furlanello, F., Giovinazzo, V. et al. J wave, QRS slurring, and ST elevation in athletes with cardiac arrest in the absence of heart disease: marker of risk or innocent bystander? *Circ Arrhythm Electrophysiol* 2010; **3**(4): 305–11.

18 Noseworthy, P.A. and Baggish, A.L. The prevalence and clinical significance of J wave patterns in athletes. *J Electrocardiol* 2013; **46**(5): 424–6.

19 Corrado, D., Pelliccia, A., Heidbuchel, H. et al. Recommendations for interpretation of 12-lead electrocardiogram in the athlete. *Eur Heart J* 2010; **31**(2): 243–59.

15 Clinical (Laboratory) Exercise Testing

Jonathan Myers and Victor Froelicher

Palo Alto Veterans Affairs Health Care System and Stanford University, Stanford, CA, USA

Introduction

Exercise testing in athletes is concerned with: (i) optimising structured training programmes; (ii) evaluating aerobic capacity; (iii) diagnosing exercise-induced symptoms; or (iv) establishing the cardiovascular risks of exercise. The latter two points are important with respect to an athlete's age, where after 35 years, coronary atherosclerosis is a predominating concern. Prior to age 35 years however, the major concern is establishing a diagnosis and cardiovascular risk for inherited cardiovascular diseases (CVDs), including both the cardiomyopathies and arrhythmic disorders.

Basic Principles

Two basic principles of exercise physiology are important to understand in regard to exercise testing. First, from a physiological perspective, total body oxygen uptake and myocardial oxygen uptake are distinct in their determinants and in the way they are measured or estimated (Table 15.1). Total body or ventilatory oxygen uptake ($\dot{V}O_2$) is the amount of oxygen that is extracted from inspired air as the body performs work. Myocardial oxygen uptake is the amount of oxygen consumed by the heart muscle. The determinants of myocardial oxygen uptake include intramyocardial wall tension, contractility and heart rate. It has been shown that myocardial oxygen uptake can be reasonably estimated by the product of heart rate and systolic blood pressure (double product). This information is clinically valuable because exercise-induced angina often occurs at the same double product, where the higher the double product achieved, the better the myocardial perfusion. When this does not hold true, the influence of other factors should be suspected, such as a recent meal, unusual ambient temperature or coronary artery spasm.

Second, from a pathophysiological perspective, the electrocardiographic (ECG) response and angina are closely related to myocardial ischaemia (and coronary artery disease, CAD). In contrast, the hemodynamic responses (exercise capacity, systolic blood pressure and heart rate) to exercise can be influenced by myocardial ischaemia, myocardial dysfunction and/or peripheral responses. The severity of ischaemia or the amount of myocardium in jeopardy is known clinically to be inversely related to the heart rate, blood pressure and exercise level achieved. However, neither resting nor exercise ejection fraction correlate well with maximal oxygen uptake. In general, coronary anomalies and myocardial bridges do not consistently create myocardial ischaemia.

Concepts of Work

As exercise testing involves the measurement of work, there are several concepts of 'work' to understand. *Work is defined as force moving through a given distance ($W = F \times D$).* If muscle contraction results in mechanical movement, then work has been accomplished. *Force is equal to mass times acceleration ($F = M \times A$).* Any weight, for example, is a force that is undergoing the resistance provided by gravity. *The basic unit of force is the newton (N).*

IOC Manual of Sports Cardiology, First Edition. Edited by Mathew G. Wilson, Jonathan A. Drezner and Sanjay Sharma.

Myocardial oxygen consumption	$\approx$ Heart rate $\times$ systolic blood pressure (determinants include wall tension $\cong$ left ventricular pressure $\times$ volume; contractility; and heart rate)
Ventilatory oxygen consumption $(\dot{V}O_2)$	$\approx$ External work performed, or cardiac output $\times$ arteriovenous O_2 difference[a]

Table 15.1 Two basic principles of exercise physiology

[a] The arteriovenous O_2 difference is approximately 15–17 vol% at maximal exercise in most individuals; therefore, $\dot{V}O_{2max}$ generally reflects the extent to which cardiac output increases

It is the force that, when applied to a 1 kg mass, gives it an acceleration of $1\,m.s^{-2}$. Since work is equal to force (*in newtons*) times distance (*in metres*), another unit for work is the newton metre (*Nm*). One Nm is equal to one joule (*J*), which is another common expression of work.

Power and Energy

Since work is nearly always expressed per unit of time (i.e. as a rate), an additional unit that is important is *power*, which is the rate at which work is performed. The body's metabolic equivalent (MET) of power is *energy*. Therefore, it is easy to think of work as anything with weight moving at some rate across time (e.g. distance).

Metabolic Equivalent

The common biologic measure of total body work is oxygen uptake, usually expressed as a rate (making it a measure of power) in litres per minute. The MET is commonly used to clinically express the oxygen requirement of the work rate during an exercise test. One MET is equated with the resting metabolic rate (approximately $3.5\,ml\ O_2.kg^{-1}.min^{-1}$), and a MET value achieved from an exercise test is a multiple of the resting metabolic rate, either measured directly (as oxygen uptake) or estimated from the maximal workload achieved using standardised equations [1].

The cardiopulmonary response to exercise requires a major redistribution of cardiac output ($\dot{Q}$) along with a number of local metabolic changes. The usual measure of the capacity of the body to deliver and utilise oxygen is the maximal oxygen uptake ($\dot{V}O_{2max}$). Thus, the limits of the cardiopulmonary system are historically defined by $\dot{V}O_{2max}$, which can be expressed by the Fick principle: $\dot{V}O_{2max} = maximal\ \dot{Q} \times maximal\ arteriovenous\ oxygen\ difference$.

Cardiac output must closely match ventilation in the lung in order to deliver oxygen to the working muscle. $\dot{V}O_{2max}$ is determined by the maximal amount of ventilation ($\dot{V}E$) moving in and out of the lung and by the fraction of this ventilation extracted by the tissues: $\dot{V}O_2 = \dot{V}E \times (FiO_2 - FeO_2)$, where $\dot{V}E$ is minute ventilation and FiO_2 and FeO_2 are the fractional amounts of oxygen in the inspired and expired air, respectively.

To accurately measure $\dot{V}O_{2max}$, CO_2 in expired air (VCO_2) must be measured. The major purpose of VCO_2 in this equation is to correct for the difference in ventilation between inspired and expired air. Consequently, the cardiopulmonary limits ($\dot{V}O_{2max}$) are defined by (i) a central component ($\dot{Q}$) that defines the pumping capacity of the heart and (ii) peripheral factors (arteriovenous oxygen difference) that define the capacity of the lung to oxygenate the blood and the capacity of the working muscle to extract this oxygen from the blood.

Methods

Safety Precautions and Risks

Everything necessary for cardiopulmonary resuscitation must be available, and regular drills should be performed to ascertain that personnel and equipment are ready for a cardiac emergency [2]. Testing athletes is generally safer than testing clinical patients, unless evaluating for new symptoms, testing master athletes or 'weekend warriors' or considering a cardiac diagnosis [3].

Athlete Preparation

The athlete should be instructed not to take any food, supplements or energy drinks or to exercise for 3 hours before the test and to come appropriately dressed. A history and physical examination should be performed to rule out any contraindications to testing. An ECG should be obtained in the supine and standing positions. The standing ECG is important in detecting individuals who develop ST-segment depression on standing and whose test results are likely to be false positives. There should be a careful explanation of the testing procedure, including its risks, and a demonstration of getting on and off the treadmill (if appropriate). Because of the effect on estimated METs and the stability of the ECG tracing, the athlete should be discouraged from holding the handrails of the treadmill unless it is necessary for balance.

Contraindications for Exercise Testing

The first step in ensuring athlete safety is to know when testing is not appropriate. Absolute contraindications for testing are listed in Table 15.2. When athletes are middle-aged or older and atherosclerotic coronary disease is suspected, it is preferable to perform the test with a physician present. The features of angina pectoris (chest pain due to myocardial ischaemia) should be well known by testing personnel. Pain due to myocardial ischaemia is typically substernal, is usually brought on by exercise, resolves with rest and often progresses to radiate to the jaw or left arm.

Heart Rate

Sympathetic and parasympathetic nervous system influences underlie the cardiovascular system's first response to exercise: an increase in heart rate. Sympathetic outflow to the heart and systemic blood vessels increases, whilst vagal outflow decreases. Vagal withdrawal is responsible for the initial 10–30 beat.min^{-1} rise, whilst further increases in heart rate are sympathetically mediated. Of the two major $\dot{Q}$ components, heart rate and stroke volume, heart rate is responsible for most of the increase in $\dot{Q}$ during exercise. Heart rate increases linearly with workload and oxygen uptake, primarily at the expense of diastolic – not systolic – time.

The heart rate response to exercise is influenced by multiple factors, including age, type of activity, body position, fitness, presence of heart disease, medications, blood volume and environment. Of these, the most important factor is age: a decline in maximal heart rate occurs with increasing age. This decline appears to be due to intrinsic cardiac changes rather than neural influences. It should be noted that there is a great deal of variability around the regression line between maximal heart rate and age; thus, age-related maximal heart rate is a relatively poor index of maximal effort. Maximal heart rate is unchanged or slightly reduced after training, whilst resting heart rate is reduced due to enhanced parasympathetic tone.

Controversy exists regarding the heart rate rise during early dynamic exercise. Based on the response to the 4-second exercise test developed by Araujo et al. [4] and our own experience, a rapid increase is normal. Individuals with the healthiest vagal tone or cardiovascular status respond to vagal withdrawal with the greatest increase at the onset of exercise. However, Falcone et al. [5,6] have reported that an excessive heart

- Unstable angina or other acute chest pain
- Serious cardiac dysrhythmias (atrial fibrillation, wide complex tachycardias)
- Pericarditis, myocarditis or endocarditis
- Aortic stenosis or valvular heart disease
- Left ventricular dysfunction or cardiomyopathy
- Acute pulmonary embolus or pulmonary infarction
- Any acute or serious noncardiac disorder
- Aortic dissection (often with chest pain radiating to the back)
- Physical impairment due to injury

Table 15.2 Absolute contraindications to exercise testing of athletes

rate response during the first minute of exercise predicts cardiovascular mortality, but we have not been able to confirm this.

Autonomic physiology during recovery from acute bouts of exercise involves reactivation of the parasympathetic system and deactivation of sympathetic activity. The decline in heart rate after cessation of exercise is commonly used to assess these mechanisms. A delay in heart rate recovery has been used as a marker of autonomic dysfunction and/or failure of the cardiovascular system to respond to the normal autonomic response to exercise [7]. A rapid heart rate recovery has been shown to be a marker of aerobic fitness since the 1940s [8]. More recently, the degree to which heart rate recovers during the first 1 or 2 minutes after cessation of exercise has been shown to be a strong prognostic marker [9].

Blood Pressure

Although numerous devices are commercially available to automate blood pressure measurement during exercise, even with ECG gating none can be recommended. The time-proven method of holding the arm with a stethoscope placed over the brachial artery remains the most reliable. The athlete's arm should be free of the handrails so that noise is not transmitted up it. An auscultatory piece or an electronic microphone can be fastened to the arm, and a device that inflates and deflates the cuff with the push of a button can be helpful. Once the athlete begins running or achieves a high level of exercise (e.g. >10 METs), it is difficult to obtain the blood pressure accurately. Thus, if all signs are stable, a final blood pressure (immediate post-exercise) is adequate. An abnormal blood pressure response at low work levels or a decrease or flat systolic response in a symptomatic individual is an ominous sign and may be the first indicator of the potential for the presence of CVD.

Indications for Treadmill Test Termination

Absolute indications for exercise test termination are listed in Table 15.3. In some athletes predicted to be at high risk by their clinical history, it may be appropriate to terminate the test at a submaximal level, since the most severe ST-segment depression or dysrhythmia may only occur in recovery.

Determinants of Maximal Effort

The measurement of maximal effort is critically important when testing athletes, because it has implications for fitness, training evaluation and performance programming. A great deal of effort has been directed towards what defines 'maximal' and how it is determined. The classic definition of an individual's maximal cardiopulmonary limits is a plateau in oxygen uptake, historically defined as the failure to increase oxygen uptake by $\geq 200\,ml.min^{-1}$ despite an increase in work rate. Whilst a plateau in oxygen uptake occurs more often in athletes than nonathletes, it is nevertheless not observed in many individuals, tends to be poorly reproducible and has been confused by the many criteria applied [10]. Although many efforts have been made to objectify maximal effort, including age-predicted maximal heart rate, exceeding the ventilatory threshold, a given blood lactate level and a respiratory exchange ratio greater than 1.10, all have considerable

- Onset of severe angina or other chest pain
- Drop in systolic blood pressure (SBP) with increasing workload, accompanied by signs or symptoms
- Marked ECG changes (e.g. $\geq 2.0\,mm$ ST-segment elevation or $\geq 2.0\,mm$ horizontal or downsloping ST-segment depression)
- Serious dysrhythmias (second- or third-degree atrioventricular (AV) block, sustained ventricular tachycardia or increasing premature ventricular contractions (PVCs))
- Signs of poor perfusion, including pallor, cyanosis and cold and clammy skin
- Central nervous system (CNS) symptoms, including ataxia, vertigo, visual or gait problems and confusion
- Technical or interpretational problems with monitoring blood pressure or the ECG
- Athlete's request

Table 15.3 Absolute indications for termination of an exercise test

6		
7	Very, very light	
8		
9	Very light	
10		
11	Fairly light	
12		
13	Somewhat hard	
14		
15	Hard	
16		
17	Very hard	
18		
19	Very, very hard	
20		

Table 15.4 Borg 20-point scale of perceived exertion

measurement error and intersubject variability. Despite being subjective, the 6-to-20 Borg perceived exertion scale is helpful in assessing exercise effort for all ages (Table 15.4). The Borg scale is a simple and valuable way of assessing the relative effort an individual exerts during exercise. When the test is being performed for a clinical reason, standard clinical criteria (Table 15.3) for stopping should supersede any physiologic criteria for maximal effort.

ECG Recording

Skin Preparation, Electrodes and Cables

Proper skin preparation for electrode placement is essential. An exercise test with an ECG signal that cannot be continuously monitored and accurately interpreted because of artefact is worthless and, worse, dangerous. Proper electrode placement for exercise testing is shown in Figure 15.1.

The general areas of electrode placement should be shaved to remove hair and cleansed with an alcohol-saturated gauze pad, with the superficial layer of skin removed by light abrasion with fine-grain emery paper. The placements are determined using anatomical landmarks found with the athlete supine, because some individuals with loose skin can have a considerable shift of electrode positions when they assume an upright position. Skin preparation is a greater problem with master athletes, since skin resistance increases with age. It is critical that electrodes for exercise testing possess a metal interface and are sunken, creating a column that is typically filled with a wet electrolyte solution. Efforts should be taken to minimise motion at the electrode–cable interface. This may be achieved by securing the cables centrally with an elastic belt worn around the waist and, if necessary, a vest designed for this purpose.

Lead Systems

Most ECG systems use the modified 12-lead system (Figure 15.1) [11]. The conventional ankle and wrist electrodes are replaced by electrodes mounted on the torso at the base of the limbs. In this way, artefact introduced by movement of the limbs is avoided. The ground electrode (right leg) can be on the lower back and the left-leg electrode should be below the umbilicus. The precordial electrodes should be placed in the appropriate interspaces.

As much as 90% of abnormal ST depression (an important consideration for middle-aged and master athletes) occurs in the lateral precordial leads (V4, V5 and V6). This does not mean that other leads should

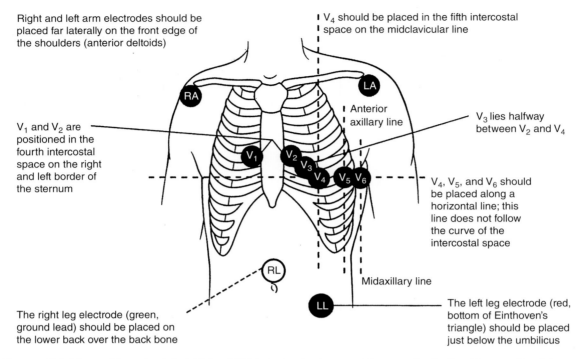

Right and left arm electrodes should be placed far laterally on the front edge of the shoulders (anterior deltoids)

I V₄ should be placed in the fifth intercostal
I space on the midclavicular line

V_1 and V_2 are positioned in the fourth intercostal space on the right and left border of the sternum

I Anterior
I axillary line

V_3 lies halfway between V_2 and V_4

V_4, V_5, and V_6 should be placed along a horizontal line; this line does not follow the curve of the intercostal space

Midaxillary line

The right leg electrode (green, ground lead) should be placed on the lower back over the back bone

The left leg electrode (red, bottom of Einthoven's triangle) should be placed just below the umbilicus

Figure 15.1 Mason–Likar simulated 12-lead ECG electrode placement for exercise testing (*Source:* Froelicher and Myers [3]. Reproduced with permission of Elsevier)

not be recorded, particularly in athletes being evaluated for chest pain, since ST elevation localises ischaemia. Arrhythmias are best diagnosed in inferior and anterior leads, where P-waves are best observed.

ECG Processing

Averaging techniques have made it possible to filter and average ECG signals to remove noise. Averaging techniques are attractive because they can produce a clean tracing when the raw data are noisy. Filtering and averaging can, however, cause false ST depression due to distortion of the raw data. The old adage 'garbage in, garbage out' holds for computerised ECG processing. For these reasons, raw ECG tracings should be recorded and averages should be used only as a supplement. Since ST measurements made by a computer can be erroneous, it is advisable to have devices mark both the isoelectric level and the beginning of the ST segment, as these determine the ST level. Computerised ST measurements require physician over-reading; errors can be made both in the choice of the isoelectric line and in the beginning of the ST segment. The standard '3 lead × 4 lead groups' print-out leaves only 2.5 seconds to assess ST changes or arrhythmias; therefore, V5 should be continuously recorded when making paper recordings for interpretation of ischaemia; leads II and aVF should be continuously recorded when making paper recordings for interpretation of arrhythmias; and, ideally, the ECG print-out created every minute should include continuous three-dimensional (3D) leads (II/AVF, V2 and V5)

Exercise Procedures

Dynamic exercise or rhythmic muscular activity resulting in movement leads to an appropriate balance between $\dot{Q}$, blood supply and oxygen exchange. Because the delivered workload can be accurately calibrated and the physiological response easily measured, dynamic, graduated and controlled exercise is preferred for exercise testing. The bicycle ergometer and the treadmill are the most commonly used dynamic exercise devices. Electronically braked bicycle ergometers keep the workload at a specified level over a wide range of pedalling speeds and have become the standard for cycle ergometer testing today.

The treadmill should have front and side rails so that athletes can steady themselves. The treadmill should be calibrated at least monthly. Some models can be greatly affected by the individual's weight and will not deliver the appropriate workload. An emergency stop button should be readily available to the staff only. The individual should not grasp the front or side rails because this decreases the work performed and the oxygen uptake and, in turn, increases exercise time, resulting in an overestimation of exercise capacity. Gripping the handrails also increases ECG muscle artefact. In most studies comparing upright cycle ergometer with treadmill exercise, maximum heart rate values have been roughly similar, but maximal oxygen uptake has been 6–25% greater during treadmill exercise. However, the specificity of exercise is an important consideration. For example, a cyclist will likely perform better on a cycle ergometer test, whilst a runner will perform better on a treadmill.

Exercise Protocols for Athletes

The appropriate protocol to use when testing athletes is quite different from those commonly used in the clinical setting. As with any exercise test, the protocol should be individualised for the participant being tested. Test duration should be targeted to fall within the range of 8–12 minutes; numerous studies over the last 3 decades have demonstrated that $\dot{V}O_{2max}$ is highest when this duration is targeted. A ramp protocol is ideal for this purpose, since the ramp rate can be individualised to the given athlete in order to achieve this duration [12].

Post-exercise Period

If maximal sensitivity for diagnosing myocardial ischaemia in a middle-aged or older individual is to be achieved, the individual should be supine during the post-exercise period. It is advisable to record about 10 seconds of ECG data whilst the athlete is motionless but still experiencing near-maximal heart rate, then have them lie down. Having the individual perform a cool-down walk after the test can delay or eliminate the appearance of ST-segment depression. However, a cool-down walk can minimise the risk of arrhythmias in this high-risk time when catecholamine levels are high. The supine position after exercise is not important when the test is not being performed for diagnostic purposes (e.g. fitness evaluation). In such cases, it may be preferable to walk slowly (e.g. ~2.0 mile.h^{-1}) or continue cycling against minimal resistance (e.g. ~25W) for several minutes after the test. Monitoring should continue for at least 5 minutes after exercise or until ECG changes stabilise. The recovery period, particularly minutes 2–4, is critical for ST analysis. Noise is generally not a problem and ST depression at that time has important implications regarding the presence and severity of CAD. A cool-down walk can delay or reduce recovery ST depression.

Ventilatory Gas-Exchange Responses

Due to the inaccuracies associated with estimating METs from work rate, it is useful to measure physiologic work directly using ventilatory gas-exchange responses, commonly referred to as *cardiopulmonary exercise testing (CPET)* [13]. Information from CPET can be particularly useful in athletes in terms of precisely measuring fitness, monitoring and optimising response to training and providing additional information concerning cardiopulmonary function during exercise. CPET adds precision to the measurement of work and permits the assessment of other parameters, including the respiratory exchange ratio, efficiency of ventilation and ventilatory threshold.

The critical measurement from CPET in the context of the athlete is the $\dot{V}O_{2max}$. $\dot{V}O_{2max}$ is a measure of the maximal amount of oxygen used by the body's cells at a given time, expressed as a rate in ml.min^{-1}. Since $\dot{V}O_2$ is related to muscle mass, it is frequently normalised for body weight in kg, and expressed in ml O_2.kg^{-1}.min^{-1}. $\dot{V}O_{2max}$ is one of the most widely applied measurements in the exercise sciences, defining the upper limits of the cardiopulmonary system, and is considered the standard for aerobic fitness. The ventilatory threshold is a submaximal parameter derived from CPET [14]. It has been defined as the highest oxygen uptake during exercise above which a sustained lactic acidosis occurs. When this level of exercise is reached, excess H$^+$ ions of lactate must be buffered to maintain physiological pH. Because bicarbonate buffering of lactate yields an additional source of CO_2 in the blood, ventilation is further stimulated; hence the term 'ventilatory' or anaerobic threshold. See Chapter 4 for further information on the cardiovascular responses to exercise.

ECG Interpretation

ST-Segment Depression

ST-segment changes, whilst critical to document, should be interpreted with caution in apparently healthy athletic individuals, as false-positive rates are high. Nevertheless, the most common manifestation of exercise-induced myocardial ischemia is ST-segment depression. Atherosclerotic CAD is extremely rare in young athletes but occurs with increasing prevalence with advancing age. CAD as a cause of sudden death generally occurs amongst individuals >35 years of age; however, chest discomfort should be evaluated thoroughly regardless of the age of the individual. Notably, other coronary anomalies and myocardial bridges are not usually associated with exercise-induced ST abnormalities.

The standard criterion for this type of abnormal response is horizontal or downward-sloping ST-segment depression of 0.1 mV or more for 60–80 ms. It appears to be caused by generalised subendocardial ischaemia. A 'steal' phenomenon is likely from ischaemic areas because of the effect of extensive collateralisation in the subendocardium. Unlike ST elevation, ST depression does not localise the area of ischaemia or help to indicate which coronary artery is occluded. It is preferable to call tests with an inadequate ST-segment slope but with ST-segment depression a 'borderline response'. Added emphasis should be placed on other clinical and exercise responses if this is observed.

ST Depression in Recovery

Abnormal ST depression occurring only in recovery provides clinically useful information and is unlikely to represent a false-positive response. When considered together with changes during exercise, changes in recovery increase the sensitivity of the exercise test without a decline in predictive value. A cool-down walk should be avoided after exercise testing for the diagnosis of CAD in athletes older than 35 years.

ST-Segment Elevation

The most common ECG abnormality seen in the exercise laboratory is ST-segment depression. ST elevation is relatively rare. Its prevalence depends upon the population tested, but it occurs more frequently in those who have had a Q-wave myocardial infarction. The degree of ST-segment elevation or depression that occurs with exercise is different depending on the resting ECG. ST-segment depression is measured from the isoelectric baseline. Alternatively, when ST-segment depression is present at rest, the amount of additional depression can be measured. Conversely, ST-segment elevation is always considered from the baseline PR interval (Figure 15.2). Resting ST-segment elevation is frequently present in athletes (*early repolarisation, ER*) because of the high vagal tone associated with training. The term 'early repolarisation' has caused confusion with an inherited arrhythmic disease, and ER is not a concern for sudden cardiac death during exercise [15].

Exercise Test-Induced Arrhythmias

The exercise test can be a very useful tool in the initial evaluation of arrhythmias associated with exercise. In general, supraventricular arrhythmias are not a risk in athletes, although they can be symptomatic if sustained. In rare cases, serious ventricular rhythm disturbances during exercise can occur in an apparently healthy person, and these should be thoroughly evaluated. Symptoms that require further evaluation include palpitations that are associated with lightheadedness, unusual shortness of breath and syncope. Any history of 'dizziness' or loss of consciousness should be thoroughly evaluated for the possibility of serious rhythm disturbances. In taking the history, be aware that many athletes use the term 'dizziness' for lightheadedness, and true vertigo is usually an inner-ear problem to be distinguished from a cardiac issue. Follow-up questions regarding direction of spinning and the presence of tinnitus or other ear problems can be very helpful in ruling out a cardiac problem. Syncope in an athlete is most often due to heightened vagal tone (termed *neurocardiogenic* or *vasovagal* syncope), and is usually a benign reflex that is common in highly trained individuals. For further information on syncope, see Chapter 35.

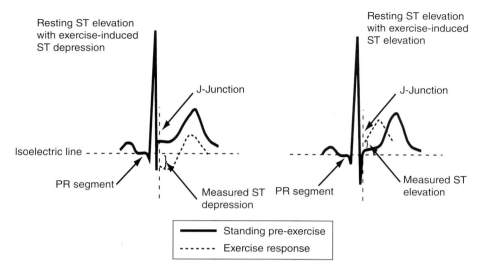

Figure 15.2 Illustration of the measurement of ST depression (left) and ST elevation (right) when there is ST elevation at rest. Often, ST elevation is present at rest in athletes because of the high vagal tone associated with training

Re-entry supraventricular tachycardias (SVTs) can be treated by catheter ablation. Isolated premature ventricular contractions (PVCs) can be common in some athletes and generally are not a concern in an otherwise healthy person. PVCs may become more frequent or may just disappear with exercise. PVCs that become frequent with exercise, are multifocal or that occur in succession (couplets or triplets) warrant further evaluation. Familial catecholaminergic polymorphic ventricular tachycardia (CPVT) is a rare arrhythmogenic disease manifesting with exercise- or stress-induced ventricular arrhythmias, syncope and even sudden death [16]. For further information on CPVT, see Chapter 29.

Diagnostic Utilisation of Exercise Testing

Diagnostic testing is indicated for those with suspected disease or to evaluate a specific complaint. American College of Cardiology (ACC)/American Heart Association (AHA) guidelines for the diagnostic use of the standard exercise test have stated that it is appropriate for testing of adult male or female individuals (including those with complete right bundle branch block (RBBB) or with <1 mm resting ST depression) with an *intermediate pre-test probability* of CAD based on gender, age and symptoms. Testing younger athletes for inherited diseases can also be helpful. Athletes with hypertrophic cardiomyopathy (HCM) can develop PVCs and chest pain and exhibit excessive systolic blood pressure and low exercise capacity. Sharma et al. [17] have described the utility of CPET in characterising subnormal functional capacity in HCM, and reported that CPET permits the differentiation of physiologic left ventricular hypertrophy (LVH) in athletes from that in patients with HCM. Athletes with inherited arrhythmic diseases can exhibit arrhythmias and prolonged QTc intervals. The concept that exercise testing is helpful in diagnosing coronary anomalies or myocardial bridging is still speculative.

Conclusion

The exercise test is a valuable tool for the evaluation of the athlete, with applications for the assessment of fitness, optimising training regimens and the evaluation of exercise-induced symptoms. Use of proper methodology is important for safety and in obtaining accurate results. Accordingly, the use of specific criteria for exclusion and termination and the paying of close attention to preparation, interaction during testing and appropriate emergency equipment are essential.

References

1 Glass, S., Dwyer, G.B. and Medicine, A.C.O.S. *ACSM's Metabolic Calculations Handbook*. Philadelphia, PA: Lippincott Williams & Wilkins, 2007.

2 Myers, J., Arena, R., Franklin, B. et al. Recommendations for clinical exercise laboratories: a scientific statement from the American Heart Association. *Circulation*, 2009; **119**: 3144–61.

3 Froelicher, V.F. and Myers, J. *Exercise and the Heart*, 5th edn. Philadelphia, PA: Saunders-Mosby, 2006.

4 Almeida, M.B.D., Ricardo, D.R. and Araújo, C.G.S.D. Validation of the 4-second exercise test in the orthostatic position. *Arq Bras Cardiol* 2004; **83**: 155–9.

5 Falcone, C., Buzzi, M.P., Klersy, C. and Schwartz, P.J. Rapid heart rate increase at onset of exercise predicts adverse cardiac events in patients with coronary artery disease. *Circulation* 2005; **112**: 1959–64.

6 Leeper, N.J., Dewey, F.E., Ashley, E.A. et al. Prognostic value of heart rate increase at onset of exercise testing. *Circulation* 2007; **115**: 468–74.

7 Okutucu, S., Karakulak, U.N., Aytemir, K. and Oto, A. Heart rate recovery: a practical clinical indicator of abnormal cardiac autonomic function. *Expert Rev Cardiovasc Ther* 2011; **9**(11): 1417–30.

8 Daanen, H.A., Lamberts, R.P., Kallen, V.L. et al. A systematic review on heart-rate recovery to monitor changes in training status in athletes. *Int J Sports Physiol Perform* 2012; 7(3): 251–60.

9 Shetler, K., Marcus, R., Froelicher, V.F. et al. Heart rate recovery: validation and methodologic issues. *J Am Coll Cardiol* 2001; **38**: 1980–7.

10 Myers, J., Walsh, D., Sullivan, M. and Froelicher, V. Effect of sampling on variability and plateau in oxygen uptake. *J Appl Physiol* 1990; **68**: 404–10.

11 Gamble, P., McManus, H., Jensen, D. and Froelicher, V. A comparison of the standard 12-lead electrocardiogram to exercise electrode placements. *Chest* 1984; **85**: 616–22.

12 Myers, J. Which exercise test in whom?. *J Cardiol Dis Prev* 1998; **1**: 13.

13 Myers, J. *Essentials of Cardiopulmonary Exercise Testing*. Champaign, IL: Human Kinetics, 1996.

14 Myers, J. and Ashley, E. Dangerous curves: a perspective on exercise, lactate, and the anaerobic threshold. *Chest* 1997; **111**: 787–95.

15 Perez, M.V., Friday, K. and Froelicher, V. Semantic confusion: the case of early repolarization and the J point. *Am J Med* 2012; **125**: 843–4.

16 Laitinen, P.J., Swan, H., Piippo, K. et al. Genes, exercise and sudden death: molecular basis of familial catecholaminergic polymorphic ventricular tachycardia. *Ann Med* 2004; **36**: 81–6.

17 Sharma, S., Elliott, P.M., Whyte, G. et al. Utility of metabolic exercise testing in distinguishing hypertrophic cardiomyopathy from physiologic left ventricular hypertrophy in athletes. *J Am Coll Cardiol* 2000; **36**: 864–70.

16 The Role of Cardiovascular Magnetic Resonance in the Assessment of Athletes

Rory O'Hanlon

Centre for Cardiovascular Magnetic Resonance, Blackrock Clinic, Dublin, Ireland

Introduction

Long-term high-intensity physical activity is associated with 'physiological' cardiac adaptive changes. Electrocardiographic (ECG) adaptations include resting bradycardia, repolarisation abnormalities and electrical changes suggestive of left ventricular hypertrophy (LVH) [1]. Morphological changes principally concern left and right ventricular enlargement. These manifestations are termed the 'athlete's heart'.

Although the benefits of regular exercise are well established, the cardiac consequences of long-term high-level competitive training are uncertain. Indeed, whilst sudden cardiac death (SCD) in athletes is rare, the rate of SCD in the athlete is 2.8 times higher than in a nonathletic matched individual. There is also a 10 times greater risk in male athletes compared with their female counterparts, and a higher risk in athletes over 35 years of age. The aetiology of SCD in athletes <35 years old is mostly attributed to inherited and structural heart disease, such as hypertrophic cardiomyopathy (HCM) or arrhythmogenic right ventricular cardiomyopathy (ARVC), but in athletes >35 years the vast majority of SCD is a consequence of acquired disease, in particular coronary artery disease (CAD). Therefore, high-level training should not be regarded as a negligible risk, and the benefits of athletic screening are well accepted.

Athletic screening usually incorporates a targeted history, physical examination and an ECG, and may include an echocardiographic study. The aim of these examinations is to detect any underlying pathology and to distinguish between normal and pathological physiological cardiac athletic remodelling. Occasionally, the ECG and echocardiographic changes seen in athletic remodelling may overlap with pathological changes seen in inherited cardiomyopathies (e.g. HCM, dilated cardiomyopathy (DCM), ARVC or left ventricular noncompaction (LVNC)) and thus confuse the diagnosis. In these cases, further noninvasive imaging with cardiovascular magnetic resonance (CMR) is required. The most common causes of SCD in an athlete is HCM, followed by anomalous coronary arteries, channelopathies, DCM and ARVC. CMR is therefore well placed to identify the majority of causes of SCD in the athlete.

CMR is an increasingly available, advanced imaging modality that helps evaluate the cardiac structure and function in an athlete. It provides very high spatial- (0.5 mm) and temporal-resolution cine images. It is the most accurate noninvasive imaging technique for the determination of left and right ventricular ejection fraction and left ventricular mass. Studies have shown that the reproducibility of CMR is excellent, which is key in assessing for any interval change in structure or function, particularly if an athlete de-trains. Furthermore, CMR allows the definition of abnormal processes occurring at the tissue level, including myocardial oedema, fatty infiltration and, importantly, myocardial fibrosis. It is the identification of these

IOC Manual of Sports Cardiology, First Edition. Edited by Mathew G. Wilson, Jonathan A. Drezner and Sanjay Sharma.
© 2017 International Olympic Committee. Published 2017 by John Wiley & Sons, Ltd.

myocardial tissue processes, as well as the unparalleled precision and reproducibility of measurement of cardiac volumes and masses, that makes CMR a unique and powerful tool for monitoring any interval change and differentiating physiological changes from disease processes.

The use of contrast agents, in particular gadolinium chelates, has revolutionised the applicability of CMR in the evaluation of cardiac disease [2]. Gadolinium-based extracellular paramagnetic contrast agents accumulate in areas of extracellular expansion and thus can be used to delineate areas of injured myocardium. Gadolinium reduces hydrogen proton T1 relaxation times in proportion to its local concentration. In areas of myocardial fibrosis, there is decreased perfusion of the fibrotic tissue and thus a prolonged wash-out time for the gadolinium. Typically, areas of gadolinium accumulation relate to areas of scar expansion due to focal myocardial replacement fibrosis, which may have both ischaemic and nonischaemic aetiologies. The pattern of fibrosis seen on late gadolinium enhancement (LGE) imaging allows for confident aetiological assessment, with greater evidence now accumulating regarding the prognostic implications of myocardial scar.

Furthermore, whilst LGE imaging typically demonstrates macroscopic replacement fibrosis to be a late stage of the pathological process, newer CMR techniques such as T1 mapping can define interstitial microscopic fibrosis and may have a role in identifying pathological changes at an earlier stage. T1 mapping has the potential to differentiate both interstitial and replacement fibrosis from normal myocardium, and allows fibrosis quantification on a standardised absolute scale. It therefore represents a more accurate means of quantifying total fibrotic burden than traditional LGE approaches [3].

Stress-perfusion CMR is an additional facet to the standard CMR study (see Figure 16.1). Adenosine, a coronary vasodilating agent, is administered, and a specific set of images is acquired. These images can demonstrate

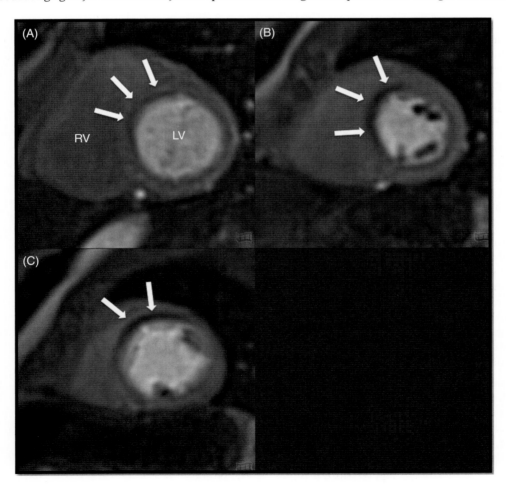

Figure 16.1 Perfusion CMR scan showing an area of decreased perfusion (increased darkness) in the anterior and anteroseptal wall of the left ventricle at (A) the basal left ventricle, (B) the mid left ventricle and (C) the apical left ventricle, which would suggest ischaemia in the territory of the left axis deviation (LAD). LV, left ventricle; RV, right ventricle

areas of impaired myocardial perfusion relating to epicardial coronary disease, but also (importantly) due to microvascular ischaemia (notable in structural cardiomyopathies such as HCM and DCM) [4].

The Athletes Heart

Athletic remodelling occurs as a result of reduced heart rate and cardiac enlargement, including increases in both left ventricular internal size (left ventricular dilation) and LVH. These changes may mimic a cardiomyopathy, but in athletic remodelling left ventricular systolic and diastolic function are normal and stroke volume is increased.

Changes in the right ventricle with high-level exercise mirror those of the left ventricle, with increases in mass, end-diastolic volumes and stroke volume. The ratio of left to right ventricular size is typically maintained, indicating that athlete's heart involves balanced remodelling of both ventricles, but right ventricular systolic function is typically normal. Notably, in athletes, right ventricular cavity enlargement involves the right ventricle inflow tract in particular. Whilst right ventricular enlargement is typically matched to left ventricular enlargement, La Gerche et al. [5] have demonstrated that intense exercise induces a right ventricular end-systolic wall stress that exceeds left ventricular end-systolic wall stress in elite athletes, which leads to greater right ventricular enlargement and greater wall thickening. Changes such as these may lead to diagnostic uncertainty regarding potential right ventricular pathology.

Atria are also affected by athletic remodelling. Moderate left atrial enlargement has consistently been shown to occur in athletes, with up to 20% of competitive athletes having left atrial enlargement >40 mm. Left atrial dilation is proportional to left ventricular dilation and the extent of endurance sport performed [6].

Who Should Have a CMR?

The question arises as to how best to proceed should pre-participation screening raise abnormal or equivocal results, and how to accurately differentiate between normal physiological changes seen in athlete's heart and the pathological changes of a previously undetected cardiomyopathy. Recent European Association of Cardiovascular Imaging (EACVI) guidelines attempt to bridge this gap [7]. Should questions remains after an echocardiogram, or if concerning symptoms are present, a CMR should be considered.

For example, in the case of HCM, the EACVI suggests that if echocardiography demonstrates a wall thickness of ≤12 mm and normal diastolic function, the changes may reliably be seen as athletic remodelling. Questions may remain, however, particularly in the context of the patient with a wall thickness on echocardiography within normal limits but a significantly abnormal ECG (specifically T-wave inversion, ST-segment depression or pathological Q waves) or of an athlete with concerning symptoms. Furthermore, peak wall-thickness measurements may be considerably greater than 12 mm, particularly in black athletes (up to 16 mm). Echocardiography may not reliably image the basal anterolateral wall or left ventricular apex, and significant ECG abnormalities in athletes may turn out to be due to basal septal HCM or apical HCM even in the absence of a family history or symptoms, or indeed occasionally in the presence of a normal ECG [8]. Therefore, in cases where questions remain following ECG and/or echocardiography, CMR would be advocated.

In this chapter, we will define how CMR can be helpful in the diagnosis – or exclusion – of a previously undetected cardiomyopathy in athletes.

Hypertrophic Cardiomyopathy

HCM is a genetic disorder characterised by myofibrillar hypertrophy, disarray and myocardial fibrosis (see Figure 16.2). The prevalence of HCM is estimated at 0.05-0.2% in the general population. HCM is the most common cause of SCD in athletes, accounting for 36% of all deaths [9]. Symptoms of HCM include dyspnea, syncope and pre-syncope, angina, and palpitations. For the majority of people, HCM remains clinically silent and does not produce symptoms and may be associated with completely normal athletic milestones. While the preponderance of patients with HCM will have an abnormal ECG, up to 5-10% of patients may have a normal ECG and therefore may not be detected through routine screening. A minority (<25%) will have evidence of left ventricular outflow tract obstruction during resting conditions and hence clinical examination may be normal. Many individuals undergoing pre-participation screening will be unaware of a family history of HCM or SCD. Indeed family history of the condition or

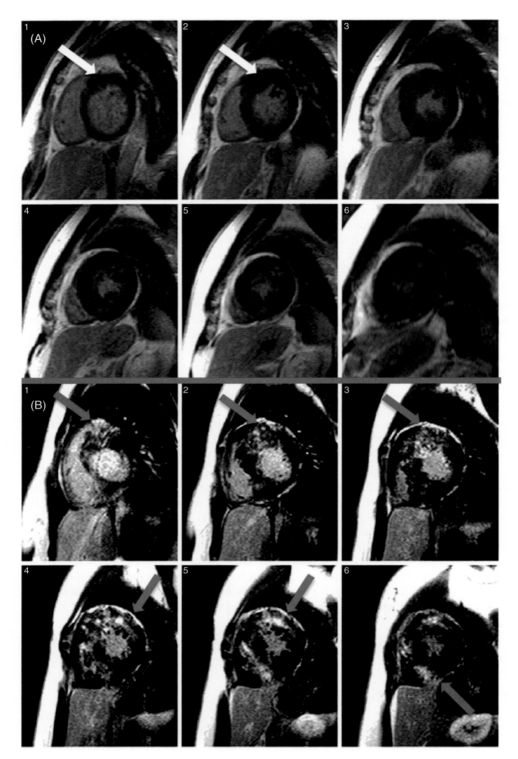

Figure 16.2 A 20-year-old male has an abnormal ECG on screening, with left-axis deviation and T-wave inversion in V1–V3. Transthoracic echocardiogram (TTE) demonstrates LVH of 14 mm. CMR is organised for further assessment. (A) Steady-state free precision (SSFP) cine CMR shows asymmetrical thickening of the anteroseptal left ventricular wall at the basal ventricular level (1,2), in addition to concentric left ventricular thickening from the mid left ventricle through to the apex (3–6). (B) LGE imaging shows evidence patchy myocardial fibrosis, notably in the maximally hypertrophied areas (1–3) and throughout the mid and basal ventricular walls (4–6)

SCD may not be present. It would be well accepted however, that the majority of HCM would be identified with ECG and echo but, as outlined previously, uncertainty may remain and in these situations, CMR is particularly useful.

Considering that a diagnosis of HCM requires disqualification from most sports in order to minimise the risk of sudden death, a misdiagnosis of athletic heart may have fatal consequences. Therefore, accurate assessment is imperative. Echocardiographic findings of HCM may overlap with other causes of LVH, including athlete's heart. Additionally, echocardiography may not entirely visualise the left ventricular anterolateral free wall and apex, so some cases of HCM may be missed. For these reasons, CMR, which allows almost complete three-dimensional (3D) reconstruction of the ventricle, is advocated for complete assessment should the diagnosis be suspected.

The differentiation between physiological LVH and HCM is essential, but often challenging. The extremes of LVH seen in athletes (beyond 13 mm in men and 12 mm in women) overlap with that seen in patients with morphologically mild HCM. Thus, an athlete with LVH beyond 13 mm represents a grey zone between physiological adaptation and mild expression of HCM, although LVH of up to 16 mm has been shown in black athletes, which again highlights the difficulty of interpreting wall-thickness measurements in distinguishing between pathological and physiological remodelling. Various criteria for making this distinction have been described, including the degree of LVH, pattern of LVH and left ventricular cavity size (see Chapter 40). However, the subtleties of differentiation between LVH and HCM may remain challenging despite extensive echocardiographic assessment, and indeed morphologically mild HCM may nonetheless be associated with significant risk of SCD.

In addition to complete anatomical and functional assessment, adenosine perfusion imaging in HCM frequently demonstrates significant microvascular disease, which may act as a nidus for fibrosis and arrhythmia generation [10]. Tissue characterisation using LGE allows for the identification of macroscopic replacement fibrosis, the presence of which strongly favours a cardiomyopathic process as opposed to athletic remodelling. Fibrosis, which occurs in 60–80% of patients with HCM, is patchy and occurs predominantly within maximally hypertrophied segments. The extent of fibrosis has been shown to be a predictor of major adverse cardiac events, including arrhythmic events, and is correlated with risk factors for SCD [11].

Should the differentiation between HCM and athlete's heart remain challenging following CMR, deconditioning may be advised. A repeat CMR following a 3-month period of de-training should show regression of LVH in athlete's heart and not in HCM, and thus allow accurate differentiation.

Other Causes of LVH

Fabry's Disease

Fabry's disease is an X-linked lysosomal disorder that results in excessive deposition of neutral glycosphingolipids in the vascular endothelium of multiple organs. It has an estimated prevalence of 1 in 40 0000. Cardiac involvement may cause palpitations, pre-syncope, syncope, chest pain and SCD.

Fabry's disease -related cardiomyopathy is characterised by concentric left ventricular remodelling which progresses over time to hypertrophy. While exceedingly rare, it remains in the differential for unexplained LVH in male athletes. Owing to partial enzyme activity in females, the condition may manifest later in life, and not infrequently without significant hypertrophy, but in both men and women it may be a consideration in the symptomatic athlete. CMR may be useful in differentiating between the physiological changes and the pathological, with LGE key to identifying any underlying fibrosis. Recently, T1 mapping has been shown to be able to detect early stages of the disease, prior to the formation of fibrosis [12].

Cardiac Amyloidosis

Cardiac amyloidosis is a rare, infiltrative cardiomyopathy caused by deposition of extracellular pathological insoluble proteins. Cardiac involvement is frequently seen in amyloid light-chain (AL) amyloidosis (primary amyloidosis) and transthyretin-related amyloidosis (ATTR amyloidosis) (amyloid deposits of an unstable variant of transthyretin). Cardiac amyloidosis presents with thickened ventricular walls and progressive heart failure.

The morphological features of cardiac amyloidosis are similar to those of other diseases (e.g. HCM, Fabry's disease), and indeed to physiological changes seen in an athlete's heart. This diagnosis is unlikely to be a significant consideration in the majority of younger athletes, but it may need to be considered in the veteran athlete with LVH who mentions a reduction in exercise capacity, for example. CMR features of cardiac amyloidosis include myocardial hypertrophy, diastolic dysfunction, a faster gadolinium blood wash-out, pleural and pericardial effusions and diffuse myocardial delayed enhancement. The pattern of LGE is very specific for amyloid on CMR.

Dilated Cardiomyopathy

Rarely, athletic remodelling may result in left ventricular cavity dimensions increasing to a degree compatible with primary DCM, especially in endurance athletes (see Figure 16.3). DCM is an important cause of SCD amongst young athletes. It is therefore essential to accurately differentiate between physiological and pathological cardiac enlargement in athletes in order to prevent exercise-related SCD.

The differentiation of athletes from potentially early DCM is addressed in the EACVI algorithm, which differentiates an left ventricular end-diastolic dimension (LVEDD) of 60 mm with and without normal ejection fraction. However, in athletic remodelling, low-normal ejection fraction is encountered in up to 12% of Tour de France athletes, and a peak LVEDD ≥60 mm is detected in up to 14% of male athletes. The role of CMR in this situation is to either rule in or rule out a diagnosis, particularly where questions remain (e.g. the symptomatic athlete or the abnormal ECG with an equivocal echo). The precise ventricular volumetric analysis offered by CMR is key to the accurate differentiation between athlete's heart and the pathological dilatation of DCM. Additionally, mid-wall fibrosis (as well as patchy focal intramyocardial fibrosis), as demonstrated by CMR LGE imaging, is a key diagnostic criterion for DCM, but it has not been demonstrated in the physiological remodelled athlete's heart [13]. The presence of mid-wall fibrosis in DCM has recently been shown to be the strongest independent predictor of major adverse cardiac events in DCM, including arrhythmic events and SCD [14].

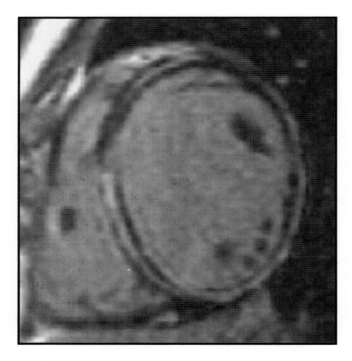

Figure 16.3 A 34-year-old professional cyclist has noted a subtle difficulty in keeping up with his team-mates on an incline over the last 3 weeks. His physical examination is noncontributory and an ECG shows left bundle branch block (LBBB). CMR shows a significantly dilated and impaired ventricle, whilst LGE shows circumferential enhancement

Arrhythmogenic Right Ventricular Cardiomyopathy

Disproportionate right ventricular changes have been shown to occur in high-level athletes, particularly after long endurance events. The question therefore arises as to whether this could reflect a right ventricular cardiomyopathy versus athletic remodelling (see Figure 16.4). Athletes with right ventricular changes may be more prone to arrhythmias of right ventricular origin, and CMR can be particularly useful in distinguishing this. ARVC is attributed to 4–22% of SCD in athletes, and involves fibro-fatty infiltration of the right ventricular myocardium, most commonly the free wall [15]. Typical right ventricular features of the athlete's heart (particularly in endurance athletes, such as cyclrs or rowers) may resemble those found in ARVC. Thus, whilst the diagnosis of right ventricular cardiomyopathy (e.g. ARVC) is not an imaging diagnosis alone, the distinction between athlete's heart and ARVC is particularly important in athletes who present with cardiac symptoms such as chest pain, syncope and palpitations.

If the diagnosis of AVRC is suspected in an athlete, a CMR should be requested. In ARVC, the enlargement of the right ventricular cavity involves both inflow and outflow and may be associated with regional right ventricular wall segmental morphological (e.g. thinning, bulging, or aneurysms) and functional (regional wall-motion) abnormalities. A recent study comparing elite athletes with anterior T-wave inversion and patients with ARVC shows that an LVED volume/RVED volume ≤1.2 supports physiological adaptation,

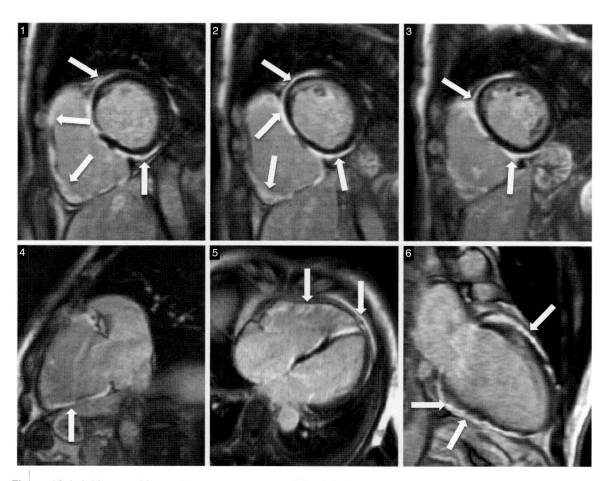

Figure 16.4 A 32-year-old marathon runner presents with palpitations and dizziness. ECG is unremarkable. Transthoracic echocardiogram (TTE) demonstrates a dilated right ventricle. CMR is performed for further assessment. LGE shows extensive fibrosis in the anterior, anteroseptal, septal and inferoseptal walls of the left ventricle, from apex to base in the short-axis stack and in the right ventricle wall (1–3). These findings correlate with findings in the right ventricle stack (4), four-chamber view (5) and two-chamber view (6)

whereas regional wall-motion abnormalities, a right ventricular ejection fraction of <45% and LGE in the right ventricle are excellent discriminators for ARVC [16].

Recent studies have documented a phenotype of ARVC characterised by a high volume of intense endurance training without evidence of a familial predisposition. This cohort may have a mild genetic risk or unrecognised gene, with intense endurance exercise accelerating the development of the ARVC phenotype [17].

It should be noted that cardiac imaging, whether by echocardiography or CMR, cannot confirm or exclude a diagnosis of ARVC on its own and that clinical features need to be considered.

Left Ventricular Noncompaction

Left ventricular noncompaction cardiomyopathy (LVNCC) is a rare cause of progressive left ventricular systolic dysfunction, thought to result from incomplete myocardial development (see Figure 16.5). It has been associated with an increased risk of SCD, especially in those with a reduced left ventricular ejection fraction. The prevalence of LVNCC is postulated to be between 0.014 and 1.260% of an unselected population, and in patients with heart failure it ranges from 3 to 4%. Up to 50% of cases have close relatives with cardiomyopathy.

LVNCC is characterised by prominent left ventricular trabeculae and deep intertrabecular recesses. However, distinguishing between pathologic LVNCC and physiologic hypertrabeculation is an increasing diagnostic challenge, particularly in the remodelled ventricles of athletes, and the current diagnostic criteria are felt to be inadequate (see Chapter 21). Athletes exhibit a higher prevalence of left ventricular trabeculation compared with controls. Even within the athletic population, differences persist, with left ventricular trabeculations more pronounced in African than Caucasian athletes.

Therefore, for the diagnosis of LVNC in this population, it is necessary to take into account other factors, such as left ventricular dilatation and dysfunction, LGE enhancement and documentation of ventricular arrhythmias. At present, however, no guidelines exist for the accurate and reproducible differentiation of LVNCC from athletic remodelling.

Myocarditis

Myocarditis is an inflammatory disease of the heart frequently resulting from viral infections or postviral immune-mediated responses (see Figure 16.6). Symptoms are nonspecific, and patients may present with chest pain, fatigue, dyspnoea or arrhythmia. Myocarditis is a relevant cause of SCD in young athletes. Task Force recommendations from 2005 have significant implications for competitive athletes, including that athletes with probable or definite evidence of myocarditis should be withdrawn from all competitive sports for at least 6 months and may return to training and competition only when left ventricular function and cardiac dimensions have returned to normal and if there are no clinically relevant arrhythmias [18]. Thus, accurate diagnosis is paramount.

CMR imaging is invaluable in the accurate diagnosis of myocarditis, and is currently regarded as the most appropriate noninvasive assessment, with a high diagnostic agreement between CMR and biopsy results. In addition to accurate assessment of left ventricular contractile function, CMR offers accurate assessment of myocardial oedema and scar burden. In the acute phase, T2-weighted oedema imaging identifies acute myocardial inflammation. LGE imaging may demonstrate two patterns of myocardial damage: either a mid-wall enhancement in the septal wall or a subepicardial (patchy) distribution in the left ventricular lateral wall. LGE imaging does not, however, allow differentiation between acute and chronic inflammation, but represents damaged myocardium.

The duration of abstinence from competitive sports after recovery from acute myocarditis is still a matter of debate.

Cardiac Sarcoid

Sarcoidosis is a heterogeneous, noncaseating, granulomatous disorder of unknown aetiology. Cardiac involvement occurs in 25% of those diagnosed. The heart may be the only organ affected, or cardiac involvement may precede, follow or occur concurrently with other organ involvement. Cardiac sarcoidosis is the most important cause of patient mortality, with a 5-year mortality rate between 25 and 60% despite immunosuppressive treatment.

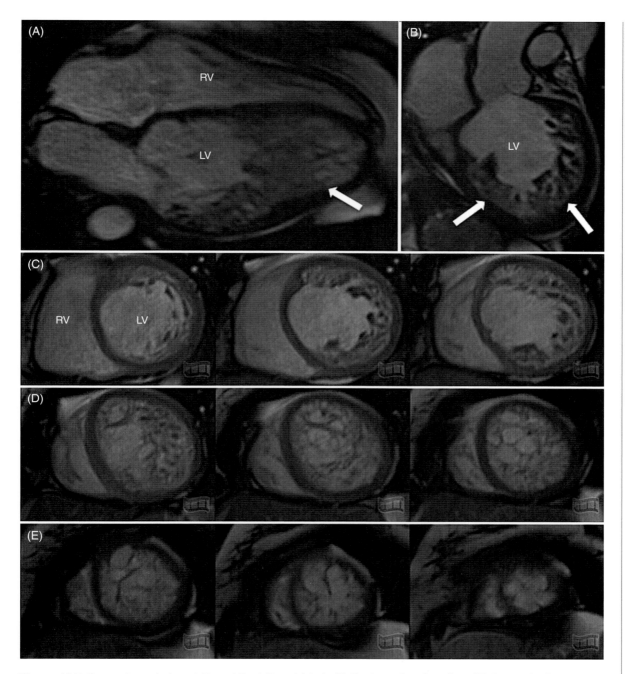

Figure 16.5 Severe hypertrabeculation of the left ventricle in (A) the four-chamber view, (B) the aortic view and the short-axis view, with increasing trabeculations from (C) the base through to (D) the mid ventricle and into (E) the apex

Cardiac sarcoid should be considered in those athletes presenting with palpitations, syncope, pre-syncope or chest pain. Should these be associated with abnormalities on ECG screening (including conduction abnormalities, ventricular arrhythmias or complete heart block), a CMR to exclude the diagnosis of cardiac sarcoid should be considered.

CMR findings consistent with a diagnosis of sarcoidosis include oedema suggestive of an acute infiltrative process on T2-weighted imaging. LGE may demonstrate fibrosis, with a typical distribution in the anteroseptal mid-myocardium and subendocardium.

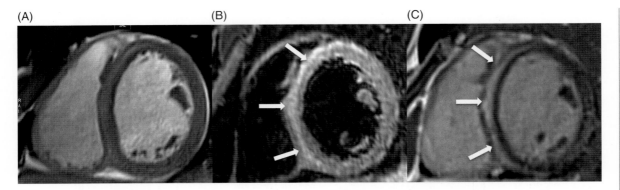

Figure 16.6 A 24-year-old female gymnast complains of intermittent chest pain on exertion. She has had a recent lower gastrointestinal infection. An ECG and transthoracic echocardiography are normal. A CMR is performed for completeness. (A) Cine images show global impairment of left ventricular systolic function. (B) STIR imaging shows significant myocardial oedema in the anteroseptal, septal and inferoseptal walls. (C) LGE imaging demonstrates extensive myocardial fibrosis in the anteroseptal, septal and inferoseptal walls. All of this is consistent with a diagnosis of severe, extensive myocarditis

Coronary Artery Disease

Congenital Coronary Artery Anomalies

Anomalous coronary arteries are implicated in approximately 17% of SCD in athletes [19]. It is postulated that high-risk coronary anomalous arteries are those which have an intra-arterial course, between the aorta and the pulmonary artery, and an associated bend at an acute angle. The most common anomalies associated with SCD are the left main stem arising from the right sinus of Valsalva and the right coronary artery arising from the left coronary sinus.

High-level athletes may be at increased risk of SCD with anomalous coronary arteries as, during training, the enlarged aorta and pulmonary artery exert external pressure, increasing the risk of a malignant cardiac arrhythmia and SCD. The 2005 Bethesda Conference recommends that an athlete with a coronary anomaly of the wrong sinus origin in which the artery passes between the great arteries be excluded from all competitive sport, regardless of symptoms [20].

Unfortunately, SCD is often the first manifestation of an anomalous coronary. In the symptomatic athlete, angina and syncope are the most common symptoms. Whilst computed tomography coronary angiography (CTCA) is the preferred imaging modality in athletes aged >35 years, in asymptomatic athletes <35 years an magnetic resonance angiography (MRA) of the proximal coronary arteries is the investigation of choice, as these individuals have low risk of CAD and CMR does not expose the younger athlete to radiation [21]. LGE images in CMR can show evidence of prior infarction. If they are present, the athlete should be investigated for coronary angiogram.

Atherosclerotic CAD

In athletes aged >35 years, the most common cause of SCD is atherosclerotic CAD [22]. SCD may result from malignant ventricular arrhythmia arising from myocardial scar, or from an acute ischaemic event. CMR is best placed as a single imaging modality by which to evaluate inducible ischaemia (adenosine perfusion CMR), rest- or stress-induced regional wall-motion abnormalities (dobutamine CMR) and the presence or absence of previous infarction.

Future Directions

It is clear the advantages that CMR provides a quick, noninvasive, often definitive investigation that can either reassure the athlete or prompt an unsuspected diagnosis. As the availability and accessibility of CMR increase, it is likely to become an increasingly commonly used tool in the sport physician's armoury. In the recent EuroCMR registry of over 27 000 patients referred for CMR [23], the CMR findings led to a direct change in management in over 60% of cases (including a new diagnosis or change in therapy) and satisfied all the imaging requirements for patients in 89% of cases.

As CMR hardware, software and contrast agents further develop, image resolution and tissue characterisation will continue to advance, which may convey new applications for CMR in the athlete. There is growing interest in the significance of myocardial fibrosis and T1 mapping of the athlete's heart. Indeed, recent research shows an association between lifelong endurance exercise and myocardial fibrosis in veteran endurance athletes, although the clinical implications of these findings are yet to be determined [24]. The potential of T1 mapping is still to be fully realised, and its advantages in the management of the athlete are untold. Studies using T1 mapping to distinguish between athlete's heart and DCM are ongoing. Further large longitudinal studies with prolonged periods of follow-up are needed to investigate the long-term outcomes of the indeterminate findings in CMR.

Conclusion

Whilst it is clear that CMR offers significant advantages over other imaging modalities in athlete evaluation, it should be stressed that the overwhelming majority of athletes can be, and are, reliably screened for sporting participation without the need for a CMR. We would suggest that CMR be reserved for the following indications:

- The athlete with concerning symptoms, such as palpitations, chest pain or syncope, and an equivocal workup.
- The asymptomatic athlete with a markedly abnormal ECG and equivocal or normal echo.
- The athlete with ventricular arrhythmias, to screening for possible ARVC or sarcoid.
- The athlete with troponin-positive events: myocarditis, missed acute coronary syndrome (ACS) (ACS and normal angiography).
- The athlete with an equivocal echo (disproportionate LVH or significant left ventricular dilatation).

Acknowledgements

I acknowledge the help of Dr Deirdre Waterhouse and Dr Theodore Murphy in the production of this chapter.

References

1 Drezner, J. Standardised criteria for ECG interpretation in athletes: a practical tool. *Br J Sports Med* 2012; **46**(Suppl. 1): i6–8.
2 Waterhouse, D., Ismail, T., Prasad, S. et al. Imaging focal and interstitial fibrosis with cardiovascular magnetic resonance in athletes with left ventricular hypertrophy: implications for sporting participation. *Br J Sports Med* 2012; **46**(Suppl. 1): i69–77.
3 Moon, J., Messroghli, D., Kellman, P. et al. Myocardial T1 mapping and extracellular volume quantification: a Society for Cardiovascular Magnetic Resonance (SCMR) and CMR Working Group of the European Society of Cardiology consensus statement. *J Cardiovasc Magn Reson*, 2013; **15**(1): 92.
4 Karamitsos, T., Dass, S., Suttie, J. et al. Blunted myocardial oxygenation response during vasodilator stress in patients with hypertrophic cardiomyopathy. *J Am Coll Cardiol* 2013; **61**(11): 1169–76.
5 La Gerche, A., Burns, A., Mooney, D. et al. Exercise-induced right ventricular dysfunction and structural remodelling in endurance athletes. *Eur Heart J* 2011; **33**(8): 998–1006.
6 La Gerche, A., Taylor, A. and Prior, D. Athlete's heart: the potential for multimodality imaging to address the critical remaining questions. *JACC Cardiovasc Imaging* 2009; **2**(3): 350–63.
7 Galderisi, M., Cardim, N., D'Andrea, A. et al. The multi-modality cardiac imaging approach to the Athlete's heart: an expert consensus of the European Association of Cardiovascular Imaging. *Eur Heart J Cardiovasc Imaging* 2015; **16**(4): 353.
8 Rowin, E., Maron, B., Appelbaum, E. et al. Significance of false negative electrocardiograms in preparticipation screening of athletes for hypertrophic cardiomyopathy. *Am J Cardiol* 2012; **110**(7): 1027–32.
9 Maron, B., Doerer, J., Haas, T. et al. Sudden deaths in young competitive athletes: analysis of 1866 deaths in the United States, 1980–2006. *Circulation* 2009; **119**(8): 1085–92.
10 Maron, M., Olivotto, I., Maron, B. et al. The case for myocardial ischemia in hypertrophic cardiomyopathy. *J Am Coll Cardiol* 2009; **54**(9): 866–75.
11 O'Hanlon, R., Grasso, A., Roughton, M. et al. Prognostic significance of myocardial fibrosis in hypertrophic cardiomyopathy using cardiovascular magnetic resonance. *J Cardiovasc Magn Reson* 2010; **12**(Suppl. 1): O50.

12 Sado, D., White, S., Piechnik, S. et al. Identification and assessment of Anderson-Fabry disease by cardiovascular magnetic resonance noncontrast myocardial T1 mapping. *Circ Cardiovasc Imaging* 2013; **6**(3): 392–8.

13 Assomull, R., Prasad, S., Lyne, J. et al. Cardiovascular magnetic resonance, fibrosis, and prognosis in dilated cardiomyopathy. *J Am Coll Cardiol* 2006; **48**(10): 1977–85.

14 Gulati, A., Jabbour, A., Ismail, T. et al. Association of fibrosis with mortality and sudden cardiac death in patients with nonischemic dilated cardiomyopathy. *JAMA* 2013; **309**(9): 896.

15 Corrado, D., Basso, C., Schiavon, M. and Thiene, G. Screening for hypertrophic cardiomyopathy in young athletes. *New Engl J Med* 1998; **339**(6): 364–9.

16 Zaidi, A., Sheikh, N., Jongman, J.K. et al. Clinical differentiation between physiological remodeling and arrhythmogenic right ventricular cardiomyopathy in athletes with marked electrocardiographic repolarization anomalies. *J Am Coll Cardiol* 2015; **65**(25): 2702–11.

17 La Gerche, A. and Heidbuchel, H. Exercise-induced arrhythmogenic right ventricular cardiomyopathy. *Cardiac Electrophysiol Clin* 2013; **5**(1): 97–105.

18 Maron, B., Ackerman, M., Nishimura, R. et al. Task Force 4: HCM and other cardiomyopathies, mitral valve prolapse, myocarditis, and Marfan syndrome. *J Am Coll Cardiol* 2005; **45**(8): 1340–5.

19 Maron, B., Thompson, P., Ackerman, M. et al. Recommendations and considerations related to preparticipation screening for cardiovascular abnormalities in competitive athletes: 2007 update: a scientific statement from the American Heart Association Council on Nutrition, Physical Activity, and Metabolism: endorsed by the American College of Cardiology Foundation. *Circulation* 2007; **115**(12): 1643–55.

20 Graham, T., Driscoll, D., Gersony, W. et al. Task Force 2: congenital heart disease. *J Am Coll Cardiol* 2005; **45**(8): 1326–33.

21 Prakken, N., Cramer, M., Olimulder, M. et al. Screening for proximal coronary artery anomalies with 3-dimensional MR coronary angiography. *Int J Cardiovasc Imaging* 2010; **26**(6): 701–10.

22 Waller, B. and Roberts, W. Sudden death while running in conditioned runners aged 40 years or over. *Am J Cardiol* 1980; **45**(6): 1292–300.

23 Bruder, O., Wagner, A., Lombardi, M. et al. European cardiovascular magnetic resonance (EuroCMR) registry – multi national results from 57 centers in 15 countries. *J Cardiovasc Magn Reson* 2013; **15**(1): 9.

24 Wilson, M., O'Hanlon, R., Prasad, S. et al. Diverse patterns of myocardial fibrosis in lifelong, veteran endurance athletes. *J Appl Physiol* 2011; **110**(6): 1622–6.

17 Genetic Testing for Cardiovascular Conditions Predisposing to Sudden Death

Colleen Caleshu and Euan Ashley

Falk Cardiovascular Research Center, Stanford, CA, USA

Introduction

Many of the conditions that cause sudden death in young athletes are genetic in origin, including inherited arrhythmias such as long QT syndrome, familial cardiomyopathies like hypertrophic cardiomyopathy (HCM), inherited aortopathies such as Marfan syndrome and dyslipidemias like familial hypercholesterolemia. Many cases of sudden death remain unexplained even after a detailed expert autopsy. However, further investigation via post mortem genetic testing and cardiac evaluations of family members reveals that a third or more of such cases are in fact due to an inherited cardiovascular condition, most frequently inherited arrhythmias [1]. Advances in both sequencing technologies and genetic knowledge raise the question of what role genetic testing might play in identifying athletes who are at increased risk of dying suddenly. This chapter will explore that question, by first reviewing the genetics of cardiovascular diseases (CVDs) that predispose to sudden death and the current state of genetic testing of these diseases, then considering the application of genetic testing to the evaluation of athletes.

Genetics of Inherited CVD

The majority of conditions that predispose to sudden cardiac death (SCD) are inherited in an autosomal-dominant manner. The genetic causes of most inherited CVDs are diverse and varied; dozens of different genes and hundreds to thousands of different variants in those genes have been associated with these diseases (Table 17.1). They tend to be disease-causing variants seen in just one family (private) or a handful of families (semi-private) with the disorder (Figure 17.1). This is in stark contrast to other genetic conditions, such as Huntington's disease, in which all cases are caused by just one genetic difference in one gene, or Tay–Sachs disease, which is caused by a handful of variants in one gene.

The diverse genetic aetiologies seen in inherited CVD are a product of the biology and pathophysiology of the conditions. For example, there are multiple ways to impair the function of several different ion channels in order to create a long QT phenotype, so hundreds to thousands of different variants in several different channel genes are implicated in long QT syndrome (Table 17.1, Figure 17.1). The clinical impact of the genetic diversity seen in inherited CVD is significant: genetic testing requires full sequencing analysis of many genes, which is more expensive and time-consuming than the focused analysis of a few specific variants required for a disease like Tay–Sachs. The clinical benefit of genetic testing to the patient and family is only realised if the genetic test can identify a variant that we are confident causes disease; as a result of the vast diversity in the genetic aetiology of these conditions, current genetic tests often find a variant that is inconclusive. Despite the long lists of disease-associated genes, the genetic cause still eludes us in many cases (Table 17.1). Identifying additional disease-associated genes has proved challenging. This is likely because each of the remaining genes is an exceptionally rare cause, accounting for a small proportion of cases. It may

IOC Manual of Sports Cardiology, First Edition. Edited by Mathew G. Wilson, Jonathan A. Drezner and Sanjay Sharma.
© 2017 International Olympic Committee. Published 2017 by John Wiley & Sons, Ltd.

Table 17.1 Genetic testing for select inherited CVDs. Genetic testing typically involves sequencing of specific genes associated with a disease. Most CVDs have been associated with many different genes. A subset are seen often and have strong evidence supporting their disease association. Others are seen very rarely. Some have very weak evidence supporting their disease association and may in fact be unrelated. Different commercial genetic tests will include different combinations of genes. Genetic tests that include additional genes beyond those most frequently implicated may have modest increases in the detection of disease-causing variants and will have significant increases in detection of variants of uncertain significance

	Hypertrophic cardiomyopathy		Arrhythmogenic right ventricular cardiomyopathy		Marfan syndrome		Long QT syndrome		Catecholaminergic ventricular tachycardia	
Detection rate*	35–60%		40–50%		70–90%		70–75%		50–55%	
Frequent and/or well validated genes^	MYH7	12–20%	PKP2	11–43%	FBN1	70–90%	KCNQ1	30–35%	RYR2	50–55%
	MYBPC3	20–28%	DSG2	12–40%			KCNH2	25–30%	CASQ2	2–5%
	TNNT2	2–5%	DSP	6–16%			SCN5A	5–10%		
	TNNI3	1–3%	DSC2	1–5%						
	TPM3	1–3%								
	MYL2	<1%								
	MYL3	<1%								
	ACTC1	<1%								
Rare and/or putative genes#	ACTN2		DES				AKAP9		KCNJ2	
	ANKRD1		JUP				ANK2		TRDN	
	BAG3		LMNA				CACNA1C		CALM1	
	CAV3		PLN				CALM1		ANK2	
	CSRP3		RYR2				CALM2			
	JPH2		SCN5A				CAV3			
	LDB3		TGFB3				KCNE1			
	MTTG		TMEM43				KCNE2			
	MTTH		TTN				KCNJ2			
	MTTI						KCNJ5			
	MTTK						NOS1AP			
	MYH6						SCN4B			
	MYLK2						SNTA1			
	MYO6									
	MYOM1									
	MYOZ2									
	MYPN									
	NEXN									
	PDLIM3									
	PLN									
	RBM20									
	RYR2									
	TCAP									
	TNNCI									
	TTN									
	VCL									

* Detection rate is frequency of rare variation in patients with the diagnosis, which usually includes variants classified as disease-causing and variants of uncertain significance

^ The most frequently implicated genes and genes with strongest evidence for involvement in the disease.

Genes that are very rarely implicated in the disease and/or with weaker evidence for involvement in disease.

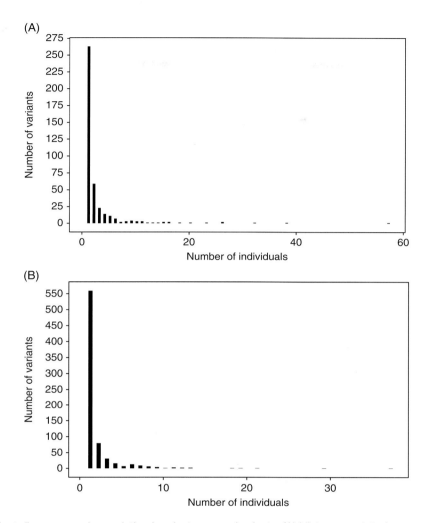

Figure 17.1 Most disease-causing variation is private or semi-private. (A) Histogram plot of sarcomere variants observed in 4349 individuals who underwent genetic testing for HCM, distributed by the number of individuals with each variant. For example, one variant, p.Arg663His in *MYH7*, was seen in 38 individuals, whilst 263 variants were seen in only one individual each (*Data sources:* Stanford (unpublished), Alfares et al. [2], Bos et al. [3]) (B) Histogram plot of potassium- and sodium-channel variants observed in 3617 individuals who underwent genetic testing for long QT syndrome Includes cohorts from two clinical genetic testing laboratories in the United States and a North American and European research cohort (*Data sources:* Kapplinger et al. [4], Lieve et al. [5], Splawski et al. [6])

also be that some cases are explained by novel genetic mechanisms that clinical genetic tests and gene-finding studies don't currently investigate. This could include variation in regulatory regions, epigenetic modification or large structural differences. It may also be that instead of being due to a single variant in a single gene, some cases are in fact caused by multiple variants in many parts of the genome. There is some emerging data to suggest that this may be the case for Brugada syndrome.

Studies of families with inherited CVD show marked intra- and interfamilial variability in severity and age of onset. Some of this may be attributed to differences in the causative variant. However, significant clinical variability is seen even amongst individuals who share the same disease-causing variant. Penetrance, a measure of the likelihood of developing a phenotype given a disease-causing genotype, is both incomplete and age-dependent. Some individuals who carry a variant predisposing to an inherited heart condition will never show any manifestation of the disease. Others will have normal cardiac evaluations for many years and then at some point develop the phenotype. The origin of this variability in clinical presentation is not well understood. A small portion of it seems to be attributable to variants in other genes and to levels of expression of the disease-causing allele. Close correlations between genotype and phenotype have been elusive in the majority of conditions. The vast number of genetic variants that underlie inherited CVD makes it hard to identify clinically meaningful correlations between genotype and phenotype. For a select few, primarily long QT syndrome, we now have an understanding of correlations between the phenotype and the specific gene, type of variant or location of the variant [7], but even then there is still considerable variability amongst patients with the same variant, and it is very difficult to predict severity based on genotype.

Genetic Testing for Inherited CVD

Advancements in the understanding of the molecular basis of rare genetic conditions, combined with marked improvements in sequencing technology, have led to the widespread availability of genetic testing for most inherited CVDs. Genetic testing is recommended as a class I (greatest consensus) indication for patients with many genetic heart conditions, including long QT syndrome, catecholaminergic polymorphic ventricular tachycardia (CPVT) and HCM [8].

The primary benefit of genetic testing for the vast majority of these conditions is in the assessment of healthy relatives. As a result of reduced and age-dependent penetrance, some family members will carry the disease-causing variant but show no evidence of disease. It is often impossible to distinguish such individuals from those who have not inherited the predisposition using cardiovascular testing. This leaves healthy family members in a prolonged state of uncertainty and in need of serial surveillance, often for the rest of their lives. If the causative variant has been identified, genetic testing can determine which family members have inherited the predisposition. Cardiac screening can be targeted to the predisposed individuals and reassurance can be provided to those who are not predisposed.

Whilst the primary benefit of genetic testing is usually in the assessment of family members, in a small minority of cases genetic testing can have direct benefit for the patient with inherited CVD, by clarifying the diagnosis, providing prognostic information or directing therapeutic choices. Genetic testing may reveal that the patient in fact has a different disease, one that mimics the initial diagnosis. One example of this is disorders of cellular metabolism that cause build-up of substances in the cardiomyocyte, leading to left ventricular hypertrophy (LVH), which can resemble HCM. In other cases, genetic testing may pinpoint a specific subtype with important management implications. Patients with a predisposition to aortic aneurysms and dissections with variants in *ACTA2*, *MYH11* or *TGFBR2* are prone to dissections at a smaller aortic diameter and thus may need earlier surgical intervention. Roughly 3–7% of individuals with inherited arrhythmias and cardiomyopathies have multiple rare variants in frequent disease-causing genes, and these individuals often have an earlier onset and a more severe phenotype.

The clinical benefit of genetic testing depends on identification of the pathogenic variant that is the cause of the patient's CVD. The sensitivity of current multigene tests for these diseases varies considerably (Table 17.1). In many cases of definite CVD with a clear familial pattern, analysis of genes associated with the condition fails to identify the underlying causative variant.

Genetic testing typically starts with a multigene-sequencing panel, ideally on the member of the family who has the most severe case of inherited CVD. The goal of this testing is to identify the variant that has caused the patient's disease. Variants are identified by comparing the patient's sequence for the genes of interest to the reference sequence for those genes. The reference is the sequence originally generated by the Human Genome Project and continuously improved upon since. Variants that are prevalent in the general population are set aside, leaving any rare variants to be considered as potential causes of the patient's disorder.

Once a candidate rare variant has been identified, its clinical significance must be carefully assessed before it is applied to care. This is necessary because not all rare variants cause disease. The genetic test interpretation process aims to distinguish benign variants from disease-causing ones. A variety of data on each variant are gathered and reviewed, including the number of patients with the variant, whether the variant tracks with disease in each family, the frequency in the general population, experimental data and the predicted effect of the variant on the gene and the protein [9]. These data are carefully synthesised and weighed in order to arrive at a classification that reflects the likelihood that the variant causes disease (Figure 17.2). Variants classified as likely pathogenic or pathogenic are considered appropriate for use in the patient's care and in assessing which family members are predisposed to disease. Variants of uncertain significance lack sufficient or consistent data to clarify whether they are benign or disease-causing. Since their status is inconclusive, they are not helpful in directing care of the patient or the patient's family.

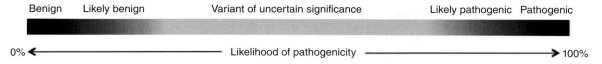

Figure 17.2 Genetic test interpretation is probabilistic. Variants found through genetic testing are classified as benign, likely benign, uncertain significance, likely pathogenic or pathogenic. These various classifications fall along a spectrum of likelihood that the variant is disease-causing, with benign at one end, pathogenic at the other, and a broad range of uncertainty in the middle

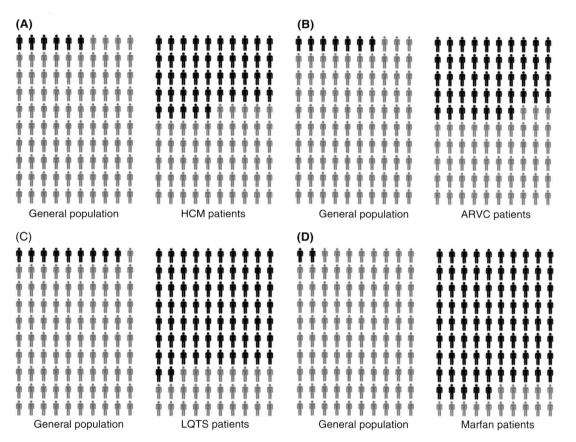

Figure 17.3 Rare genetic variation in inherited CVD genes in the general population and in patients for (A) HCM, (B) arrhythmogenic right ventricular cardiomyopathy (ARVC), (C) long QT syndrome, (D) Marfan syndrome. Black-shaded figures represent individuals who carry a rare variant that would be identified on a typical clinical genetic test and would be noted on the results report as a variant of uncertain significance or as a disease-causing variant

Changes in our understanding of genetic variation have led to shifts in the interpretation of genetic tests. The difficulty inherent in interpreting genetic testing in cardiology stems from the fact that rare variation is seen in both patients and healthy individuals (Figure 17.3). As previously noted, the majority of causative variants are either unique to a given family or seen in just a handful of families (Figure 17.1). Application of new high-throughput sequencing technologies to tens of thousands of individuals from the general population has revealed that rare genetic variation is far more abundant, and presumably better tolerated, than previously suspected. Sequencing of individuals unselected for rare genetic heart disease has shown that 4–16% have a rare variant in one of the genes included on current genetic tests for these diseases (Figure 17.3) [8]. Considering this on an individual level, genome sequencing reveals that any one person has ~100 rare or private genetic variants in disease-associated genes. If identified on a clinical genetic test, any one of these might be considered as a candidate for a disease-causing variant, leading to a 'positive' or 'variant of uncertain significance' result. Yet, the vast majority of these do not in fact cause genetic disease. Thus, it has become clear that rare and private variation is common, and likely mostly benign. Historically, the thinking in the field was that rare variation is most likely disease-causing and is limited to individuals with rare genetic disease. One impact of this old paradigm is that some genes have been erroneously associated with disease; the only evidence supporting their association is the rarity of the variant and the biological plausibility of the relationship.

Taken together, these findings inspire a certain amount of humility and warrant caution in the interpretation of genetic test results. When a rare variant is found with a genetic test, we must consider two competing hypotheses: that the variant causes genetic disease or that the variant is one of the many presumably benign rare variants all humans have. The interpretation of the genetic test arises from a careful analysis that weighs the evidence supporting each hypothesis, the pre-test probability of finding a pathogenic variant and the rate of rare variation in healthy individuals in all the genes on the panel. We must also consider the strength of evidence that the gene itself is truly associated with disease. Instead of being binary (positive or negative), genetic test results reflect a spectrum of likelihood that a given variant causes disease (Figure 17.2). As new data come to light, the classification may change.

When genetic testing identifies a variant that has a sufficiently high likelihood of being disease-causing, that variant can be applied to clinical care. Identification of no variant or a variant of uncertain significance is unfortunately not clinically useful. It does little to affect the patient's care and genetic testing cannot be used to assess healthy relatives. For most inherited cardiovascular conditions, such a result cannot rule out a diagnosis in the patient, because the test is positive in those who truly have the disease significantly less than 100% of the time (Table 17.1). In contrast, when a pathogenic variant is found, the diagnosis in the patient is further supported and disease risk in healthy family members can be assessed by testing specifically for that variant alone, with a targeted, faster and cheaper genetic test.

Genetic testing is just one tool used in a comprehensive cardiovascular genetics evaluation (Figure 17.4). Guidelines and consensus statements from many different professional organisations recommend that a cardiovascular genetics evaluation include genetic counselling, thorough family history analysis, consultation with clinicians with expertise in inherited heart disease, careful interpretation of genetic test results and cardiac screening of family members [1,8]. Comprehensive genetic evaluation is recommended for individuals diagnosed with inherited CVD.

Many cardiovascular genetics centres include genetic counsellors, master's-level trained health care professionals with expertise in genetic assessment, genetic test interpretation, communication of genetic information to families and psychological support. Genetic counselling provided prior to genetic testing prepares the patient and broader family for possible results, their clinical application and potential psychological responses. Once the genetic test results have been received, genetic counselling helps the patient and family understand, emotionally adapt to and apply the new information. An important distinction between the care of a patient with inherited CVD and typical medical care is in the broadening of focus to include the entire family. A diagnosis of genetic disease or an abnormal genetic test result has implications for the entire family. A comprehensive genetics evaluation ensures that the needs of both the patient and their family are addressed (Figure 17.4).

Genetic Testing in Sudden Death Risk Assessment

Much work has been done to try to improve sudden death risk stratification in inherited CVD. Since the genetic variant causing the disease is the very origin of the condition, it has been tempting to expect that genetic data will reveal sudden death risk. Unfortunately, for most diseases, this has not been the case. As previously noted, these conditions show marked variability, even amongst individuals with the same pathogenic variant – even within the same family. Many early case reports described particular variants as more severe or associated with a higher risk of sudden death. However, subsequent studies using broader samples and more robust statistical analyses have suggested the picture is more complex. One notable example is the long-suspected association between troponin variants in HCM and a higher risk of sudden death, based on case reports. A recent study comparing a multicentre sample of patients with such variants to other HCM patients found no difference in arrhythmic outcomes [10]. Thus, for the majority of conditions, genetic testing does not play a role in sudden death risk assessment. There are, however, a few notable – and clinically useful – exceptions.

Genetics-guided sudden death risk assessment has been most fruitful in long QT. Individuals with type 1 long QT syndrome (due to variants in *KCNQ1*) are more likely to have events with exercise than individuals

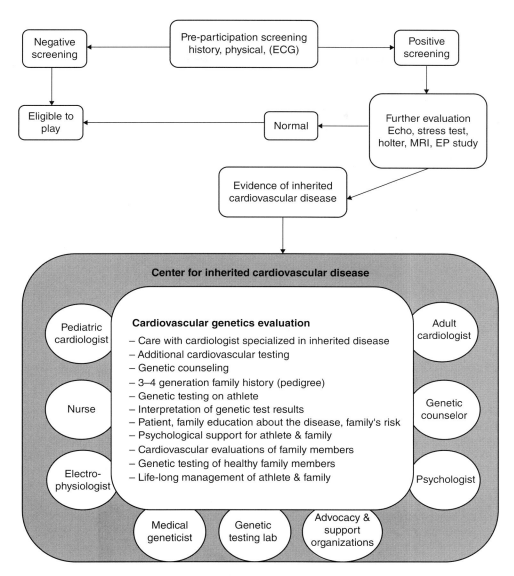

Figure 17.4 Role of comprehensive genetics evaluation in athlete screening. When pre-participation screening shows evidence of inherited CVD, athletes should be referred to a centre specialising in inherited CVD, where an interdisciplinary team will perform a comprehensive genetics evaluation of the athlete and their family members

with type 2 (*KCNH2*) or 3 (*SCN5A*), although arrhythmias can happen with exercise in all three. Specific subsets of variants in long QT have been associated with a higher risk of events, including variants in the cytoplasmic loops in *KCNQ1*, variants in *KCNQ1* with dominant-negative effects and variants in the pore region of *KCNH2* [7]. Patients with the *LMNA*-associated constellation of dilated cardiomyopathy, atrial and ventricular ectopy and conduction-system disease have a higher, and earlier, risk of sudden death than patients with other forms of familial dilated cardiomyopathy. A multicentre European study of *LMNA* patients found that having a non-missense variant was one of several factors associated with higher arrhythmic risk [11].

Even when the patient has one of these genotypes that seem to confer a higher risk of sudden death, it is not recommended that implantable cardioverter-defibrillator (ICD) decisions be made based on the genetic data alone [1]. Sudden death risk stratification remains a multifactorial endeavour, based primarily on clinical parameters, with either minimal or, in most cases, no input from genetic testing.

Genetic Testing in the Athlete

When Genetic Testing is Abnormal but Cardiovascular Testing is Normal

If interpretation challenges could be overcome, the advantage of adding genetic testing to the pre-participation screening regimen would be in the ascertainment of individuals who harbour a predisposition to an inherited CVD that is missed on history, physical and, where applicable, ECG. We must then consider whether these individuals are in fact at significantly increased risk for SCD. A subset of these individuals will have active disease process. Unfortunately, this is an understudied subgroup and the data needed to guide practice are not available. Studies on families with long QT syndrome have demonstrated that individuals who carry the disease-causing variant but have a normal ECG do indeed have increased risk of arrhythmic events, albeit a lower one than their relatives with abnormal ECGs [12]. Similarly, individuals predisposed to catecholaminergic polymorphic ventricular tachycardia (CPVT) have undergone normal exercise testing and then gone on to have cardiac events [13]. These data have led experts to recommend consideration of medical therapy for individuals with a genetic predisposition to these channelopathies but normal cardiovascular tests (so-called 'genotype-positive, phenotype-negative individuals') [1,13]. Revised diagnostic criteria for long QT syndrome suggest that the presence of a pathogenic variant is sufficient to make the diagnosis, even in the absence of symptoms or QT prolongation [1]. These data fit with the very nature of these disorders: they entail an increased risk to arrhythmias that is somewhat paroxysmal in nature.

In contrast to the paroxysmal nature of inherited arrhythmias, inherited cardiomyopathies have a more discrete onset. Most individuals with familial cardiomyopathy had morphologically normal hearts at birth and for the first years or decades of life. Then, at some point, morphological changes became evident. Some individuals predisposed to familial cardiomyopathies will never develop an overt myopathy. Robust data on the risk of sudden death prior to overt cardiomyopathy are not available. Rare cases of sudden death in such individuals have been reported.

To date, there has been inconsistency in the activity recommendations for individuals who carry a predisposition to inherited CVD but show no signs of that disease. The 2015 American College of Cardiology and American Heart Association recommendations allowing individuals with predisposition to long QT or HCM to participate in competitive athletics (with the exception of competitive swimming when the predisposition is to long QT type 1) [14]. In contrast, the European Society of Cardiology (ESC) recommendations advise that such individuals should not participate in competitive sports [15]. The authors of these documents have attributed the inconsistencies to the lack of available data and the need to rely heavily on expert opinions.

An important subgroup is genetic predispositions that may be potentiated by athletic activity. There is growing evidence that the likelihood of developing arrhythmogenic right ventricular cardiomyopathy (ARVC) increases with the predisposed individual's volume of exercise [16]. Haemodynamic stress on a genetically compromised aorta can similarly hasten the development of dilatation and dissection. It may be prudent to recommend individuals with such predispositions refrain from high-volume and high-intensity training. The joint ACC/AHA eligibility recommendations for competitive sport suggests that athletes with Marfan syndrome and normal aortic root dimensions can participate in 'low and moderate/low dynamic competitive sports', whilst the European recommendations advise against all competitive sports [14,15].

There is also the question of how disease risk conferred by pathogenic variants differs in families with known inherited CVD and in healthy individuals from the general population. There is a long-recognised temporal pattern of selection bias in genetics: early reports of a genetic disease describe severe cases with high risk conferred by the genetic variant, in contrast to later studies of more broadly ascertained cases, which reveal that the phenotype is often milder and the risk lower. Emerging data from exome and genome sequencing suggest that genetic predisposition to CVD may be more common than previously thought and that the disease risk associated with such predispositions may be lower than expected. Essentially, all of the data available on risk of sudden death in inherited CVD come from families with at least one individual with overt clinical disease. These data may not be generalisable to a healthy athlete with a known pathogenic variant but an unremarkable family history and normal cardiovascular testing.

The question of how to manage athletes with a disease-associated genotype but no overt phenotype must be considered within the context of growing debate about whether current participation guidelines for individuals with inherited CVD are overly restrictive. There are preliminary data in long QT which suggest that looser recommendations may not lead to significant harm [17]. A 2013 international expert consensus statement on the management of inherited arrhythmias left room for select low-risk patients with long QT to be permitted to compete after expert consultation and with automated external defibrillators (AEDs) and life support professionals available [1]. Individuals with a predisposition to inherited CVD but no signs of that disease likely fall into the lowest risk strata, especially if they were discovered through broad population screening.

Even if genetic testing is never introduced as a frontline test in pre-participation screening, teams and physicians will encounter individuals who know they carry a predisposition to inherited CVD. Some athletes will have a family history of genetic heart disease that prompts them to learn about their predisposition. Others may learn their genetic status after undergoing exome or genome sequencing. The American College of Medical Genetics and Genomics (ACMG) recommended in 2013 that anyone undergoing clinical exome or genome sequencing be informed of disease-associated variants in a list of 56 genes considered to have high medical impact. The list includes genes associated with HCM, long QT syndrome and Marfan syndrome and related aortopathies.

Genetic Testing after an Abnormal Physical or ECG

As highlighted in Chapters 11, 14 and 40, determining whether borderline findings on ECG or echocardiogram are signs of CVD or normal variants is a challenging task, with weighty medical, psychological and financial implications for the athlete. Athletes, physicians and teams may turn to genetic testing to help clarify ambiguous clinical scenarios. Interpretation of genetic testing depends on the pre-test probability of the diagnosis. As the probability of the diagnosis decreases, the likelihood that an identified rare variant is pathogenic also decreases, with a corresponding increase in the likelihood the variant is one of the many benign rare variants we all have. Thus, when genetic testing is performed on an athlete with ambiguous cardiovascular findings, there is a high likelihood that it will be inconclusive or uninformative. This is not to say that there is no role for genetic testing in the clarification of ambiguous cardiovascular findings. When genetic testing identifies a variant with strong evidence supporting pathogenicity, it can solidify a diagnosis of a genetic disease and clarify management, including participation recommendations. When genetic testing on an ambiguous case does not identify a variant, it can decrease the likelihood of inherited CVD – but it cannot rule it out, since the sensitivity of current genetic tests is far less than 100% (Table 17.1). Thus, genetic testing can only rarely act as an arbiter in ambiguous cases, and interpretation of results is particularly challenging when the diagnosis is unclear.

After an athlete has been diagnosed with a genetic heart condition, genetic testing may help determine which other family members are predisposed and need screening or treatment. Since sudden death can occur in nonathletes and there can be important clinical manifestations unrelated to sudden death, the diagnosis of an inherited heart condition in an athlete should prompt an evaluation of the entire family, including genetic counselling and family screening (Figure 17.4). Thus, when pre-participation screening reveals evidence of inherited CVD, the athlete and their family should be referred to a centre with expertise in that condition for a comprehensive genetics evaluation. In addition to meeting their medical needs, a specialised centre can often also address the significant psychological needs that arise when a diagnosis takes an athlete out of sport.

Cascade Screening of Families

An alternative and perhaps complementary method of identifying athletes genetically predisposed to sudden death is a more thorough evaluation of families already known to have inherited CVD. The term 'cascade screening' describes the stepwise evaluation of family members at risk of genetic disease. The index patient's diagnosis prompts evaluation of all immediate relatives. Molecular or clinical diagnosis in an immediate relative then leads to evaluation of that person's immediate relatives, and so forth. In one such programme, a Dutch group evaluated 130 families with inherited arrhythmias, identifying 509 relatives with the genetic predisposition, including 249 who needed drug treatment, 26 who needed a pacemaker and 14 who needed a defibrillator [18]. Genetic counselling interventions are integral to these approaches and help to increase the number of family members who present for evaluation. These data underscore the importance of referral to cardiovascular genetics centres and pursuit of family evaluations (Figure 17.4). Even more compelling are the data from another Dutch group on a more aggressive form of cascade screening that has identified over

9000 patients with familial hypercholesterolemia [19]. In the first 5 years, the programme tested 5442 relatives of 237 patients with familial hypercholesterolemia, identifying 2039 carriers. What makes this programme distinct from the cascade screening performed in most cardiovascular genetics clinics is the use of a direct-contact model and 'genetic fieldwork'. The immediate relatives of index cases are contacted by the health care team directly and a specialised nurse visits their home to evaluate them, including drawing blood for genetic testing. This active and direct approach contrasts with the inactive and passive approach used in most clinics, in which the patient is given information to share with their family and the family has to contact the clinic and come in for an appointment. Direct-contact programmes can be challenging in countries, like the United States, with strict privacy laws. However, efforts are underway to develop compliant versions of such programmes. The Dutch experience shows that identification of new cases through families, instead of through general-population screening, can be both powerful and cost-effective.

Genetic Testing for Performance and Injury

Whilst the primary focus of this chapter is on cardiovascular genetic testing, the sports medicine community now faces the prospect of genetic testing to predict performance and injury. A variety of companies and institutions offer genetic tests for a handful of common variants purportedly associated with athletic ability (e.g. *ACTN3*, *ACE*, *NOS3*) or injury (e.g. *COL5A1*, *COL1A1*, *MMP3*) [20]. The scientific validity of such claims and the ethics of basing genetic testing services on them have been the focus of significant criticism, with commentaries in the literature using such terms as 'preposterous' and 'snake oil' [21].

The genetic underpinnings of injury susceptibility and athletic performance are quite different from those of diseases like familial hypercholesterolemia and long QT syndrome. Whilst rare genetic diseases are driven predominantly by one rare variant in one gene, most diseases and traits are influenced by a multitude of variants throughout the genome, most of them common. Each individual common variant makes only a minor contribution to disease risk, with odds ratios typically in the range of 1.05–1.20. Diseases such as diabetes and coronary artery disease (CAD) and traits such as height and athletic ability are of course also influenced by lifestyle and environment. They are ultimately determined by a complex interplay of multiple genetic variants and multiple nongenetic factors (Figure 17.5).

There was hope that completion of the Human Genome Project and advances in genetic technologies would provide deep insights into the genetic basis of most diseases, which would in turn allow us to use genetic

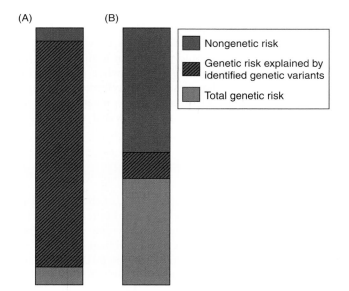

Figure 17.5 Proportion of disease or trait risk explained by identified genetic variants. (A) For rare genetic diseases like HCM and long QT syndrome, the majority of the disease risk is genetic and almost all of that genetic risk is attributable to a single rare variant in a single gene. (B) For most diseases and traits, such as CAD and athletic performance, both genetic and nongenetic factors make substantial contributions. The genetic risk is attributable to multiple variants, mostly common, and only a small portion is explained by the variants identified to date

testing to predict a wide range of diseases in the general population. A decade of work and thousands of publications have revealed that the genetic basis of most human diseases and traits is far more elusive than we had hoped. Whilst insights have been gained, the bulk of the genetic aetiology of most diseases and traits remains unexplained. One of the most thoroughly investigated diseases is CAD, which has been subject to multiple large studies, including an international consortium studying hundreds of thousands of individuals [22]. These large sample sizes are needed to ensure sufficient power to detect multiple small effects, to allow for correction for multiple-hypothesis testing and to ensure accurate estimation of effect sizes. Approximately 100 locations in the genome have been implicated in CAD, yet in combination they only explain a quarter of the genetic portion of the aetiology and only a tenth of the aetiology overall [22]. This same inability to explain the majority of the genetic aetiology has been seen for the vast majority of diseases and traits (Figure 17.5). As a result, genetic tests of common variants for most diseases have disappointingly low positive and negative predictive values (NPVs and PPVs). This is in contrast to genetic testing to assess disease risk in families with rare genetic diseases: when a healthy relative undergoes genetic testing for the variant that causes HCM in their family, for example, the PPV is high and the NPV approaches 100%.

The genetics of injury susceptibility and athletic performance have been subject to far less robust investigation than diseases like CAD. In contrast to the hundreds of thousands of individuals studied in CAD genetics, most sports genetics studies include several dozen or, at best, a few hundred subjects. Many associations have only been reported once, whilst others have been refuted [23]. Experience with studies of the genetics of a variety of diseases and traits has shown that early findings, especially with small sample sizes and candidate gene approaches, tend to overestimate effect sizes and identify trait–variant associations that do not replicate. Optimal study designs identify putative trait–variant associations in a large discovery cohort using hypothesis-free genome-wide methods that correct for multiple-hypothesis testing, then replicate those findings in a large replication cohort. In contrast, nearly all of the studies of injury and performance genetics carried out to date have been on small samples, focusing on gene(s) of interest, with no replication [23]. Many of the reported associations are likely erroneous, and those that are real are likely overestimated.

Thus, the data on the genetics of injury and performance are not robust or mature enough to accurately translate to individual assessment [23]. Given the limited contribution of identifiable genetic factors to the aetiology of most diseases and traits (Figure 17.5), we may never have a meaningful genetic test for performance and injury, even once robust studies have been carried out in large samples. Even if such a test could be developed, it is unclear how such information should be used in the selection and training of athletes.

Ethics of Genetic Testing in Athletes

The potential for making participation decisions based on genetic information must be considered in the context of concerns about genetic discrimination and the vulnerable status of the athlete. Such concerns stem from the predictive and uncontrollable nature of genetic information and the value placed on privacy and justice. It has been noted that laws protecting against genetic discrimination likely do not apply to collegiate athletes, since they are not employees, and may be made irrelevant for professional athletes by collective bargaining agreements [20]. Some athletes with a family history of heart problems defer genetic testing because of fear of disqualification based on genotype alone. In 2005, an American professional basketball team requested that one of their players, Eddy Curry, have genetic testing for HCM after he missed several games due to cardiovascular symptoms. Curry refused genetic testing and was signed by another team. The incident sparked heated debate, reflecting the ethical conflicts surrounding genetic testing on athletes.

Conclusion

Genetic testing for conditions predisposing to sudden death is valuable in the care of the family once a diagnosis of such a condition has been made. This is true both in the cardiovascular genetics clinic and in pre-participation screening programmes. Careful interpretation of genetic tests is critical, and interpretation is particularly difficult when the diagnosis is uncertain or when testing is applied to the general population. Athletes with a likely diagnosis of inherited CVD should be referred to interdisciplinary cardiovascular genetics centres, where they and their family can undergo a comprehensive genetics evaluation. Participation decisions for individuals who carry a genetic predisposition to CVD but are not manifesting that disease should be made carefully, balancing any increased risk of sudden death against the possibility that a clinically significant phenotype may never develop. It remains unclear what role, if any, genetic testing should play as a frontline test in pre-participation screening. Another avenue by which to improve identification of athletes with inherited CVD is through more aggressive family-based screening programmes that aim to identify all family members with a disease once one family member has been diagnosed.

References

1 Priori, S.G., Wilde, A.A., Horie, M. et al. HRS/EHRA/APHRS expert consensus statement on the diagnosis and management of patients with inherited primary arrhythmia syndromes: document endorsed by HRS, EHRA, and APHRS in May 2013 and by ACCF, AHA, PACES, and AEPC in June 2013. *Heart Rhythm* 2013; **10**(12): 1932–63.

2 Alfares, A., Kelly, M., McDermott, G. et al. Results of clinical genetic testing of 2912 probands with hypertrophic cardiomyopathy: expanded panels offer limited additional sensitivity. *Genet Med* 2015; **17**(11): 880–8.

3 Bos, J.M., Will, M.L., Gersh, B.J. et al. Characterization of a phenotype-based genetic test prediction score for unrelated patients with hypertrophic cardiomyopathy. *Mayo Clin Proc* 2014; **89**(6): 727–37.

4 Kapplinger, J.D., Tester, D.J., Salisbury, B.A. et al. Spectrum and prevalence of mutations from the first 2500 consecutive unrelated patients referred for the FAMILION long QT syndrome genetic test. *Heart Rhythm* 2009; **6**(9): 1297–303.

5 Lieve, K.V., Williams, L., Daly, A. et al. Results of genetic testing in 855 consecutive unrelated patients referred for long QT syndrome in a clinical laboratory. *Genet Test Mol Biomarkers* 2013; **17**(7): 553–61.

6 Splawski, I., Shen, J., Timothy, K.W. et al. Spectrum of mutations in long-QT syndrome genes. KVLQT1, HERG, SCN5A, KCNE1, and KCNE2. *Circulation* 2000; **102**(10): 1178–85.

7 Giudicessi, J.R. and Ackerman, M.J. Genotype- and phenotype-guided management of congenital long QT syndrome. *Curr Probl Cardiol* 2013; **38**(10): 417–55.

8 Ackerman, M.J., Priori, S.G., Willems, S. et al. HRS/EHRA expert consensus statement on the state of genetic testing for the channelopathies and cardiomyopathies this document was developed as a partnership between the Heart Rhythm Society (HRS) and the European Heart Rhythm Association (EHRA). *Heart Rhythm* 2011; **8**(8): 1308–39.

9 Richards, S., Aziz, N., Bale, S. et al. Standards and guidelines for the interpretation of sequence variants: a joint consensus recommendation of the American College of Medical Genetics and Genomics and the Association for Molecular Pathology. *Genet Med* 2015; **17**(5): 405–24.

10 Coppini, R., Ho, C.Y., Ashley, E. et al. Clinical phenotype and outcome of hypertrophic cardiomyopathy associated with thin-filament gene mutations. *J Am Coll Cardiol* 2014; **64**(24): 2589–600.

11 van Rijsingen, I.A., Arbustini, E., Elliott, P.M. et al. Risk factors for malignant ventricular arrhythmias in lamin a/c mutation carriers a European cohort study. *J Am Coll Cardiol* 2012; **59**(5): 493–500.

12 Goldenberg, I., Horr, S., Moss, A.J. et al. Risk for life-threatening cardiac events in patients with genotype-confirmed long-QT syndrome and normal-range corrected QT intervals. *J Am Coll Cardiol* 2011; **57**(1): 51–9.

13 Hayashi, M., Denjoy, I., Extramiana, F. et al. Incidence and risk factors of arrhythmic events in catecholaminergic polymorphic ventricular tachycardia. *Circulation* 2009; **119**(18): 2426–34.

14 Maron, B.J., Zipes, D.P. and Kovacs, R.J. Eligibility and disqualification recommendations for competitive athletes with cardiovascular abnormalities: Preamble, principles, and general considerations: A scientific statement from the American Heart Association and American College of Cardiology. *J Am Coll Cardiol* 2015; **66**(21): 2343–9.

15 Pelliccia, A., Fagard, R., Bjørnstad, H.H. et al. Recommendations for competitive sports participation in athletes with cardiovascular disease: a consensus document from the Study Group of Sports Cardiology of the Working Group of Cardiac Rehabilitation and Exercise Physiology and the Working Group of Myocardial and Pericardial Diseases of the European Society of Cardiology. *Eur Heart J* 2005; **26**(14): 1422–45.

16 James, C.A., Bhonsale, A., Tichnell, C. et al. Exercise increases age-related penetrance and arrhythmic risk in arrhythmogenic right ventricular dysplasia/cardiomyopathy-associated desmosomal mutation carriers. *J Am Coll Cardiol* 2013; **62**(14): 1290–7.

17 Sweeting, J., Ingles, J., Ball, K. and Semsarian, C. Challenges of exercise recommendations and sports participation in genetic heart disease patients. *Circ Cardiovasc Genet* 2015; **8**(1): 178–86.

18 Hofman, N., Tan, H.L., Alders, M. et al. Active cascade screening in primary inherited arrhythmia syndromes. Does it lead to prophylactic treatment? *J Am Coll Cardiol* 2010; **55**(23): 2570–6.

19 Umans-Eckenhausen, M.A., Defesche, J.C., Sijbrands, E.J. et al. Review of first 5 years of screening for familial hypercholesterolaemia in the Netherlands. *Lancet* 2001; **357**(9251): 165–8.

20 Wagner, J.K. Playing with heart and soul…and genomes: sports implications and applications of personal genomics. *PeerJ* 2013; **1**: e120.

21 Collier, R. Genetic tests for athletic ability: science or snake oil? *CMAJ* 2012; **184**(1): e43–4.

22 Teslovich, T., Musunuru, K., Smith, A et al. Biological, clinical and population relevance of 95 loci for blood lipids. *Nature* 2010; **466**: 707–13.

23 Wang, G., Padmanabhan, S., Wolfarth, B. et al. Genomics of elite sporting performance: what little we know and necessary advances. *Adv Genet* 2013; **84**: 123–49.

Part 3
Cardiac Conditions Predisposing to Sudden Cardiac Death

Section 1
Introduction

18 Causes of Sudden Cardiac Death in Sport: The Importance of Autopsy and Specialist Examination of the Heart

Mary N. Sheppard

Department of Cardiovascular Pathology, St George's University of London, London, UK

Introduction

Sudden cardiac death (SCD) in young competitive athletes (<35 years old) is a tragic event that receives widespread media attention. As early as 1975, sudden death in sport was highlighted with an emphasis on ischaemic heart disease [1] and in marathon runners [2]. The majority of deaths in athletes are due to underlying cardiovascular disease (CVD), which is often not diagnosed during life. However, by the 1980s it was apparent that death was due not just to ischaemic heart disease, but also to diseases of heart muscle, cardiomyopathies and valvular heart disease [3]. The investigation of these deaths in previously very fit individuals calls for a detailed autopsy, with an emphasis on examination for structural disorders associated with SCD in young athletes [4].

Disorders of the Coronary Arteries

Abnormalities of the coronary arteries associated with SCD in young athletes represent a diverse group of atherosclerotic, nonatherosclerotic and structural anomalies.

Coronary Artery Disease

Most sudden death in athletes over the age of 35 is due to coronary artery atheroma with significant blockage (>75% narrowing of main vessel, usually the left anterior descending coronary artery) (Figure 18.1). There may be a substrate for sudden death, such as acute or chronic infarction, but the cardiac muscle may be normal, so the presumed mode of death is a cardiac arrhythmia due to increased demands made on the myocardium by exercise. Thus, significant atheroma alone, without plaque rupture, thrombosis or acute or chronic infarction, may be present. Exercise can lead to transient activation of the coagulation system and left ventricular contractile dysfunction due to post-exercise stunning as a result of coronary artery disease (CAD). The typical case is the weekend footballer or the person who decides to run a marathon in middle age. Premature CAD can also occur, especially related to familial hypercholesterolemia, as evidenced by the

---

IOC Manual of Sports Cardiology, First Edition. Edited by Mathew G. Wilson, Jonathan A. Drezner and Sanjay Sharma.

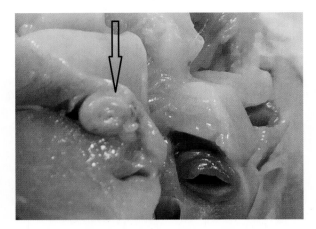

Figure 18.1 Coronary artery atheroma. Blocked coronary artery (arrow) and more proximal patent vessel with eccentric plaque

death of an 11-year-old whilst on a cross-country run, who had widespread diffuse atheroma in all coronary arteries. This athlete had been totally asymptomatic until sudden death, but significantly she had a strong family history of hypercholesterolaemia. Usually precocious atheroma in those under the age of 35 has surface endothelial erosion of the vessel with thrombosis. Family screening is advised in these cases. Ischaemic heart disease is not covered further in this review. Pathologists should be conservative in attributing death to CAD, unless there is significant atheroma in the left main stem, left anterior descending coronary artery or right coronary artery (RCA), or there is evidence of corresponding myocardial infarction. Significant atheroma in the diagonal/marginal branches or left circumflex is open to interpretation when there is no rupture, thrombosis or evidence of ischaemic damage in the ventricle. Most people in Western cultures have some atheroma in their coronary arteries, so caution is advised in order to avoid overinterpretation of insignificant CAD. Histologic sampling of coronary artery lesions in young people is recommended, because not all blocked coronary vessels are caused by atheroma.

Coronary Artery Spasm on Exercise

Myocardial ischaemia may also be caused by coronary vasospasm (in the microvasculature, as well as in epicardial coronary segments). Exercise-induced ischaemia and/or a pathological exercise test result is usually caused by severe coronary stenosis, but may also be due to reduced coronary perfusion reserve secondary to microvascular dysfunction. Proatherogenic cardiovascular risk factors are associated not only with atheromatous CAD, but also with a coronary vasomotility disorder. Coronary artery spasm is a controversial topic for pathologists, as it is impossible to detect at autopsy. It is presumed to be the cause of SCD if there is transmural myocardial ischaemic damage, usually in the anterolateral wall of the left ventricle (region of distribution of the left coronary artery (LCA)), with normal coronary arteries. The ischaemic damage in this area points to a regional arterial transient blockage/spasm. Thrombotic/embolic disease with lysis is a possibility in such cases, but there is no source for thrombosis or emboli found at autopsy [5].

Drugs and CAD

Androgenic-anabolic steroid (AAS) use is associated with SCD, myocardial infarction, altered serum lipoproteins and cardiac hypertrophy in humans who habitually use these drugs. There are at least four hypothetical models of AAS-induced adverse cardiovascular effects: (i) an atherogenic model, involving the effects of AAS on lipoprotein concentrations; (ii) a thrombosis model, involving the effects of AAS on clotting factors and platelets; (iii) a vasospasm model, involving the effects of AAS on the vascular nitric oxide system; and (iv) a direct myocardial injury model, involving the effects of AAS on individual myocardial cells. Systematic toxicology indicates that 3.1% of SCDs are cocaine-related and are mainly due to left ventricular hypertrophy (LVH), small-vessel disease and premature coronary artery atheroma, with or without lumen thrombosis. Smoking of cannabis is also related to coronary thrombosis and infarction.

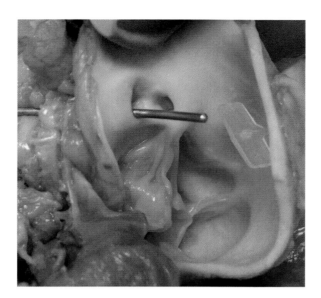

Figure 18.2 Anomalous LCA. Both coronary arteries originate in one aortic sinus, with the anomalous LCA having an intramural course and crossing between the aorta and pulmonary trunk (probe)

Toxicology is thus essential in all cases of sudden death in athletes, to rule out atheroma, thrombosis, infarction or hypertrophy being related to these drugs [6–8].

Nonatheromatous Coronary Causes of SCD

There are many nonatheromatous abnormalities of the coronary arteries that can cause sudden death. In a review of 50 cases of nonatherosclerotic CAD associated with SCD, 24% of SCD occurred during or immediately after physical exertion. Anomalous origin of coronary artery occurred in 48%, coronary artery dissection in 16%, coronary artery vasculitis in 12% and coronary artery spasm in 12%. Only 20 of the 50 patients (40%) were documented to have experienced cardiac symptoms such as syncope, chest pain on exertion or breathlessness before SCD [9].

Anomalous Coronary Arteries

Most SCDs related to coronary abnormalities in young athletes are caused by an anomalous origin of the left coronary system from the right coronary sinus (Figure 18.2). The sudden death is from ventricular arrhythmia triggered by myocardial ischaemia during exercise. Coronary blood flow is impaired by the abnormal ostium of the anomalous vessel, compression of the anomalous artery as it courses between the pulmonary artery and ascending aorta and/or coronary spasm triggered by endothelial dysfunction. Victims of SCD due to these anomalous coronary arteries are often asymptomatic before presentation, although chest pain associated with syncope should raise suspicion of the disorder [10]. Dangerous anomalies are one artery taking origin from the pulmonary trunk [11] or both arteries taking origin in one aortic sinus, with the anomalous artery having an intramural aortic component and crossing between the aorta and pulmonary trunk. An anomalous LCA originating from the right coronary sinus is considered more dangerous than the RCA originating from the left coronary sinus. High take-off of the coronary artery (>10 mm above the sinotubular junction) has been associated with SCD. It is well established that there is normal anatomical variation in the location of coronary ostia at, below and above the sinotubular junction. Muriago et al. [12] proposed that a measurement of 120% or more of the depth of the sinus should be used as the criterion for pathological high take-off. It was the combination of a high take-off, a slit-like opening, an intramural course and ischaemic damage in the ventricle that established this entity as a cause of SCD.

Coronary Artery Dissection

Spontaneous dissection of the coronary arteries is a rare cause of SCD and can be missed unless looked for carefully [13]. The process is distinct from aortic dissection. It starts as an intramural haematoma, which compresses the vessel lumen from outside and can lead to SCD or myocardial infarction. This haematoma may rupture into the lumen, creating a dissection track. Cases of spontaneous coronary artery dissection occurring after intense exercise have been described in the literature around SCD and infarction [14]. They can also occur with drug use – especially cocaine. The pathogenesis is not clear. Previously, it was considered a vasculitis, because of the presence of adventitial inflammatory eosinophils and basophils, but this is now seen as a response to the dissection itself. It is also seen rarely in connective-tissue disorders such as Marfan syndrome.

Myocardial Bridging

Myocardial bridging is a congenital coronary anomaly whose clinical relevance is debated [15]. It is a condition in which a band of cardiac muscle overlies the coronary artery along its course for a varying length. Compression of the coronary artery lumen in systole, extending into diastole, is the main functional consequence of this anatomic abnormality. It has been reported that this anomaly is of clinical and pathological significance when it involves the left anterior coronary artery and has a long (20–30 mm) and deep (5 mm) intramyocardial course. An association between coronary artery spasm and myocardial bridging has been reported, as has an association with hypertrophic cardiomyopathy (HCM). Thus, finding a significant muscle bridge over the left anterior coronary artery should alert the pathologist to this potential cardiomyopathy.

Disorders of the Heart Muscle

All studies on SCD in sport emphasise that cardiomyopathies are an important cause of sudden death during athletic activity.

Hypertrophic Cardiomyopathy

HCM is a primary myocardial disorder with an autosomal-dominant pattern of inheritance, characterised by LVH in the absence of abnormal loading conditions. The hypertrophy can be concentric, eccentric or regional (e.g. apical) and is often associated with scarring in the left ventricle (Figure 18.3). There can be an impact lesion due to anterior motion of the mitral valve leaflet with hypertrophy of the interventricular septum and left ventricular outflow obstruction. This impact lesion is a focal thickening on the left side of

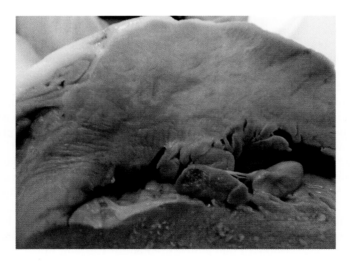

Figure 18.3 HCM. The heart weighs 600 g, with an increase in left ventricular wall thickness to above 15 mm in the anterior wall of the left ventricle. Note the pale focal areas of scarring, which are common in HCM. Coronary arteries are normal

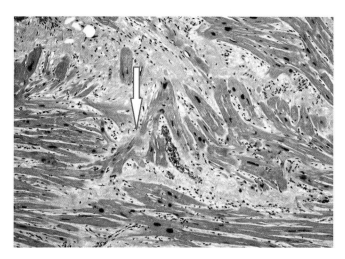

Figure 18.4 Myocyte disarray in HCM. Myocyte cellular disarray in the left ventricle (arrow) seen on haematoxylin and eosin staining of the myocardium

the interventricular septum. Microscopic examination shows myocardial disarray to confirm the diagnosis (Figure 18.4). Sudden death is often the first clinical manifestation of the disease. Deaths caused by HCM are common in start–stop sports (e.g. football and basketball) but rare in endurance events (e.g. rowing, long-distance cycling and running). It is hypothesised that the combination of myocardial hypertrophy, impaired myocardial relaxation, myocardial ischaemia and dynamic left ventricular outflow obstruction impede augmentation of stroke volume for prolonged periods, and individuals with HCM are therefore usually selected out of endurance sports.

HCM is caused by mutations in genes encoding proteins of the cardiac sarcomere (components of thick or thin filaments with contractile, structural or regulatory functions). It has a prevalence of 1 : 500 in the adult population and is one of the most common cardiac genetic diseases. Several high-profile footballers/athletes have died suddenly in the past 5 years, many of whom had HCM, as reflected in some US studies. HCM is disproportionately prevalent in African-American athletes. Factors which increase the risk of sudden death include a family history of sudden death, extreme left ventricular wall thickness (≥30 mm), nonsustained ventricular tachycardia on Holter monitoring, unexplained (non-neurocardiogenic) syncope (particularly in young patients) and a hypotensive blood-pressure response to exercise.

At autopsy, the heart weight typically exceeds 500 g, with an increase in left ventricular wall thickness to above 15 mm, with or without myocardial scarring. However, absolute left ventricular wall thickness should be interpreted with caution, as death in systole (or from rigor mortis) can increase wall thickness in a normal heart but leave the heart weight within normal limits (<500 g). Impact lesions on the left side of the upper interventricular septum due to imprint of the anterior mitral leaflet are found only in a small number of cases. Some cases of HCM may have normal heart weight and ventricular wall thickness but pathognomonic microscopic myocyte disarray, particularly in mutations in troponin T. Microscopic myocyte cellular disarray can be widely distributed, occupying substantial portions of the left ventricular wall. It is more extensive in young patients who die suddenly. Left ventricular scarring is prominent in most athletes who die suddenly with HCM, usually in the inner third of the left ventricle. Myocyte disarray may occur in the anteroseptal and posteroseptal wall of a normal heart, so these areas are to be avoided in sampling. Focal myocyte disarray is noted in subendocardium around trabeculae and around intramural blood vessels, where it is a common finding in the normal heart. It is recommended that that the diagnosis be made only if 7–10 blocks of myocardium are seen from the left ventricle, with myocyte disarray present in at least 3 out of 10. Myocyte disarray should be present in order to make the specific pathological diagnosis of HCM at autopsy.

Idiopathic LVH

In a study of UK athletes, LVH without myocyte disarray was the predominant finding (31%), as opposed to HCM and arrhythmogenic right ventricular cardiomyopathy (ARVC), which predominate in the US and Italy, respectively [16]. LVH is defined as an increase in heart weight to above 500 g and an increase in left ventricular wall thickness to above 15 mm. There may be fibrosis present, but not always in the left ventricle. Idiopathic LVH is becoming increasingly recognised, and although it has been reported in previous studies, this is the first athlete series in which it predominates. It is unclear whether idiopathic LVH is part of the HCM spectrum, a separate inherited entity or an acquired pathological variant of the physiological LVH exhibited as part of the athlete's heart on certain predisposing genetic backgrounds. Among highly trained black athletes, 3% exhibit substantial LVH ($\geq$15 mm), and it is plausible in such athletes that marked LVH predisposes to exercise-related fatal ventricular arrhythmias. LVH has also been linked to the use of anabolic steroids.

Myocardial Fibrosis

Myocardial fibrosis, with or without LVH, is prominent in more recent studies of athlete deaths. The aetiology of cardiac fibrosis remains unclear. The coronary arteries are normal and the fibrosis is scattered throughout the left ventricular wall and does not have a regional or subendocardial distribution. The left ventricular wall is normal in thickness, and the heart weight is also normal. It is possible that in some athletes, prolonged arduous physical activity may result in myocardial fibrosis [17]. Transient myocardial damage has been detected in athletes in the post-race setting. This pathology may represent an acquired, exercise-related cardiomyopathy and/or genetic predisposition leading to a fatal arrhythmia.

Arrhythmogenic Right Ventricular Cardiomyopathy

ARVC is the most recently described cardiomyopathy, and unlike the other types it predominantly involves the right ventricle. It is the second most common, accounting for 13% of SCD cases in UK athletes [16]. It is characterised by loss of myocytes, with fatty or fibro-fatty replacement of the right ventricle, ventricular arrhythmias, congestive heart failure and SCD. The prevalence of ARVC in young athletes experiencing sudden or aborted cardiac death in the US and France is about 3–4%. In the UK, ARVC is the primary cause of death in 10% of athletes younger than 35 years and 24% of those older than 35 years [16]. In Italy, ARVC accounts for nearly one-quarter of all sudden cardiovascular deaths in young athletes. In the early 'concealed' stage of the disease, patients are usually asymptomatic but can be at risk of life-threatening ventricular arrhythmias.

ARVC has recently been characterised as involving both ventricles in the majority of cases. The left ventricle is so frequently involved as to support the adoption of the broad term 'arrhythmogenic cardiomyopathy'. It is characterised by progressive replacement of right ventricular myocardium by either segmental or diffuse fibro-fatty tissue, which extends on to the right side of the interventricular septum and the epicardial surface of the left ventricle (Figures 18.5 and 18.6). Rarely, involvement of the left ventricle alone can occur, with distribution of the fat and fibrous tissue on the epicardial surface. This fibro-fatty replacement leads to ventricular arrhythmias.

ARVC is an inherited heart-muscle disease in most cases, caused by mutations in genes encoding desmosomal proteins. There is a wide spectrum of macroscopic findings in ARVC, ranging from normal and focal involvement of the right ventricular outflow tract (RVOT) to a dilated, thin-walled appearance mimicking dilated cardiomyopathy (DCM). Both the right and left ventricle show dilatation and thinning of the wall, with replacement by fat and fibrosis. Usually, the fat and scar tissue are on the epicardial aspect of the ventricle and extend in to replace the full thickness of the wall (Figure 18.5). Microscopically, fibrosis is present, as is fat in the wall, with degenerative features in the residual myocytes (Figure 18.6) [18]. Fat in the right ventricle is a normal finding, especially in obese middle-aged females, so it should be interpreted with caution [19]. High wall stress of the right ventricle during intense sports may lead to cellular disruption and leaking of cardiac enzymes and may explain observed B-type natriuretic peptide (BNP) elevations immediately after a race. It can even result in transient right ventricular dilatation and dysfunction, which can lead over time to chronic remodelling and a proarrhythmic state, resembling ARVC in some cases. ARVC in high-endurance athletes may develop in the absence of underlying desmosomal abnormalities, probably as a result of excessive right ventricular wall stress during exercise. This has been labelled 'exercise-induced ARVC'.

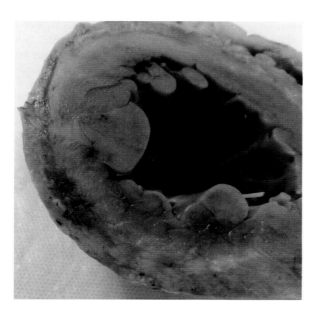

Figure 18.5 Arrhythmogenic cardiomyopathy. Wall of the left ventricle, showing fibrosis and thinning of the wall, with replacement by fat and fibrous tissue on the epicardial surface, extending into the interventricular septum

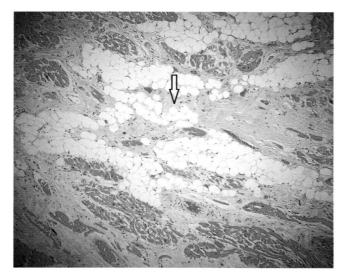

Figure 18.6 Arrhythmogenic cardiomyopathy. Microscopic picture of myocytes (pink) admixed with fat and fibrous tissue in the ventricle (arrow), seen on haematoxylin and eosin staining

Dilated Cardiomyopathy

DCM is an unusual cause of sudden death in athletes, due to the fact that most patients with this entity are symptomatic and have cardiac dysfunction, limiting their engagement in sport. The disease is inherited in 20–48% of cases. Autosomal-dominant forms are caused by mutations in cytoskeletal, sarcomeric protein/ Z-band, nuclear-membrane and intercalated disk protein genes. X-linked diseases associated with DCM include muscular dystrophies (e.g. Becker and Duchenne) and X-linked DCM. DCM may also occur in patients with mitochondrial cytopathies and inherited metabolic disorders (e.g. haemochromatosis). Examples of acquired causes of DCM include nutritional deficiencies, endocrine dysfunction and the administration of cardiotoxic drugs. Dilated cardiomyopathies caused by lamin gene defects are highly penetrant, adult-onset, malignant diseases characterised by a high rate of heart failure and life-threatening arrhythmias during sport [20]. The heart is heavy, weighing over 500 g, with a thin-walled left ventricle measuring <10 mm. There is usually fine interstitial fibrosis in the wall of the left ventricle, which is scattered throughout the wall. Coronary arteries are normal in all cases. There is no difference between congenital and acquired DCM on histology.

Myocarditis

All series of SCD record cases in which acute lymphocytic myocarditis is present at autopsy. Myocarditis, typically caused by viral infections (e.g. Coxsackie B), may lead to ventricular arrhythmias and accounts for up to 7% of SCD in athletes [16]. Athletes diagnosed with myocarditis should refrain from sports activity for a 6-month convalescent period in order to reduce the risk of SCD. Previously unsuspected cardiac sarcoidosis is also a cause of sudden death, but patients are usually older [21].

Stress Cardiomyopathy

Takotsubo syndrome is a reversible neuromyocardial failure that is thought to be related to acute catecholamine toxicity of the myocardium brought upon by a stressful event. It is also known as 'apical ballooning syndrome' and is a transient cardiomyopathy that can mimic an acute myocardial infarct. Patients present with clinical evidence of infarction and echocardiographic findings of apical ballooning with hypokinesia. The pathogenesis of this disorder is likely to be catecholamine-mediated myocyte damage and microvascular dysfunction; however, a number of possible alternative theories have been suggested, including oxidative stress, transient coronary obstruction and oestrogen deficiency, the last of which explains the high prevalence of Takotsubo cardiomyopathy in postmenopausal women. It can be triggered by hyponatraemia but is usually nonfatal, with recovery within days to weeks. It has been reported in sport and can be fatal. At autopsy in fatal cases, contraction-band necrosis has been described in myocytes at the apex of the left ventricle; alternatively, there may be infarction with normal coronary arteries [5].

Cardiac Valve Disease

There is increasingly awareness of bicuspid aortic valve (BAV) amongst young athletes. A normally functioning BAV usually does not represent a limit for practising sport, but the stress of regular and intense exercise on an abnormal aortic valve may favour its early deterioration and accelerate the development of complications. Such valves usually calcify early, leading to stenosis. Therefore, athletes with BAV warrant regular follow-up. Whilst non-existent in elite athletes, undiagnosed severe congenital aortic bicuspid stenosis may cause sudden death when undertaking unaccustomed exercise. In aortic stenosis, progressive LVH accounts for myocardial ischaemia and subendocardial scarring. Asymptomatic young people with BAV are at risk of a significantly dilated aortic root, supporting the concept of a BAV 'syndrome' (aortopathy), with increased risk of aortic aneurysm and dissection.

Mitral valve prolapse (MVP) is defined as thickening and hooding of the mitral valve leaflets, particularly the posterior one, involving chordae elongation and prolapse of the leaflets with lack of coaptation into the left atrium. The natural history of a floppy mitral valve is usually benign, but a number of patients have ventricular arrhythmias. The origin of arrhythmias is in the left ventricular myocardium and papillary muscles, where replacement fibrosis is observed. Sudden death may occur in this subgroup, but it is rare and usually occurs in young females who do not have significant regurgitation.

Morphologically Normal Heart

Recently, electrical conduction abnormalities of the heart, such as the channelopathies, have risen in prominence in the context of negative autopsy in athletes [16,22]. The identification of a morphologically normal heart is of great importance, since studies indicate that more than 50% of SCD in such cases is caused by malignant arrhythmias secondary to the presence of inherited ion-channel disorders, usually affecting the potassium, sodium and calcium ion channels of the myocardial cells, which will not be seen morphologically at autopsy. The first presentation of such disorders may be life-threatening cardiac arrhythmias occurring at rest or during exercise. Sudden unexpected death during exercise can in many families reveal a previously unsuspected cardiac condition that can be diagnosed by screening first-degree family members. These electrical faults, which cannot be detected by gross autopsy but may be identified by post-mortem genetic testing, are inherited, as are the cardiomyopathies, usually in an autosomal-dominant fashion. The role of the pathologist is pivotal in the screening process, in providing a definitive cause of SCD. Thus, a pathologist needs to carefully examine the heart and must do a microscopic analysis before concluding it is normal. A heart may look normal to the naked eye but still have microscopic abnormalities, and histological cardiac examination is essential in all such deaths. Overinterpretation of pathological findings and missed or wrong diagnoses can have catastrophic consequences for families in which other members are at risk of sudden death [23].

Conduction System

Conduction-system abnormalities have been described as premature ageing, sclerosis of the left side of the cardiac skeleton fat and mononuclear cell infiltration and thrombosis of the sinoatrial (SA) node artery in sudden death in young athletes. The significance of these findings and the lack of normal controls make a detailed study of the conduction system extremely time-consuming and unsatisfactory in the investigation of most sudden-death cases. Two variants of ventricular pre-excitation, namely Wolff–Parkinson–White (WPW) and Lown–Ganong–Levine (LGL) syndromes are linked to sudden death in athletes. In WPW cases, with a short refractory period of the anomalous atrioventricular (AV) pathway, the occurrence of atrial fibrillation and 1 : 1 conduction of the atrial electrical impulse to the ventricles may trigger ventricular fibrillation. This is considered the usual mechanism accounting for arrhythmic SCD in these patients. In the Italian experience, 6% of SCD cases are due to ventricular pre-excitation, proved both at the electrocardiogram (ECG) and on histology [24]. Histologic findings suggestive of ventricular pre-excitation include an abnormal muscle bundle connecting the atrium to the ventricle, usually at the left AV junction.

Aortic Dissection

Acute aortic dissection (Figure 18.7) can occur during exercise, particularly with weightlifting. The aortic dissection may occur in the setting of a congenital and/or hereditary–familial condition. Four inherited disorders known to affect major arteries include Marfan syndrome, Ehlers–Danlos syndrome (EDS), BAV (with or without aortic isthmic coarctation) and nonsyndromic familial aortic dissection. Marfan syndrome affects approximately 1 in 5000 of the general population and is caused by a mutation in the fibrillin gene involved in elastin production in connective tissues. People who have this medical condition are usually tall, slender and loose-jointed and may be volleyball or basketball players. Nonsyndromic familial thoracic aortic aneurysms and dissections (TAADs) are inherited in families as an autosomal-dominant disorder through

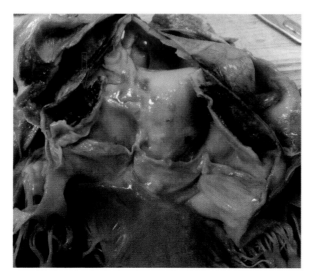

Figure 18.7 Aortic dissection. Aortic wall showing acute dissection, with separation of layers and intramural haematoma in the ascending aorta (arrow)

mutations in collagen genes, including TAAD1, TAAD2, FAA1 and ACTA2. These loci overlap a second locus for Marfan syndrome, termed the MFS2 locus. The aortic-wall fragility invovles severe disruption/loss of elastic fibres and smooth-muscle cells of the tunica medias. Acute aortic dissection can occur at the time of intense physical exertion in strength-trained athletes, such as weightlifters, bodybuilders, throwers and wrestlers. A rapid rise in blood pressure and a history of hypertension are the most common causes of aortic dissection in these athletes.

Blunt Chest Trauma

Commotio Cordis

A blow to the chest in the area of the heart causing ventricular fibrillation, called commotio cordis (or cardiac concussion), is a rare cause of sudden death in athletes. This condition often occurs in children or adolescents upon receiving a nonpenetrating and usually innocent-appearing blow to the middle of the chest, such as when struck by a baseball, hockey puck, lacrosse ball, softball or karate blow. It is amongst the most frequent cardiovascular causes of sudden death in young US athletes, after HCM and congenital coronary artery anomalies, but is rarely reported elsewhere. Most victims are adolescent boys and are white. Although cardiovascular collapse is virtually instantaneous, 20% of victims remain physically active for a few seconds after the blow (e.g. continuing to walk, run, skate, throw a ball or even speak), which may reflect individual tolerance for sustained ventricular tachyarrhythmias. Commotio cordis is a primary arrhythmic event that occurs when the mechanical energy generated by a blow is confined to a small area of the precordium and profoundly alters the electrical stability of the myocardium, resulting in ventricular fibrillation. The first of these determinants involves the location of the blow, which must be directly over the heart (particularly at or near the centre of the cardiac silhouette). This finding is consistent with clinical observations that precordial bruises representing the imprint of a blow are frequently evident in victims. There is no evidence in humans or in experimental models that blows sustained outside the precordium (e.g. the back, the flank or the right side of the chest) cause sudden death.

The second determinant concerns the timing of the blow, which must occur within a narrow window of 10–20 ms on the upstroke of the T-wave, just before its peak (accounting for only 1% of the cardiac cycle) – that is, the blow must occur during an electrically vulnerable period, when inhomogeneous dispersion of repolarisation is greatest, creating a susceptible myocardial substrate for provoked ventricular fibrillation. At autopsy, the heart is normal, and there may be bruising over the chest area. The history and circumstances are vital in coming to the conclusion that death is due to commotio cordis.

Contusio Cordis

Contusio cordis is also rare. It is defined by damage from a violent kinetic force resulting from blunt trauma to the precordial region. Syncope is almost always the first clinical manifestation observed, and commonly precedes death. It is often seen in high-impact accidents, such as car accidents. The kinetic force usually affects other organs, such as the lungs, trachea, oesophagus and costal arches, leading to pulmonary contusion and costal arch fractures. The right ventricle and tricuspid valve are most commonly affected, because of their anterior anatomical position in the chest. Myocardial contusion may be evident at autopsy, and tricuspid regurgitation can result from rupture of the papillary muscle or of the anterior cusp.

Sickle-Cell Disease

Fatal rhabdomyolysis during intense training can occur in athletes with sickle-cell trait who develop fulminant rhabdomyolysis, profound lactic acidosis, acute myoglobinuric renal failure, hyperkalemia and disseminated intravascular coagulation. Sustained exercise evokes four forces that can foster sickling: hypoxemia, acidosis, hyperthermia and red-cell dehydration. Whilst most commonly reported in American football players [25], sudden death in military recruits with sickle-cell trait appears to be related to hyperthermia during exercise, with vaso-occlusion due to sickling noted in both the heart and the lungs. Usually, the sickling of the red blood cells is noted in very dilated blood vessels, and it is associated with capillary leakage and haemorrhage into the myocardium when it is significant.

Conclusion

Sudden death in fit young athletes generates widespread public attention, as this group is seen as the epitome of health and fitness. The autopsy needs to address issues of toxicology in view of drug use. Detailed examination of the heart including histological study, ideally by an expert cardiac pathologist, is essential, since most cases result from structural CVD. Post-mortem genetic testing should be considered in autopsy-negative cases. Standardised methods, universal pathological criteria for entities and wider reporting of cases will provide a better understanding of the causes of sudden death in athletes.

References

1 Opie, L.H. Sudden death and sport. *Lancet* 1975; **1**: 263–6.
2 Noakes, T., Opie, L., Beck, W. et al. Coronary heart disease in marathon runners. *Ann N Y Acad Sci* 1977; **301**: 593–619.
3 Sugishita, Y., Matsuda, M., Iida, K. et al. Sudden cardiac death at exertion. *Jpn Circ J* 1983; **47**: 562–72.
4 Sheppard, M.N. Approach to the cardiac autopsy. *J Clin Pathol* 2012; **65**: 484–95.
5 Silvanto, A., de Noronha, S.V. and Sheppard, M.N. Myocardial infarction with normal coronaries: an autopsy perspective. *J Clin Pathol* 2012; **65**: 512–16.
6 Martinez-Quintana, E., Saiz-Udaeta, B., Marrero-Negrin, N. et al. Androgenic anabolic steroid, cocaine and amphetamine abuse and adverse cardiovascular effects. *Int J Endocrinol Metab* 2013; **11**: e8755.
7 Furlanello, F., Bentivegna, S., Cappato, R. et al. Arrhythmogenic effects of illicit drugs in athletes. *Ital Heart J* 2003; **4**: 829–37.
8 Sullivan, M.L., Martinez, C.M., Gennis, P. et al. The cardiac toxicity of anabolic steroids. *Prog Cardiovasc Dis* 1998; **41**: 1–15.
9 Hill, S.F. and Sheppard, M.N. Non-atherosclerotic coronary artery disease associated with sudden cardiac death. *Heart* 2010; **96**: 1119–25.
10 Hill, S.F. and Sheppard, M.N. A silent cause of sudden cardiac death especially in sport: congenital coronary artery anomalies. *Br J Sports Med* 2014; **48**: 1151–6.
11 Krexi, L. and Sheppard, M.N. Anomalous origin of the left coronary artery from the pulmonary artery (ALCAPA), a forgotten congenital cause of sudden death in the adult. *Cardiovasc Pathol* 2013; **22**: 294–7.
12 Muriago, M., Sheppard, M.N., Ho, S.Y. et al. Location of the coronary arterial orifices in the normal heart. *Clin Anat* 1997; **10**: 297–302.
13 Desai, S. and Sheppard, M.N. Sudden cardiac death: look closely at the coronaries for spontaneous dissection which can be missed. A study of 9 cases. *Am J Forensic Med Pathol* 2012; **33**: 26–9.
14 Kalaga, R.V., Malik, A. and Thompson, P.D. Exercise-related spontaneous coronary artery dissection: case report and literature review. *Med Sci Sports Exerc* 2007; **39**: 1218–20.
15 Biggs, M.J.P., Swift, B. and Sheppard, M.N. Myocardial bridging: is it really a cause of sudden death? In: Tsokos, M. (ed.) *Forensic Pathology Reviews*, Vol. **5**. Totowa, NJ: Springer, 2008. pp. 115–27.
16 de Noronha, S.V., Sharma, S., Papadakis, M. et al. Aetiology of sudden cardiac death in athletes in the United Kingdom: a pathological study. *Heart* 2009; **95**: 1409–14.
17 Whyte, G.P., Sheppard, M.N., George, K. et al. Post-mortem evidence of idiopathic left ventricular hypertrophy and idiopathic interstitial myocardial fibrosis: is exercise the cause? *Br J Sports Med* 2008; **42**: 304–5.
18 Fletcher, A., Ho, S.Y., McCarthy, K.P. et al. Spectrum of pathological changes in both ventricles of patients dying suddenly with arrhythmogenic right ventricular dysplasia. Relation of changes to age. *Histopathology* 2006; **48**: 445–52.
19 Tansey, D.K., Aly, Z. and Sheppard, M.N. Fat in the right ventricle of the normal heart. *Histopathology* 2005; **46**: 98–104.
20 Pasotti, M., Klersy, C., Pilotto, A. et al. Long-term outcome and risk stratification in dilated cardiolaminopathies. *J Am Coll Cardiol* 2008; **52**: 1250–60.
21 Bagwan, I.N., Hooper, L.V.B. and Sheppard, M.N. Cardiac sarcoidosis and sudden death. The heart may look normal or mimic other cardiomyopathies. *Virchows Archiv* 2011; **458**: 671–8.
22 Asif, I.M., Yim, E.S., Hoffman, J.M. and Froelicher, V. Update: Causes and symptoms of sudden cardiac death in young athletes. *Phys Sportsmed* 2015; **45**(1): 44–53.
23 de Noronha, S.V., Behr, E.R., Papadakis, M. et al. The importance of specialist cardiac histopathological examination in the investigation of young sudden cardiac deaths. *Europace* 2014; **16**: 899–907.
24 Thiene, G. Sudden cardiac death and cardiovascular pathology: from anatomic theater to double helix. *Am J Cardiol* 2014; **114**: 1930–6.
25 Harmon, K.G., Drezner, J.A., Klossner, D. et al. Sickle cell trait associated with a RR of death of 37 times in national collegiate athletic association football athletes: a database with 2 million athlete-years as the denominator. *Br J Sports Med* 2012; **46**: 325–30.

Section 2
Inherited and Congenital Cardiovascular Pathologies

19 Hypertrophic Cardiomyopathy

David S. Owens

Division of Cardiology, University of Washington, Seattle, WA, USA

Introduction

In 1958, British pathologist Donald Teare described a series of eight young individuals who experienced sudden death and were found on autopsy to have asymmetric left ventricular hypertrophy (LVH) [1]. This was the first characterisation of a disease entity that has gone by many names, but is now termed 'hypertrophic cardiomyopathy' (HCM). This account is of historical interest, but it also represents an early perspective that saw HCM as a severe disease entity with a high risk of sudden death, which continues to linger today.

Over the past 50 years, as the full spectrum of HCM has become apparent, the medical perception of the disease has changed dramatically. Rather than considering HCM a rare and debilitating disease, it is now recognised that it is not uncommon and is compatible with a full lifespan, with only minor symptoms in up to half of affected individuals. For those with more severe symptoms, modern medical therapies, including medications, septal reduction therapies, implantable cardioverter-defibrillators (ICDs) and heart transplantation, have improved the quality of life dramatically.

This chapter will discuss the prevalence of HCM, its diagnostic criteria, its common clinical presentations, evaluation of suspected HCM, sudden death risk stratification, disease management and considerations in the context of exercise, including physical activity recommendations.

One point of clarification is needed before we begin. The US and Europe remain divided over how HCM should be defined. The recent European Society of Cardiology (ESC) guidelines define it as the presence of increased left ventricular wall thickness that is not solely explained by abnormal loading conditions [2]. Under this definition, HCM can have multiple familial and nonfamilial aetiologies, including metabolic (e.g. Fabry disease), infiltrative (e.g. amyloidosis) and neuromuscular (e.g. Friedrich's ataxia) disorders. In contrast, the American Heart Association (AHA)/American College of Cardiology Foundation (ACCF) guidelines define HCM as only LVH due to (or suspected to be due to) an underlying sarcomeric gene mutation [3]. For the purposes of this chapter, the narrowed AHA/ACCF definition will be utilised, because the other aetiologies of LVH have distinct risks and prognoses and are less likely to present in an athletic population.

Epidemiology

The commonly accepted prevalence of HCM in the general population is 0.20–0.23% (1 in 500); this is thought to be similar across sex and ethnicities. This estimate is derived from a number of population-based studies that define HCM as idiopathic LVH on echocardiography, and thus capture asymptomatic individuals without clinically apparent disease. These data agree with clinical experience of a disease that is uncommon but not rare.

However, this estimate of the point-prevalence of the HCM phenotype may underestimate the lifetime HCM prevalence for several important reasons. First, individuals with HCM who experienced early mortality

IOC Manual of Sports Cardiology, First Edition. Edited by Mathew G. Wilson, Jonathan A. Drezner and Sanjay Sharma.
© 2017 International Olympic Committee. Published 2017 by John Wiley & Sons, Ltd.

were not counted in these studies. Second, the penetrance of HCM is age-dependent, and LVH may occur late in life. Third, with improvements in imaging, there is greater recognition that HCM patients can manifest atypical patterns or lesser degrees of hypertrophy. Extrapolating from existing genetic-testing, population and imaging data, it has been estimated that the true prevalence of HCM in the community may be as high as 0.5% (1 in 200) [4].

The prevalence of HCM in a young, athletic population is likely to be lower than that in the general population, in part due to the age-dependent penetrance of hypertrophy. Additionally, although half of HCM patients are asymptomatic or minimally symptomatic [5], most are unable to achieve high aerobic workloads due to the presence of obstruction or other limitations to cardiac performance. Thus, individuals with HCM are less likely to be able to perform and compete at elite levels. Basavarajaiah et al. [6] examined 3500 high-performance athletes and found three possible (<0.1%) and no definite cases of HCM after diagnostic evaluation, suggesting the prevalence of HCM in elite athletes is rare. The exact prevalence of the disease likely depends on the age of the athlete and the cardiac demands of the particular sporting discipline. It is also important to recognise that some patients with HCM – particularly those with nonobstructive HCM – may still be able to achieve high workloads, and that athletes are capable of adapting their performance to compensate for aerobic limitations.

Genetics

Studies as far back as the 1960s identified HCM as a familial disease with an autosomal-dominant pattern of inheritance, implying that a single gene defect is capable of causing disease [7,8]. It has been subsequently shown that HCM is caused by genetic mutations within the cardiac sarcomere, the main contractile apparatus within the heart [9,10]. With the dramatic advances in genetic-testing technologies in recent years, genetic testing for the diagnosis and management of HCM has become economically and clinically feasible [11].

To date, thousands of different genetic mutations involving a variety of sarcomeric and sarcomere-related proteins have been identified as causing HCM. Amongst patients with a clinical diagnosis of HCM, 50–70% carry a pathogenic mutation in these genes. Mutations in beta-myosin (*MYH7*) and myosin-binding protein C (*MYBPC3*) account for 70–80% of these gene-positive cases. Other genes that have been implicated in HCM include alpha-tropomyosin (*TPM1*), troponin T (*TNNT*) and troponin I (*TNNI*), each of which accounts for 1–5% of cases. Because our understanding of the genetics of HCM is incomplete, a negative genetic test result does not necessarily exclude the diagnosis of HCM. On occasion, it is unclear whether an identified change in an individual's genetic code is benign or disease-causing. If such a 'variant of uncertain significance' (VUS) is identified, the patient should be referred to a genetics provider for evaluation, and it is often helpful to phenotype family members in order to determine whether the VUS tracks with disease expression.

At present, there is a limited role for genetic testing in managing HCM patients, other than to confirm a diagnosis and assist with family screening. HCM is a genetically heterogeneous disorder and many mutations are found only within individual families and thus have not been previously described. There is also considerable variability in the HCM phenotype even within individual families, and gene–gene and gene–environment interactions likely play an important role in phenotypic expression.

Diagnosis

The AHA/ACCF guidelines define HCM as 'unexplained [LVH] with non-dilated ventricular chambers in the absence of another cardiac or systemic disease that itself would be capable of producing the magnitude of hypertrophy evident in a given patient' [3]. Thus, by its nature, HCM is a diagnosis of exclusion, and metabolic, infiltrative, neuromuscular and syndromic causes of LVH are not deemed to represent HCM under this definition.

Although any degree of LVH is potentially compatible with the presence of an underlying sarcomeric gene mutation, HCM patients often manifest substantial LVH, and HCM is usually clinically recognised by maximal wall thickness ≥15 mm (or two or more Z-scores in children). Wall thickness of 13–14 mm is considered borderline, but in the presence of additional clinically supportive data (e.g. family history of HCM, marked repolarisation changes on electrocardiogram (ECG), arrhythmias or other pathologic findings), this degree of hypertrophy may be sufficient to warrant an HCM diagnosis. Notably, the definition of HCM *does not* require asymmetric or septal hypertrophy or the presence of left ventricular outflow obstruction.

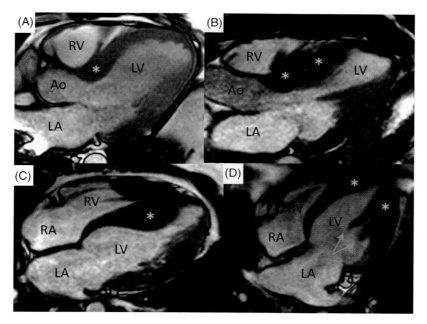

Figure 19.1 Cardiac magnetic resonance imaging (MRI) of patients with HCM, demonstrating morphologic spectrum of hypertrophy. Areas of involvement are indicated by asterisks. (A) Asymmetric hypertrophy isolated to the basal anterior septum. (B) Reverse curvature septal morphology. (C) Midventricular septal hypertrophy resulting in midventricular obstruction. (D) Apical HCM with an aberrant, bifid papillary muscle (arrows). LV, left ventricle; RV, right ventricle; LA, left atrium; RA, right atrium; Ao, aorta

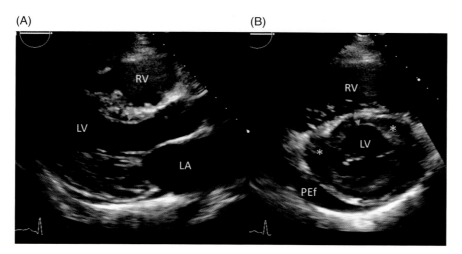

Figure 19.2 Patient with genetically confirmed HCM due to *MYH7* missense mutation, showing (A) normal thickness of the anterior septum on parasternal long-axis view (arrows) but (B) asymmetric hypertrophy in the anterior and inferior walls (asterisks) on parasternal short-axis view. Maximal wall thickness is 27 mm by cardiac MRI. LV, left ventricle; RV, right ventricle; LA, left atrium; PEf, pericardial effusion

Several morphologic subtypes of HCM have been described (Figure 19.1). Most commonly, HCM results in asymmetric hypertrophy involving (but not limited to) the basal anterior septum. HCM may also present as concentric hypertrophy or hypertrophy of the distal left ventricular cavity, including the midventricular or apical segments. The 'apical variant' of HCM often presents with few symptoms but markedly abnormal ECG findings. Additionally, a subset of patients manifest hypertrophy in regions other than the septum or apex (Figure 19.2).

Noninvasive imaging – both echocardiography and cardiac magnetic resonance imaging (MRI) – plays a critical role in the diagnosis of HCM, and it is important to recognise the limitations of these technologies. Echocardiography is the first diagnostic test under most circumstances and is generally well suited to identifying

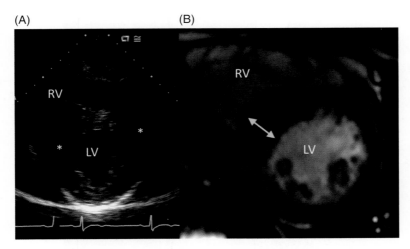

Figure 19.3 An echocardiogram is nondiagnostic in a 19-year-old high-level athlete with abnormal ECG (A) due to inadequate endocardial and epicardial definition in the inferior septum and anterior wall on parasternal short axis views (asterisks). (B) Follow-up cardiac MRI provides a diagnosis of HCM, with maximal wall thickness of 23 mm (arrows). LV, left ventricle; RV, right ventricle

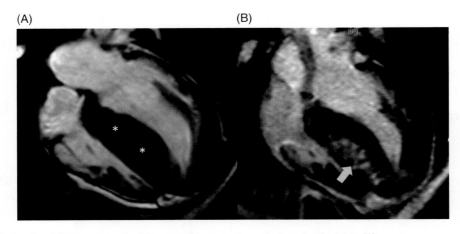

Figure 19.4 Cardiac MRI images of a 22-year-old asymptomatic female showing (A) severe, reverse curvature septal hypertrophy (asterisks) with (B) extensive intramyocardial late gadolinium enhancement (LGE) due to interstitial fibrosis. Based on a wall thickness >30 mm and extensive LGE, an ICD is recommended

hypertrophy affecting the basal anterior septum. However, echocardiography has some limitations. Image quality is dependent on sonographer experience, patient factors and the availability of adequate sonographic windows. Regions of the heart that are tangential to the ultrasound beam are less reflective, providing fewer data points for image reconstruction. As a result, the anterior wall, inferior septum and left ventricular apex are often not optimally visualised, which can cause a failure to make the diagnosis (Figure 19.3).

Cardiac MRI is a tomographic imaging technique that improves the detection of myocardial borders in all segments, and is the gold standard for assessing the presence and severity of LVH [12,13]. There are numerous examples in which HCM was not detected on echocardiography but was readily apparent on cardiac MRI. Cardiac MRI may also provide additional supporting evidence of HCM beyond assessment of maximal wall thickness. Abrupt segmental changes in wall thickness and/or noncontiguous hypertrophy are better seen by cardiac MRI and are highly suggestive of HCM. Additionally, the use of gadolinium as a contrast agent allows the identification of regions of myocardial fibrosis or scarring. About 50–70% of HCM patients have some degree of late gadolinium enhancement (LGE), often involving the regions of right ventricular insertion and the intramyocardial layer of hypertrophied segments (Figure 19.4). The presence of LGE is neither necessary nor sufficient for the diagnosis of HCM, but severe LGE in a patient with HCM may be a marker for worse prognosis [14].

Electrocardiogram Abnormalities

Although ECG findings are not part of the diagnostic algorithm for HCM, the majority of HCM patients have abnormalities on ECG. In one study by Rowin et al. [15], 90% of asymptomatic HCM patients had at least one HCM finding, with the most common abnormalities being nonvoltage criteria for LVH (60%), ST-segment deviation (27%), T-wave inversions (62%) and pathologic Q-waves (48%), representing aberrant septal depolarisation. Axis deviation (19%), left atrial enlargement (21%) and intraventricular conduction delay (13%) were other common findings.

The number and severity of ECG changes may be related to the severity of HCM phenotype, with greater hypertrophy and LGE in patients with more ECG abnormalities [16, 17]. The apical variant of HCM, which can produce markedly abnormal ECGs with minor degrees of hypertrophy, is a notable exception to this. Conversely, HCM patients with normal ECGs appear to have less LVH and an overall good prognosis [18].

When ECG is performed as part of a pre-participation screening programme, the finding of any ST-segment depression, T-wave inversion in the inferolateral leads or pathologic Q-waves should raise suspicion for HCM [19]. Schnell et al. [20] evaluated 155 athletes with pathologic T-wave inversion and found cardiomyopathy in 44.5%, of whom 81% had HCM. Of the athletes diagnosed with cardiomyopathy, 54% were identifiable by echocardiography and 89% by cardiac MRI, with the remainder identifiable by Holter and stress testing. One ECG pattern is particularly noteworthy. The finding of deep T-wave inversions across the precordial leads (V3–V6) is highly suspicious for the apical variant of HCM (Figure 19.5), and a cardiac MRI should be considered in all patients with this ECG pattern when standard echocardiography is negative or nondiagnostic.

ECG abnormalities may also precede the development of hypertrophy. A study of sarcomeric gene carriers showed pathologic Q-waves were present in 18% of cases (versus 3% of controls) even before the onset of LVH [21]. In a longitudinal study of 81 athletes with markedly abnormal ECGs (deeply inverted T-waves in three or more leads), 5 (6%) developed cardiomyopathy over a mean follow-up of 9 ± 7 years. Additionally, in the study by Shnell and colleagues [20], an additional 7% of athletes with deep T-wave inversion on the ECG developed cardiomyopathy over a mean follow-up of 12 months. For this reason, individuals with marked repolarisation changes should be followed longitudinally, and at least annually if they are engaged in vigorous or competitive exercise.

Left Ventricular Outflow Tract Obstruction

Left ventricular outflow tract (LVOT) obstruction, defined as a resting gradient >30 mmHg or a provocable gradient >50 mmHg, is common in HCM, occurring in about one-third of patients at rest and an additional third during exercise [22]. The clinical importance of LVOT obstruction was the subject of a longstanding and passionate debate, but it is now clear that it is a common and central cause of symptoms. The mechanism of LVOT obstruction in HCM is complex, but generally requires both a hypertrophied anterior interventricular septum that alters the systolic flow vectors and primary abnormalities in mitral valve leaflets and/or leaflet tethering. These factors increase the systolic drag forces across the valve and result in anterior displacement of the mitral valve towards the interventricular septum, which results in progressive narrowing of the LVOT during systole. Reductions in preload or afterload and increases in contractility or heart rate can increase the amount of obstruction.

On physical exam, obstruction usually produces a late-peaking systolic murmur along the left sternal border, and a holosystolic murmur at the apex may also be apparent due to concurrent mitral regurgitation. Provocative manoeuvres that decrease preload, such as Valsalva or a squat-to-stand manoeuvre, may increase the intensity of the murmur. Conversely, hand grip may increase afterload and reduce the intensity of the murmur. In the third of HCM patients with provocable LVOT obstruction, a murmur may not be apparent at rest, becoming manifest only with one of these physical exam manoeuvres.

Differentiation from Athlete's Heart

The diagnosis of HCM in an athlete presents unique challenges. In response to repetitive exercise, the heart can remodel and manifest both eccentric and concentric hypertrophy. Moreover, some degree of asymmetric hypertrophy can be seen in athletes, and many athletes may have occult hypertension, which may contribute to hypertrophy. There is no single test that can distinguish between pathologic and

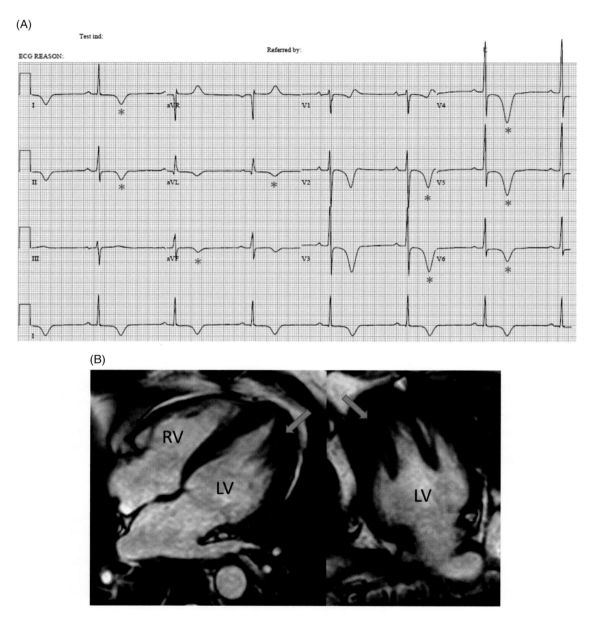

Figure 19.5 (A) ECG from a patient with apical HCM, showing characteristic deep T-wave inversions across the inferior, lateral and precordial leads (arrows). (B) The same patient had echocardiography, which was interpreted as normal, followed by cardiac MRI, which showed apical hypertrophy (arrows)

physiologic remodelling, and the distinction between these entities relies on assessment of chamber dimensions, diastolic function and functional status, the presence of scarring or arrhythmias and family history. It is recommended that athletes with LVH that falls within the 'grey zone' of 13–16 mm be evaluated by cardiologists with expertise is sports cardiology and HCM. This topic is detailed more extensively in Chapter 40.

Natural History and Clinical Course

The clinical manifestations of HCM are heterogeneous and somewhat unpredictable. Nearly half of HCM patients have few or no clinical symptoms and survive to advanced age without major cardiovascular complications. With improvements in noninvasive imaging and genetic testing, more of these asymptomatic patients are being identified. However, the absence of clinical symptoms does not exclude the possibility of life-threatening arrhythmias, and the risk of these arrhythmias should be assessed in all HCM patients regardless of symptom status.

The most common symptom seen in HCM patients is exercise limitation due to dyspnoea on exertion and/ or anginal chest discomfort. This exercise limitation is thought to be principally due to reduced stroke volume augmentation at peak exercise and, to a lesser degree, to a reduction in peak heart rate. Both contractility and heart rate increase during exercise, which can worsen or provoke LVOT obstruction. This results in a significant increase in afterload and myocardial work. Aggravating this, many patients with HCM have an element of microvascular narrowing due to perivascular fibrosis, which limits myocardial oxygen delivery and contributes to oxygen supply–demand mismatch.

Other clinical manifestations of more advanced HCM include atrial fibrillation and the development of overt heart-failure symptoms. This may be seen in patients with both obstructive and nonobstructive HCM, due to diastolic dysfunction and elevated left ventricular filling pressures. A small (~5%) but important subset of HCM patients develop 'end-stage' HCM, characterised by progressive myocardial fibrosis and a reduction in left ventricular contractile function, with or without associated left cavity dilatation.

Management Considerations

Once a diagnosis of HCM has been established, subsequent management should focus on improvement of symptoms, risk stratification for sudden cardiac death (SCD), counselling on sports and exercise and family screening. A detailed description of the management of symptomatic HCM is beyond the scope of this chapter, but general principles will be discussed.

For symptomatic HCM patients, it is important to determine whether LVOT obstruction is present during exercise. This generally requires a stress echocardiogram focused on the motion of the mitral valve, the magnitude of obstruction and the severity of mitral regurgitation during or immediately following stress. If LVOT obstruction is present, medical and procedural therapies are available to help reduce the amount of obstruction.

Medical therapy for LVOT obstruction is primarily aimed at reducing left ventricular contractility and maximising diastolic filling. Treatment with cardioselective beta blockers (e.g. metoprolol) is generally first-line therapy, titrating the dose to a heart rate of 55–65 beats.min^{-1}. Beta blockers have little effect on resting LVOT gradients but improve exertional symptoms by restricting peak heart rate. For patients who are refractory to or intolerant of beta blockers, nondihydropyradine calcium channel blockers (e.g. verapamil) are considered next-line therapy. Verapamil reduces contractility and resting gradients and improves diastolic filling. However, it should be avoided in patients with severe obstruction and high left ventricular filling pressure because arterial vasodilation could potentially worsen obstruction. Disopyramide is a highly potent negative inotropic agent and has been shown to reduce LVOT gradient by about 50%. The drug may be considered as additive drug therapy in patients who remain symptomatic due to large LVOT gradients despite taking either a beta blocker or a nondidydropyridine calcium channel blocker. However, its utility is often limited by anticholinergic side effects and it frequently causes urinary retention in males with prostatism.

For patients who have refractory symptoms despite maximal medical therapy, septal reduction procedures can be considered. Surgical septal myectomy is the gold standard for relief of obstruction and should be considered the preferred option in young HCM patients. Alcohol septal ablation, in which alcohol is injected into a septal perforator to cause an iatrogenic myocardial infarction, is an alternative procedure that may be appropriate for individuals at higher operative risk. It is recommended that all HCM patients being considered for septal reduction procedures be evaluated at an HCM centre of excellence by clinicians experienced in these procedures.

Sudden Cardiac Death

The most feared complication of HCM is SCD, which is most commonly caused by ventricular arrhythmias, but may also be precipitated by myocardial ischemia, AF with rapid ventricular rate or severe LVOT obstruction. SCD is most common in adolescent and young-adult patients and can occur without antecedent cardiovascular symptoms and without resting or provocable LVOT obstruction, striking individuals who appear outwardly healthy. SCD in athletes with HCM has garnered a lot of public and media attention, and with early reports focusing on patients with severe phenotype, the risk of SCD in HCM is often overestimated.

The overall risk of SCD in all HCM patients is about 0.5–0.8% per year, but individual patients may have substantially increased risk. Clinical research studies have identified a number of clinical risk factors for SCD, including a family history of SCD in a first-degree relative, wall thickness ≥30 mm and recent unexplained syncope. Other factors that appear to increase risk to a lesser degree include recurrent, nonsustained ventricular tachycardia (NSVT) on 24-hour rhythm monitoring and an abnormal blood-pressure response to exercise (amongst patients <45 years of age), as well as the presence of LVOT obstruction, AF, myocardial ischemia or a high-risk mutation. There is a current, ongoing debate as to whether extensive LGE is an independent risk factor for SCD.

The US and European consensus guidelines recommend SCD risk stratification for all HCM patients regardless of symptoms or the presence of obstruction, but they differ in the methods used to assess risk [2, 3]. In the US guidelines, the presence of any one of the three 'major' risk factors (family history of SCD, wall thickness ≥30 mm, recent unexplained syncope) merits consideration of an ICD. In contrast, the European guidelines adopt a more quantitative risk-assessment model, derived from 3675 HCM patients [23]. This model incorporates age, wall thickness, extent of LVOT obstruction, left atrial size and the presence of NSVT or syncope to give an estimated 5-year risk of SCD. A version of the calculator used can be found at: http://doc2do.com/hcm/webHCM.html. Patients who are deemed to be at high risk of SCD (5-year mortality ≥6%) by this model may benefit from placement of an ICD.

Exercise and HCM

There are currently few objective data on the risks and benefits of exercise in patients with HCM. Regular, moderate levels of exercise are known to have myriad health benefits and to promote weight loss, combat hypertension, hypercholesterolemia and dysglycaemia, maintain bone density and improve sleep, self-esteem and mental outlook [24]. Withdrawal from an active lifestyle may therefore have negative implications for health. However, in what is known as the 'paradox of sport', exercise can increase the risk of SCD in individuals with susceptible cardiac substrate (either known or occult), including HCM. Indeed, HCM and possible HCM are amongst the leading causes of SCD in athletes and young adults [25].

There are a number of mechanisms by which exercise may serve as an arrhythmogenic trigger for patients with HCM. Exercise increases catecholamine levels and may cause dehydration and electrolyte imbalances, unmask LVOT obstruction and induce myocardial ischaemia [26]. In one analysis of HCM-related death, 15–20% of sudden death events occurred in the setting of moderate or vigorous exercise [27]. Although it is difficult to quantify the risk associated with these activities, acute exercise likely increases it.

Several professional guidelines make recommendations on the type and intensity of exercise appropriate for patients with HCM [28,29]. These guidelines distinguish between competitive sports and recreational exercise. In competitive sports, there are often external motivators in the form of a coach or personal or monetary rewards. Athletes train intensively and may disregard their short-term physical health to break limits or achieve victory. In contrast, recreational activities are generally less intense and usually self-regulated, and have the primary goal of maintaining fitness.

The 2015 joint ACC/AHA recommendations adopt a stringent standard and restrict HCM patients from most sports participation [28]. Patients with a 'probable or unequivocal' diagnosis of HCM are excluded from all competitive sports, with the possible exception of low-intensity sports. These recommendations apply to all HCM patients, regardless of age, sex or race, the presence of LVOT obstruction, clinical assessment of SCD risk, the use of medications or the presence of an ICD. This guidelines recommend that HCM patients only participate in class IA competitive sports that have both low static and low dynamic components, such as billiards, bowling, cricket, curling or golf. The ESC consensus statement on competitive sports participation is largely in agreement with the 2015 joint ACC/AHA recommendations (Table 19.1) [29], although the two societies differ in their recommendations for carriers of pathogenic gene variants who have yet to manifest LVH (see Chapter 34).

There is a common misconception amongst medical providers that these restrictions on competitive sports also apply to recreational activities. In fact, there is growing recognition that stringent activity restrictions

	US	Europe
Overt HCM		
Competitive sports	Class IA only	Class IA, if low risk profile. Otherwise, none
Recreational activities	Some restrictions	Some restrictions
Preclinical HCM[a]		
Competitive sports	No restrictions	None
Recreational activities	No restrictions	No restrictions

Table 19.1 Comparison of US and European guideline recommendations for participation is competitive sports and recreational exercise

[a] Gene carrier without HCM phenotype.

Sports not recommended	Sports permitted on an individual basis	Sports permitted
Baseball	Moderate-intensity weights	Stationary bicycle
Basketball	Cross-country skiing (flat)	Bowling
Road cycling	Horseback riding[a]	Brisk walking
Ice hockey[a]	Jogging	Golfing
Rowing/canoeing	Running	Moderate hiking
Rock climbing	Motorcycling[a]	Skating
Scuba diving	Sailing[b]	Tennis (doubles)
Sprinting	Stationary rowing	Treadmill
Football	Swimming[b]	Low-intensity weights
Squash[a]		
Tennis (singles)		
Track events		
High-intensity weights		
Windsurfing[b]		

Table 19.2 ESC recommendation for amateur and leisure-time sport activities in patients with HCM (*Source*: Based on recommendations provided in Pelliccia et al. [29])

[a] These sports involve the potential for traumatic injury, which should be taken into consideration for individuals with a risk for impaired consciousness.

[b] The possibility of impaired consciousness occurring during water-related activities should be taken into account with respect to the clinical profile of the individual patient.

are potentially detrimental to long-term health and well being and may have a profound psychological impact on patients. In one survey, 60% of HCM patients felt that exercise restrictions had a negative impact on their emotional health, whilst 71% expressed anxiety towards exercise, although this was generally mild and correlated poorly with physical activity levels [30].

Both US and European expert panels have provided recommendations on the intensities and types of recreational activity that might be appropriate for patients with HCM [26, 29, 31]. Acknowledging the health benefits of regular, low- to moderate-intensity exercise, these recreational activity guidelines are less restrictive than those for competitive sports. European consensus recommendations divide activities into categories of 'not recommended', 'allowed on an individual basis' or 'permitted' (Table 19.2). In general, vigorous activities, burst activities (e.g. basketball) and activities where a transient loss of consciousness would have profound impact (e.g. scuba diving) are to be avoided.

The AHA guidelines are similar in their scope and purpose, but grade activities on a 0–5-point scale of 'permissibility': activities with a score of 0–1 are 'not advisable', those with 2–3 are 'intermediate' and those with 4–5 are 'probably permitted' [26]. The US guidelines are more lenient towards biking/cycling and baseball (intermediate) and swimming (probably permitted), but are more strict towards running (not advisable), although both sets of guidelines categorise jogging as a medium-risk activity. Additionally, the US guidelines do not comment on rowing sports and track events, and divide weightlifting into machine weights (probably permitted) and free weights (not advisable).

In practice, these recommendations appear to have only a limited impact on patient activity levels. In a study by Reineck et al. [30], HCM patients were more likely to be engaged in moderate or vigorous activities than were controls, and 10% of HCM patients were engaged in one or more competitive sports. This may be due in part to inadequate education, as only 46% of patients had discussed exercise restrictions with their doctor, and only 29% were aware of professional guideline recommendations. However, amongst those who knew about exercise restrictions, only 59% reported being adherent. Thus, it is clear that HCM patients value exercise as a contributor to their sense of well being.

The safety of exercise in HCM patients with ICDs has not been established, and currently the same restrictions apply whether or not these devices are fitted. To better understand the risks of exercise in patients with ICDs, the SPORT-ICD registry followed patients with ICDs who elected to participate in sports against guideline recommendations [32]. Over a median 31-month follow-up period, 13 and 11% of participants experienced appropriate and inappropriate shocks, respectively. Shocks were equally likely to occur in the setting of recreational activities as in competitive sports. Amongst the 65 subject in the registry who had HCM, 13 participated in competitive sports, and there was one event that required multiple appropriate ICD shocks prior to return of spontaneous circulation. With very limited data, the safety of exercise in HCM patients with ICDs remains uncertain.

Ultimately, the proper balance between the risks and benefits of exercise is not a one-size-fits-all recommendation but involves a conversation with individual patients. Some general considerations may guide this discussion. The goal of exercise for patients with HCM should be health maintenance and not competition. Patients should be in a position to stop exercising if they experience symptoms and should not put themselves in precarious situations where a transient change in consciousness would have catastrophic effects. Whenever possible, patients should exercise with a partner or in a group to allow for a quick response should an event occur. Finally, high-intensity activities and those that involve intermittent bursts (e.g. basketball, football) appear to confer the most risk and should be avoided.

Family Screening

A diagnosis of HCM is a family diagnosis. HCM is an autosomal-dominant disorder with a lifetime penetrance >90%, and thus immediate family members are at risk of developing HCM. The US and European guidelines recommend that all HCM patients undergo counselling regarding the genetic basis of their condition and that all first-degree relatives undergo screening for HCM. This screening traditionally consists of both ECG and echocardiography, but screening can be guided by genetic testing. If a pathogenic mutation is identified in the index patient, this can be used to screen family members in a cascade manner. Individuals who test negative for the family variant are not at risk of developing HCM or passing along the mutation. For gene (+) individuals or individuals whose genetic status is unknown, a single normal phenotypic evaluation does not exclude the future development of HCM, and serial evaluations are recommended (Table 19.3). These recommendations are age-dependent, with annual screening in the pubertal period and less frequent screening thereafter.

AHA/ACCF		ESC	
Age	**Recommendation**	**Age**	**Recommendation**
<12	Screen only if there are red flags or symptoms	<10	Screen only if there are red flags or symptoms
12 to (18–20)	Screen every 12–18 months	10–20	Screen every 1–2 years
>18–20	Screen at onset of symptoms and at least every 5 years	>20	Screen every 2–5 years

Table 19.3 Comparison of the US and European guideline recommendations for family screening of first-degree relatives of patients with HCM

Conclusion

HCM is a heterogeneous genetic disorder that is characterised by LVH, impairment of cardiac performance and an increased risk of potentially fatal arrhythmias, especially in young individuals, including athletes. Importantly, this increased risk of sudden death is independent of symptom status, but may be minimised by appropriate lifestyle modifications and the implantation of an ICD in those deemed to be at high risk. Participation in competitive sport of moderate to high intensity is generally not recommended for HCM patients, but lower-intensity recreational exercise may be appropriate to reduce the burden of acquired cardiovascular risk factors.

References

1   Teare, D. Asymmetrical hypertrophy of the heart in young adults. *Br Heart J* 1958; **20**: 1–8.
2   Elliott, P.M., Anastasakis, A., Borger, M.A. et al. 2014 ESC Guidelines on diagnosis and management of hypertrophic cardiomyopathy: the Task Force for the Diagnosis and Management of Hypertrophic Cardiomyopathy of the European Society of Cardiology (ESC). *Eur Heart J* 2014; **35**: 2733–79.
3   Gersh, B.J., Maron, B.J., Bonow, R.O. et al. 2011 ACCF/AHA guideline for the diagnosis and treatment of hypertrophic cardiomyopathy: a report of the American College of Cardiology Foundation/American Heart Association Task Force on Practice Guidelines. *Circulation* 2011; **124**: e783–831.
4   Semsarian, C., Ingles, J., Maron, M.S. and Maron, B.J. New perspectives on the prevalence of hypertrophic cardiomyopathy. *J Am Coll Cardiol* 2015; **65**: 1249–54.
5   Maron, B.J. and Maron, M.S. Hypertrophic cardiomyopathy. *Lancet* 2013; **381**: 242–55.
6   Basavarajaiah, S., Wilson, M., Whyte, G. et al. Prevalence of hypertrophic cardiomyopathy in highly trained athletes: relevance to pre-participation screening. *J Am Coll Cardiol* 2008; **51**: 1033–9.
7   Braunwald, E., Lambrew, C.T., Rockoff, S.D. et al. Idiopathic hypertrophic subaortic stenosis. I. A description of the disease based upon an analysis of 64 patients. *Circulation* 1964; **30**(Suppl. 4): 3–119.
8   Clark, C.E., Henry, W.L. and Epstein, S.E. Familial prevalence and genetic transmission of idiopathic hypertrophic subaortic stenosis. *N Engl J Med* 1973; **289**: 709–14.
9   Geisterfer-Lowrance, A.A., Kass, S., Tanigawa, G. et al. A molecular basis for familial hypertrophic cardiomyopathy: a beta cardiac myosin heavy chain gene missense mutation. *Cell* 1990; **62**: 999–1006.
10 Watkins, H., MacRae, C., Thierfelder, L. et al. A disease locus for familial hypertrophic cardiomyopathy maps to chromosome 1q3. *Nat Gen* 1993; **3**: 333–7.
11 Ho, C.Y. Genetic considerations in hypertrophic cardiomyopathy. *Prog Cardiovasc Dis* 2012; **54**: 456–60.
12 Maron, M.S., Maron, B.J., Harrigan, C. et al. Hypertrophic cardiomyopathy phenotype revisited after 50 years with cardiovascular magnetic resonance. *J Am Coll Cardiol* 2009; **54**: 220–8.
13 Maron, M.S. Clinical utility of cardiovascular magnetic resonance in hypertrophic cardiomyopathy. *J Cardiovasc Magnetic Res* 2012; **14**: 13.
14 Chan, R.H., Maron, B.J., Olivotto, I. et al. Prognostic value of quantitative contrast-enhanced cardiovascular magnetic resonance for the evaluation of sudden death risk in patients with hypertrophic cardiomyopathy. *Circulation* 2014; **130**: 484–95.
15 Rowin, E.J., Maron, B.J., Appelbaum, E. et al. Significance of false negative electrocardiograms in preparticipation screening of athletes for hypertrophic cardiomyopathy. *Am J Cardiol* 2012; **110**: 1027–32.
16 Chen, X., Zhao, T., Lu, M. et al. The relationship between electrocardiographic changes and CMR features in asymptomatic or mildly symptomatic patients with hypertrophic cardiomyopathy. *Int J Cardiovasc Imaging* 2014; **30**(Suppl. 1): 55–63.
17 Delcre, S.D., Di Donna, P., Leuzzi, S. et al. Relationship of ECG findings to phenotypic expression in patients with hypertrophic cardiomyopathy: a cardiac magnetic resonance study. *Int J Cardiol* 2013; **167**: 1038–45.
18 McLeod, C.J., Ackerman, M.J., Nishimura, R.A. et al. Outcome of patients with hypertrophic cardiomyopathy and a normal electrocardiogram. *J Am Coll Cardiol* 2009; **54**: 229–33.
19 Drezner, J.A., Ashley, E., Baggish, A.L. et al. Abnormal electrocardiographic findings in athletes: recognising changes suggestive of cardiomyopathy. *Br J Sports Med* 2013; **47**: 137–52.
20 Schnell, F., Riding, N., O'Hanlon, R. et al. Recognition and significance of pathological T-wave inversions in athletes. *Circulation* 2015; **131**: 165–73.
21 Lakdawala, N.K., Thune, J.J., Maron, B.J. et al. Electrocardiographic features of sarcomere mutation carriers with and without clinically overt hypertrophic cardiomyopathy. *Am J Cardiol* 2011; **108**: 1606–13.
22 Maron, M.S., Olivotto, I., Zenovich, A.G. et al. Hypertrophic cardiomyopathy is predominantly a disease of left ventricular outflow tract obstruction. *Circulation* 2006; **114**: 2232–9.
23 O'Mahony, C., Jichi, F., Pavlou, M. et al. A novel clinical risk prediction model for sudden cardiac death in hypertrophic cardiomyopathy (HCM risk-SCD). *Eur Heart J* 2014; **35**: 2010–20.
24 Thompson, P.D., Franklin, B.A., Balady, G.J. et al. Exercise and acute cardiovascular events placing the risks into perspective: a scientific statement from the American Heart Association Council on Nutrition, Physical Activity, and Metabolism and the Council on Clinical Cardiology. *Circulation* 2007; **115**: 2358–68.
25 Maron, B.J., Doerer, J.J., Haas, T.S. et al. Sudden deaths in young competitive athletes: analysis of 1866 deaths in the United States, 1980–2006. *Circulation* 2009; **119**: 1085–92.

26 Maron, B.J., Chaitman, B.R., Ackerman, M.J. et al. Recommendations for physical activity and recreational sports participation for young patients with genetic cardiovascular diseases. *Circulation* 2004; **109**: 2807–16.

27 Maron, B.J., Olivotto, I., Spirito, P. et al. Epidemiology of hypertrophic cardiomyopathy-related death: revisited in a large non-referral-based patient population. *Circulation* 2000; **102**: 858–64.

28 Maron, B.J., Zipes, D.P. and Kovacs, R.J. Eligibility and disqualification recommendations for competitive athletes with cardiovascular abnormalities: Preamble, principles, and general considerations: A scientific statement from the American Heart Association and American College of Cardiology. *J Am Coll Cardiol* 2015; **66**(21): 2343–9.

29 Pelliccia, A., Fagard, R., Bjornstad, H.H. et al. Recommendations for competitive sports participation in athletes with cardiovascular disease: a consensus document from the Study Group of Sports Cardiology of the Working Group of Cardiac Rehabilitation and Exercise Physiology and the Working Group of Myocardial and Pericardial Diseases of the European Society of Cardiology. *Eur Heart J* 2005; **26**: 1422–45.

30 Reineck, E., Rolston, B., Bragg-Gresham, J.L. et al. Physical activity and other health behaviors in adults with hypertrophic cardiomyopathy. *Am J Cardiol* 2013; **111**: 1034–9.

31 Gersh, B.J., Maron, B.J., Bonow, R.O. et al. 2011 ACCF/AHA guideline for the diagnosis and treatment of hypertrophic cardiomyopathy: executive summary: a report of the American College of Cardiology Foundation/American Heart Association Task Force on Practice Guidelines. *Circulation* 2011; **124**: 2761–96.

32 Lampert, R., Olshansky, B., Heidbuchel, H. et al. Safety of sports for athletes with implantable cardioverter-defibrillators: results of a prospective, multinational registry. *Circulation* 2013; **127**: 2021–30.

20 Arrhythmogenic Right Ventricular Cardiomyopathy

Alessandro Zorzi and Domenico Corrado

Department of Cardiac, Thoracic and Vascular Sciences, University of Padua Medical School, Padua, Italy

Introduction

Arrhythmogenic right ventricular cardiomyopathy (ARVC) is an inherited heart muscle disease with an incidence of 1 in 2500–5000 and male predominance [1]. The disease is characterised pathologically by fibro-fatty myocardial replacement of the ventricular myocardium and clinically by ventricular electrical instability, which may lead to arrhythmic cardiac arrest, mostly in young people [2]. Life-threatening ventricular arrhythmias are triggered by physical exercise, and participation in competitive athletics has been associated with an increased risk for sudden cardiac death (SCD) (Figure 20.1) [3,4]. In addition, physical sport activity has been implicated as a factor promoting acceleration of disease progression [5–7]. This chapter will examine the pathophysiology, natural history, diagnosis, prognosis and clinical management of ARVC, with particular reference to affected athletes and relevance to risk of SCD during sports.

Pathophysiology and Natural History

Disease Mechanism

The pathological hallmark of the disease is the progressive loss of myocytes due to a genetically determined defect in the intercellular junction structures (desmosomes), with subsequent fibro-fatty replacement, which first involves the right ventricle and then the left. It has been postulated that the genetically determined impairment of myocyte cell-to-cell adhesion may lead to tissue and organ fragility that is sufficient to promote myocyte death and subsequent fibro-fatty repair, especially under conditions of mechanical stress, such as those occurring during physical activity [1,2]. The resulting alterations in the myocardial structure not only can impair the mechanical function of the ventricles, but render affected individuals vulnerable to life-threatening ventricular arrhythmias via three different mechanisms. First, patients with overt disease may experience scar-related monomorphic ventricular tachycardia, which is the result of re-entrant circuits related to underlying fibro-fatty ventricular scars [9]. Second, ventricular fibrillation and SCD may occur in young patients during the so-called 'hot phases', characterised by myocarditis-mediated bouts of acute myocyte death and marked electrical instability [2]. Third, loss of expression of desmosomal proteins might 'per se' induce electrical myocardial instability via secondary ion-channel dysfunction, which predisposes to lethal ventricular arrhythmias even prior to the expression of an overt structural abnormality [10].

Natural History

The natural history of the disease is typically characterised by four different phases: (i) 'concealed', characterised by the absence of or subtle right ventricular structural changes, with or without minor ventricular arrhythmias, during which SCD may occasionally be the first manifestation of the disease, mostly in young

IOC Manual of Sports Cardiology, First Edition. Edited by Mathew G. Wilson, Jonathan A. Drezner and Sanjay Sharma.
© 2017 International Olympic Committee. Published 2017 by John Wiley & Sons, Ltd.

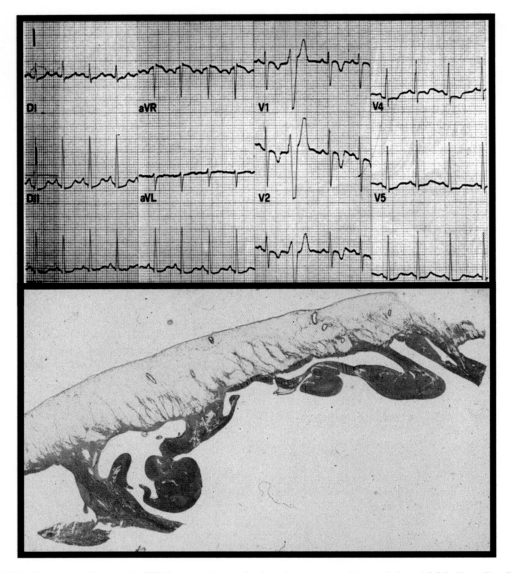

Figure 20.1 Electrocardiographic (ECG) and autopsy findings in a young athlete victim of SCD. Top: The ECG showed negative T-waves in V1–V4 and a ventricular ectopic beat with a left bundle branch block (LBBB) configuration (suggesting a right ventricular origin). Bottom: Post-mortem investigation revealed near transmural myocyte loss with fibro-fatty scar in the right ventricular free wall, consistent with the diagnosis of ARVC (*Source*: Corrado et al. [8]. Reproduced with permission of Oxford University Press)

people during competitive sports or intense physical exercise; (ii) 'overt electrical disorder', in which symptomatic right ventricular arrhythmias possibly leading to sudden cardiac arrest are associated with overt right ventricular functional and structural abnormalities; (iii) 'right ventricular failure', caused by the progression and extension of right ventricular muscle disease, which provokes global right ventricular dysfunction with relatively preserved left ventricular function; and (iv) 'biventricular pump failure', caused by pronounced left ventricular involvement. At this stage, ARVC mimics biventricular dilated cardiomyopathy of other causes, leading to congestive heart failure. A minority of ARVC patients are characterised by early and greater left ventricular involvement, which may either parallel ('biventricular') or exceed ('left dominant') the severity of right ventricular disease [1,2].

Role of Exercise in the Development of the Disease

Exercise has been implicated as a factor in promoting the development and progression of the ARVC phenotype, because physical activity acutely increases the right ventricular afterload and causes cavity enlargement, which may elicit the death of genetically defective myocytes by stretching the diseased right ventricular myocardium [1,2]. In an animal model of plakoglobin-deficient mice, endurance training accelerated the development of right ventricular dilatation, dysfunction and ventricular ectopy, suggesting that chronically increased ventricular load might contribute to worsening of the ARVC phenotype [11]. Studies in genetically affected humans have confirmed that endurance sports and frequent exercise increase age-related penetrance, risk of ventricular tachycardia/ventricular fibrillation and occurrence of heart failure in ARVC desmosomal-gene carriers. Moreover, in affected individuals, physical activity is a strong proarrhythmic factor, due to adrenergic and mechanical stimulation of the diseased myocardium (Figure 20.2) [5–7].

Recently, it has been postulated that intense physical exertion may cause an ARVC phenocopy (i.e. alterations in right ventricular structure and function mimicking ARVC in the absence of a pathological genetic substrate) via an alteration of the myocardial interstitial matrix secondary to strenuous and repeated exercise [13]. The theory is supported by a study in a group of endurance athletes with ventricular arrhythmias originating from the right ventricle with clinical features of ARVC. Genetic analysis revealed the presence of a desmosomal gene mutation in 12.8%, a proportion that is significantly lower than the ~30–50% prevalence of desmosomal gene mutations in series describing familial ARVC probands [14]. However, although strenuous physical exercise may itself cause an acquired form of ARVC, affected athletes may have unrecognised genes and/or polymorphisms which predispose them to develop an ARVC-like phenotype as a result of participation in intensive endurance sports.

Diagnosis

The diagnosis of ARVC is based on a series of criteria – including histopathological manifestations, alterations in cardiac structure and function, electrocardiographic (ECG) abnormalities, arrhythmic manifestations and the identification of disease-causing genetic mutations (Figure 20.3) – elaborated by an international task force of experts (Table 20.1) [15]. As no single criterion is sufficiently accurate, the diagnosis requires a combination of criteria (classified as minor or major according to their specificity). More precisely, the diagnosis of 'definite' ARVC is fulfilled in the presence of two major criteria, one major and two minor criteria or four minor criteria from different categories. The diagnosis is considered 'borderline' in the presence of one major and two minor criteria or three minor criteria, and 'possible' when two minor criteria are met.

Classic ARVC Phenotype

The classic ARVC phenotype is characterised by prevalent right ventricular involvement with progressive fibro-fatty replacement of the ventricular myocardium, particularly in the so-called 'triangle of dysplasia' (outflow tract, apex and inflow). Demonstration of fibrous or fibro-fatty replacement on endomyocardial biopsy is the most specific diagnostic criterion [16].

The pathophysiological process of progressive myocyte loss causes a gradual dilation and systolic dysfunction of the right ventricle, initially at a regional level, then, as the disease progresses, at a global level. The regional distribution of right ventricular wall-motion abnormalities (bulging, akinesis or diskinesis) is highly specific for ARVC and allows differentiation from other right ventricular diseases (e.g. congenital heart diseases (CHDs) or pulmonary hypertension), characterised by uniform dilation/dysfunction of the entire right ventricle. Hence, the morphofunctional diagnostic criteria for ARVC are based on the demonstration of global dilation/dysfunction of the right ventricle associated with regional wall-motion abnormalities [17].

Electrical abnormalities secondary to the fibro-fatty scarring process are also the basis for the typical ECG changes of ARVC, including depolarisation (delayed intraventricular conduction with widening/slurring of the S-wave in V1–V3, epsilon waves and late potentials) and/or repolarisation (T-wave inversion) abnormalities. Such features usually involve the right precordial leads (V1–V3/V4) [18].

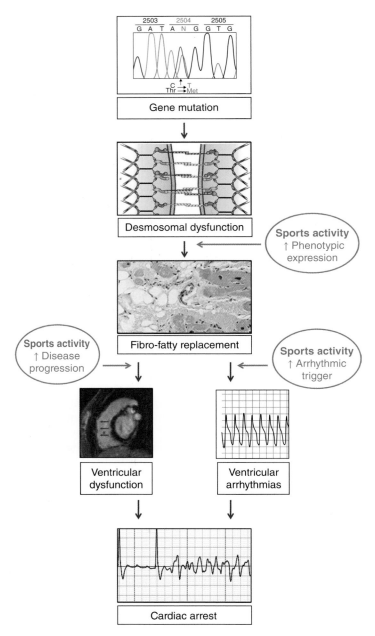

Figure 20.2 Schematic representation of the course of ARVC, from desmosomal gene mutation to phenotypic expression and cardiac arrest due to ventricular fibrillation. Sports activity may promote development of phenotypic expression, accelerate disease progression and trigger life-threatening ventricular arrhythmias (*Source*: Corrado et al. [12]. Reproduced with permission of Oxford University Press)

Ventricular arrhythmias with a left bundle branch block (LBBB) morphology (negative QRS complex in V1), suggestive of a right ventricular origin, are another key feature of ARVC [9]. However, arrhythmias originating from the right ventricular outflow tract (RVOT) (negative QRS complex in V1 and inferior QRS axis in the limb leads) are less specific for ARVC compared to those arising from other right ventricular regions, because in the majority of cases they are benign, nonfamilial and not related to an underlying cardiomyopathy ('idiopathic' RVOT ventricular tachycardia) [19].

Finally, because of the hereditary nature of the disease, a positive family history for SCD and/or ARVC and the demonstration of a pathogenetic mutation in the genes encoding for desmosomal proteins represent major diagnostic criteria.

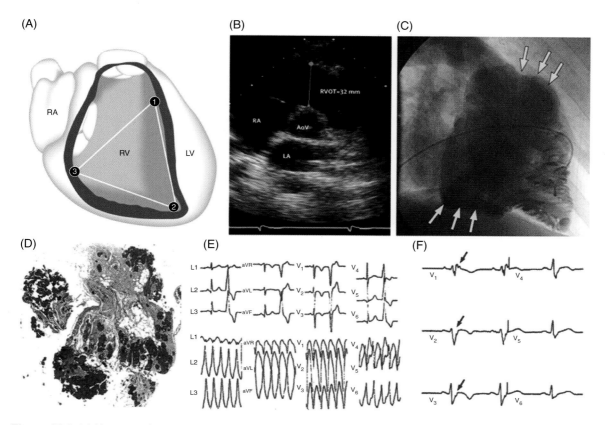

Figure 20.3 Multiparametric approach to the diagnosis of ARVC. (A) ARVC is characterised by fibro-fatty replacement of the ventricular myocardium, particularly in the so-called 'triangle of dysplasia' (right ventricular outflow tract (RVOT), inflow and apex). These regions typically show dilation and wall-motion abnormalities on (B) echocardiogram, (C) ventriculography or magnetic resonance. (D) Endomyocardial biopsy reveals myocyte loss with fibro-fatty replacement. The disease is characterised by arrhythmias with (E) a left bundle branch block (LBBB) configuration (suggesting a right ventricular origin) and ECG depolarisation (delayed intraventricular conduction with widening/slurring of the S-wave in V1–V3, epsilon waves and late potentials) and/or (F) repolarisation (T-wave inversion) abnormalities (*Source*: Basso et al. [1]. Reproduced with permission of Elsevier)

Left-Dominant ARVC

The classic ARVC phenotype mostly involves the right ventricle, whilst morphofunctional abnormalities of the left ventricle become evident only in the late stages of the disease. However, the 'left dominant' ARVC variant is characterised by an early and predominant left ventricular involvement, as a result of a specific genetic substrate (e.g. mutations of the gene encoding for desmoplakin). The phenotype is the counterpart of the classic variant, with T-wave inversion in the left precordial leads (V4–V6) and left ventricular arrhythmias (right bundle branch block (RBBB) pattern, i.e. positive QRS complex in V1) [1]. In contrast with the classic variant, the diagnostic power of echocardiography is limited because left ventricular systolic dysfunction, whether regional or global, is identified in only a minority of patients with this variant. The reason for this is that the fibro-fatty scarring process initially involves the subepicardial myocardial layers, which contribute marginally to the development of the contractile power, and does not translate into prominent wall-motion abnormalities. As a consequence, the left-dominant ARVC phenotype is difficult to diagnose, and its incidence is probably underestimated. Contrast-enhanced cardiac magnetic resonance (CMR) increases the diagnostic sensitivity because it allows identification of nontransmural left ventricular scars (areas of late gadolinium enhancement) at a subepicardial and/or midmural level. However, it must be emphasised that subepicardial left ventricular scarring is not specific for ARVC and may also be the hallmark of other left ventricular diseases, such as dilated cardiomyopathy and myocarditis; therefore, its presence should not be considered diagnostic for left-dominant ARVC [20].

1. Endomyocardial biopsy

Major:

- The total amount of the residual myocytes is <60% by morphometric analysis (or <50% if estimated), and the remainder of the free wall myocardium is replaced by fibrous tissue with or without fatty changes in more than one sample

Minor:

- The total amount of the residual myocytes is 60–75% by morphometric analysis (or 50–65% if estimated), and the remainder of the free wall myocardium is replaced by fibrous tissue with or without fatty changes in more than one sample

2. Right ventricular structural and functional abnormalities

A. Echocardiography

Major:

- Regional wall akinesis, diskinesis or aneurismal dilatation of the right ventricle
    1. Plus one of the following:
    2. RVOT >19 mm.m^{-2} in parasternal long-axis view at the end diastole, or >21 mm.m^{-2} in parasternal short-axis view at the end diastole
- Right ventricular fractional area change <33%

Minor:

- Regional wall akinesis or diskinesis

Plus one of the following:

1. Right ventricular outflow tract of 16–19 mm.m^{-2} in parasternal long-axis view at the end diastole, or 18–21 mm.m^{-2} in parasternal short-axis view at the end diastole
2. Right ventricular fractional area change 33–40%

B. Cardiac magnetic resonance (CMR)

Major:

- Regional wall akinesis or diskinesis, or dyssynchronous contraction

Plus one of the following:

1. Ejection fraction <40%
2. End-diastolic volume >110 ml.m^{-2} in males or >100 ml.m^{-2} in females

Minor:

- Regional wall akinesis or diskinesis, or dyssynchronous contraction

Plus one of the following:

1. Ejection fraction <45%
2. End-diastolic volume >110 ml.m^{-2} in males or >100 ml.m^{-2} in females

C. Right ventricular angiography

Major:

- One or more diskinetic, akinetic or aneurismatic right ventricular regions

3. ECG repolarisation abnormalities

Major:

- Inverted T-waves in right precordial leads (V1–V3) or beyond in individuals >14 years of age (in the absence of complete right bundle branch block (RBBB) QRS >120 ms)

Minor:

- Inverted T-waves in leads V1 and V2 in individuals >14 years of age (in the absence of complete RBBB), or in V4, V5 or V6
- Inverted T-waves in leads V1–V4 in individuals >14 years of age in the presence of complete RBBB

4. ECG depolarisation abnormalities

Major:

- Epsilon wave (reproducible low-amplitude signals between end of QRS complex and onset of the T-wave) in the right precordial leads (V1–V3)

Minor:

- Late potentials by signal-averaged ECG in one or more of three parameters, in the absence of a QRS duration >110 ms on the standard ECG:
    - Filtered QRS duration (fQRS) >114 ms
    - Duration of terminal QRS 40 mV (low-amplitude signal duration) >38 ms
    - Root-mean-square voltage of terminal 40 ms <20 mV
- Terminal activation duration of QRS >55 ms, measured from the nadir of the S-wave to the end of the QRS, including R0, in V1, V2 or V3, in the absence of complete RBBB

Table 20.1 International task force criteria for the diagnosis of ARVC

5. Arrhythmias

Major:

- Nonsustained or sustained ventricular tachycardia of LBBB morphology with superior axis (negative or indeterminate QRS in leads II, III and aVF and positive in lead aVL)

Minor:

- Nonsustained or sustained ventricular tachycardia of right ventricular outflow configuration, LBBB morphology with inferior axis (positive QRS in leads II, III and aVF and negative in lead aVL) or of unknown axis
- >500 premature ventricular beats per 24 hours (Holter)

6. Family history/genetics

Major:

- Positive family history in a first-degree relative, confirmed by current task force criteria
- Pathological confirmation of the disease in a first-degree relative, either by autopsy or by surgery
- Discovery of a DNA pathogenic mutation that has been recognised to be associated or probably associated with ARVC in a patient evaluated for ARVC

Minor:

- Positive family history of a first-degree relative in whom the diagnosis cannot feasibly be confirmed by current task force criteria
- Positive family history of a young (<35 years) first-degree relative with sudden death due to suspected ARVC
- Positive family history of disease in a second-degree relative who has been confirmed to have the disease either by current task force criteria or pathologically

7. Diagnosis

Established

At least two major criteria, one major criterion and three minor criteria, or four minor criteria from different categories.

Borderline

One major criterion and two minor criteria, or three minor criteria from different categories.

Possible

One major criterion or two minor criteria from different categories.

Table 20.1 (Continued)

Diagnosis of ARVC in Athletes

The ultimate diagnosis of cardiomyopathy in a young competitive athlete may be problematic due to physiologic (and reversible) structural and electrical adaptations of the cardiovascular system to long-term athletic training. This condition, known as 'athlete's heart', is characterised by an increase in ventricular cavity dimension and wall thickness, which may overlap with cardiomyopathies. An accurate diagnosis is crucial, both because of the potentially adverse outcome associated with cardiomyopathy in an athlete but also due to the possibility of an erroneous diagnosis leading to unfair disqualification from sport, with financial and psychological consequences.

A sizable proportion of highly trained athletes have increased right ventricular cavity dimensions, raising the spectre of ARVC. Morphologic criteria that indicate a physiologic right ventricular enlargement consist of preserved global and regional ventricular function without evidence of wall-motion abnormalities such as dyskinetic regions or diastolic bulging [21]. During the last 2 decades, advances in molecular genetics have allowed the identification of a growing number of defective genes involved in the pathogenesis of ARVC. The hope is that molecular genetic tests will be clinically available in the near future for definitive differential diagnosis between ARVC and training-related physiologic right ventricular changes.

Prevention of ARVC-Related Sudden Death

ARVC as a Cause of Sudden Death in Athletes

Systematic monitoring and pathologic investigation of sudden death in young people and athletes of the Veneto region of Italy showed that ARVC is the most common pathologic substrate, accounting for nearly a quarter of fatalities in young athletes, and that the risk of sudden death from ARVC was five times higher during competitive sports than during sedentary activity. The incidence of sudden death from ARVC in athletes was estimated to be 0.5 per 100 000 person-years. Sudden-death victims with ARVC were all males, with a mean age of 22.6 ± 4.0 years [4].

Although ARVC has been demonstrated to be the leading cause of SCD in athletes of the Veneto region, previous studies from other countries show a higher prevalence of other pathologic substrates, such as hypertrophic cardiomyopathy (HCM), anomalous coronary arteries and myocarditis [22]. This discrepancy may be explained by several factors, including the experience of the pathologists or coroners performing the post mortem investigations. ARVC is rarely associated with cardiomegaly and usually spares the left ventricle, so that affected hearts may be erroneously diagnosed as normal hearts. Therefore, a number of SCDs in young people and athletes, in which the routine pathologic examination discloses a normal heart, may in fact be due to an unrecognised ARVC. On the other hand, the high incidence of ARVC in the Veneto region may be due to a genetic factor in the population of northeastern Italy, although ARVC can no longer be considered a peculiar 'Venetian disease', since there is growing evidence that it is ubiquitous and largely underdiagnosed, both clinically and at post mortem [23].

Role or Pre-participation ECG Screening

The risk of dying suddenly from ARVC has been estimated to be 5.4 times greater during competitive sports than during sedentary activity, and early identification of athletes with arrhythmogenic right ventricular cardiomyopathy/dysplasia (ARVC/D) plays a crucial role in the prevention of SCD during sport (Figure 20.4) [4].

By reviewing clinical and ECG findings of 22 young competitive athletes who died suddenly from arrhythmogenic right ventricular cardiomyopathy/dysplasia (ARVC/D) proven at autopsy, it has been demonstrated that the majority of SCD victims exhibit ECG changes, ventricular arrhythmias or both (Figure 20.5). Right precordial T-waves were recorded in 88%, right precordial QRS duration >110 ms in 76% and ventricular arrhythmias with an LBBB pattern in the form of isolated/coupled premature ventricular beats or nonsustained ventricular tachycardia (NSVT) in 76%. Limited exercise testing induced ventricular arrhythmias in 50%. Thus, the majority of young competitive athletes who died suddenly from ARVC showed ECG abnormalities that could raise the suspicion of the underlying cardiovascular disease (CVD) at pre-participation evaluation, leading to further testing for a definitive diagnosis [1].

For more than 20 years, a systematic pre-participation screening, based on 12-lead ECG in addition to history and physical examination, has been the practice in Italy. A time-trend analysis of the incidence of SCD in young competitive athletes aged 12–35 years in the Veneto region between 1979 and 2004 provides

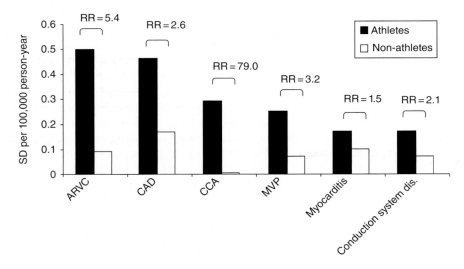

Figure 20.4 Incidence and relative risk (RR) of sudden death (SD) for specific cardiovascular causes among athletes and nonathletes. ARVC, arrhythmogenic right ventricular cardiomyopathy; CAD, coronary artery disease; CCA, congenital coronary artery anomaly; MVP, mitral valve prolapse (*Source*: Corrado et al. [4]. Reproduced with permission of Elsevier)

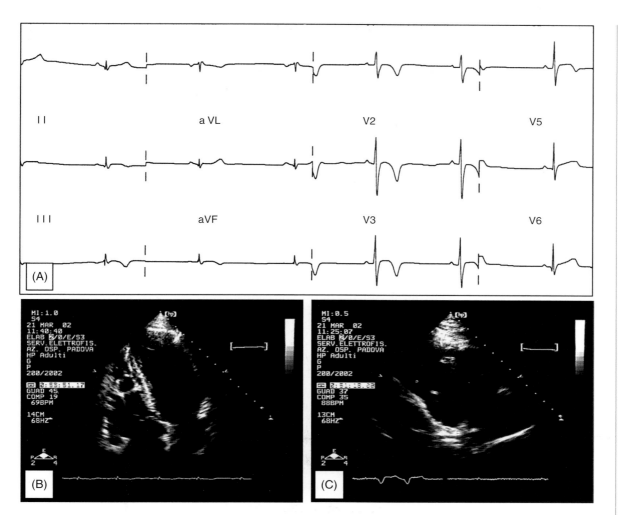

Figure 20.5 Diagnosis of ARVC at pre-participation screening. (A) Pre-participation ECG of a young athlete, showing T-wave inversion in right precordial leads V1–V4. The echocardiogram reveals right ventricular dilation with akinesis of the (B) lateral and (C) inferior right ventricular regions (*Source*: Corrado et al. [24]. Reproduced with permission of Oxford University Press)

compelling evidence that ECG screening is a lifesaving strategy. The analysis demonstrates a 90% decrease in SCD among athletes following the introduction of the nationwide screening programme. By comparison, the incidence of SCD in the unscreened nonathletic population of the same age did not change significantly over the same time. Most of the mortality reduction is attributable to fewer deaths from HCM and ARVC. A parallel analysis of the causes of disqualifications from competitive sports at the Center for Sports Medicine in the Padua area shows that the proportion of athletes identified and disqualified for cardiomyopathies doubled from the early to the late screening period. This indicates that mortality reduction was a reflection of a lower incidence of SCD from cardiomyopathies, as a result of increasing identification over time of affected athletes at ECG pre-participation screening [3].

Interpretation of Repolarisation Abnormalities in Athletes

The 12-lead ECG is one of the most important tools for the diagnosis, follow-up and risk stratification of ARVC, and inversion of T-waves in the right precordial leads V1–V3/V4 is the most common ECG sign of ARVC. The persistence of T-wave inversion in the right precordial leads (known as persistence of the juvenile pattern of repolarisation) may be observed in healthy athletes, but whilst the incidence of benign persistence of the juvenile pattern of repolarisation declines sharply following puberty, the clinical manifestations of

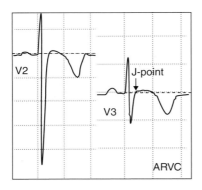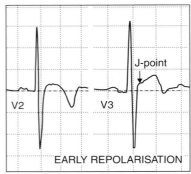

Figure 20.6 Differential diagnosis between cardiomyopathic negative T-waves and early repolarisation of athlete's heart. Left: Right-precordial leads V2–V3 of a patient with ARVC, showing no J-point elevation and negative T-wave. Right: Right precordial leads V2–V3 of an Afro-Caribbean athlete, showing an early repolarisation pattern characterised by J-point elevation, domed ST elevation and a negative T-wave (*Source*: Zorzi et al. [26]. Reproduced with permission of Elsevier)

ARVC usually occur after puberty. Hence, the persistence of right precordial T-wave inversion in the post-pubertal age should raise the problem of an underling ARVC and prompt further investigation [25].

Another cause of benign negative T-waves in healthy athletes, especially of Afro-Caribbean descent, is an anterior early repolarisation variant characterised by domed ST-segment elevation followed by a negative T-wave in anterior leads V1–V3. The differential diagnosis requires careful analysis of the ST-segment morphology preceding the negative T-wave. Athletes exhibit J-point elevation (the hallmark of early repolarisation) followed by an upsloping ST-segment elevation with a domed morphology, whilst ARVC patients usually show no J-point elevation and no or minimal ST-segment elevation (Figure 20.6) [24].

The clinical workup for differential diagnosis between pathologic and nonpathologic negative T-waves traditionally includes ECG exercise testing. The current perception is that negative T-waves usually revert to normal with exercise in healthy subjects but persist in patients with structural heart muscle disease. However, the available data in favour of this concept are very limited. In fact, on comparing ARVC patients with healthy athletes with right precordial T-wave inversion, the prevalence of complete or partial normalisation of T-wave polarity with exercise is observed in the majority of both groups (Figure 20.7) [26].

Clinical Management of Athletes with ARVC

Risk Stratification and Therapy

Patients with ARVC should undergo lifelong clinical *follow-up* (every 6–24 months, depending on age, symptoms and disease severity), including echocardiography, 24-hour Holter monitoring and exercise testing, to periodically evaluate new-onset or worsening symptoms, progression of morphological and/or functional ventricular abnormalities and risk of SCD. Due to the age-related penetrance of ARVC, healthy gene carriers and family members should also be offered repeat clinical assessment, mostly during adolescence and young adulthood.

Lifestyle changes include restriction from sports, with the possible exception of low-intensity activities. Both patients with overt ARVC and asymptomatic patients and healthy gene carriers should be prudently advised to avoid vigorous exercise, not only in order to reduce the risk of ventricular arrhythmias and SCD, but also to prevent disease progression.

Drug therapy in ARVC may include antiarrhythmic agents, beta blockers and heart-failure drug therapy. Beta-blocker drugs should be offered to all patients with a definite diagnosis of ARVC and evidence of morphostructural ventricular abnormalities or ventricular arrhythmias, because of their proven efficacy in preventing effort-induced ventricular arrhythmias, their proven efficacy in heart-failure management and their potential but unproven ability to hinder myocardial disease progression by lowering right ventricular wall stress. Adjunctive antiarrhythmic drug therapy is indicated to reduce the arrhythmia burden in patients with frequent premature ventricular beats and/or complex ventricular arrhythmia. For patients who have developed heart failure, standard pharmacologic treatment with angiotensin-converting enzyme (ACE) inhibitors, angiotensin II receptor blockers (ARBs), beta blockers and diuretics is prescribed as appropriate.

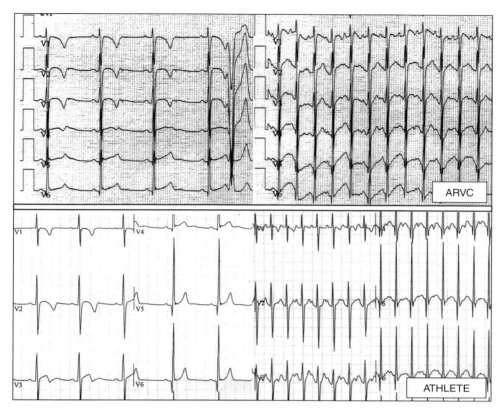

Figure 20.7 Stress test findings in a patient with ARVC (top) and in a young athlete with benign persistence of the juvenile repolarisation pattern (bottom). Both subjects exhibit right precordial negative T-waves at baseline ECG (left), which normalise during exercise (right) (*Source*: Zorzi et al. [26]. Reproduced with permission of Elsevier)

Catheter ablation is a therapeutic option for ARVC patients who have recurrent ventricular tachycardia despite antiarrhythmic drug therapy. However, catheter ablation has not been proven to prevent SCD and should not be considered as an alternative to implantable cardioverter-defibrillator (ICD) therapy. Also, because of the progressive nature of the disease, repeated ablation procedures may be required to provide clinical control of ventricular arrhythmias.

Implantation of an ICD is the most logical therapeutic strategy for patients with ARVC, whose natural history is primarily characterised by the risk of arrhythmic cardiac arrest.

There is general agreement that patients who have survived an episode of ventricular fibrillation or sustained ventricular tachycardia most benefit from ICD implantation, because of their high incidence of malignant arrhythmia recurrences.

Other risk factors identified by studies on ARVC patients include unexplained syncope; NSVT on 24-hour Holter monitoring; systolic dysfunction of the right or left ventricle, or both; male gender; compound and digenic heterozygosity of desmosomal-gene mutations; young age at the time of diagnosis; proband status; inducibility at programmed ventricular stimulation; electroanatomic scar and electroanatomic scar-related fractionated electrograms; high T-wave inversion across precordial and inferior leads; low QRS amplitude; and QRS fragmentation. The decision to implant an ICD in a patient with one or more of these risk factors should be made on an individual basis, by assessing the overall clinical profile, the age, the strength of the risk factor identified, the level of SCD risk that is acceptable to the patient and the potential risk of inappropriate interventions and complications.

Finally, asymptomatic patients with no risk factors have a favourable long-term outcome regardless of familial history of SCD and electrophysiologic (EP) study findings. These results are particularly relevant for clinical management of the growing cohort of asymptomatic ARVC patients and desmosomal gene mutation carriers (Figure 20.8) [27].

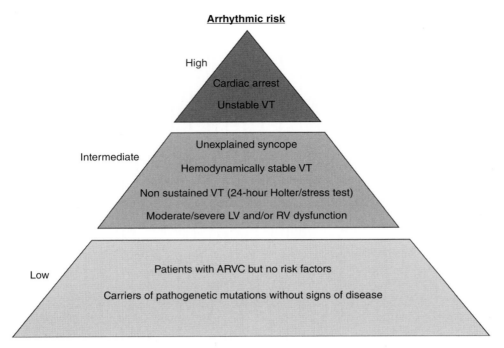

Arrhythmic risk

High

Cardiac arrest

Unstable VT

Intermediate

Unexplained syncope

Hemodynamically stable VT

Non sustained VT (24-hour Holter/stress test)

Moderate/severe LV and/or RV dysfunction

Low

Patients with ARVC but no risk factors

Carriers of pathogenetic mutations without signs of disease

Figure 20.8 Pyramid of ARVC risk stratification. LV, left ventricular; VT, ventricular tachycardia; RV, right ventricular; ARVC, arrhythmogenic right ventricular cardiomyopathy (*Source*: Migliori et al. [27]. Reproduced with permission of Bentham Science Publishers)

Sports Eligibility

According to current recommendations for sports eligibility, athletes with a clinical diagnosis of ARVC should be excluded from all competitive sports [28]. This recommendation is independent of age, gender and phenotypic appearance, and does not differ for those athletes without symptoms or for those being treated with drugs, surgery, catheter ablation or ICD. The presence of a free-standing automated external defibrillator at sporting events should not be considered absolute protection against sudden death, nor a justification for participation in competitive sports in athletes with previously diagnosed ARVC.

Patients with ARVC may wish to participate in recreational and leisure-time exercise activity, given the recognised beneficial effects of a physically active lifestyle. A recent study suggests that the absolute risk of ventricular tachyarrhythmia/death in ARVC patients practising recreational sports does not significantly differ from that of physically inactive ARVC patients [7]. However, the conclusion that the recreational sports activity does not increase the risk of SCD or disease progression is not supported by adequate statistical power, because of the small subgroup size. In addition, the intensity of the physical exercise was not quantified in this study, and recreational sportspeople – particularly those engaged in long-distance running or cycling – often exercise more than competitive athletes, such as football players. Further studies in larger ARVC patient populations over longer follow-up periods are required before the definitive conclusion that ARVC patients can safely participate in recreational sports can be drawn. In the meantime, patients with ARVC should be restricted from participation in all sports, with the possible exception of leisure-time sports activities with low cardiovascular demand [12,29].

ICD and Sports

The accurate prediction of the performance of ICD in athletes remains a challenging subject. Successful ICD therapy depends on a well-functioning device that is capable of both appropriately sensing the malignant arrhythmia and delivering an adequate amount of energy to depolarise a critical myocardial mass and so overcome the ongoing arrhythmic state. Sports may hinder the success of ICD therapy in many aspects. First, sinus tachycardia and other supraventricular tachyarrhythmias that are often present during sports activity represent an obstacle to the appropriate differentiation of malignant ventricular arrhythmias. Second, physical trauma, whether due to direct or indirect contact, may lead to device damage and malfunction. Third, physiological changes associated with exertion, such as high catecholamine levels, electrolyte imbalance, metabolic acidosis and cardiac loading alterations, can lead to persistent arrhythmogenic states in which defibrillation may not be successful (electrical storms) or – even worse – to SCD due to electromechanical dissociation, where defibrillation will not be of any benefit.

Recently, Lampert et al. [30] reported on a series of 372 US athletes with ICDs (age 10–60 years), including 53 with ARVC, participating in competitive (n = 328) or dangerous (n = 44) sports. During a median follow-up of 31 months, there were no occurrences of death, resuscitated arrest or arrhythmia- or shock-related injury during sports. During this period, 46 athletes received appropriate therapies (25 during sports or other physical exertion), whilst 29 received inappropriate ones (25 during sports or other physical exertion). Freedom from lead malfunction was 97% at 5 years (from implant) and 90% at 10 years. The authors concluded that these data are similar to previously published data on nonathletic ICD patients and therefore do not support competitive sports restriction for all athletes with ICDs.

Despite these reassuring data, it must be emphasised that the reasons for restricting young athletes with ICDs from taking part in competitive sports go beyond the increased risk of inappropriate intervention, injury to the patient and damage of the system. Sports participation plays a major role in the progression of the disease, worsening the substrate and leading to adverse outcomes. Although evidence has emerged in support of the safety of competitive sports in selected individuals carrying ICD, it is still prudent to restrict participation in competitive sports in ARVC patients.

Acknowledgments

This work was funded by a TRANSAC Research Grant of the University of Padua, Italy and by the Federazione Italiana Gioco Calcio (Research Grant to Dr Zorzi).

References

1 Basso, C., Corrado, D., Marcus, F. et al. Arrhythmogenic right ventricular cardiomyopathy. *Lancet* 2009; **373**: 1289–300.

2 Basso, C., Bauce, B., Corrado, D. and Thiene, G. Pathophysiology of arrhythmogenic cardiomyopathy. *Nat Rev Cardiol* 2012; **9**(4): 223–33.

3 Corrado, D., Basso, C., Pavei, A. et al. Trends in sudden cardiovascular death in young competitive athletes after implementation of a preparticipation screening program. *JAMA* 2006; **296**(13): 1593–601.

4 Corrado, D., Basso, C., Rizzoli, G. et al. Does sports activity enhance the risk of sudden death in adolescents and young adults? *J Am Coll Cardiol* 2003; **42**(11): 1959–63.

5 James, C.A., Bhonsale, A., Tichnell, C. et al. Exercise increases age-related penetrance and arrhythmic risk in arrhythmogenic right ventricular dysplasia/cardiomyopathy-associated desmosomal mutation carriers. *J Am Coll Cardiol* 2013; **62**(14): 1290–7.

6 Saberniak, J., Hasselberg, N.E., Borgquist, R. et al. Vigorous physical activity impairs myocardial function in patients with arrhythmogenic right ventricular cardiomyopathy and in mutation positive family members. *Eur J Heart Fail* 2014; **16**(12): 1337–44.

7 Ruwald, A.C., Marcus, F., Estes, N.A. 3rd et al. Association of competitive and recreational sport participation with cardiac events in patients with arrhythmogenic right ventricular cardiomyopathy: results from the North American multidisciplinary study of arrhythmogenic right ventricular cardiomyopathy. *Eur Heart J* 2015; **36**(27): 1735–43.

8 Corrado, D., Basso, C., Pelliccia, A. and Thiene, G. Sports and heart disease. In: Camm, J., Luscher, T.F. and Serruys, P.W. (eds) *The ESC Textbook of Cardiovascular Medicine*. New York: Oxford University Press, 2009. pp. 1215–37.

9 Lemola, K., Brunckhorst, C., Helfenstein, U. et al. Predictors of adverse outcome in patients with arrhythmogenic right ventricular dysplasia/cardiomyopathy: long term experience of a tertiary care centre. *Heart* 2005; **91**(9): 1167–72.

10 Cerrone, M., Lin, X., Zhang, M. et al. Missense mutations in plakophilin-2 cause sodium current deficit and associate with a brugada syndrome phenotype. *Circulation* 2014; **129**(10): 1092–103.

11 Kirchhof, P., Fabritz, L., Zwiener, M. et al. Age- and training-dependent development of arrhythmogenic right ventricular cardiomyopathy in heterozygous plakoglobin-deficient mice. *Circulation* 2006; **114**(17): 1799–806.

12 Corrado, D. and Zorzi, A. Arrhythmogenic right ventricular cardiomyopathy and sports activity. *Eur Heart J* 2015; **36**(27): 1708–10.

13 La Gerche, A., Burns, A.T., Mooney, D.J. et al. Exercise-induced right ventricular dysfunction and structural remodelling in endurance athletes. *Eur Heart J* 2012; **33**(8): 998–1006.

14 La Gerche, A., Robberecht, C., Kuiperi, C. et al. Lower than expected desmosomal gene mutation prevalence in endurance athletes with complex ventricular arrhythmias of right ventricular origin. *Heart* 2010; **96**(16): 1268–74.

15 Marcus, F.I., McKenna, W.J., Sherrill, D. et al. Diagnosis of arrhythmogenic right ventricular cardiomyopathy/dysplasia: proposed modification of the task force criteria. *Circulation* 2010; **121**(13): 1533–41.

16 Basso, C., Ronco, F., Marcus, F. et al. Quantitative assessment of endomyocardial biopsy in arrhythmogenic right ventricular cardiomyopathy/dysplasia: an in vitro validation of diagnostic criteria. *Eur Heart J* 2008; **29**(22): 2760–71.

17 Yoerger, D.M., Marcus, F., Sherrill, D. et al. Echocardiographic findings in patients meeting task force criteria for arrhythmogenic right ventricular dysplasia: new insights from the multidisciplinary study of right ventricular dysplasia. *J Am Coll Cardiol* 2005; **45**(6): 860–5.

18 Steriotis, A.K., Bauce, B., Daliento, L. et al. Electrocardiographic pattern in arrhythmogenic right ventricular cardiomyopathy. *Am J Cardiol* 2009; **103**(9): 1302–8.

19 O'Donnell, D., Cox, D., Bourke, J. et al. Clinical and electrophysiological differences between patients with arrhythmogenic right ventricular dysplasia and right ventricular outflow tract tachycardia. *Eur Heart J* 2003; **24**(9): 801–10.

20 Sen-Chowdhry, S., Syrris, P., Prasad, S.K. et al. Left-dominant arrhythmogenic cardiomyopathy: an under-recognized clinical entity. *J Am Coll Cardiol* 2008; **52**(25): 2175–87.

21 Bauce, B., Frigo, G., Benini, G. et al. Differences and similarities between arrhythmogenic right ventricular cardiomyopathy and athlete's heart adaptations. *Br J Sports Med* 2010; **44**(2): 148–54.

22 Maron, B.J. Sudden death in young athletes. *N Engl J Med* 2003; **349**(11): 1064–75.

23 Elmaghawry, M., Alhashemi, M., Zorzi, A. and Yacoub, M.H. A global perspective of arrhythmogenic right ventricular cardiomyopathy. *Glob Cardiol Sci Pract* 2013; **2012**(2): 81–92.

24 Corrado, D., Pelliccia, A., Heidbuchel, H. et al. Recommendations for interpretation of 12-lead electrocardiogram in the athlete. *Eur Heart J* 2010; **31**(2): 243–59.

25 Migliore, F., Zorzi, A., Michieli, P. et al. Prevalence of cardiomyopathy in Italian asymptomatic children with electrocardiographic T-wave inversion at preparticipation screening. *Circulation* 2012; **125**(3): 529–38.

26 Zorzi, A., ElMaghawry, M., Rigato, I. et al. Exercise-induced normalization of right precordial negative T waves in arrhythmogenic right ventricular cardiomyopathy. *Am J Cardiol* 2013; **112**(3): 411–15.

27 Migliore, F., Zorzi, A., Silvano, M. et al. Clinical management of arrhythmogenic right ventricular cardiomyopathy: an update. *Curr Pharm Des* 2010; **16**(26): 2918–28.

28 Pelliccia, A., Fagard, R., Bjornstad, H.H. et al. Recommendations for competitive sports participation in athletes with cardiovascular disease: a consensus document from the Study Group of Sports Cardiology of the Working Group of Cardiac Rehabilitation and Exercise Physiology and the Working Group of Myocardial and Pericardial Diseases of the European Society of Cardiology. *Eur Heart J* 2005; **26**(14): 1422–45.

29 Corrado, D., Wichter, T., Link, M.S. et al. Treatment of arrhythmogenic right-ventricular cardiomyopathy/dysplasia: an international task force consensus statement. *Eur Heart J* 2015; **132**(5): 441–53.

30 Lampert, R., Olshansky, B., Heidbuchel, H. et al. Safety of sports for athletes with implantable cardioverter-defibrillators: results of a prospective, multinational registry. *Circulation* 2013; **127**(20): 2021–30.

21 Dilated Cardiomyopathy, Left Ventricular Hypertrabeculation and Noncompaction

Sabiha Gati and Sanjay Sharma

Department of Cardiovascular Sciences, St George's University of London, London, UK

Introduction

Regular physical exercise is associated with physiological alterations in cardiac structure and function, which permit the generation of a fivefold increase in cardiac output for prolonged periods. The promotion of a large stroke volume is facilitated by a benign and reversible cardiac remodelling process, comprising ventricular hypertrophy, an increase in cardiac chamber size and enhanced diastolic ventricular filling. Such changes are a major component of the 'athlete's heart'.

In general, athletes exhibit a 10–20% increase in left ventricular wall thickness and a 10–15% increase in left and right ventricular cavity size. The magnitude of this increase is governed by several demographic factors, and some large male athletes engaging in endurance sports reveal ventricular cavity dimensions that may be consistent with either dilated cardiomyopathy (DCM) or arrhythmogenic right ventricular cardiomyopathy (ARVC). More recently, advances in tissue harmonics have led to better characterisation of myocardial architecture and have revealed some athletes to exhibit increased left ventricular trabeculations, which overlap with yet another cardiomyopathy: notably isolated left ventricular noncompaction (LVNC). The distinction between a physiological increase in cardiac size and cardiomyopathy is crucial when one considers that the cardiomyopathies are frequently implicated in exercise-related sudden cardiac death (SCD) in young athletes. An erroneous diagnosis has potentially sinister consequences, ranging from unfair disqualification from sport at one end to false reassurance of a young person with a life-threatening condition at the other.

The differentiation between athlete's heart and left ventricular enlargement resembling DCM or trabeculations of the myocardium suspicious of LVNC is a well-recognised diagnostic challenge in sports cardiology. This chapter focuses on differentiation of athlete's heart from DCM and LVNC.

Dilated Cardiomyopathy

DCM is defined as a dilated and poorly functioning left ventricle in the absence of significant ischaemic heart disease, hypertension or valvular disease. At least 25% of cases of DCM are familial, inherited as an autosomal-dominant trait [1]. Most patients have a relatively poor prognosis, with a 5-year survival of just over 50%. The clinical presentation of patients with DCM varies considerably, with most patients typically exhibiting symptoms of low cardiac output and pulmonary congestion, but others presenting with systemic embolism and sudden death. A small but significant proportion of affected individuals may remain completely asymptomatic despite markedly impaired systolic function.

Echocardiography is the gold-standard investigation for the diagnosis of DCM. The most widely applied criteria are based on the Henry formula, which defines left ventricular enlargement as a left ventricular cavity >112% of predicted normal values and an ejection fraction (EF) of <45% and/or fractional shortening

IOC Manual of Sports Cardiology, First Edition. Edited by Mathew G. Wilson, Jonathan A. Drezner and Sanjay Sharma.
© 2017 International Olympic Committee. Published 2017 by John Wiley & Sons, Ltd.

of <25% (to define abnormal systolic function) [2]. Recent European guidelines suggest a more liberal cut-off of a left ventricular cavity >117% of predicted values (2 SD + 5%). Late enhancement following gadolinium on the cardiac magnetic resonance imaging (MRI) scan is almost pathognomonic of an underlying cardiomyopathic process in a patient with an increased left ventricular volume and reduced EF, but the absence of late gadolinium enhancement does not exclude a DCM.

Exercise testing is useful for assessing functional capacity in patients with DCM. Metabolic exercise testing provides an objective measure of exercise capacity and response to pharmacological therapies and has prognostic value. 24-hour Holter electrocardiogram (ECG) may demonstrate arrhythmias at a very early stage of the disease, including supraventricular and ventricular tachyarrhythmias, as well as major conduction delays [3].

The primary aims of treatment are to control symptoms, prevent disease progression and improve prognosis. Diuretics are the mainstay of therapy, to relieve peripheral oedema and pulmonary congestion. Angiotensin-converting enzyme (ACE) inhibitors and beta blockers have revolutionised the prognostic outlook in DCM and are recommended in all patients with left ventricular systolic dysfunction. Patients in New York Heart Association (NYHA) class II or more despite ACE inhibitors and beta blockers benefit both symptomatically and in terms of prognosis from the addition of an aldosterone antagonist.

An implantable cardioverter-defibrillator (ICD) is recommended for patients with an NYHA class II or more who have a baseline EF <35%. Biventricular pacing provides symptomatic relief in patients with an interventricular conduction defect and is recommended in patients with symptomatic heart failure despite optimal medical therapy, left ventricular EF <35% and QRS >120 ms, in addition to an ICD.

DCM in Athletes

DCM is a rare but recognised cause of SCD in athletes. In the majority of athletes with DCM, the inability to generate a satisfactory cardiac output during exercise selects them out of competitive sports.

It is well established that endurance athletes, such as swimmers, rowers and cyclists, may develop significant chamber dilatation due to long-term volume and pressure overload, which overlaps with DCM. Profound left ventricular cavity changes are particularly observed in professional cyclists who compete in ultra-endurance events.

Pelliccia et al. [4] assessed 1309 elite athletes and observed that the left ventricular end-diastolic dimension (LVEDD) exceeded the normal limits (≥55 mm) in 584 (45%). Furthermore, 185 (14%) of these athletes had an LVEDD of ≥60 mm. In another study, one-third of highly trained American football players were noted to exhibit an LVEDD >55 mm, and 10 (6%) had an LVEDD >60 mm [5]. An echocardiographic study by Abergel et al. [6] of 286 elite professional cyclists (and 52 sedentary controls) competing in the Tour de France showed that 214 (75%) had an LVEDD outside the normal range (cut-off of 57.4 mm as the upper limit of normal (ULN)), 147 (51%) had an LVEDD >60 mm and 4 (1.4%) showed a markedly enlarged LVEDD >70 mm.

A common misconception amongst physicians is that the resting left ventricular EF should be normal in athletes – in fact, in some highly trained endurance athletes, the resting EF can appear suppressed during resting conditions, due to a combination a large end-diastolic volume and profound bradycardia. In the group of 286 elite cyclists studied by Abergel et al. [6], 111 (37%) had an EF ≤60%, 38 (15%) had an EF of 52–56% and, interestingly, 20 (11%) had an EF <52%.

The combination of a dilated left ventricle and suppressed left ventricular EF poses a diagnostic challenge, and the distinction between physiological left ventricular enlargement and DCM can be difficult in such circumstances. As the number of athletes engaging in gruelling endurance sports rises, the issue becomes an ever more common conundrum for sports cardiologists. Although cardiac magnetic resonance (CMR) is increasingly used to confirm the diagnosis of DCM, the conventional cardiac parameters used to derive EF using CMR in the general population frequently lead to an underestimation of cardiac performance in athletes at rest. As a result, a combination of electrical, structural and haemodynamic investigations may prove useful in facilitating the correct diagnosis in athletes (Figure 21.1).

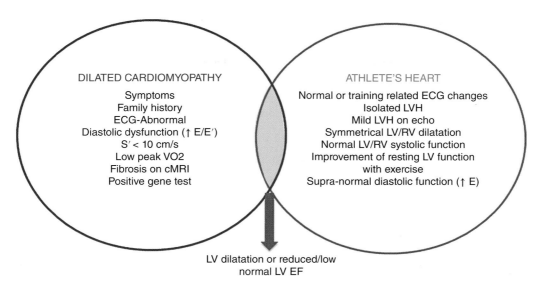

Figure 21.1 Algorithm to distinguish athlete's heart from DCM. ECG, electrocardiogram; E, early diastolic velocity; S', longitudinal systolic velocity; cMRI, cardiac magnetic resonance imaging; LVH, left ventricular hypertrophy; LV, left ventricle; RV, right ventricle; EF, ejection fraction

Evaluation of DCM in Athletes

Clinical History As with any patient, a comprehensive history is paramount. Specifically, a history of syncope or pre-syncope, reduced exercise capacity or a past history of a flu-like illness (which can lead to a myocarditis) should be ascertained. In addition, a family history of SCD, DCM or heart failure should be sought. The presence of any of these features in an athlete with a dilated left ventricle and reduced EF makes the diagnosis of DCM more likely.

Electrocardiography It is well established that athletes have normal ECGs or training-related ECG changes such as sinus bradycardia and isolated Sokolow–Lyon voltage criteria for left ventricular hypertrophy (LVH). However, our own experience suggests that up to 10% of patients with DCM have isolated Sokolow–Voltage criteria for LVH. Nonetheless, the presence of an ECG showing training-unrelated changes such as ST-segment depression, T-wave inversion (particularly in the lateral leads), interventricular conduction defects or left bundle branch block (LBBB) should raise suspicion of a myocardial disorder.

Echocardiography In addition to assessing left ventricular cavity dimension and systolic function, diastolic parameters prove valuable in differentiating DCM from structural changes associated with athletic training in the absence of symptoms. Enhanced diastolic function at high heart rates is an essential mechanism of stroke-volume augmentation during exercise. The ability to maintain adequate stroke volume for prolonged periods is particularly important in endurance exercise. Studies have shown that endurance athletes have higher peak E waves and E' than sedentary controls [7–11]. It is well acknowledged that patients with DCM have abnormal myocardial relaxation; in fact, this may be one of the only abnormal features in a patient with a morphologically mild/early stage of a cardiomyopathic process. Furthermore, a majority of athletes in the absence of pathology show normal indices of longitudinal function with systolic velocity >10 cm.s⁻¹ [12].

Exercise Echocardiography Exercise echocardiography can be helpful in cases where athletes exhibit the combination of left ventricular dilatation and suppressed or low–normal resting EF. Abernethy et al. [5] demonstrated normal left ventricular function with exercise in all athletes with reduced resting systolic function included in their study. In contrast, patients with DCM rarely demonstrate the ability to augment cardiac output in response to increased metabolic demands.

Cardiopulmonary Exercise Testing Simultaneous measurement of gas exchange during cardiopulmonary exercise testing can prove useful in the diagnosis of DCM. A high peak VO_2 can be utilised as another useful tool in distinguishing physiological left ventricular dilation from a morphologically mild DCM. Pluim et al. [13] performed a meta-analysis and documented the peak VO_2 of endurance athletes (runners) (53 ± 3 to 75 ± 1 ml.min^{-1}.kg^{-1}) and mixed endurance and strength athletes (rowers and cyclists) (55.6 ± 8.0 to 72 ± 6 ml. min^{-1}.kg^{-1}). Their results were far superior to the level of oxygen consumption that could be expected of patients with DCM, who are unlikely to reach the cut-off for normality of >84% of age-predicted VO_2 and rarely achieve values exceeding 40 ml.min^{-1}.kg^{-1}.

One limitation of the studies examining cardiopulmonary exercise testing is the bias towards Caucasian cohorts. Peak VO_2 values in athletes of African or Afro-Caribbean decent are less well established. As a result, caution must be taken when extrapolating normal peak VO_2 values to black athletes until further studies are undertaken in this cohort.

Cardiac Magnetic Resonance CMR can underestimate overall cardiac function in athletes, but it has the ability to look for myocardial fibrosis. The presence of scar is almost pathognomonic of an underlying myocardial disorder.

Exercise Recommendations for Athletes with DCM

The current European Society of Cardiology (ESC) recommendation for athletes with a definite diagnosis of DCM is complete restriction from competitive sport [3].

Left Ventricular Noncompaction

LVNC is an intriguing novel and as yet unclassified cardiomyopathy. The condition is characterised by prominent myocardial trabeculations and deep recesses. The precise stage of development and the natural history of the disorder are not fully understood, but preliminary data suggest that it is a morphologically and clinically heterogeneous disorder. As with DCM, some individuals present with overt heart failure and potentially fatal arrhythmias, whilst others may remain asymptomatic. There is no specific treatment to retard the cardiomyopathic process in LVNC. Patients with left ventricular systolic dysfunction are treated with conventional heart-failure therapy and anticoagulation. Those with severe symptoms or ventricular arrhythmias are implanted with a prophylactic cardiovertor defibrillator.

Diagnosis of LVNC

Echocardiography The clinical diagnosis is predominantly reliant on three proposed echocardiographic criteria (Table 21.1) [14]. All three rely on the presence of increased left ventricular trabeculations and a double myocardial layer (an outer thin compacted area and an inner noncompacted layer), differing with respect to the precise area and the timing of the measurement of the compacted and noncompacted layers within the cardiac cycle. Chin et al. [15] were the first to propose echocardiographic criteria. They calculated the ratio of the distance from the epicardial surface to the trough of the trabeculae (X) to the distance from the epicardial surface to the peak of the trabeculae (Y), measured at end diastole (Table 21.1). A ratio of ≤0.5 based on measurements acquired in the parasternal short-axis views is best for establishing a diagnosis of LVNC.

The Jenni criteria [16] are the most commonly used in clinical practice: a noncompaction to compaction ratio >2.0 in end systole on short-axis views; the absence of other cardiac abnormalities; and colour Doppler demonstrating perfusion of the intertrabecular recesses (Table 21.1). Jenni et al. [16] showed that noncompacted segments are frequently found in the mid-lateral and inferior walls and apex.

Stöllberger et al. [17] defined LVNC as more than three individual trabeculations protruding from the left ventricular wall apical to the papillary muscle in one imaging plane (Table 21.1). Stöllberger's criteria were further refined to include a two-layered myocardium with a ratio of noncompacted to compacted myocardium >2.0 in end diastole.

	Chin criteria [15]	Jenni criteria [16]	Stollberger criteria [17]	Petersen criteria [18]	Jacquier criteria [19]
Number of patients forming the basis for the criteria	8	34	62	7	16
Description	Two-layered structure with an epicardial compacted and endocardial noncompacted layer	Two-layered structure with a compacted epicardial (C) and noncompacted endocardial (NC) layer Colour Doppler evidence of intertrabecular recesses supplied by intraventricular blood Absence of coexisting cardiac structural abnormalities	More than three trabeculations protruding from the left ventricular wall apically to the papillary muscle in one imaging plane	Two-layered structure with a compacted epicardial (C) and noncompacted endocardial (NC) layer Images from horizontal and long-axis views at points of prominent trabeculations	Calculated total left ventricular trabeculated mass from steady-state free precession (SSFP) short-axis papillary muscles excluded from myocardial mass
Cardiac phase	End diastole	End systole	End diastole	End diastole	End diastole
Ratio	X/Y ≤0.5	NC/C ≥2	NC/C ≥2	NC/C >2.3	Left ventricular trabecular mass >20%

Table 21.1 Summary of LVNC criteria (*Data Sources:* Chin et al. [15], Jenni et al. [16], Stöllberger et al. [17], Petersen et al. [18], Jacquier et al. [19])

Cardiac Magnetic Resonance Alternative imaging modalities, particularly CMR, are increasingly used to confirm the diagnosis of LVNC. Two sets of CMR criteria are in use, the first proposed by Petersen et al. in 2005 [18] and the second by Jacquier et al. in 2010 [19] (Table 21.1).

Petersen et al. [18] tested the precision of CMR in the diagnosis of LVNC in 177 individuals with and without cardiac disease. They were able to identify a distinct two-layered appearance of trabeculated and compacted myocardium on the horizontal, vertical long-axis and left ventricular outflow tract (LVOT) views at end diastole in 7 patients with a clinical diagnosis of LVNC and, interestingly, in patients with normal and athlete's hearts and known cardiac disease (aortic stenosis, hypertension, hypertrophic cardiomyopathy (HCM)). Based on these findings, Petersen proposed a noncompaction to compaction ratio >2.3 in diastole as a cut-off point for LVNC. The sensitivity and specificity of the Petersen criteria are 86 and 99%, respectively.

Jacquier et al. [19] calculated the left ventricular trabecular mass using steady-state free precession short-axis views (Table 21.1). Based on an assessment of 16 patients (12 known and 4 suspected) with LVNC, compared with patients with DCM, HCM and healthy controls, a left ventricular trabecular mass >20% of the total left ventricular mass was predictive of LVNC. The sensitivity and specificity of the Jacquier criteria [19] are both 93.7% based on the Jenni criteria [16] for LVNC.

Controversies in the Pathogenesis of LVNC and Issues with Current Diagnostic Criteria

The main problem with all of these criteria for LVNC is that they have been derived from small cohorts and have not been validated in large populations. There are also increasing reports that they lack specificity in low-risk populations. The initial prevalence of LVNC was estimated to be less than 0.3%, but over the past 2 decades improvement in tissue harmonics has led to an improvement in the characterisation of the myocardial architecture and an increasing number of reported cases of LVNC. In a study from the UK, LVNC was considered in almost 25% of patients in a dedicated heart-failure clinic. This figure is several hundredfold greater than the prevalence of all the other primary cardiomyopathies and suggests that myocardial trabeculation may be a physiological response to an increased wall stress (an epiphenomenon) resulting from a high left ventricular preload. Data from patients with chronic anaemia, who are subject to an increased cardiac preload, support this concept. In a recent study by our group, 10% of patients with sickle-cell anaemia fulfilled echocardiographic criteria for LVNC.

Gati et al. [20] performed a longitudinal study assessing the impact of a physiological increase in cardiac loading conditions on left ventricular trabeculations. They used a pregnancy model associated with a 50% increase in blood volume (preload) by the 24th week and demonstrated that of 102 women with a morphologically normal left ventricle, 25% developed de novo trabeculations and 8% fulfilled echocardiographic criteria for LVNC as pregnancy progressed. The data support the theory that increased preload may promote left ventricular trabeculations in some individuals and that most low-risk individuals fulfilling criteria for LVNC are unlikely to have a cardiomyopathy.

LVNC and Athletic Training

There are few reports relating to LVNC in athletes. A recent meta-analysis identified just 18 cases of LVNC in the context of sport and exercise, 10 reported in athletes and 8 in nonathletic individuals participating in regular exercise (the type of exercise was not reported) [21]. The mean age of patients was 29 ± 17 years. All 18 cases appeared to be at high risk, judged by the fact that 50% experienced unheralded syncope, 44% had a family history of sudden death, 22% showed nonsustained ventricular tachycardia (NSVT) and 11% (2 cases) revealed impaired left ventricular systolic function.

Our own observations suggest that the increased left ventricular trabeculations or even criteria for LVNC are not uncommon in asymptomatic athletes. In a recent study of over 1000 asymptomatic athletes, 18% exhibited increased left ventricular trabeculation (this phenomenon was more common in black athletes) and 8% (76) fulfilled echocardiographic criteria for LVNC [22]. Most athletes fulfilling echocardiographic criteria for LVNC exhibited recognised manifestations of the athlete's ECG, such as sinus bradycardia, early repolarisation or the voltage criterion for LVH. Echocardiography revealed normal or increased left ventricular size and normal systolic and diastolic function.

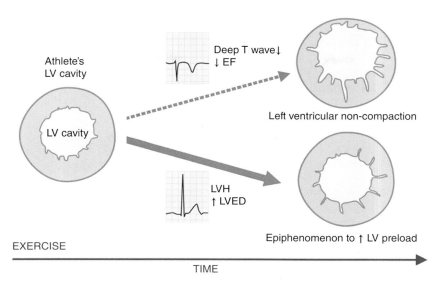

Figure 21.2 Potential significance of increased left ventricular trabeculation in young individuals engaging in intensive physical training. EF, ejection fraction; LV, left ventricle; LVH, left ventricular hypertrophy; LVED, left ventricular end-diastolic dimension (*Source:* Gati et al. [22]. Reproduced with permission of BMJ)

A minority of those studied (0.9%) demonstrated concomitant T-wave inversion and reduced indices of systolic function, which may be suggestive of LVNC. Alternatively, these manifestations may represent extreme features of cardiac adaptation to exercise or may denote an incomplete expression of LVNC that is unmasked through intensive exercise in certain predisposed young athletes (Figure 21.2).

Evaluation of Athletes Fulfilling Criteria for LVNC

A multimodal diagnostic approach is the current recommendation for the assessment of athletes presenting with increased left ventricular trabeculations consistent with LVNC, impaired resting left ventricular function and T-wave inversion on ECG (Figure 21.3) [14,22]. This algorithm is designed to aid the sports physician in taking a pragmatic approach to low-risk athletes fulfilling criteria for LVNC.

The proposal is based on our own experience of comparing athletes with features of LVNC and actual patients diagnosed with the condition [22]. Patients with LVNC frequently (75%) express symptoms of left ventricular dysfunction, whereas athletes are asymptomatic. Patients also frequently (66%) demonstrate a left ventricular cavity >64 mm, an EF <45%, suppressed longitudinal left ventricular function (Sa <9 cm.s^{-1}) and impaired left ventricular filling. In contrast, athletes with increased left ventricular trabeculation and reduced EF usually show an EF range of 45–50%, normal indices of longitudinal left ventricular function and normal diastolic function. The pattern of T-wave inversion is different between the two groups: patients with noncompaction show T-wave inversion in the inferolateral leads, whereas the majority of athletes show T-wave inversion in V1–V3. In our experience, a cardiopulmonary exercise stress test followed by a peak exercise echo is useful in the differentiation between the two groups. Athletes reveal a high peak VO$_2$ (>120% predicted for age and size) and dynamic left ventricular contraction, whereas patients with LVNC show low peak VO$_2$ and persistently reduced left ventricular function on exercise echo. The identification of NSVT during exercise in athletes with criteria for LVNC would favour pathology. Abnormal myocardial strain patterns are in the experimental phase for this condition, but abnormal parameters may imply disease. The presence of late gadolinium enhancement on CMR is suggestive of a myopathic process. A family history of premature SCD and heart failure in such athletes is an indication for long-term follow-up. In such circumstances, we also recommend screening of first-degree relatives for features of LVNC; the detection of another member with a similar phenotype would favour a diagnosis of LVNC.

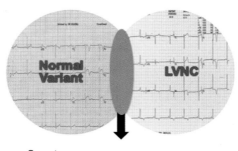

–	Symptoms	+
–	Family history	+
–	T wave inversion	+
–	LBBB	+
–	E' lateral < 9 cm/sec	+
–	Peak VO2 < 85%	+
–	↓ LVEF on exercise echo	+
–	Exercise induced VT/AF	+
–	Abnormal myocardial strain	+
–	Late gadolinium enhancement on CMR	+
–	Family member with similar features	+

Figure 21.3 Differentiating physiological increased left ventricular trabeculation from pathological LVNC. LBBB, left bundle branch block; LVEF, left ventricular ejection fraction; VT, ventricular tachycardia; AF, atrial fibrillation; CMR, cardiac magnetic resonance (*Source:* Gati et al. [14]. Reproduced with permission of Elsevier)

Risk Stratification and Exercise Recommendations

Based on the available literature, we would not consider an asymptomatic athlete with incidental features of noncompaction to necessarily harbour a cardiomyopathy in the absence of symptoms, family history, abnormal ECG patterns and impaired left ventricular function, as outlined in this section. In athletes with features to indicate a diagnosis of LVNC, we would propose abstinence from competitive sports involving medium- or high-intensity exercise, as for all other cardiomyopathies.

Conclusion

Differentiating physiological left ventricular dilatation from DCM or deep left ventricular invaginations from LVNC is not straightforward; however, by adopting a systematic and pragmatic approach, the distinction of physiological training-related changes from pathology can be achieved by utilising several noninvasive investigations.

References

1 Elliott, P. Cardiomyopathy. Diagnosis and management of dilated cardiomyopathy. *Heart* 2000; **84**: 106–12.
2 Mestroni, L., Maisch, B., Mckenna, W.J. et al. Guidelines for the study of familial dilated cardiomyopathies. Collaborative Research Group of the European Human and Capital Mobility Project on Familial Dilated Cardiomyopathy. *Eur Heart J* 1999; **20**: 93–102.
3 Pelliccia, A., Fagard, R., Bjornstad, H.H. et al. Recommendations for competitive sports participation in athletes with cardiovascular disease: a consensus document from the Study Group of Sports Cardiology of the Working Group of Cardiac Rehabilitation and Exercise Physiology and the Working Group of Myocardial and Pericardial Diseases of the European Society of Cardiology. *Eur Heart J* 2005; **26**: 1422–45.
4 Pelliccia, A., Culasso, F., Di Paolo, F.M. and Maron, B.J. Physiologic left ventricular cavity dilatation in elite athletes. *Ann Intern Med* 1999; **130**: 23–31.
5 Abernethy, W.B., Choo, J.K. and Hutter, A.M. Jr. Echocardiographic characteristics of professional football players. *J Am Coll Cardiol* 2003; **41**: 280–4.
6 Abergel, E., Chatellier, G., Hagege, A.A. et al. Serial left ventricular adaptations in world-class professional cyclists: implications for disease screening and follow-up. *J Am Coll Cardiol* 2004; **44**: 144–9.
7 Baggish, A.L., Yared, K., Weiner, R.B. et al. Differences in cardiac parameters among elite rowers and subelite rowers. *Med Sci Sports Exerc* 2010; **42**: 1215–20.

8 Caso, P., D'Andrea, A., Galderisi, M. et al. Pulsed Doppler tissue imaging in endurance athletes: relation between left ventricular preload and myocardial regional diastolic function. *Am J Cardiol* 2000; **85**: 1131–6.

9 Naylor, L.H., Arnolda, L.F., Deague, J.A. et al. Reduced ventricular flow propagation velocity in elite athletes is augmented with the resumption of exercise training. *J Physiol* 2005; **563**: 957–63.

10 Prasad, A., Popovic, Z.B., Arbab-Zadeh, A. et al. The effects of aging and physical activity on Doppler measures of diastolic function. *Am J Cardiol* 2007; **99**: 1629–36.

11 Tumuklu, M.M., Ildizli, M., Ceyhan, K. and Cinar, C.S. Alterations in left ventricular structure and diastolic function in professional football players: assessment by tissue Doppler imaging and left ventricular flow propagation velocity. *Echocardiogr* 2007; **24**: 140–8.

12 D'Ancrea, A., Cocchia, R., Riegler, L. et al. Left ventricular myocardial velocities and deformation indexes in top-level athletes. *J Am Soc Echocardiogr* 2010; **23**: 1281–8.

13 Pluim, B.M., Zwinderman, A.H., Van Der Laarse, A. and Van Der Wall, E.E. The athlete's heart. A meta-analysis of cardiac structure and function. *Circulation* 2000; **101**: 336–44.

14 Gati, S., Rajani, R., Carr-White, G.S. and Chambers, J.B. Adult left ventricular noncompaction: reappraisal of current diagnostic imaging modalities. *JACC Cardiovasc Imaging* 2014; **7**: 1266–75.

15 Chin, T.K., Perloff, J.K., Williams, R.G. et al. Isolated noncompaction of left ventricular myocardium. A study of eight cases. *Circulation* 1990; **82**: 507–13.

16 Jenni, R., Oechslin, E., Schneider, J. et al. Echocardiographic and pathoanatomical characteristics of isolated left ventricular non-compaction: a step towards classification as a distinct cardiomyopathy. *Heart* 2001; **86**: 666–71.

17 Stollberger, C., Finsterer, J. and Blazek, G. Left ventricular hypertrabeculation/noncompaction and association with additional cardiac abnormalities and neuromuscular disorders. *Am J Cardiol* 2002; **90**: 899–902.

18 Petersen, S.E., Selvanayagam, J.B., Wiesman, F. et al. Left ventricular non-compaction: insights from cardiovascular magnetic resonance imaging. *J Am Coll Cardiol* 2005; **46**: 101–5.

19 Jacquier, A., Thuny, F., Jop, B. et al. Measurement of trabeculated left ventricular mass using cardiac magnetic resonance imaging in the diagnosis of left ventricular non-compaction. *Eur Heart J* 2010; **31**: 1098–104.

20 Gati, S., Papadakis, M., Papamichael, N.D. et al. Reversible de novo left ventricular trabeculations in pregnant women: implications for the diagnosis of left ventricular noncompaction in low-risk populations. *Circulation* 2014; **130**: 475–83.

21 Ganga, H.V. and Thompson, P.D. Sports participation in non-compaction cardiomyopathy: a systematic review. *Br J Sports Med* 2014; **48**(20): 1466–71.

22 Gati, S., Chandra, N., Bennett, R.L. et al. Increased left ventricular trabeculation in highly trained athletes: do we need more stringent criteria for the diagnosis of left ventricular non-compaction in athletes? *Heart* 2013; **99**: 401–8.

22 Marfan Syndrome and Aortopathies

Anne H. Child and Bethan Davies

Cardiovascular and Cell Sciences Research Institute, St George's University of London, London, UK

What is Marfan Syndrome?

Marfan syndrome is an inherited connective-tissue disorder that affects many organ systems, including the skeleton, lungs, eyes, heart and blood vessels [1]. This condition can affect both men and women of any race or ethnic group, with a population incidence of approximately 1 in 3300 to 1 in 5000 [2]. It is estimated that around 18 000 people in the UK have Marfan syndrome.

Salient Features

Skeletal

Common physical findings of Marfan syndrome include a tall, thin physique, long limbs and fingers, scoliosis, narrow chest with pigeon or funnel deformity, joint hypermobility [3] and dislocations. Dural ectasia occurs in 65% of patients [4]. This body build – with long arms and legs – is important for selection into certain sports, including volleyball, hockey, basketball, swimming and rowing.

Cardiovascular

Abnormalities in the cardiovascular system include dilatation of the ascending (and sometimes descending) aorta, incompetence of aortic and mitral valves, and aneurysm and dissection of the aorta which can be the cause of sudden death in patients with Marfan syndrome.

Respiratory

The respiratory system is at risk of pneumothorax, bronchiectasis, emphysema, fibrosis and asthma [5,6].

Ocular

Subluxation or dislocation of the lens, myopia and unstable refraction, detachment of the retina, strabismus and glaucoma are found in patients with Marfan syndrome [7,8].

Dental

A high, arched palate and crowding of teeth are additional features found in Marfan syndrome [9].

IOC Manual of Sports Cardiology, First Edition. Edited by Mathew G. Wilson, Jonathan A. Drezner and Sanjay Sharma.
© 2017 International Olympic Committee. Published 2017 by John Wiley & Sons, Ltd.

Genetic

Marfan syndrome is an autosomal-dominant disorder that affects males and females with equal frequency. Each child of an affected parent has a 50% chance of inheriting Marfan syndrome. In 25% of cases, neither parent is affected; however, apparently unaffected parents should be screened carefully as the severity and pattern of disease are variable, even within a single family.

Diagnosis

Diagnosis of Marfan syndrome is based on the revised Ghent nosology [10] and is made after careful physical examination and echocardiography [11,12]. Diagnosis can be made by demonstrating classical features in two out of three major systems (eyes, heart, skeletal), and is supported by a family history in 75% of cases (Figure 22.1) [10]. There are many genes which can cause familial thoracic aortic aneurysm and dissection

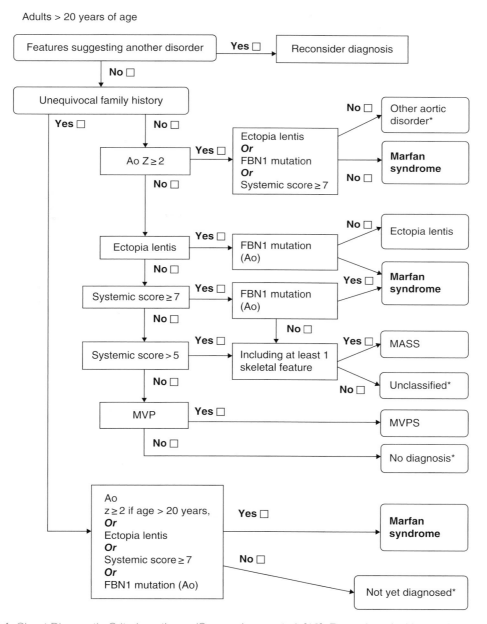

Figure 22.1 Ghent Diagnostic Criteria pathway (*Source*: Loeys et al. [10]. Reproduced with permission of BMJ)

Gene (protein)	Phenotypic characteristics	Pathway
Extracellular matrix protein		
FBN1 (fibrillin-1)	Marfan syndrome; highly penetrant ascending aortic aneurysm; ectopia lentis; scoliosis; dolichostenomelia (marfanoid habitus)	TGF-β
COL 3 A1(collagen α-1(III))	EDS type 4; arterial dissection with infrequent aneurysm; thin skin; large eyes; beaked nose; thin lips, lobeless ears; acrogeria (aged appearance in extremities)	Collagen Metabolism
Transmembrane protein		
TFGBR1 (TGF-β receptor type I)	LDS; TAAD with other arterial involvement (cerebral, carotid, abdominal); marfanoid but no ocular disease; early age of onset (30s); bifid uvula; hypertelorism; craniosynostosis; congenital heart defects; mental retardation	TGF-β
TGFBR2 (TGF-β receptor type 2)	LDS; TAAD with marfanoid appearance; cerebral artery involvement; onset in 40s; dissection at low aortic root diameter; operation by 4.5 cm	TGF-β
Cytoplasmic protein		
SMAD3 (SMAD family member 3)	LDS; TAAD with osteoarthritis (AOS); risk of involvement of cerebral arteries; entire aorta extending into iliac arteries	TFG-β
ACTA2 (α-smooth-muscle actin)	Association with PDA, BAV, early CAD and stroke; livedo reticularis; iris floccule; smooth-muscle cell dysfunction leading to gut immobility; pulmonary hypertension	IGF-1, Ang II
MYH11 (smooth-muscle myosin)	Association with PDA	IGF-1, Ang II

Table 22.1 Genotype–phenotype correlation of selected genetic mutations involved in familial thoracic aortic aneurysm and dissection (FTAAD)

TGF-β, transforming growth factor beta; EDS, Ehlers–Danlos syndrome; LDS, Loeys–Dietz syndrome; TAAD, thoracic aortic aneurysm and dissection; PDA, patent ductus arteriosus; BAV, bicuspid aortic valve; CAD, coronary artery disease; IGF-1, insulin-like growth factor 1.

(TAAD) [13]. Mutations can be found in the fibrillin-1 gene in 97% of Marfan syndrome patients, which assists with screening of family members and pregnancies (Table 22.1).

In competitive athletes with aortic dilatation, if no genetic cause can be found and aortic measurements are just outside the normal upper limits of 4.0 cm in the sinus of Valsalva (no greater than 4.2 cm) and are non-progressive based on serial echocardiogram measurements in the same centre, the athlete may be allowed to continue sporting activity, subject to ongoing annual echocardiographic surveillance.

Cardiac Problems

The most serious problems occur in the heart and blood vessels. The aorta is usually wider than expected for a given body surface area and is more fragile due to deficiency in the amount of fibrillin-1 present. The dilatation tends to be progressive, leading to aortic dissection with or without aortic regurgitation. Surgical repair is recommended when the aortic root becomes widened to 4.8 cm, or earlier in cases with a family history of early dissection. Beta-blocker therapy and strict blood-pressure control can delay dilatation.

Mitral valve prolapse (MVP) is also often present on echocardiogram. Antibiotic prophylaxis is recommended for dental procedures involving bleeding, if a heart valve is leaking sufficiently to produce an audible heart murmur or if a heart valve has been replaced.

Impact on Physical Activity

For people with Marfan syndrome, certain activities are thought to increase the risk of serious complications [3, 14, 15]. In addition, some of the physical manifestations of Marfan syndrome may limit a person's ability to fully participate in exercise [16]. For example, those with eye problems may have difficulty playing sports involving hand–eye coordination, such as racquet sports. People with Marfan syndrome are affected in different ways, so what is suitable for one person may not be for another.

Guidelines

In general, most people living with Marfan syndrome should exercise regularly through low-intensity, low-impact activities adapted to meet their specific needs. They should avoid contact sports, because of the risk of damaging the aorta or loose ligaments and joints and of injuring the eyes. Strenuous activities, such as competitive sports and weightlifting, should also be avoided, because of the stress placed on the aorta.

The Marfan Association (UK) (www.marfan-association.org.uk) and the Marfan Foundation (US) (www.marfan.org) provide guidelines on what exercise is suitable for people with Marfan syndrome (Table 22.2) and what is best avoided (Table 22.3) [17]. There is currently very limited evidence on how exercise affects people with Marfan syndrome [18], so recommendations are based on consensus guidelines issued by the Marfan Association and Marfan Foundation.

As a point of emphasis in formulating physical activity recommendations, it is important to remember that each patient is affected differently and that general recommendations need to be discussed with the patient's medical attendants and parents. Children should be allowed to stop any activity when tired.

Other considerations regarding physical activity to prevent damage to the heart (H), joints (J), or eyes (E):

- Heavy lifting is not advised (H).
- Basketball should be carefully discussed, because if played as a contact or competitive sport, it can lead to repeated falls or excessive stress to the aortic wall (H).

Archery	Cycling (on the level)	Field hockey
Shotput	Badminton	Discus
Javelin	Skating	Bowls
Fencing	Netball	Swimming
Canoeing	Football (no heading, not in goal position)	Racketball
Table tennis	Cricket	Golf
Sailing	Tennis	Yoga
Walking/jog-walking	Dancing	Light weightlifting

Table 22.2 Recommended exercises for people with Marfan syndrome (not high-level competition, minimal contact)

Boxing	E
Rugby	H, J
Deep-sea diving	L
Rowing	H, J
Distance running	H, J
Skydiving	L
Hang gliding	L
High-altitude mountaineering	L
Trampolining	J
High-diving	E
Weightlifting	H, J
Karate/judo	H, J
Wrestling	H, J
Squash	E, H

Table 22.3 Contraindicated exercises for people with Marfan syndrome (to prevent damage to: E, eyes; H, heart; J, joints; L, lungs)

243

- Horse riding on a quiet horse is best. Jumping may cause falls (H, J).
- For those who do not have heart problems, squash can be played wearing goggles, to protect the eyes (E, H).
- Participation in aerobics (H, J) or abseiling (J) should be governed by the patient's limitations.
- Prolonged exertion at peak capacity should be avoided. In the gym, short stints of low or moderate intensity across a number of activities are recommended.

Children can engage in light activities such as swimming in the school pool whilst their class is performing more stressful physical education (PE) activities. If this is not possible, then the child should be given another task, such as refereeing (and the necessary instruction to complete it properly); this gives them a position of importance without involving them in the physical activity. Some children are given an individual fitness routine to work through in the corner of the gym.

Medication Impact on Physical Activity

Many people with Marfan syndrome take a beta-blocker medication to reduce stress on the aorta. This medication lowers the pulse at rest and during exercise and makes it somewhat more difficult to achieve a given level of physical fitness for the amount of physical work performed. It does not, however, enable a person with Marfan syndrome or another aortic aneurysm syndrome to perform very strenuous exercises or play contact sports. Some patients with Marfan syndrome take other blood-pressure medications, such as an angiotensin receptor blocker (ARB) or an angiotensin-converting enzyme (ACE) inhibitor. These do not protect the aorta against strenuous exercise.

People who have artificial heart valves usually take an anticoagulant medication, which interferes with blood clotting and increases the chances of bruising and internal haemorrhages. Anyone taking this medication should avoid contact sports and any activity with a moderate risk of a blow to the head or abdomen.

Final advice should come from the patient's own doctor.

Problems Encountered by Patients

In a survey of the exercise habits of 70 UK patients with Marfan syndrome aged between 18 and 65, the following results emerged:

- 72% said that their exercise habits had been affected by having Marfan syndrome. Reasons (most common first) included joint pain, shortness of breath, medical advice, fatigue, palpitations, dislike of exercise and overheating.
- By far the most popular exercise activity was walking, followed by gym, swimming, jogging, cycling and yoga/pilates. Only a handful of people participated in activities that are considered unsuitable (long-distance running, heavy weightlifting).
- Only 44% had received information about exercise. The most common sources (most common first) were hospital consultation, the Marfan Association, family physician, the Internet and occupational therapists/ physiotherapists.
- The advice given seems to have corresponded with the published guidelines.
- 17% said that they had received conflicting advice.
- Of the 25 people who had cardiac surgery, only 13 had been offered subsequent rehabilitation. Of these, nine took up the offer. In only four cases was the person in charge of the programme definitely aware of Marfan syndrome.
- A number of those engaging in rehabilitation programmes found that they were not tailored to their needs, but to the needs of an older population with different conditions (e.g. coronary artery disease, CAD).
- Many patients commented that although they had been given general exercise advice, they were still unclear about what it actually meant in practice. In addition, they often found that doctors, other health care professionals and employees of gyms/fitness centres were not able to give accurate and appropriate advice.
- Worryingly, two people had been turned away from gyms once they disclosed that they had Marfan syndrome. A letter from the doctor to the gym instructor indicating suitable sports is therefore recommended.
- Some found the exercise advice frustrating and demoralising; for those who were keen to improve their fitness, positive suggestions on how to achieve this were limited – much of the advice focussed on what not to do.

- A number of people commented on their negative experiences of sport at school and their distress at being told that they could no longer do their favourite sport or compete. Tapering unsuitable sports, such as long-distance running, and gradually replacing them with more suitable sports, such as jog-walking, is recommended.

Who Should be Aware?

Hospital doctors, family physicians, physiotherapists, physical education teachers, sports coaches and those working in the fitness industry should be aware of the nature of Marfan syndrome and how it relates to exercise ability. A letter from the hospital doctor to a PE teacher or other programme supervisor is helpful.

What Advice is Needed?

- A system should be in place to ensure that all people with Marfan syndrome receive information about exercise as soon as possible after diagnosis.
- Patients should be encouraged to exercise as much as possible within their capabilities. They should be recommended limits in order to improve and maintain their general health.
- When giving advice to patients, the advice should be tailored to the needs of the individual, taking into account how they are affected by Marfan syndrome, their age and their general health.
- Patients need more than a couple of activity suggestions (e.g. walking and swimming). They need to know what level they should exercise at, how long and how often to exercise and how they can maximise their fitness. Where possible, the patient's own sporting and exercise preferences should be accommodated.
- For those who are involved in exercise considered a risk to their health, the advice should be to taper down the activity over a period of time, rather than stop it suddenly. This is more acceptable to the patient and gives time to develop an interest in an alternative sport.
- As a general rule, the patient should be able to converse whilst exercising.

After Surgery

Following heart surgery, the patient should be offered a cardiac rehabilitation programme suitable to their needs and age.

Other Aortopathies

The younger a patient at the time of discovery of an ascending aortic aneurysm or actual dissection, the more likely it is that there is an underlying genetic predisposition. A positive family history for TAAD signals an increased risk. Each offspring of an affected parent has up to 50% risk of also developing an aortic aneurysm, at approximately the same age. There are many predisposing dominantly inherited genes reported [13], and the list is growing annually. Some have associated phenotypic features; many do not (Table 22.1).

An athlete with an ascending aortic dimension ≥4.0 cm, no matter how tall, should be referred to a cardiovascular genetic screening clinic, where a family history can be taken, snapshots of affected family members can be reviewed (for phenotypic features such as height, body build, facial features and joint hypermobility), a careful past medical history can be taken and a physical examination performed. If increased risk is confirmed, a 5 ml ethylenediamine tetraacetic acid (EDTA) blood sample should be taken for TAAD gene screening or exome sequencing to study reported causative genes and search for unidentified genes. The athlete should have three consecutive annual echocardiograms to assess progression. If progression is shown, they should be placed on medication, such as a beta blocker or ARB, and referred for elective aortic root surgery between aortic root diameters 4.5 and 4.8 cm, depending on the gene and the family history. Affected athletes should not be allowed to compete at high level and should be advised to limit sporting activities to moderate exercise in order to keep fit.

First-degree relatives (siblings, parents and offspring) should be screened by echocardiogram. An affected patient should be counselled that there may be up to a 50% risk of genetic predisposition to aortic aneurysm for each offspring, regardless of sex.

Conclusion

Each patient with Marfan syndrome or another genetic aortopathy is unique. The symptoms and signs are determined by how the genotype (gene mutation) affects the phenotype (body build). Frank dialogue between physician, patient, family and sports coach will determine what level of suitable sporting activity will maintain fitness without jeopardising future health. Competitive sport at high levels involving prolonged exertion at peak capacity or collision sports should be discouraged unless the individual is mildly affected and is kept under careful, regular echocardiographic surveillance.

References

1 Dietz, H.C. In: Pagon R.A., Adam M.P., Ardinger H.H. et al. (eds) *GeneReviews®. Marfan Syndrome.* Seattle, WA: University of Washington, Seattle, 1993–2014.

2 Arslan-Kirchner, M., Arbustini, E., Boileau, C. et al. Clinical utility gene card for: Marfan syndrome type 1 and related phenotypes [FBN1]. *Eur J Hum Genet.* 2010; **18**(9).

3 Abid, N., Davies, K., Grahame, R. et al. Joint hypermobility syndrome in childhood. A not so benign multisystem disorder? *Rheumatology (Oxford)* 2005; **44**(6): 744–50.

4 Jones, K.B., Sponsellor, P.D., Erkula, G. et al. Symposium on the musculoskeletal aspects of Marfan syndrome: meeting report and state of the science. *J Orthop Res* 2007; **25**(3): 413–22.

5 Wood, J., Bellamy, D., Child, A. and Citron, K.M. Pulmonary disease in patients with Marfan syndrome. *Thorax* 1984; **39**: 780–4.

6 Giske, L., Stanghelle, J.K., Rand-Hendrikssen, S. et al. Pulmonary function, working capacity and strength in young adults with Marfan syndrome. *J Rehabil Med* 2003; **35**(5): 221–8.

7 Loewenstein, A., Barquet, I.S., De Juan, E. Jr and Maumenee, I.H. Retinal detachment in Marfan syndrome. *Retina* 2000; **20**(4): 358–63.

8 Traboulsi, E., Whittum-Hudson, J.A., Mir, S.H. and Maumenee, I.H. Microfibril abnormalities of the lens capsule in patients with Marfan syndrome and ectopia lentis. *Ophthalmic Genet* 2000; **21**(1): 9–15.

9 Crosher, R. and Holmes, A. Marfan syndrome: dental problems and management. *Dent Update* 1988; **15**(3): 120–2.

10 Loeys, B.L., Dietz, H.C., Braverman, A.C. et al. The revised Ghent nosology for the Marfan syndrome. *J Med Genet* 2010; **47**(7): 476–85.

11 Dean, J.C. Marfan syndrome: clinical diagnosis and management. *Eur J Hum Genet* 2007; **15**(7): 724–33.

12 Stout, M. The Marfan syndrome: implications for athletes and their echocardiographic assessment. *Echocardiogr* 2009; **26**(9): 1075–81.

13 Milewicz, D.M. Thoracic aortic aneurysms and aortic dissections. In: Regalado, E., Pagon, R.A., Adam, M.P. et al. (eds) *GeneReviews®.* Seattle, WA: University of Washington, Seattle, 1993–2014.

14 Maron, B.J., Chaitman, B.R., Ackerman, M.J. et al. Recommendations for physical activity and recreational sports participation for young patients with genetic cardiovascular diseases. *Circulation* 2004; **109**(22): 2807–16.

15 Yim, E.S. Aortic root disease in athletes: aortic root dilation, anomalous coronary artery, bicuspid aortic valve, and Marfan's syndrome. *Sports Med* 2013; **43**(8): 721–32.

16 Crilley, J.G., Bendahan, D., Boehm, E.A. et al. Investigation of muscle bioenergetics in the Marfan syndrome indicates reduced metabolic efficiency. *J Cardiovasc Magn Reson* 2007; **9**(4): 709–17.

17 Boodhwani, M., Andelfinger, G., Leipsic, J. et al. Canadian Cardiovascular Society position statement on the management of thoracic aortic disease. Canadian Cardiovascular Society. *Can J Cardiol* 2014; **30**(6): 577–89.

18 Peres, P., Bernardelli, G.F., Mendes, C.C. et al. Immediate effects of submaximal effort on pulse wave velocity in patients with Marfan syndrome. *Braz J Med Biol Res* 2010; **43**(4): 397–402.

23 Valvular Disease

Kathleen E. Kearney and Catherine M. Otto

Division of Cardiology, University of Washington School of Medicine, Seattle, WA, USA

Basic Principles

Prevalence and Causes

Valvular heart disease is common in older adults but also may present in young and middle-aged adults who are interested in participating in athletic activities and competitive sports [1–3]. A congenital bicuspid aortic valve (BAV) occurs predominantly in men (70–80% of cases) and is estimated to affect about 1% of the entire population [4]. Nearly all BAV patients will need aortic valve replacement, either for severe regurgitation as young adults or for calcific valvular stenosis at an older age [1,2]. BAV disease is also associated with an aortopathy and increased risk of aortic dissection. Calcific stenosis of a congenitally bicuspid or anatomically normal trileaflet valve is usually diagnosed in older adults, with mild valve changes affecting about 25% and severe stenosis seen in up to 2% of those aged 65 years and older in the US and Europe [5].

Mitral valve prolapse (MVP), likely an inherited disorder resulting in primary changes of the valve leaflets, is the most common cause of primary mitral regurgitation (MR), with an estimated prevalence of 2.4%. MVP often presents in young adults, with a male predominance, and is associated with an increased risk of cardiac arrhythmias [1,2]. Arrhythmias predominantly occur in patients with significant MR, including atrial premature beats, paroxysmal supraventricular tachycardia (SVT), ventricular premature beats and complex ventricular ectopy. The relationship between MVP and sudden cardiac death (SCD) remains unclear.

Worldwide, rheumatic heart disease remains the most common cause of valvular disease, with an estimated prevalence of over 15 million patients, mostly in underdeveloped countries, where streptococcal pharyngitis is common and antibiotic therapy is not always available [6]. Rheumatic valvular disease typically presents years after an episode of acute rheumatic fever, with a shorter interval between rheumatic fever and symptomatic valvular disease in patients with recurrent episodes. Mitral stenosis (MS) is the most common sequela of rheumatic disease, but isolated MR may be seen in younger patients. Concurrent aortic valve involvement is present in 20–30% of patients.

Pathophysiology

The pathophysiology of valve dysfunction varies according to whether the predominant abnormality is valve narrowing (e.g. stenosis), backflow across the valve (e.g. regurgitation) or combined stenosis and regurgitation. The specific valve affected also determines the pathophysiology and clinical features of each valve lesion (Table 23.1).

In patients with stenotic valves, the reduction in leaflet motion due to leaflet thickening, fusion or calcification results in a smaller blood flow orifice and an increased blood flow velocity, with the magnitude of the increase

IOC Manual of Sports Cardiology, First Edition. Edited by Mathew G. Wilson, Jonathan A. Drezner and Sanjay Sharma.
© 2017 International Olympic Committee. Published 2017 by John Wiley & Sons, Ltd.

Valve lesion	Clinical presentation	Anatomy	Haemodynamics	Consequences	Interventions
Aortic stenosis (AS)	• Dyspnoea • Chest pain • Decreased exercise tolerance • Syncope • Systolic murmur • Delayed and diminished carotid upstroke	• Calcified, thickened leaflets with decreased mobility, causing a small orifice • Congenital BAV in 60%	• Increased transaortic velocity and pressure gradient • Decreased valve area	• Increased left ventricular workload to maintain cardiac output • Concentric left ventricular hypertrophy	• Cardiovascular risk factor reduction • Surgical AVR for severe symptomatic AS • TAVR, if not a surgical candidate
Aortic regurgitation (AR)	• Decreased exercise tolerance • Diastolic murmur • Wide pulse pressure	• Aortic sinus root enlargement • Congenital BAV	• Increased transaortic volume flow • Left ventricular pressure and volume overload	• Left ventricular enlargement • Eventual decline in left ventricular EF	• AVR for symptoms or for progressive left ventricular dilation or fall in left ventricular EF
Mitral stenosis (MS)	• Dyspnoea • Decreased exercise tolerance • AF • Diastolic murmur	• Commissural fusion and chordal thickening	• Reduced mitral orifice area • Increased left atrial pressure • Small, underfilled left ventricle	• AF • Pulmonary hypertension	• BMV for severe MS • Anticoagulation, if AF • Surgical MVR for severe symptomatic MS, if BMV is not feasible
Mitral regurgitation (MR)	• Dyspnoea • Left heart failure • Systolic murmur • Midsystolic click with MVP	• MVP (primary MR) • Left ventricular dilation and dysfunction (secondary MR)	• Increased total left ventricular stroke volume due to backflow across the mitral valve	• Left ventricular dilation and systolic dysfunction • Elevated left atrial pressure • Pulmonary hypertension • AF	• Valve repair or MVR in primary MR • Heart failure or coronary disease therapies in secondary MR
Tricuspid regurgitation (TR)	• Right heart failure • Prominent V-wave jugular pulsation	• Congenital leaflet abnormality • Secondary to left heart disease or pulmonary hypertension and right ventricular failure	• Right ventricular volume overload and dilation	• Right heart failure, in severe cases	• Tricuspid annuloplasty

Table 23.1 Valvular disease characteristics

AF, atrial fibrillation; BAV, bicuspid aortic valve; AVR, aortic valve replacement; TAVR, transcatheter aortic valve replacement; EF, ejection fraction; BMV, balloon mitral valvotomy; MVR, mitral valve replacement; MVP, mitral valve prolapse.

in velocity proportional to the severity of the reduction in valve area. The transvalvular pressure gradient (ΔP) can be calculated from velocity (v) using the Bernoulli equation, as:

$$\Delta P = 4v^2 \qquad \text{(Equation 23.1)}$$

Maximum velocity is used to calculate the maximum transvalvular gradient and instantaneous pressure gradients are integrated over the flow period to calculate mean pressure gradients. Valve area can be calculated by measuring the volume flow rate proximal to and in the narrowed orifice, in an approach known as the 'continuity equation', or by the time course of the velocity curve across the valve, known as the 'pressure half-time method'. With stenosis of the semilunar valves (aortic and pulmonic), transvalvular velocities and

Valvular disease	Mild to moderate	Severe
Aortic stenosis (AS)	Bicuspid valve or calcified valve leaflets Aortic V_{max} 2.0–2.9 m.s^{-1}	Severely calcified or thickened leaflets Severely reduced systolic opening of valve Aortic V_{max} ≥4 m.s^{-1} or ΔP ≥40 mmHg, typically aortic valve area ≤1.0 cm^2 Low-flow low-gradient AS may be present in older adults
Aortic regurgitation (AR)	Colour Doppler vena contracta <0.3 cm; Rvol <30 ml.beat^{-1} RF <30% ERO <0.10 cm^2	Abnormal aortic valve anatomy or dilated aorta Colour Doppler vena contracta >0.6 cm RVol >60 ml.beat^{-1} RF ≥50% ERO ≥0.3 cm^2
Mitral stenosis (MS)	Rheumatic or congenital valve changes MVA >1.5 cm^2	Severe restricted diastolic leaflet opening Very severe: MVA ≤1.0 cm^2 Severe: MVA ≤1.5 cm^2
Mitral regurgitation (MR) (primary)	Mitral prolapse or abnormal valve leaflets Vena contracta <0.7 cm Regurgitant volume <60 ml RF <50% ERO <0.4 cm^2	Mitral prolapse or abnormal valve leaflets Vena contracta ≥0.7 cm Regurgitant volume ≥60 ml RF ≥50% ERO ≥0.4 cm^2

Table 23.2 Haemodynamic severity of valvular heart disease

Moderate disease is classified as mixed features between mild and severe disease.

V_{max}, maximum transvalvular velocity; RF, regurgitant fraction; ERO, effective regurgitant orifice; RVol, regurgitant volume; MVA, mitral valve area.

pressure gradients are markedly elevated, because ventricular pressures are relatively high and blood is actively ejected into the great vessels. In contrast, stenosis of the atrioventricular (AV) valves (mitral and tricuspid) results in much lower velocities and pressure gradients, reflecting the low-pressure difference and passive flow between the atrial and ventricular chambers in diastole (Table 23.2).

Valve regurgitation, or backflow of blood across the closed valve, may be caused by either restriction of leaflet motion, limiting adequate coaptation of the valve leaflets, or excessive leaflet motion, for example with mitral prolapse, resulting in lack of apposition of the leaflets. In either case, the total amount of blood pumped by the ventricular chamber increases to compensate for the volume of back flow across the incompetent valve [7]. Regurgitant severity is measured as the volume of back flow (regurgitant volume in ml), the percentage of the total stroke volume ejected backwards (regurgitant fraction as a percentage) or the size of the regurgitant orifice area.

Secondary cardiac changes in patients with valvular heart disease include left ventricular hypertrophy (LVH) due to pressure overload from aortic stenosis (AS), left ventricular enlargement due to volume overload from aortic regurgitation (AR) or MR and left atrial enlargement and pulmonary hypertension with MS. These chronic changes in myocardial function and intracardiac pressures also predispose patients to cardiac arrhythmias, particularly atrial fibrillation, and are associated with an increased risk of atrial thrombi and cardioembolic events.

Diagnostic Approach to Valvular Heart Disease

Echocardiography is the primary diagnostic modality for all patients with known or suspected valvular disease (Figure 23.1). Although many patients are initially detected based on the finding of a murmur, physical examination is not reliable for identification of the type or severity of valve dysfunction, and it can be challenging to distinguish a benign flow murmur from abnormal valve function. An electrocardiogram (ECG) may show changes associated with chamber enlargement, including criteria for LVH, left atrial enlargement or atrial arrhythmias. However, ECG findings are not adequate for diagnosis or risk stratification, and a normal ECG does not exclude the possibility of valvular disease. Similarly, chest radiography is not helpful for diagnosis or risk stratification.

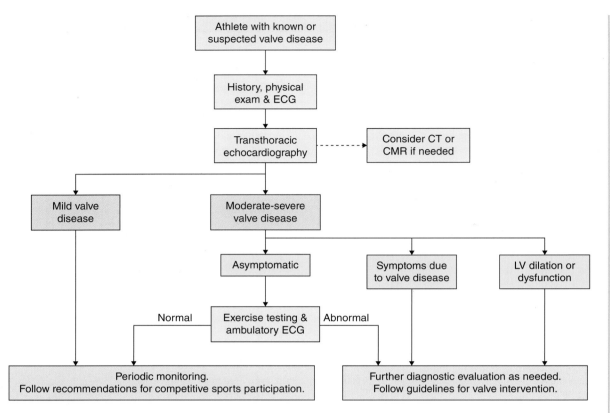

Figure 23.1 Practical clinical approach. A suggested framework for evaluation of the athlete with known or suspected valvular disease. The key diagnostic elements are transthoracic echocardiography (TTE), exercise testing and ambulatory ECG monitoring. Guideline timings for valve intervention are given in Table 23.1 and recommendations for periodic monitoring and sports participation are given in Table 23.3. ECG, electrocardiogram; CT, computed tomography; CMR, cardiac magnetic resonance; LV, left ventricle

Transthoracic echocardiography (TTE) is recommended for a systolic murmur grade 3 of 6 or louder, any diastolic murmur or a murmur associated with symptoms or other physical examination findings [1–3]. In asymptomatic patients with a soft, midsystolic, ejection-type murmur with no other findings on physical examination, TTE is not mandatory, but, given the absence of adverse effects of diagnostic ultrasound, may be prudent if there is any doubt about the diagnosis of valvular disease. The goals of TTE are to determine valve morphology and quantify function, assess left ventricular size and function, measure aortic size, estimate pulmonary systolic pressure and evaluate right heart function (see Chapter 14). If valvular disease is present, periodic monitoring is recommended, with the interval determined by the severity of valve dysfunction, any evidence of disease progression and family history (Table 23.2). Along with clinical symptoms, TTE findings are the key elements in optimising the timing of intervention in patients with valvular heart disease.

When TTE data are inadequate or there is a discrepancy between clinical and echocardiographic findings, transoesophageal echocardiography (TOE) provides improved image quality and better quantitation of disease severity. Cardiac magnetic resonance (CMR) allows quantitation of regurgitant severity and more accurate measurement of left ventricular volumes and ejection fraction (EF). Additional imaging with chest computed tomography (CT) or CMR is recommended if the ascending aorta cannot be adequately visualised by echocardiography. CT imaging may also be useful for evaluation of prosthetic valve dysfunction.

Exercise testing is not routinely indicated in adults with asymptomatic valvular disease but may be helpful when symptom status is unclear, when it can objectively measure exercise capacity and the blood-pressure and heart-rate response to exercise, and can detect exercise-induced symptoms or arrhythmias [8]. Exercise testing is also appropriate before participation in sports when more than mild valve dysfunction is present, to ensure the patient tolerates the level of exertion expected from the specific type of activity.

Valve lesion	Periodic monitoring	Allowed participation in competitive sports[b]
Aortic stenosis (AS)	• Annual clinical exam • Echocardiography every 3–5 years (mild AS), 1–2 years (moderate AS) or 6–12 months (severe AS) • Exercise testing and Holter monitor prior to participation in competitive sports (moderate or severe AS)	• Mild AS: all competitive sports • Moderate AS and normal exercise test: low to moderate static and dynamic sports only • Severe asymptomatic AS: no competitive sports
Aortic regurgitation (AR)	• Annual clinical exam • Echocardiography every 3–5 years (mild AR), 1–2 years (moderate AR) or 6–12 months (severe AR) • Exercise testing and Holter monitor prior to participation in competitive sports	• Mild to moderate AR and normal or mildly dilated left ventricle: all competitive sports • AR with moderate left ventricular enlargement (EDD 60–65 mm) and normal exercise test: low to moderate static and all dynamic sports • AR with asymptomatic NSVT: only low-intensity sports • AR and dilated aorta (diameter >45 mm): only low-intensity sports • Severe AR and left ventricular enlargement (EDD >65 mm): no competitive sports
Mitral stenosis (MS)	• Annual clinical exam • Echocardiography every 3–5 years (mild MS), 1–2 years (moderate MS) or annually (severe MS) • Close monitoring during times of haemodynamic stress	• Mild MS in NSR with exercise PASP <50 mm: all sports • Moderate MS and exercise PASP <50 mmHg: low to moderate static and dynamic competitive sports • Severe MS or exercise PASP >50 mmHg: no competitive sports • MS of any severity with atrial fibrillation on anticoagulation: no sports with risk of bodily contact
Mitral regurgitation (MR)	• Annual clinical exam • Echocardiography every 3–5 years (mild MR), 1–2 years (moderate MR) or 6–12 months (severe MR) • Exercise testing and Holter monitor prior to participation in competitive sports	• Mild to moderate MR in NSR with normal left ventricle size, function and PASP: all competitive sports • Mild to moderate MR in NSR with mild left ventricular enlargement <60 mm at end diastole: low to moderate static and all dynamic competitive sports • Severe MR and left ventricular enlargement or elevated PASP: no competitive sports • MR of any degree with atrial fibrillation on anticoagulation: no sports with risk of bodily contact • MVP with unexplained syncope; SVT, ventricular tachycardia or prolonged QT interval; severe MR or family history of sudden death: no competitive sports

Table 23.3 Periodic monitoring[a] and exercise recommendations for patients with valvular heart disease

[a] A baseline complete transthoracic echocardiogram is recommended in all patients with valvular heart disease.

[b] Based on European Society of Cardiology (ESC) and American College of Cardiology (ACC)/American Heart Association (AHA) 2005 Bethesda Conference recommendations [9–11].

EDD, end-diastolic dimension; NSVT, nonsustained ventricular tachycardia; PASP, pulmonary artery systolic pressure; NSR, normal sinus rhythm; MVP, mitral valve prolapse; SVT, supraventricular tachycardia.

In addition, ambulatory ECG monitoring to detect asymptomatic arrhythmias during typical athletic activities is recommended before participation in competitive sports.

Haemodynamic Changes with Exercise

Most patients with valvular heart disease remain asymptomatic, with no exercise limitations, until very late in the disease course. To some extent, this is due to the normal physiologic changes of exercise, particularly in patients with valvular regurgitation. Systemic vascular resistance decreases with exercise and diastole shortens as heart rate rises. With AR, these changes may reduce the amount of regurgitation on each cardiac

Valve lesion	Heart rate	Stroke volume	Pulmonary artery pressure	Valve area	Valve gradient	Regurgitation	Cardiac output
Aortic stenosis (AS)	↑	→ or ↓	↑	↑	↑		↑ or →
Aortic regurgitation (AR)	↑	↑↑	→	→		→	↑↑
Mitral stenosis (MS)	↑	↓	↑↑	→	↑		↑
Mitral regurgitation (MR)	↑	↓ (antegrade)	↑↑	→		↑ (ischaemic or MVP) → if secondary	↓ (effective)

Table 23.4 Effect of exercise in asymptomatic patients with moderate to severe valvular disease compared to the normal physiologic state

Compensatory changes may occur to preserve cardiac output, with decline in this reserve with severe disease progression. Once cardiac output during exercise falls, the patient develops decreased exercise tolerance or dyspnoea.

↑, increased; →, no significant change from normal state; ↓, decreased. Double arrows indicate a higher magnitude of change. MVP, mitral valve prolapse.

cycle, although the total regurgitation per minute is unchanged, due to the increase in heart rate. MR may also improve with systemic afterload reduction during exercise.

With severe valvular disease, symptom onset is often insidious, with the initial symptoms only occurring during exertion or with a gradual decline in exercise capacity that is not always fully appreciated by the patient. Symptom onset with severe valvular disease results from a reduced ability to increase cardiac output with exercise, resulting in limited exercise capacity and an imbalance in myocardial oxygen demand and supply, with the potential for ischaemia and arrhythmias (Table 23.4). The maximal age-appropriate increase in heart rate with exercise is usually not affected by valvular disease, assuming the individual is not on pharmacotherapy that limits heart-rate response and in the absence of underlying conduction disease. However, stroke volume may not increase appropriately, due to a narrowed valve orifice or to a stiff ventricular chamber, resulting in decreased exercise capacity. MS limits left ventricular stroke volume due to decreased diastolic filling of the left ventricle, whilst severe AS results in a fixed stroke volume when the left ventricle can no longer overcome the valve obstruction. This obstruction creates a state of pressure overload and increased wall stress on the left ventricle. With a fixed stroke volume, cardiac output is reliant on a rapid rise in heart rate, which may be experienced as early dyspnoea by the patient. Any drop in systemic vascular resistance, such as occurs with high vagal tone following intense exercise, is poorly tolerated in these patients. In addition, left ventricular end-diastolic and left atrial pressure may increase excessively with exercise, leading to pulmonary congestion and exertional dyspnoea.

In some types of valvular disease, there is concern that exercise may directly worsen disease severity. High-intensity isometric exercise may be less well tolerated, as the sudden rise in systemic vascular resistance may transiently increase regurgitant severity, and has been associated in case reports and anecdotal clinical experience with acute severe regurgitation due to mitral chordal rupture or an aortic leaflet fenestration.

Medical Therapy

Currently, there are no known medical therapies that directly prevent progression of valvular heart disease. Guideline recommendations for secondary prevention of rheumatic fever should be followed in patients with rheumatic valvular disease. In all patients, standard cardiovascular risk factors are associated with an increased prevalence of calcific valve changes and it is desirable to prevent superimposed coronary disease. Thus, evaluation and treatment of cardiovascular risk factors is mandatory in patients with valvular heart disease. Patients should be encouraged to eat a healthy diet, maintain a normal body weight and avoid smoking. Hypercholesterolemia, hypertension and diabetes should be treated based on standard guideline recommendations.

Valve-disease patients, particularly those with a BAV or MVP, are at higher risk of endocarditis than the general population. Optimal dental hygiene is important in preventing endocarditis, although antibiotic prophylaxis is no longer recommended.

Atrial fibrillation (AF) frequently occurs as a consequence of valvular disease, particularly with involvement of the mitral valve. Patients with valvular disease and AF are at higher risk of thromboembolic complications than patients without valvular disease, and standard risk scores, such as CHADS$_2$, are not applicable. When indicated, a vitamin K antagonist (e.g. warfarin) is recommended for anticoagulation, as the efficacy of the newer oral anticoagulants has not been studied in patients with valvular heart disease. Athletes requiring anticoagulation should not participate in contact or collision sports.

Asymptomatic patients with mild to moderate valvular disease should be encouraged to be physically active and to maintain fitness, although many experts suggest that high-intensity isometric exercise be avoided due to concerns that a sudden increase in afterload might excessively stress the abnormal tissue of the aortic wall, aortic valve leaflets or mitral chords. In patients with significant valvular disease, recommendations about exercise and participation in competitive sports are based on an assessment of disease severity, exercise capacity, ambulatory ECG monitoring and other parameters, depending on the specific valve lesion (see Table 23.3).

Aortic Valvular Disease

Bicuspid Aortic Valve Disease

A congenital BAV is an important cause of valvular disease in the athlete and is twice as common in men as in women [4]. About 10% of BAV patients have an associated aortic coarctation; conversely, a BAV is present in about 50% of patients with coarctation of the aorta. Echocardiography in BAV patients should include evaluation of the flow pattern in the descending thoracic aorta, which has a high sensitivity for diagnosis of coarctation, particularly if the patient is hypertensive. BAV disease appears to be an inherited disorder with variable penetrance, although a specific gene mutation has not been identified and only about one-third of families have more than one affected individual.

Pathophysiology BAV anatomy results from congenital fusion of two cusps of the normally trileaflet aortic valve, resulting in two asymmetric cusps (Figure 23.2), with fusion of the right and left coronary cusps in 70–80% of cases. In some patients, excess leaflet tissue results in AR, but most patients have relatively normal valve function until late in life, when superimposed calcific changes result in reduced leaflet opening and eventual severe stenosis. Some patients classified as having BAV disease actually have a unicuspid valve with a single commissure, resulting in a more distorted morphology, with one free edge of the leaflet failing to communicate with the aortic annulus. These patients may present with severe stenosis at a younger age.

Clinical Presentation The adolescent or young-adult athlete with a BAV is most likely to present with an asymptomatic diastolic murmur or the finding of a BAV on echocardiography requested for other reasons. Some patients present with symptomatic AR, an aortic dissection or bacterial endocarditis. A few present with symptomatic severe AS, most likely with a congenital unicuspid valve. However, most young patients do not have significant AS or AR and remain asymptomatic until developing AS, typically after age 50 years.

Outcomes and Management Most young athletes have a normally functioning BAV that is unlikely to need intervention for many years. Current guidelines recommend periodic monitoring of aortic size, valve and ventricular function, along with education about symptoms of aortic valvular disease and aortic dissection.

In asymptomatic patients with normal BAV function, survival rates are no different than in the general population. Long term, approximately 25% require surgery over a 20-year period, either for AR in young adulthood or, most often, for AS later in life, and nearly all will require valve surgery over their lifetime. About 50% of BAV patients have an associated aortopathy, defined as an aortic diameter greater than expected for age and body size, with tissue abnormalities resulting in larger aortic dimensions and a faster rate of progressive aortic dilation compared to the normal population (Figure 23.3). BAV patients have an estimated five to nine times higher risk of developing an aortic dissection than the general population. However, the absolute risk of aortic dissection in a BAV patient is low, estimated at 3 per 10 000 patient-years [12,13]. Imaging with CT or CMR is recommended for evaluation of the aortic sinuses and ascending aorta, if they are not adequately visualised on echocardiography. Current recommendations for timing of surgical indications for ascending aorta replacement in BAV patients are the same as for the general population, but because BAV patients are at higher risk, closer follow-up of aortic size is needed (see Chapter 20). In BAV patients under age 30 years or with an aortic diameter >4.0 cm, and in those participating in competitive sports, we generally perform annual echocardiography to evaluate aortic size, as some of these

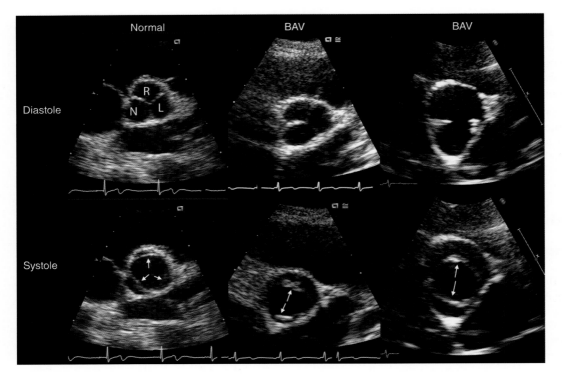

Figure 23.2 BAV anatomy. A short-axis echocardiographic view of the aortic valve in diastole (upper left) shows the right, left and noncoronary cusps of the closed trileaflet wave in diastole (top) and the open leaflets (arrows) in systole (bottom). In a patient with a bicuspid valve (centre panels), the valve may look trileaflet in diastole but systolic images show only two open leaflets, with a raphe in the anterior larger leaflet. In a different patient (right panels), the bicuspid valve and sinuses are more asymmetric, with associated aortic dilation

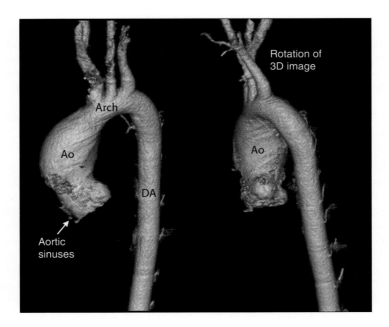

Figure 23.3 Aortopathy in BAV disease. In the same patient as in the right panels of Figure 23.2, three-dimensional (3D) CT imaging shows relatively normal aortic sinuses, with moderate to severe enlargement of the mid-ascending aorta

patients will have progressive aortic dilatation. In older patients with stable aortic dimensions, imaging is performed at intervals recommended for the predominant valve lesion (stenosis or regurgitation) [1,2].

Exercise Recommendations Exercise recommendations for BAV patients with significant AS or AR are provided in the following sections. In BAV patients with aortic involvement, there is a theoretical concern that increased aortic wall stress due to an increased stroke volume and blood pressure during high-intensity exercise may increase the risk of aortic dilation and dissection. Although firm clinical data are lacking, current guidelines suggest that BAV patients with an ascending aortic diameter >45 mm participate only in low-intensity sports [11]. In those with an aortic diameter of 40–45 mm, participation in low and moderate static and dynamic competitive sports is reasonable, but high-intensity isometric exercise such as heavy weight training and sports with higher trauma risk or high-impact collisions should be avoided. In BAV patients with an aortic sinus and ascending aortic diameter <40 mm (or equivalent size indexed to body size in younger patients), there is no limitation on competitive sports unless there is concomitant significant valve dysfunction.

Aortic Stenosis

Pathophysiology The severity of AS is defined by the increase in transaortic velocity and gradient and decrease in valve area [14]. Severe AS is present when the aortic velocity is $4\,\mathrm{m.s^{-1}}$ or higher, corresponding to a mean gradient of 40 mmHg or higher (Figure 23.4). Some patients have severe AS with a lower velocity and gradient in the setting of a low cardiac output due to left ventricular systolic dysfunction or a small hypertrophied left ventricle chamber. AS results in LVH and diastolic dysfunction, but most patients have normal systolic function until very late in the disease course. Coronary blood flow is reduced in AS, likely as a result

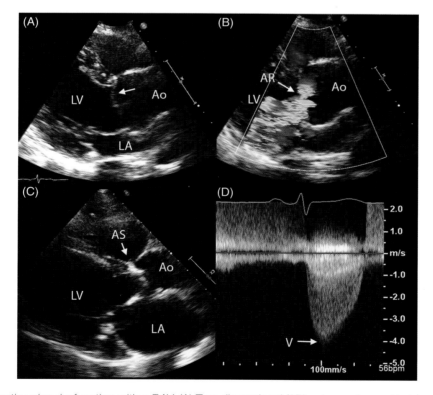

Figure 23.4 Aortic valve dysfunction with a BAV. (A) Two-dimensional (2D) echocardiographic images showing sagging (arrow) of the anterior leaflet of a bicuspid valve. (B) Colour Doppler showing severe AR (arrow). In a different patient, (C) the long-axis echocardiographic view shows a severely calcified aortic valve that opens very little on this systolic frame and (D) continuous-wave Doppler shows an aortic velocity (V) $>4\,\mathrm{m.s^{-1}}$, consistent with severe stenosis. LV, left ventricle; LA, left atrium; Ao, aorta; AR, aortic regurgitation

of a combination of thickened myocardium, decreased diastolic filling times and increased myocardial oxygen demand. About 50% of adults with AS also have significant coronary artery disease (CAD).

Clinical Presentation A systolic murmur is likely the only finding in the asymptomatic patient. Factors suggestive of AS, as opposed to a benign 'flow murmur', include a murmur grade 3 or louder, radiation to the carotids, a single second heart sound and an associated diastole murmur. The murmur of AS may diminish with Valsalva and manoeuvres that decrease venous return, and the carotid upstroke is typically delayed and diminished. Echocardiography is indicated if there is a clinical history of valvular disease or for any of these physical examination findings. Symptoms are often understated in the trained athlete, as a gradual decline in exercise tolerance and even angina can be ignored by the athlete who can still outperform peers. If symptom status is unclear, standard treadmill exercise testing is reasonable – provoked symptoms, a reduced exercise capacity and a failure of blood pressure to rise normally with exercise are all consistent with symptomatic disease. ECG changes on exercise testing are not helpful, as ST-segment depression is seen in 80% of adults with AS, even when coronary disease is not severe. Exercise testing is also useful in recommending a safe exercise regimen for the casual athlete with moderate disease.

Outcomes and Management The most common initial symptoms of severe AS are exertional dyspnoea and reduced exercise tolerance. Late symptoms include angina, syncope and heart failure. Any symptom due to AS is an indication for prompt valve replacement. Transcatheter balloon aortic valvotomy may also be an option in young adults [15]. Valve replacement is indicated in asymptomatic patients with severe AS and left ventricular systolic dysfunction (EF <50%) and is reasonable in patients with very severe valve obstruction (velocity >5 m.s^{-1}), rapidly progressive disease or an abnormal stress test.

In patients with asymptomatic severe AS, progression to symptoms is seen in about 80% of cases within 2 years. The risk of sudden death with asymptomatic severe AS is low, estimated as <1% per year, which is lower than the risk of valve replacement surgery. With mild to moderate AS, haemodynamic progression is inevitable, with an average rate of increase in aortic velocity of 0.3 m.s^{-1}.year^{-1}, an increase in mean gradient of 5–10 mmHg.year^{-1} and a decline in valve area of about 0.1 cm^2.year^{-1}. Timing of follow-up in the asymptomatic patient is defined by AS severity: echocardiography is recommended every 6–12 months for severe AS (aortic velocity 4 m.s^{-1} or higher), every 1–2 years for moderate AS (velocity 3.0–3.9 m.s^{-1}) and every 3–5 years for mild AS (velocity 2.0–2.9 m.s^{-1}).

The goals of medical therapy for asymptomatic AS are to optimise cardiovascular health and prevent complications. Unfortunately, there is currently no known therapy to prevent progression of leaflet thickening and calcification. Screening and treatment for conventional cardiovascular risk factors help avoid concurrent CAD. Hypertension is treated with standard therapy, although it may be prudent to avoid diuretics in the setting of LVH with a small left ventricular chamber, and medications may need to be started at low doses and titrated slowly upwards to avoid a sudden drop in systemic vascular resistance.

Exercise Recommendations In the asymptomatic AS patient, the flexible valve leaflets allow valve area to increase slightly (on average 0.2 cm^2) along with the modest increase in stroke volume with exercise, but the increase in cardiac output is largely driven by a higher heart rate. Symptom onset correlates with progressive valve leaflet rigidity, resulting in a fixed valve area with exercise, preventing an increase in stroke volume. Changes in left ventricular diastolic function contribute to exercise limitations, with an excessive rise in left ventricular diastolic pressure on any increase in volume or flow rate.

Patients with symptomatic severe AS should undergo valve replacement, as there is a high risk of sudden death, particularly with exercise. Competitive sports should be avoided in patients with asymptomatic severe AS as well, due to the high risk of a fall in cardiac output, myocardial ischaemia or an arrhythmia with strenuous exercise. With asymptomatic moderate AS, athletes may participate in low to moderate static or dynamic sports if exercise stress testing is normal. The patient with mild AS may participate in all sports if they have no concerning symptoms or arrhythmias and have otherwise normal cardiac testing (see Table 23.3).

Aortic Regurgitation

Pathophysiology The cause of AR may be primary leaflet abnormalities, most often a BAV, or may be secondary to dilation of the aortic sinuses or ascending aorta, with stretching of the valve apparatus preventing normal leaflet coaptation (see Figure 23.4). Other causes of chronic primary AR include rheumatic disease and leaflet fenestrations (Bonow). Secondary AR in the setting of dilated aortic sinuses is commonly seen in Marfan syndrome but can be seen with any aortopathy, including those due to a systemic inflammatory disease. Acute AR is a medical emergency, occurring in the setting of aortic dissection or aortic valve endocarditis [16].

Clinical Presentation AR is most commonly diagnosed based on the finding of a murmur in an asymptomatic patient. The diastolic decrescendo murmur along the left sternal board is best appreciated with the sitting patient leaning forward in held expiration. However, the murmur is not always audible and may be overshadowed by a systolic-flow murmur due to the increased forward transaortic flow. With severe AR, pulse pressure is increased, peripheral pulses are bounding, a head bob may be present and auscultations reveals a diastolic murmur over the femoral arteries due to retrograde flow. In contrast, with acute severe AR, many of these findings are absent.

Outcomes and Management Patients with chronic AR typically remain asymptomatic for many years [17,18]. Long-term outcomes are related to the effect of chronic pressure and volume overload on the left ventricle. Slowly progressive left ventricular enlargement allows for maintenance of a normal forward cardiac output, even with exercise. Most patients with severe AR eventually develop symptoms of decreased exercise tolerance or dyspnoea, which is an indication for surgical aortic valve replacement. In about 25% of patients, excessive left ventricular dilation or a decline in systolic function occurs, even in the absence of symptoms. Overall, in asymptomatic patients with severe AR and normal left ventricular size and function, only about 4% per year progress to symptoms or a decrease in left ventricular function.

Excessive left ventricular dilation or a fall in EF is associated with an increased risk of sudden death and a higher likelihood of long-term heart failure after valve replacement. Thus, in the asymptomatic patient with severe AR, valve replacement is recommended when left ventricular end-systolic dimension is >50 mm or when left ventricular EF falls below 50%.

Exercise Recommendations Asymptomatic patients with severe AR and a left ventricular diastolic diameter >65 mm should not participate in any competitive sports, due to the risk of sudden death. Asymptomatic patients with moderate AR and normal left ventricular size and function may participate in sports with low to moderate static exercise or any degree of dynamic exercise, but only if exercise testing is normal at the degree of activity required for the specific sport. Ambulatory ECG monitoring is recommended to screen for nonsustained ventricular tachycardia (NSVT), which limits an athlete to low-intensity sports. In athletes with AR, there is often concern that left ventricular dilation is partly attributable to high-intensity training rather than solely to AR. A prudent approach is to quantitate AR severity by echocardiography or CMR. If AR is severe, standard indications for valve replacement should be followed, regardless of the level of physical activity.

Mitral Valvular Disease

Mitral Valve Prolapse

Pathophysiology MVP is most likely a genetic condition resulting in myxomatous changes of the mitral valve leaflets. Thickening and redundancy of the valve leaflets and chords result in sagging of the leaflets into the left atrium in systole, with loss of leaflet apposition and consequent MR. MVP often primarily affects the central scallop of the posterior leaflet with an anatomy that is amendable to surgical valve repair, without valve replacement (Figure 23.5).

Clinical Presentation Age of presentation is variable, due to both a long asymptomatic period and limited detection on physical exam in asymptomatic subjects, but most cases are diagnosed at between 20 and 60 years of age. Diagnosis may be made incidentally based on the presence of the characteristic late-systolic murmur at the apex, radiating to the axilla, often with a midsystolic click [19]. As the disease progresses, the murmur becomes holosystolic, with lack of leaflet apposition occurring earlier and earlier in systole. Some patients initially present with palpitations due to AF, symptoms of exertional dyspnoea, endocarditis or, rarely, resuscitated ventricular fibrillation [20].

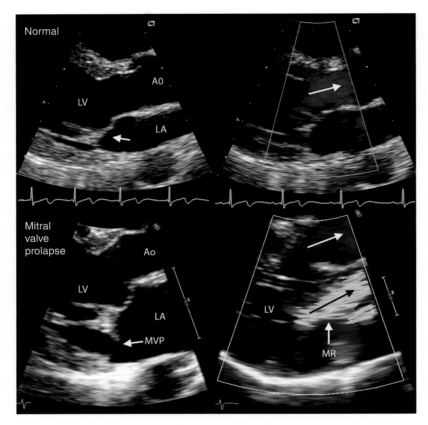

Figure 23.5 MVP and regurgitation. In a long-axis echocardiographic view, a normal mitral valve (top) is compared with MVP (bottom). The normal mitral closure in systole (arrow) contrasts with the sagging and prolapse of the posterior mitral leaflet (arrow). In the normal patient, colour Doppler shows normal left ventricular ejection into the aortic valve in red, with no systolic flow in the left atrium (top right). With mitral prolapse, left ventricular ejection is seen in red (white long arrow), but MR is also present, with a jet directly anteriorly (black arrow) due to posterior mitral leaflet prolapse

Outcomes and Management Overall outcomes in patients with MVP without severe MR are excellent [21]. Many patients will eventually require surgical intervention for severe MR, but surgical valve repair is feasible in most, at a low surgical risk and with excellent long-term outcomes, durable valve function and no need for chronic anticoagulation. Surgical intervention is recommended for severe MR in all symptomatic MVP patients and in asymptomatic patients with a left ventricular EF of 30–60% or with a left ventricular end-systolic diameter of ≥40 mm. Mitral valve surgery is reasonable with severe MR and normal left ventricular size and systolic function if the likelihood of a successful valve repair is >95% and estimated surgical mortality is <1% [22,23].

In patients with mild or moderate MR, the severity may increase gradually over many years, with a slow increase in leaflet redundancy and prolapse, or it may suddenly increase with spontaneous chordal rupture. Most patients develop symptoms of exercise intolerance or dyspnoea once MR is severe, but some develop irreversible left ventricular systolic dysfunction in the absence of symptoms. Thus, periodic monitoring of left ventricular size and function, as well as MR severity and pulmonary pressures, is essential in the management of patients with MVP. In some patients with MVP, the severity of MR increases with exercise due to increased leaflet prolapse, with increased afterload and a reduction in left ventricular size. These patients often have symptoms out of proportion to the severity of MR at rest. Exercise testing with TTE measurement of pulmonary pressures at rest and peak exercise can be helpful in elucidating the cause of symptoms in these patients.

Complications of MR due to MVP include pulmonary hypertension, right heart disease and an increased likelihood of AF. MVP patients may be at higher risk for cardioembolic events, likely due to the increased risk of AF. Endocarditis occurs more often than in the general population and may be the initial presentation.

MVP may be associated with an increased risk of SCD compared to the normal population, with an estimated incidence of 0.2–0.4% per year. However, it remains unclear whether this risk is primarily due to the haemodynamic effects of severe MR or if there is an underlying genetic predisposition. Ventricular arrhythmias may be the initial presentation of previously undiagnosed severe MR and left ventricular dysfunction, but ventricular arrhythmias have also been reported without severe MR or after valve surgery [24]. Clinical factors that may indicate a higher risk of sudden death in MVP patients include a history of syncope with a documented arrhythmia, a family history of sudden death, severe MR, left ventricular systolic dysfunction, a prior embolic event and an ambulatory ECG showing significant arrhythmias.

Exercise Recommendations In patients with MVP who do not meet criteria for surgical intervention, participation in all sports is allowed only if left ventricular function and ambulatory ECG monitoring are normal and there is no family history of SCD. If any of these risk factors are present, exercise is restricted to low-intensity competitive sports.

Mitral Regurgitation

Pathophysiology Chronic primary MR is most often caused by MVP, rheumatic disease or age-related changes of the valve leaflets. MR may also be secondary to disease of the left ventricle, most often dilated cardiomyopathy or ischaemic disease, with tethering of the valve leaflets by the dilated left ventricle and displaced papillary muscles resulting in incomplete leaflet coaptation. In patients with hypertrophic cardiomyopathy (HCM), significant MR may be seen due to abnormal mitral leaflet anatomy and dynamics (see Chapter 17).

Left ventricular volume overload due to chronic severe MR results in progressive left ventricular dilation and eventual systolic dysfunction, and some patients develop irreversible left ventricular systolic dysfunction in the absence of symptoms. MR is an isolated volume overload, as compared to the combined pressure and volume overload of AR, so that more subtle (and less severe) changes in left ventricular size and EF signify early left ventricular systolic dysfunction. Regurgitation into the left atrium also results in elevated left atrial size and pressure, predisposing to AF and pulmonary hypertension.

The pathophysiology of acute severe MR (e.g. due to spontaneous chordal rupture or endocarditis) is characterised by a sudden increase in left atrial pressure, resulting in pulmonary edema. Left ventricular EF increases acutely but, with insufficient time for compensatory left ventricular dilation, forward cardiac output falls, resulting in cardiogenic shock. Acute severe MR is often mistaken for an acute pulmonary process; TTE provides the correct diagnosis.

Clinical Presentation Most patients with primary MR present with an asymptomatic systolic murmur or at the time of symptom onset with dyspnoea or an atrial arrhythmia. Patients with secondary MR present with the symptoms and signs of the primary disease process: either a cardiomyopathy or CAD. TTE provides accurate diagnosis of the cause and severity of MR, left ventricular size and systolic function and an estimate of pulmonary pressures. In patients being considered for surgical intervention when severity measures are borderline, TOE with 3D imaging of valve anatomy and precise quantitation of regurgitant severity are recommended.

Outcomes and Management The clinical outcomes with MR due to MVP have already been discussed. In patients with secondary MR, clinical outcomes are primarily driven by the underlying disease process. Surgical or transcatheter intervention for severe secondary MR is reserved for patients with refractory symptoms after optimal therapy for heart failure and coronary disease [25].

Exercise Recommendations Athletes with mild to moderate primary MR, normal left ventricular size and function and normal pulmonary artery pressures can participate in all competitive sports. No restrictions are necessary in patients with mild to moderate MR and only mild left ventricular enlargement considered consistent with athletic conditioning. However, the presence of severe MR and left ventricular enlargement, pulmonary hypertension or any decrease in left ventricular systolic function precludes participation in any competitive sports, and these patients should be considered for mitral valve surgery. In patients with secondary MR, recommendations for exercise are based on the underlying cardiac condition (see Chapters 19, 21 and 24).

Mitral Stenosis

Pathophysiology Obstruction at the mitral valve level results in elevated left atrial and pulmonary arterial pressures. Initially, the increase in pulmonary pressures is passive, equivalent to the increase in left atrial pressure, but over time pulmonary vascular changes develop, with irreversible pulmonary hypertension and eventual right heart failure. As with MR, it is important to consider exercise-induced pulmonary hypertension when symptoms are present despite only moderate disease on the resting TTE. Patients with isolated MS have a small, underfilled left ventricular chamber, with normal systolic function. However, multivalve involvement is typical with rheumatic MS, and left ventricular changes due to concurrent MR or aortic valve involvement may be present.

Clinical Presentation In underdeveloped countries, patients present with rheumatic MS as teenagers or young adults, but in Europe and North America, rheumatic MS primarily affects older women, typically in the 40–60-year age group. In the elderly, nonrheumatic mitral annular calcification can become severe and can encroach on the mitral orifice, resulting in functional obstruction to left ventricular filling. The loud S1, an opening snap in early diastole and the holodiastolic, rumbling murmur of MS are best heard with the patient in a steep left lateral decubitus position, but physical examination has a low sensitivity for diagnosis. Many patients with MS present in the setting of a superimposed haemodynamic stress, such as pregnancy or an acute febrile illness, or with new-onset AF.

Outcomes and Management Rheumatic MS is a slowly progressive disease, with leaflet fibrosis and calcification superimposed on the commissural fusion due to rheumatic fever, and patients remain asymptomatic until severe valve obstruction is present. If AF develops, rate control and anticoagulation are appropriate. In MS patients with cardiovascular decompensation due to a superimposed condition, beta blockers may be considered even with sinus rhythm, because a slower heart rate allows increased left ventricular diastolic filling. However, intervention is recommended early in the disease course, because transcatheter balloon mitral commissurotomy provides a significant increase in mitral orifice area, resulting in relief of symptoms and a decrease in pulmonary pressures in most patients. Balloon commissurotomy is recommended for symptomatic patients with a mitral valve area of $1.5\,cm^2$ or less if valve anatomy is favourable, there is no left atrial thrombus and there is no or mild MR. In asymptomatic patients, balloon commissurotomy may be considered with a valve area of $1.5\,cm^2$ or less and new-onset AF or in those with less severe MS at rest but a significant increase in pulmonary pressures with exercise. Surgical mitral valve replacement is appropriate for symptomatic severe MS when the transcatheter approach is not feasible or is high-risk.

Exercise Recommendations Unrestricted participation is allowed in patients with mild MS if peak pulmonary systolic pressure is <50 mmHg with exercise. Severe MS or a pulmonary systolic pressure >50 mmHg precludes participation in any competitive sports, although these patients may be eligible after an effective intervention. Those with moderate MS and acceptable pulmonary pressures during exercise can participate in low to moderate dynamic competitive sports.

Right Heart Valvular Disease

Primary right heart valvular disease is caused by congenital disease in young adults, such as pulmonic regurgitation after repair of tetralogy of Fallot or tricuspid regurgitation due to Ebstein's anomaly (see Chapter 24). Causes of acquired right-sided primary valvular disease are rheumatic disease, endocarditis and carcinoid syndrome. Tricuspid valve regurgitation occurs secondary to left-sided valvular disease in association with elevated pulmonary pressures and consequent right ventricular dilation and systolic dysfunction. Secondary tricuspid regurgitation presents and is treated as a component of the underlying left heart valvular disease.

Prosthetic Valves

Young adults may require, or may have previously undergone, prosthetic heart valve replacement. Whenever possible, prosthetic valve implantation is avoided with transcatheter approaches, such as balloon valvotomy, or with surgical valve repair to relieve stenosis or prevent regurgitation. When valve replacement is necessary, two categories of prosthetic valve can be used: mechanical valves, which are very durable but require lifelong vitamin K antagonist anticoagulation, and bioprosthetic valves, which avoid chronic anticoagulation but are subject to leaflet degeneration and the need for recurrent surgical interventions. Both types of prosthetic valve have a high risk for endocarditis, so antibiotic prophylaxis at the time of dental and other procedures is recommended. Long-term treatment with 75–100 mg of aspirin daily is recommended for both types. Currently, the novel oral anticoagulants are contraindicated in patients with prosthetic heart valves. The optimal choice of prosthetic valve in the young patient is controversial, with patient values and preferences becoming important with respect to the risk of reoperation versus long-term anticoagulation. In the athlete, the limitations imposed by chronic anticoagulation may be the determining factor.

Prosthetic heart valves are evaluated using the same assessments (by echo and exercise testing) used for native valvular disease, with a similar standard for disease severity. Prosthetic valve haemodynamics are suboptimal compared to a normal native valve and may impact athlete performance. In addition, the prosthetic valve may be too small for the patient's body size, particularly if valve replacement is performed before full growth, resulting in a condition known as 'patient–prosthesis mismatch': effectively a type of valve stenosis. Exercise testing may be helpful in patients with prosthetic valves who wish to engage in high levels of physical activity, to evaluate the haemodynamic response at the level of exertion expected in competition.

Bioprosthetic valve leaflets are prone to calcification, resulting in slowly progressive prosthetic valve stenosis or regurgitation (often acute, where there is a leaflet tear adjacent to an area of calcification). Severe valve dysfunction is unlikely before 10 years after implantation, but valve durability is inversely proportional to age, so periodic monitoring is especially important in younger patients. A baseline postoperative TTE is recommended, with subsequent studies if there is any concern over early valve dysfunction. After 10 years, annual TTE is reasonable for bioprosthetic valves. Indications for intervention for prosthetic valve stenosis or regurgitation are the same as for native valvular disease. In addition, transcatheter options may be available for paravalvular regurgitation or bioprosthetic valve stenosis.

Conclusion

Prompt diagnosis and evaluation of valvular heart disease allow appropriate counselling about the risks of competitive athletics and optimal timing of surgical or transcatheter intervention. Aortic and mitral valve stenosis limit the normal increase in cardiac output with exercise and may result in poor coronary perfusion, myocardial ischaemia and hypotension during intense exercise. Conversely, AR and MR result in left ventricular dilation, adverse remodelling and eventual systolic dysfunction, and if untreated place the athlete at increased risk of ventricular arrhythmias and sudden death. MVP patients may be at higher risk for SCD, particularly if there is a positive family history, severe MR or left ventricular systolic dysfunction. Atrial arrhythmias are also common, especially with mitral valvular disease. However, most athletes with valvular heart disease can participate safely in competitive sports until valve dysfunction is severe, symptoms of valvular disease are present or there is evidence of early left ventricular systolic dysfunction. Periodic non-invasive monitoring and clinical follow-up to monitor for progressive valvular disease, treat conventional cardiovascular risk factors and assess exercise capacity allow for optimal timing of interventions and thus prevention of adverse outcomes.

References

1 Nishimura, R.A., McGoon, M.D., Shub, C. et al. Echocardiographically documented mitral-valve prolapse. Long-term follow-up of 237 patients. *N Engl J Med* 2985; **313**: 1305–9.

2 Nishimura, R.A., Otto, C.M., Bonow, R.O. et al. AHA/ACC guideline for the management of patients with valvular heart disease: executive summary: a report of the American College of Cardiology/American Heart Association Task Force on Practice Guidelines. *J Am Coll Cardiol* 2014; **63**: 2438–88.

3 Vahanian, A., Alfieri, O., Andreotti, F. et al. Guidelines on the management of valvular heart disease (version 2012). *Eur Heart J* 2012; **33**: 2451–96.

4 Siu, S.C. and Silversides, C.K. Bicuspid aortic valve disease. *J Am Coll Cardiol* 2010; **55**: 2789–800.

5 Eveborn, G.W., Schirmer, H., Heggelund, G. et al. The evolving epidemiology of valvular aortic stenosis. the Tromso study. *Heart* 2013; **99**: 396–400.

6 Nkomo, V.T., Gardin, J.M., Skelton, T.N. et al. Burden of valvular heart diseases: a population-based study. *Lancet* 2006; **368**: 1005–11.

7 Gaasch, W.H. and Meyer, T.E. Left ventricular response to mitral regurgitation: implications for management. *Circulation* 2008; **118**: 2298–303.

8 Pierard, L.A. and Lancellotti, P. Stress testing in valve disease. *Heart* 2007; **93**: 766–72.

9 Maron, B.J., Ackerman, M.J., Nishimura, R.A. et al. Task Force 4: HCM and other cardiomyopathies, mitral valve prolapse, myocarditis, and Marfan syndrome. *J Am Coll Cardiol* 2005; **45**: 1340–5.

10 Pelliccia, A., Fagard, R., Bjornstad, H.H. et al. Recommendations for competitive sports participation in athletes with cardiovascular disease: a consensus document from the Study Group of Sports Cardiology of the Working Group of Cardiac Rehabilitation and Exercise Physiology and the Working Group of Myocardial and Pericardial Diseases of the European Society of Cardiology. *Eur Heart J* 2005; **26**: 1422–45.

11 Bonow, R.O., Cheitlin, M.D., Crawford, M.H. and Douglas, P.S. Task Force 3: valvular heart disease. *J Am Coll Cardiol* 2005; **45**: 1334–40.

12 Eleid, M.F., Forde, I., Edwards, W.D. et al. Type A aortic dissection in patients with bicuspid aortic valves: clinical and pathological comparison with tricuspid aortic valves. *Heart* 2013; **99**: 1668–74.

13 Verma, S. and Siu, S.C. Aortic dilatation in patients with bicuspid aortic valve. *N Engl J Med* 2014; **370**: 1920–9.

14 Otto, C.M. and Prendergast, B. Aortic-valve stenosis–from patients at risk to severe valve obstruction. *N Engl J Med* 2014; **371**: 744–56.

15 Warnes, C.A., Williams, R.G., Bashore, T.M. et al. ACC/AHA 2008 guidelines for the management of adults with congenital heart disease: a report of the American College of Cardiology/American Heart Association Task Force on Practice Guidelines (Writing Committee to Develop Guidelines on the Management of Adults with Congenital Heart Disease). *Circulation* 2008; **118**: e714–833.

16 Stout, K.K. and Verrier, E.D. Acute valvular regurgitation. *Circulation* 2009; **119**: 3232–41.

17 Bonow, R.O. Aortic regurgitation: time to reassess timing of valve replacement? *JACC Cardiovasc Imaging* 2011; **4**: 231–3.

18 Bonow, R.O. Chronic mitral regurgitation and aortic regurgitation: have indications for surgery changed? *J Am Coll Cardiol* 2013; **61**: 693–701.

19 Topilsky, Y., Michelena, H., Bichara, V. et al. Mitral valve prolapse with mid-late systolic mitral regurgitation: pitfalls of evaluation and clinical outcome compared with holosystolic regurgitation. *Circulation* 2012; **125**: 1643–51.

20 Enriquez-Sarano, M., Avierinos, J.F., Messika-Zeitoun, D. et al. Quantitative determinants of the outcome of asymptomatic mitral regurgitation. *N Engl J Med* 2005; **352**: 875–83.

21 Freed, L.A., Benjamin, E.J., Levy, D. et al. Mitral valve prolapse in the general population: the benign nature of echocardiographic features in the Framingham Heart Study. *J Am Coll Cardiol* 2002; **40**: 1298–304.

22 Otto, C.M. Surgery for mitral regurgitation: sooner or later? *JAMA* 2013; **310**: 587–8.

23 Otto, C.M. and Nishimura, R.A. New ACC/AHA valve guidelines: aligning defintions of aortic stenosis severity with treatment recommendations. *Heart* 2014; **100**(12): 902–4.

24 Zuppiroli, A., Mori, F., Favilli, S. et al. Arrhythmias in mitral valve prolapse: relation to anterior mitral leaflet thickening, clinical variables, and color Doppler echocardiographic parameters. *Am Heart J* 1994; **128**: 919–27.

25 Otto, C.M. and Salerno, C.T. Timing of surgery in asymptomatic mitral regurgitation. *N Engl J Med* 2005; **352**: 928–9.

24 Congenital Heart Disease

Guido E. Pieles[1] and A. Graham Stuart[2]

[1] National Institute for Health Research (NIHR) Cardiovascular Biomedical Research Unit, Congenital Heart Unit, Bristol Royal Hospital for Children and Bristol Heart Institute, Bristol, UK
[2] Congenital Heart Unit, Bristol Royal Hospital for Children and Bristol Heart Institute, Bristol, UK

Introduction

The long-term follow-up of the athlete with corrected or palliated congenital heart disease (CHD) can be challenging. For most CHD patients, regular physical activity and sport should be encouraged, but long-term complications can occur, such as heart failure, arrhythmias and the need for reoperation. The sports cardiologist must be alert to the presence of underlying CHD, as intervention may be necessary before the onset of major symptoms. Although the athlete population with CHD is small, there is a wide range of diagnoses, and individualised assessment is essential. This requires detailed knowledge of CHD, which can be a challenge to the sports physician and cardiologist. Although consensus management guidelines for adults with CHD patients are available, there is very little lesion-specific advice on sports and exercise. General guidelines for sport and exercise participation in children with CHD are available, but in both children and adults, recommendations for individual evaluation of unrepaired, palliated and repaired CHD are needed.

Epidemiology of CHD

CHD represents the commonest birth defect, with a worldwide prevalence of 9.1 per 1000 live births [1]. Due to advances in diagnosis and intervention, most CHD patients survive to adulthood, including over 85% with complex disease. As a result, the adult population with CHD has increased significantly to 4 per 1000 adults [1], and 1 in 150 young adults will have some form of CHD – an increase of over 50% in the last 10 years [2]. This makes it likely that sports cardiologists will be confronted with athletes who have been diagnosed with CHD. In addition, some types of CHD may present for the first time in adult life and may be detected during routine examination or screening. Underdiagnosis of CHD is particularly prevalent in Africa, and with the rising number of African athletes competing in European and American professional and college sport, CHD in athletes is likely to be encountered with increasing frequency [1].

Aetiology of CHD

CHD is defined as a 'gross structural abnormality of the heart or intra-thoracic great vessels present at birth that is actually or potentially of functional significance' [3]. Genes, environmental factors and maternal infections all contribute to a multifactorial aetiology [4]. A genetic origin for many forms of CHD has been established, and this is associated with a familial recurrence risk of 2–5%. CHD can occur as a chromosomal syndrome (12%) or a heritable syndrome with Mendelian pattern (8%), or it may be sporadic (80%), with variable penetrance and heritability. In many cases, the complex genetic mechanisms remain undefined. Environmental factors include maternal diabetes, prescribed and recreational maternal drugs (e.g. diphenylhydantoin or alcohol/cocaine) and infective embryopathies (rubella, cytomegalovirus (CMV), coxsackie,

IOC Manual of Sports Cardiology, First Edition. Edited by Mathew G. Wilson, Jonathan A. Drezner and Sanjay Sharma.
© 2017 International Olympic Committee. Published 2017 by John Wiley & Sons, Ltd.

human immunodeficiency virus (HIV)). Approximately 25% of patients with CHD have an additional non-cardiac abnormality. Whilst this may make sports participation more challenging, it does mean that occult cardiac disease may feature in Paralympic athletes with noncardiac anomalies.

CHD in the Athlete Population

In Western health care systems, over 90% of CHD [1] is diagnosed in the first year of life, with most palliative and corrective surgery performed in early childhood. The adolescent and adult CHD population consists of mild unrepaired lesions, palliated and repaired CHD and a small number of undiagnosed lesions, particularly in individuals from the developing world. The precise number of professional and recreational athletes with underlying CHD is unknown. However, it is likely exercise participation will increase as knowledge of the multiple benefits of exercise in patients with CHD is disseminated [5]. Overall, 90% of adults with CHD are in New York Heart Association (NYHA) class I or II [6] and can participate in some form of recreational sports and exercise. A small number of high-profile competitive athletes have CHD.

Mortality Risks of Sudden Cardiac Death in CHD

Cardiovascular mortality accounts for 75% of all deaths in CHD – predominantly due to sudden cardiac death (SCD) (26%) and heart failure (21%) [7]. Important risk factors may include arrhythmias, heart failure, coronary ischaemia, outflow or prosthetic conduit obstructions and aneurysms. Despite this, the annual incidence of SCD in CHD is only 0.09% [8], and only 8% of deaths occur during exercise. Data on high-risk lesions and diagnosis independent risk factors for SCD in CHD are available (Table 24.1) [8,9]. The most common CHDs associated with SCD in competitive athletes are abnormal coronary artery origin (which is challenging to diagnose on screening), aortic stenosis, mitral valve prolapse (MVP) and aortic aneurysms [10]. SCD in other conditions is usually caused by a ventricular arrhythmia occurring in a patient who has undergone surgical intervention. Cardiac arrhythmias are the most common cause of emergency hospital admission in adults with CHD, and it is likely that extreme exercise can unmask an underlying arrhythmic tendency. This emphasises the need for individual patient assessment, including exercise stress testing. It is not known whether the intensity of exercise is an SCD risk factor in CHD.

Cause of SCD in all CHD	Arrhythmias (ventricular tachycardia and ventricular fibrillation) (80%)
	Aortic dissection (9%)
	Cerebrovascular events and pulmonary haemorrhage (8%)
	Myocardial infarct (2%)
	Other (1%)
Conditions at highest risk for SCD in CHD	Tetralogy of Fallot
	Transposition of the great arteries (TGA)
	Congenitally corrected transposition of the great arteries (ccTGA)
	Aortic stenosis
	Univentricular (Fontan) circulation
	Coronary artery anomalies
	Eisenmenger syndrome
Risk factors for SCD in CHD (diagnosis independent)	Supraventricular tachycardia (SVT) (mostly atrial flutter and atrial fibrillation)
	Ventricular tachycardia
	Increased QRS duration
	QT dispersion
	Moderate to severe systemic and/or subpulmonary ventricular dysfunction
	Moderate to severe tricuspid regurgitation

Table 24.1 General risk stratification for SCD in CHD

Activity and Sports in CHD

Exercise in Athletes with CHD – Current Guidelines and Recommendations

The first published guidelines for athletes with cardiovascular abnormalities did not include eligibility recommendations for patients with CHD. However, the unique challenge of sports participation in CHD was addressed subsequently [11,12]. The later consensus guidelines were based primarily on anatomic diagnosis and parameters such as severity of underlying lesion, nature of intervention and known or identified complications. In general, they state that many patients with CHD can participate in competitions and that most should engage in recreational exercise activities, whilst acknowledging that few objective outcome data exist. Exercise intolerance in CHD is a strong predictor of both outcome and SCD [6]. Most sports participation recommendations are based on evidence of reduced exercise capacity in CHD and accumulating evidence that exercise training is beneficial. General recommendations on the type and intensity of physical activity in adults and children with CHD differentiate between physical activity and exercise training but do not give explicit training recommendations [5]. A further general aid is the classification of sports [13] on which lesion-specific recommendations have been based. The challenges posed by the wide variation in physiology and function in adults with CHD led to the introduction of individualised algorithms for physical activity participation and exercise prescription in adults (>16 years) with CHD [14]. Although complex, these five-step guidelines recognise that underlying cardiovascular physiology is more important than the historical anatomic diagnosis. In summary, current guidelines classify sports participation according to type of sport, congenital lesion and risk factors, and provide a starting point for assessment and exercise recommendations in athletes with CHD. However, a detailed individual patient assessment is essential before specific sports participation can be recommended. Moreover, although some athletes with CHD may be able to participate in high-intensity exercise, if a thorough assessment has not identified any risk factors then assessment will have to be repeated regularly due to the potential for subsequent deterioration.

Exercise and Sports Participation in Patients with CHD

Children and Adolescents In the past, few children with CHD were encouraged to participate in competitive sports, as there was a poor understanding of the risks and benefits of exercise amongst health care professionals, patients and their families [15]. However, this attitude has changed, and a recent scientific statement from the American Heart Association (AHA) proposed that counselling to encourage daily participation in exercise should be a core component of every patient encounter [5]. Moreover, children with CHD should be encouraged to reach published activity guidelines (60 minutes of moderate-intensity exercise daily) in order to overcome the recognised risks of a sedentary lifestyle [15]. Current recommendations for participation in noncompetitive sports give diagnosis-specific general advice and conclude that it is safe for most children with CHD to compete at an amateur level [16]. Additionally, exercise and training as a therapeutic intervention in children with CHD can provide clear and sustained benefits [5].

Exercise-related death in children with CHD is extremely rare. Most children with fully repaired CHD can engage in sporting activities with minimal restriction if individual risk factors have not been identified. Few studies have investigated the effects of competitive training in children with CHD on cardiac morphology, physiology and cardiovascular risk. Exercise training programmes in children with CHD should be tailored to take account of an individual's disease subtype, the medical intervention used to treat them and their current fitness level, as well as deficiencies in other organ systems (pulmonary, musculoskeletal, neurological and nutritional).

A recently published document from the European Association for Cardiovascular Prevention and Rehabilitation (EACPR) on physical activity and exercise prescription for adolescents and adults with CHD is a first step towards an evidenced-based approach to the assessment of sports eligibility, and this ought to be translated to the paediatric population with CHD [14].

Adults Exercise capacity is significantly reduced in most forms of adult CHD, leading to an impaired quality of life and poor long-term outcomes [17]; however, the level of exercise limitation is extremely variable. Cardiopulmonary exercise testing (CPET) has been used to risk-stratify the adult with CHD and can predict outcome in many patient groups with CHD [18]. Exercise is also an effective tool by which to reduce general cardiovascular risk factors in adults with CHD. There is increasing scientific evidence for the sustained benefits of exercise in rehabilitation in adults with CHD [19], but, surprisingly, only 10% of all adult CHD candidates receive structured exercise training. A further problem is that cardiovascular exercise rehabilitation guidelines in the disease context often use protocols at low rehabilitational intensity levels [16]. Whilst these levels are safe, they have a low training effect.

Pathophysiological Mechanisms of Exercise Intolerance in CHD

Many factors contribute to reduced exercise capacity in patients with CHD, and all may occur in the athlete. A blunted chronotropic response can occur secondary to sinus-node disease, conduction delay or an abnormal force–frequency relationship. Reduced metabolic parameters, such as $\dot{V}O_{2max}$ and peak oxygen pulse, can indicate a reduced stroke-volume response and are found in most forms of complex CHD, but also in repaired tetralogy of Fallot, aortic regurgitation and postoperative coarctation of the aorta. In some lesions, the ventilatory anaerobic threshold is lower in CHD than in the normal population, impairing gas-exchange efficiency in many dynamic and endurance sports. This may relate to previous thoracotomy or lung disease. Similarly, there may be an elevated VE/VCO_2 slope, indicating inadequacy of the pulmonary vascular bed [18]. Besides cardiopulmonary factors, skeletal muscle weakness and reduced muscle mass are common in adults with CHD, contributing to decreased tissue oxygen uptake.

Assessment Tools in CHD

Electrocardiogram

Due to congenital or postoperative changes, many athletes with CHD will fail the standard screening guidelines for athlete electrocardiogram (ECG) interpretation [20]. The ECG assessment in CHD should be interpreted in light of known lesion-specific ECG changes by a cardiologist experienced in the normal findings in CHD. The assessment of the athlete with CHD and symptoms of potential arrhythmias requires close collaboration between a congenital heart specialist and sports cardiologist.

Transthoracic Echocardiography

Transthoracic echocardiography (TTE) is the first-line imaging modality in the assessment of the athlete with CHD. Guidelines for the performance of paediatric and adult echocardiograms should be followed, but the assessment of the athlete with CHD requires considerable experience and an understanding of both sports cardiology and CHD. In the majority of cases, TTE will provide detailed information on cardiac anatomy, the connection of extracardiac vessels to the heart, ventricular function, valves and shunt lesions. Athletes with CHD should undergo regular echocardiographic examination, particularly if increasing or changing standard training activities.

Exercise Stress Echocardiography

In the athlete with CHD, stress echocardiography can unmask subclinical ventricular dysfunction and valvar stenosis or regurgitation, which may not be apparent at rest. Although detailed normative data have not been established, load independent parameters, such as isovolumic acceleration time and exercise-related deformation assessment, can provide information on the force–frequency relationship and contractility reserve during exercise stress. Exercise stress is superior to dobutamine stress in the assessment of the athlete with CHD, as it assesses ventricular function in relation to other physiological exercise adaptations and can be combined with CPET.

Cardiac Magnetic Resonance and Computed Tomography

The relevance and application of cardiac magnetic resonance (CMR) in CHD is rapidly increasing [9]. CMR allows window-independent imaging, accurate delineation of detailed anatomy (including three-dimensional (3D) reconstruction and tissue characterisation) and is the gold standard in ventricular and regurgitant volume quantification. The main use of CMR is in the assessment of right and left ventricular volumes, myocardial mass, myocardial scar (which may act as a surrogate for arrhythmia risk), regurgitation fraction, visualisation of prosthetic materials (conduits) and inherent myocardial pathologies using contrast and detailed morphological studies (e.g. pulmonary veins, coronary arteries). The use of exercise imaging during CMR is in its infancy but promises to have considerable utility in the future assessment of the athlete with CHD.

Cardiac computed tomography (CT) is the imaging modality of choice in the delineation of small anatomical structures, such as coronary arteries and collateral arteries, and for imaging parenchymal lung pathology. The main disadvantages of CT are its low temporal resolution and exposure to radiation, but modern techniques have reduced the latter.

CMR and CT imaging in the CHD patient should be performed in specialist CHD centres.

Cardiac Catheterisation

Diagnostic cardiac catheterisation should be reserved for specific anatomical and physiological indications, such as coronary angiography, extracardiac collateral vessel angiography, shunt calculation, measurement of pressure gradients and pulmonary vascular resistance. Cardiac catheterisation is the investigation of choice if suspicion of pulmonary arterial hypertension (PAH) has been raised by echocardiography, and it is an essential prerequisite for transcatheter interventions, such as interventional stent and valve implantation. Cardiac catheterisation should only be performed in CHD centres with congenital surgical back-up facilities.

Cardiopulmonary Exercise Testing

CPET is a formidable tool in risk stratification for the determination of morbidity and mortality, timing of intervention and correlation of anatomic findings and physiological function in CHD. Reference values for the adult CHD population are available [17]. Longitudinal CPET assessment enables the monitoring of disease progression and of the consequences of exercise training progression. CPET should always be combined with exercise 12-lead ECG testing to allow assessment of underlying exercise-related arrhythmias. It is advisable that CPET and exercise 12-lead ECG testing be performed annually in the athlete with CHD. Additionally, they are indicated if significant changes in exercise performance, symptoms or echocardiographic parameters are noted.

General Considerations in Athletes with CHD

Assessment

The primary assessment of the athlete with CHD should follow general guidelines for a periodic health evaluation. In addition, athletes with CHD require a lesion-specific and individualised assessment that takes into account the nature of the defect, mode of corrective (or palliative) surgical and catheter interventions, residual lesions, haemodynamic state, arrhythmia risk and exercise capacity. A knowledge of potential complications for each lesion is paramount.

Equally important, and often neglected, is the age-specific pathophysiology in patients with CHD, irrespective of lesions, corrective or palliative procedures and pathophysiology. Children over 10 years of age and adults with CHD who participate in regulated training and recreational and competitive sports should undergo a comprehensive annual assessment that includes clinical examination, 12-lead ECG, transthoracic echocardiography and a CPET, including exercise stress 12-lead ECG.

The recent EACPR recommendations on exercise prescription can help risk-stratify individuals [14]. The asymptomatic athlete with CHD may have residual intracardiac shunts (atrial septal defect (ASD), patent ductus arteriosus (PDA) or ventricular septal defect (VSD)) or valve dysfunction, but, in most cases, exercise participation can be recommended with minimal or no restriction.

Undiagnosed structural lesions in the child athlete are rare, with the exception of anomalous coronary arteries, which are the main risk for SCD. In young-adult athletes with CHD sequelae of previous surgery, valvular incompetence and arrhythmias are the predominant problems, with ventricular dysfunction encountered less often. Arrhythmias and heart-failure risk increase significantly after 35 years of life in CHD, and it is in the master athlete with CHD that problems secondary to corrective or palliative procedures become a significant burden. These include cardiac arrhythmias, left and particularly right systemic ventricular dysfunction, valvar incompetence and obstruction of prosthetic conduits. Secondary interventions, such as valve and conduit surgery and arrhythmia ablation procedures, are frequent in this age group and should be performed at the earliest point in time, ideally before significant symptoms occur.

Undiagnosed CHD in Adulthood

Most CHD lesions will be identified, corrected or palliated in childhood, and it is unusual to encounter an athlete with undiagnosed complex CHD. Simple lesions of borderline haemodynamic significance can present during adulthood, however. Prime examples include athletes with a small ASD, PDA and small VSD, but also mild outflow-tract obstructions. In cases of shunt lesions (ASD, VSD, PDA), the decision to close these defects depends on resting haemodynamics. Recent studies have suggested that even mild ventricular dysfunction – subclinical at rest – can lead to impaired exercise performance. European Society of Cardiology (ESC) and AHA guidelines should be followed for treatment of valvar lesions.

Assessment and Prevention of Arrhythmias

Arrhythmias are the most common cause of emergency hospital admissions in adult patients with CHD [9]. They are normally the result of lesion-specific and surgical sequelae. They may be caused by areas of focal scar, but can also be a sign of occult haemodynamic deterioration or subclinical heart failure. Guidelines for the assessment and treatment of arrhythmias in CHD have been published [21], but antiarrhythmic prevention and therapy are often hampered by the negative chronotropic effects of antiarrhythmic treatment, and expert assessment and careful follow-up are essential. Assessment of arrhythmias in athletes with CHD should be performed at rest (12-lead ECG, Holter) and during exercise (stress 12-lead ECG), and in individual cases electrophysiology (EP) studies or loop-recorder implantation should be considered.

Heart Failure

In general, the treatment of heart failure in CHD should follow recommendations for non-CHD heart failure, but the aetiology, pathophysiology and management in CHD may differ significantly. There are few scientific data available, so treatment should be guided by individual patient pathophysiology [9]. Heart-failure assessment in CHD needs to concentrate on detailed left and right ventricular assessment, as many forms of CHD present with right ventricular pathology (e.g. Fallot, Fontan, congenitally corrected transposition of the great arteries (ccTGA), Eisenmenger). Right ventricular failure occurs secondary to pressure or volume loading, and right–left ventricle interaction in this setting has recently been recognised as a common cause of ventricular dysfunction [22]. Subclinical dysfunction can be accentuated during exercise in this patient group, particularly in the setting of systemic right ventricular dysfunction.

Pulmonary Arterial Hypertension

PAH may be idiopathic, but it is also an uncommon but severe complication of CHD. It can occur in the setting of a longstanding intra- or extracardiac communication (e.g. VSD, PDA, atrioventricular septal defect (AVSD)), which allows unrestricted volume and pressure overload, leading over time to fixed supranormal pulmonary artery pressures and reversal of shunting (Eisenmenger syndrome). The increase in right ventricular afterload and right ventricular pressure restricts the right ventricle's ability to increase cardiac output through enhanced stroke volume, and also impairs left ventricular filling and systemic cardiac output via right–left ventricle interaction. The result is a severely reduced exercise tolerance [17]. Moderate to severe PAH is therefore unlikely to be encountered even in recreational athletes.

Pulmonary artery pressures can rise beyond the defined normal range during exercise in healthy athletes, although the clinical importance of this is still uncertain. Even mildly raised pulmonary artery pressures can unbalance haemodynamics in complex CHD, and the new onset of exercise dyspnoea should prompt investigation. In the first instance, echocardiography should evaluate right ventricular pressure, intracardiac shunts (where right-to-left shunting should raise suspicion) and valves and pulmonary veins. Secondary assessment should include lung function tests, CPET and a catheter pulmonary vascular resistance study.

As PAH can also be a late postoperative complication after surgical correction of CHD, assessment for underlying PAH should be part of every echocardiographic examination in athletes with CHD and of precompetition screening. Patients with PAH are not eligible for any competitive sport but can engage in light dynamic and static exercise.

High Altitudes

No current guidelines address sports activities at moderate altitudes (1500–2500 m above sea level) in patients with CHD. Hypobaric hypoxia leads to decreased oxygen consumption, decreased cardiac output, tachycardia, hypocapnia-mediated stroke-volume decrease and a rise in pulmonary artery pressures in the acclimatisation phase. These mechanisms can significantly reduce oxygen tissue uptake in patients with complex CHD. Left ventricular dysfunction is very rare, but exacerbation of right ventricular heart failure has been described. Myocardial ischaemia is not observed in the healthy population but can present an additional problem in patients with CHD. Patients with cyanosis and complex CHD should be advised not to engage in moderate- or high-intensity sporting activities at moderate altitude (1500–2500 m) and should be told that they might become symptomatic even at rest. Air travel is well tolerated, but travel to moderate altitude should follow an assessment by CPET and echocardiography, and travel beyond 2500 m is not recommended in complex CHD. There is also a reported risk of exacerbation of arrhythmia at moderate and high altitudes.

Endocarditis Prophylaxis

The endocarditis risk is significantly higher in patients with CHD than in the general population, varying between specific lesions. The risk is lower in repaired CHD, but implantation of prosthetic conduits and valves poses an endocarditis risk in itself. Although antibiotic prophylaxis is no longer recommended, primary prevention with good dental hygiene and appropriate treatment of skin infections is vital. In our view, high-risk groups (prosthetic valves, residual shunts, previous endocarditis) should still receive antibiotic prophylaxis for invasive dental procedures.

The Child Athlete

The number of children and teenagers participating in organised sports has increased recently, and the intensity and frequency of training in this group can be compared to that of elite adult athletes. This development has been recognised by the International Olympic Committee (IOC), with a call for guidelines targeting the unique challenges faced by child and teenage athletes – as well as the professionals looking after these young talents [23].

At present, there are few scientific data on cardiac screening for the under-16-year-old athletic population. Adult normative data and current cardiological precompetition screening guidelines cannot be adapted to the still-developing heart, which differs in size and function. Inherited cardiac diseases may not manifest in childhood and may not be detectable with existing screening tools. The cardiac adaptation to elite training in children has not been fully investigated. Preliminary recommendations for ECG interpretation in the screening of child athletes have been published recently [24], but a concerted effort is necessary to emulate the advances in adult sports cardiology and athlete screening.

An even greater challenge is children with CHD who participate in competitive sport. A lack of scientific data and of expertise and informed advice amongst health care professionals has led to overprotection, which has had a negative effect on physical-activity goals, quality of life and long-term health [15]. Future research should focus on the development of gender, growth and age-specific normative 12-lead ECG and echocardiographic criteria; this will require synergistic approaches between paediatric and adult sports cardiologists and exercise physiologists.

Athletic Performance and Complications in Common Specific Lesions

Simple Shunt Lesions with Volume Loading

Simple shunt lesions, such as ASD, VSD and PDA, are usually diagnosed and corrected in childhood. In the adult athlete, haemodynamically significant unrepaired lesions will cause significant exercise intolerance, dyspnoea and recurrent respiratory infections, but also palpitations (particularly ASD). Atrial fibrillation, atrial flutter, paroxysmal intra-atrial re-entry tachycardias and first-degree atrioventricular (AV) block are common in unrepaired ASD but also occur in repaired defects, although life-threatening ventricular arrhythmias are rare. Late-onset complete heart block can occur occasionally post VSD repair. Residual lesions can lead to left-sided volume loading. Exercise capacity is reduced in unrepaired simple shunt lesions, including patients without overt clinical exercise symptoms [6]. Symptoms should prompt urgent reassessment and closure of defect unless there is a specific contraindication.

Atrioventricular Septal Defects

Exercise capacity in repaired AVSD can be moderately impaired as a result of left and right ventricular dysfunction, elevated pulmonary pressures, aortic valve regurgitation or progressive subaortic stenosis. These residual lesions often warrant surgical reintervention. Atrial arrhythmias and AV conduction defects can develop even years after repair. Life-threatening ventricular arrhythmias are rare, but do occur.

Right Ventricular Outflow Tract Obstruction (Tetralogy of Fallot)

Most complications in tetralogy of Fallot are sequelae of primary or secondary surgical intervention. Arrhythmias cause significant morbidity, and atrial flutter, AF and sustained ventricular tachycardia are observed in approximately 10% of patients 35 years after repair; the prevalence increases with age (Figure 24.1). Predictors for arrhythmias and associated SCD are moderate pulmonary or tricuspid incompetence, ventricular dysfunction, transannular patch repair, older age at repair and QRS >180 ms [25]. Exercise performance, which can be moderately reduced [17], is determined by right ventricular dysfunction and resulting right–left ventricle interaction [22]. Residual bioprosthetic conduit or valve stenosis or regurgitation is common and is well tolerated if mild, but will cause decreased exercise performance. In athletes, pulmonary valve replacement should be performed before symptoms occur. Aortic and pulmonary artery aneurysms are rare and serious complications and are often clinically silent. Aortic aneurysms can rupture and pulmonary artery aneurysms may cause symptoms of angina or dyspnoea during exercise secondary to coronary artery compression. Isolated pulmonary stenosis, even if mild, will reduce exercise performance.

Congenital Aortic Stenosis

Aortic stenosis is a cause of SCD in athletes [24]. Mild and moderate lesions have a low risk, but disease can progress fast. The key is symptom assessment during rest and exercise (ischaemia, arrhythmias, reduced cardiac reserve). Severe or moderate aortic stenosis with symptoms is not eligible for competitive sports. Treated congenital aortic stenosis often shows residual stenosis and regurgitation, and a dilated aortic sinus or ascending aorta is seen in 45% of patients after a decade of follow-up. Performance is mildly reduced in palliated lesions, due to regurgitation and residual left ventricular hypertrophy (LVH) with subclinical diastolic function.

Coarctation of Aorta

Coarctation is part of a generalised aortopathy. Problems persist post-intervention. Left ventricular remodelling and systemic hypertension, as well as collaterals and premature coronary artery disease (CAD), cause impaired exercise performance. Aortic or cerebral aneurysms are a serious and progressive complication

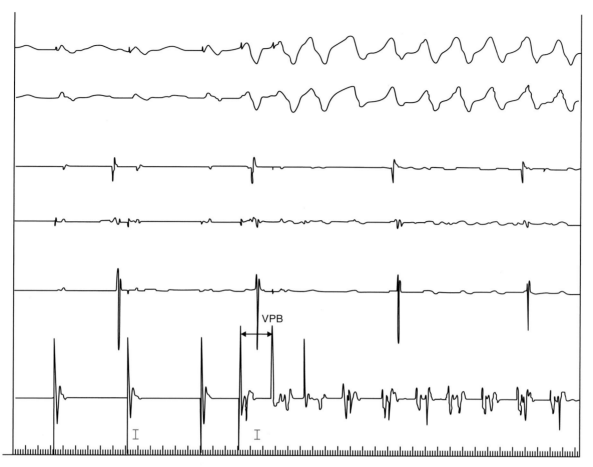

Figure 24.1 Presentation with collapse during exercise. A 28-year-old man with tetralogy of Fallot who had undergone surgical correction at the age of 9 years was discharged from follow-up in early adulthood. He had recently retired from competitive kickboxing but remained a keen recreational athlete. He collapsed whilst playing football, without having previously experienced significant symptoms. The 12-lead ECG recorded during resuscitation showed ventricular fibrillation. After successful resuscitation, he was transferred to the tertiary congenital heart centre, where he underwent an EP study. The image shows an ECG recorded during the diagnostic EP study: a single ventricular premature beat (VPB) induced a very rapid ventricular tachycardia. A full haemodynamic study was also performed, which demonstrated that he had excellent haemodynamics. The diagnosis was focal scar-mediated ventricular arrhythmia. An ablation procedure was not performed in this case, but a defibrillator was implanted and a beta blocker was commenced. The patient continued with moderate dynamic non-impact recreational exercise, but his exercise capacity was reduced secondary to beta-blocker medication

(Figure 24.2). New diagnosis should prompt early intervention to reduce left ventricular remodelling. Arrhythmias are rare. Undiagnosed coarctation of the aorta may present with hypertension, and it is important to exclude this diagnosis.

Cyanotic Lesions

In CHD, cyanosis is caused by right-to-left shunting, leading to deoxygenated blood entering the systemic circulation. Cyanotic patients require specialist follow-up in CHD centres. Their exercise capacity is moderately to severely reduced, and 30% of adults with cyanotic heart disease will be in New York Heart Association (NYHA) class III [6]. This may be due to ventricular dysfunction and significantly reduced oxygen availability, and reduced exercise function is a strong outcome predictor [18]. In general, patients are only eligible for competitive sport of low static and dynamic intensity but should be encouraged to participate in light to

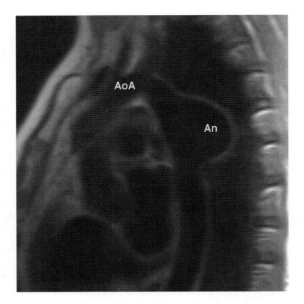

Figure 24.2 Acute presentation with haemoptysis. A young active woman who had undergone coarctation repair in early childhood presented after discontinuation of long-term follow-up. There had been no previous symptoms at rest or during exercise. CMR showed a large aortic aneurysm at the repaired coarctation site, a potentially fatal complication. The aneurysm was treated with a covered stent in the catheter laboratory. This case demonstrates that absence of symptoms is a poor indicator of individual risk and that regular assessment is needed in all athletes with CHD

moderate dynamic exercise after comprehensive assessment. General exercise advice should take into account the mechanisms of adaptation to cyanosis, such as a low cardiac exercise reserve due to high resting cardiac output, polycythaemia and coagulopathy, which requires optimal hydration at all times.

Transposition of the Great Arteries In the modern era, corrective surgery is performed in infancy by the arterial switch operation. In an earlier surgical epoch, the atrial switch operation (Mustard or Senning operation) was used. This had significant complications, which resulted in moderate to severe exercise intolerance. The most severe complication is progressive dysfunction of the systemic right ventricle, aggravated by tricuspid regurgitation and residual shunts. Tachyarrhythmias, including sustained atrial and ventricular arrhythmias, are also seen, and the risk for SCD is significant.

Following the prognostically favourable arterial switch operation, exercise capacity may be reduced secondary to left ventricular dysfunction and there is a potential for significant coronary artery stenosis. Arrhythmias are less common.

Congenitally Corrected Transposition of the Great Arteries Often, no operation is required in early childhood, unless there is coexistence of lesions such as VSD, pulmonary stenosis or tricuspid valve abnormalities. Progressive systemic right ventricular dysfunction, tricuspid regurgitation and AV conduction defects and progressive AV block are associated with a high morbidity in adulthood. Right ventricular failure and atrial and ventricular arrhythmias are the most serious complications during exercise. Exercise capacity may be moderately to severely limited. This diagnosis may present for the first time in adult life.

Fontan Circulation A univentricular (Fontan) circulation is the result of a staged surgical approach to create a direct connection between the systemic venous return and the pulmonary arteries, in which a single right or left ventricle supports the systemic circulation. This is the final surgical pathway for many of the most complex forms of CHD, characterised by an absent cardiac chamber or valve. The inability to increase stroke volume, a blunted chronotropic response, residual shunting with cyanosis and ventilatory and musculoskeletal impairment usually result in significantly reduced exercise capacity. However, some Fontan patients have managed to compete in significant endurance events, albeit at a low level of competition. Progressive sinus-node dysfunction and intra-atrial re-entry tachycardias are common. The risk of exercise-induced life-threatening arrhythmias is relatively low, but it increases with the degree of ventricular dysfunction.

Ebstein's Anomaly Ebstein's anomaly is represented by displacement of the tricuspid valve, leading to 'atrialisation' of the right ventricle. Exercise performance in Ebstein's anomaly is determined by the severity of tricuspid valve dysplasia, right ventricular dysfunction and interatrial shunting with cyanosis, and can vary from near-normal to severe incapacity. Ebstein's anomaly is often associated with the presence of AV accessory pathways. In combination with atrial dilatation, this can lead to a significant arrhythmia risk.

Conclusion

Athletes with significant CHD are still relatively uncommon, but their numbers are increasing. They represent a wide spectrum of functional variation, with a variable risk of cardiac dysfunction and arrhythmias. The key message for the sports cardiologist is to be aware of the underlying diagnosis, the potential for change in functional impairment with time, the relatively high arrhythmia risk and the need to ensure individualised assessment at rest and during exercise. Close collaboration with congenital heart specialists is recommended.

References

1 Van Der Linde, D., Konings, E.E., Slager, M.A. et al. Birth prevalence of congenital heart disease worldwide: a systematic review and meta-analysis. *J Am Coll Cardiol* 2011; **58**: 2241–7.

2 Marelli, A.J., Ionescu-Ittu, R., Mackie, A.S. et al. Lifetime prevalence of congenital heart disease in the general population from 2000 to 2010. *Circulation* 2014; **130**: 749–56.

3 Mitchell, S.C., Korones, S.B. and Berendes, H.W. Congenital heart disease in 56 109 births. Incidence and natural history. *Circulation* 1971; **43**: 323–32.

4 Pierpont, M.E., Basson, C.T., Benson, D.W. Jr et al. Genetic basis for congenital heart defects: current knowledge: a scientific statement from the American Heart Association Congenital Cardiac Defects Committee, Council on Cardiovascular Disease in the Young: endorsed by the American Academy of Pediatrics. *Circulation* 2007; **115**: 3015–38.

5 Longmuir, P.E., Brothers, J.A., De Ferranti, S.D. et al. Promotion of physical activity for children and adults with congenital heart disease: a scientific statement from the American Heart Association. *Circulation* 2013; **127**: 2147–59.

6 Inuzuka, R., Diller, G.P., Borgia, F. et al. Comprehensive use of cardiopulmonary exercise testing identifies adults with congenital heart disease at increased mortality risk in the medium term. *Circulation* 2012; **125**: 250–9.

7 Oechslin, E.N., Harrison, D.A., Connelly, M.S. et al. Mode of death in adults with congenital heart disease. *Am J Cardiol* 2000; **86**: 1111–16.

8 Koyak, Z., Harris, L., De Groot, J.R. et al. Sudden cardiac death in adult congenital heart disease. *Circulation* 2012; **126**: 1944–54.

9 Baumgartner, H., Bonhoeffer, P., De Groot, N.M. et al. ESC guidelines for the management of grown-up congenital heart disease (new version 2010). *Eur Heart J* 2010; **31**: 2915–57.

10 Maron, B.J., Doerer, J.J., Haas, T.S. et al. Sudden deaths in young competitive athletes: analysis of 1866 deaths in the United States, 1980–2006. *Circulation* 2009; **119**: 1085–92.

11 Graham, T.P. Jr, Driscoll, D.J., Gersony, W.M. et al. Task Force 2: congenital heart disease. *J Am Coll Cardiol* 2005; **45**: 1326–33.

12 Pelliccia, A., Zipes, D.P. and Maron, B.J. Bethesda Conference #36 and the European Society of Cardiology Consensus Recommendations revisited a comparison of US and European criteria for eligibility and disqualification of competitive athletes with cardiovascular abnormalities. *J Am Coll Cardiol* 2008; **52**: 1990–6.

13 Mitchell, J.H., Haskell, W., Snell, P. and Van Camp, S.P. Task Force 8: classification of sports. *J Am Coll Cardiol* 2005; **45**: 1364–7.

14 Budts, W., Borjesson, M., Chessa, M. et al. Physical activity in adolescents and adults with congenital heart defects: individualized exercise prescription. *Eur Heart J* 2013; **34**: 3669–74.

15 Pieles, G.E., Horn, R., Williams, C.A. and Stuart, A.G. Paediatric exercise training in prevention and treatment. *Arch Dis Child* 2014; **99**(4): 380–5.

16 Takken, T., Giardini, A., Reybrouck, T. et al. Recommendations for physical activity, recreation sport, and exercise training in paediatric patients with congenital heart disease: a report from the Exercise, Basic and Translational Research Section of the European Association of Cardiovascular Prevention and Rehabilitation, the European Congenital Heart and Lung Exercise Group, and the Association for European Paediatric Cardiology. *Eur J Prev Cardiol* 2012; **19**: 1034–65.

17 Kempny, A., Dimopoulos, K., Uebing, A. et al. Reference values for exercise limitations among adults with congenital heart disease. Relation to activities of daily life – single centre experience and review of published data. *Eur Heart J* 2012; **33**: 1386–96.

18 Dimopoulos, K., Okonko, D.O., Diller, G.P. et al. Abnormal ventilatory response to exercise in adults with congenital heart disease relates to cyanosis and predicts survival. *Circulation* 2006; **113**: 2796–802.

19 Dua, J.S., Cooper, A.R., Fox, K.R. and Graham Stuart, A. Exercise training in adults with congenital heart disease: feasibility and benefits. *Int J Cardiol* 2010; **138**: 196–205.

20 Drezner, J.A., Ackerman, M.J., Anderson, J. et al. Electrocardiographic interpretation in athletes: the 'Seattle criteria'. *Br J Sports Med* 2013; **47**: 122–4.

21 Khairy, P., Van Hare, G.F., Balaji, S. et al. PACES/HRS expert consensus statement on the recognition and management of arrhythmias in adult congenital heart disease: developed in partnership between the Pediatric and Congenital Electrophysiology Society (PACES) and the Heart Rhythm Society (HRS). Endorsed by the governing bodies of PACES, HRS, the American College of Cardiology (ACC), the American Heart Association (AHA), the European Heart Rhythm Association (EHRA), the Canadian Heart Rhythm Society (CHRS), and the International Society for Adult Congenital Heart Disease (ISACHD). *Heart Rhythm* 2014; **11**: e102–65.

22 Apitz, C., Webb, G.D. and Redington, A.N. Tetralogy of Fallot. *Lancet* 2009; **374**: 1462–71.

23 Mountjoy, M., Armstrong, N., Bizzini, L. et al. IOC consensus statement: 'training the elite child athlete'. *Br J Sports Med* 2008; **42**: 163–4.

24 Maron, B.J., Friedman, R.A., Kligfield, P. et al. Assessment of the 12-lead electrocardiogram as a screening test for detection of cardiovascular disease in healthy general populations of young people (12–25 years of age): a scientific statement from the American Heart Association and the American College of Cardiology. *J Am Coll Cardiol* 2014; **64**: 1479–514.

25 Gatzoulis, M.A., Balaji, S., Webber, S.A. et al. Risk factors for arrhythmia and sudden cardiac death late after repair of tetralogy of Fallot: a multicentre study. *Lancet* 2000; **356**: 975–81.

25 Congenital Coronary Artery Anomalies

Cristina Basso and Gaetano Thiene

Cardiovascular Pathology Unit, Department of Cardiac, Thoracic and Vascular Sciences, University of Padua Medical School, Padua, Italy

Introduction

Despite the low prevalence in the overall population, congenital coronary artery anomalies (CCAAs) are frequently found to be the cause of sudden death in the young, particularly during effort and/or on the athletic field [1–5]. The estimated prevalence of CCAA in the general population is based upon several sources, including angiography, computed tomography (CT), cardiac magnetic resonance (CMR) and autopsy databanks. Each of these has limitations due to entry biases and a lack of clear diagnostic criteria regarding an abnormality versus a normal variant. Thus, the prevalence of CCAA is quite variable, ranging from to 0.21 to 5.79% [4].

Older classification schemes divided CCAA into 'major' and 'minor', on the basis of the presence or not of haemodynamic consequences [1]. Those CCAAs connecting to the aorta (i.e. anomalies of number, size, orifices and course) were referred to as 'minor'. However, since even so-called 'minor' CCAA may be associated with ischaemia or life-threatening arrhythmias, this terminology was been abandoned. Subsequently, CCAAs with potential clinical implications (such as connection of a coronary artery to the pulmonary artery, coronary artery from the opposite sinus with an interarterial course, coronary artery fistulae, single coronary artery and certain variants of a myocardial bridge) were labelled as 'malignant', whilst all other anomalies were designated 'benign' CCAAs. Currently, the most commonly used classification of CCAA is based on pure anatomical considerations, recognising three categories: (i) anomalies of origin and course; (ii) anomalies of intrinsic coronary artery anatomy; and (iii) anomalies of termination [6].

This chapter reviews CCAAs considered at risk of sudden death during physical exertion.

Anomalous Origin of a Coronary Artery from the Pulmonary Trunk

This CCAA is usually highly symptomatic in infancy. Typically, the left coronary artery connects to the pulmonary artery or trunk (anomalous origin of the left coronary artery from the pulmonary artery, ALCAPA) and the right coronary artery connects normally to the aorta (so-called 'Bland–White–Garland (BWG) syndrome'). Coronary blood steal from the aorta to the pulmonary artery may occur, accounting for extensive myocardial infarction with either sudden death or congestive heart failure. The extent of the acquired collateral circulation between the two coronary arteries is the major determinant of the degree of ischaemia and clinical outcome. This explains why patients with well-established collaterals have the 'adult type' of ALCAPA, and those without or with few collaterals have the 'infant type', with early onset of symptoms. The availability of less invasive diagnostic modalities, such as CT and CMR, has resulted in a more frequent identification of this CCAA in older people [7]. However, this anomaly is only rarely observed in athletes or reported as a cause of sudden death in young adults.

IOC Manual of Sports Cardiology, First Edition. Edited by Mathew G. Wilson, Jonathan A. Drezner and Sanjay Sharma.
© 2017 International Olympic Committee. Published 2017 by John Wiley & Sons, Ltd.

Anomalous Coronary Artery Origin from a Wrong Aortic Sinus

Anomalous coronary artery origin, either the left main coronary artery from the right sinus of Valsalva or the right coronary artery from the left sinus, represents a rare congenital defect, found in 0.17% of patients undergoing autopsy, in 1.2% of all patients undergoing coronary angiography and in 0.17% of 2388 children and adolescents prospectively evaluated by transthoracic echocardiography (TTE) [4,8]. However, the clinical populations cannot be considered truly 'normal', since they comprise people referred for cardiovascular investigation. Thus, the prevalence in a large and unselected population is likely lower [9].

Usually, either the right coronary artery origin from the left coronary sinus or the left coronary artery origin from the right coronary sinus is a hidden condition, at risk of sudden death. The proximal anomalous coronary artery may run anterior to the pulmonary trunk (prepulmonic), posterior to the aorta (retroaortic), septal (subpulmonic) or, more frequently, between the pulmonary artery and the aorta (interarterial). Those with interarterial course are regarded as hidden conditions at risk of ischaemia and even sudden death (Figure 25.1) [1,2,4]. Several mechanisms of ischaemia, particularly during exercise, have been postulated: (i) increased cardiac output with expansion of the great arteries, accounting for compression of the anomalous vessel coursing between the aorta and the pulmonary artery; (ii) acute-angle take-off of the anomalous vessel, with further stretch during exercise; (iii) a spasm or kinking of the anomalous vessel; and (iv) intramural course of the proximal tract of the anomalous vessel within the aortic wall [4,6]. This intramural aortic course, originally documented in pathology reports [4], can explain the imaging feature (angiography and echocardiography) of coronary artery intussusception into the aortic wall, the narrowing of the proximal segment of the anomalous coronary segment (segmental hypoplasia) and the asymmetrical lateral compression of the anomalous vessel with a slit-like or ovoid rather than circular lumen, particularly during systole and stress [6].

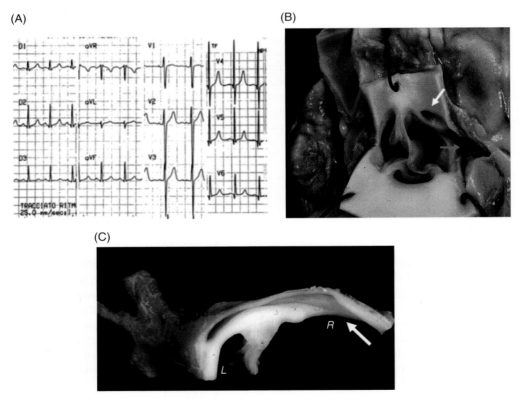

Figure 25.1 A 15-year-old soccer player with a history of exertional syncope died suddenly during the second half of a game. (A) Normal 12-lead ECG performed 10 months before death, as part of routine pre-participation screening. (B) View of the aortic root: note the right coronary artery arising normally from the right aortic sinus (red arrow) and the left main coronary artery arising anomalously from the right sinus, with an acute angle take-off producing a slit-like lumen (white arrow). (C) The transverse section of the aortic root at the commissural level, showing the intramural course of anomalous coronary artery just behind the commissure between the two coronary cusps. R, right cusp; L, left cusp

In anomalous coronary arteries from the wrong sinus, our findings typically demonstrate normal resting and stress ECG patterns but associated pathologic evidence of acute myocardial ischaemic damage and/or chronic ischaemic injury with replacement-type fibrosis [4], suggesting that myocardial ischaemia is episodic in nature and probably occurs in infrequent bursts, which may be cumulative with time. In a study comparing the various cardiovascular diseases (CVDs) accounting for sudden death in athletes versus nonathletes, congenital anomalies of coronary artery occurred more frequently in athletes than in nonathletes (12.2 vs 0.5%), confirming that they are particularly prone to causing cardiac arrest during exercise and physical exertion [5].

Although both right and left coronary artery anomalous origins from the wrong sinus pose a risk of sudden death, the anomalous left coronary artery from the right is considered higher-risk because ischaemia occurs in a larger amount of left ventricular myocardium. By contrast, an anomalous right coronary artery origin from the left sinus may be incidental at autopsy or at angiographic observation, and until recently has been considered a minor congenital anomaly of no clinical significance. Notably, we found that all our autopsy cases with anomalous left coronary artery died suddenly, as compared to 43% of cases with anomalous right coronary artery, suggesting the possibility of death from other causes [2].

Anomalous origin of the left coronary artery from the posterior aortic sinus is a rare coronary malformation and is infrequently associated with sudden death [2].

Other CCAAs from the Aorta: Variants of Uncertain Significance

An *anomalous origin of the left circumflex branch from the right coronary artery or right sinus*, itself with a separate ostium, is considered the most frequent CCAA, with an estimated prevalence of 0.67% [10]. This anomaly was regarded as a benign condition, having been observed incidentally at autopsy or angiography or in association with obstructive coronary atherosclerosis, until cases were reported with left circumflex branch-related myocardial infarction or sudden death in the absence of any disease other than the anomaly itself (Figure 25.2) [1,2]. The left circumflex branch usually shows an anomalous take-off and a retroaortic course to the left atrioventricular (AV) groove, crossing the mitroaortic fibrous continuity. At present, it is recommended that the clinical significance of this CCAA be judged using a case-by-case integrated approach, after exclusion of all other possible causes of ischaemia in patients with symptoms or signs. Importantly, in our series of sudden death in competitive athletes, anomalous left circumflex from the right has never been found amongst structural causes at autopsy.

Another variant is an *anomalous left anterior descending (LAD) coronary artery arising from the right coronary artery*. In coronary angiography studies, the prevalence of this anomaly was noted in 0.006% of patients. It can be classified based on the course of the LAD: preaortic (interarterial), prepulmonic (anterior), retroaortic, intraseptal or a combination. The anterior type is the most common, and is generally thought to be benign.

The *single coronary artery* is a very rare CCAA, seen in only 0.0024–0.0440% of the population [11]. There is only one coronary artery originating from the aorta, with a single ostium, taking the course of either the right or the left coronary artery and dividing into two or three of the main coronary branches. A single coronary artery is compatible with a normal life expectancy, but when a major coronary artery branch courses between the pulmonary artery and the aorta, patients are at increased risk of myocardial ischaemia, with a mechanism similar to that of wrong sinus CCAA. Moreover, atherosclerotic lesions may be devastating due to the obvious inability to develop collaterals.

High take-off of a coronary artery consists in the origin of a coronary artery from the tubular portion of the aorta and is considered a variant of normal, without consequences unless surgical procedures are performed. However, there are some case reports of this anomaly (both clinical and at autopsy; i.e. otherwise unexplained myocardial infarction or sudden death cases) perhaps supporting a role for this anomaly in precipitating myocardial ischaemia [2]. In some instances, a funnel-like ostium and a vertical intramural aortic course of the first tract of the anomalous vessel have been described, before the aortic root. The clinical significance of this variant remains controversial.

Hypoplastic coronary artery is amongst the rare CCAAs that bring a risk of sudden death and which are characterised by underdevelopment of at least one of the major epicardial coronary arteries [12]. Coronary artery hypoplasia can manifest as a narrowed luminal diameter or a shortened course, and is typically present in one or two of the three major epicardial branches. A luminal diameter <1.5 mm with no nearby compensatory branches has been proposed as a criterion for diagnosis. In a post mortem analysis of athletes who died suddenly, hypoplastic coronary arteries were identified in less than 5% [3].

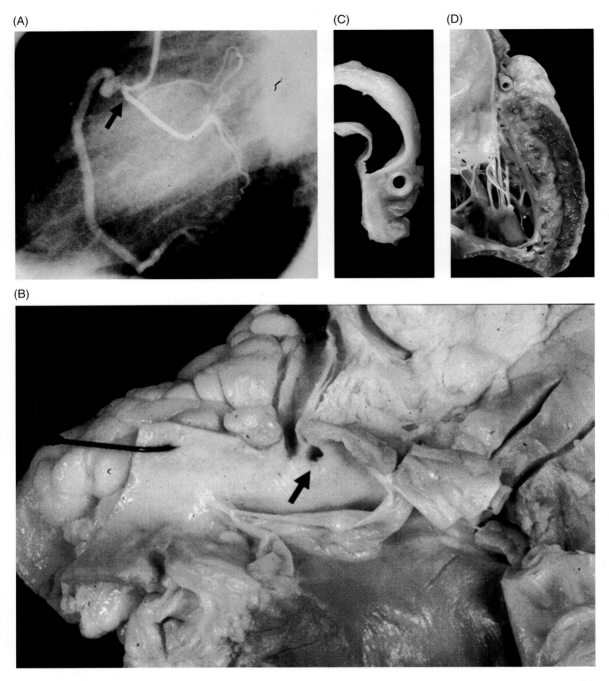

Figure 25.2 Anomalous origin of the left circumflex branch form the right aortic sinus with a retroaortic course in a 52-year-old patient with acute myocardial infarction. (A) Selective coronary angiography with contrast medium in both the right coronary artery and left circumflex branch (arrow). (B) Aortic root. Note the presence of two ostia in the right coronary sinus, with the left circumflex on the right side (arrow). (C) Longitudinal section of the aortic root, showing the retroaortic course of the anomalous left circumflex branch. (D) Extensive subendocardial fibrosis of the lateral left ventricular wall

Myocardial bridge or tunnelled epicardial coronary artery consists of a major epicardial coronary artery, usually the LAD, coursing deep within the myocardium, with an intramural course [13]. The pathognomonic angiographic sign is the so-called 'milking effect': a transient systolic vessel constriction due to myocardial compression. A significant vessel constriction is present when there is a ≥70% luminal reduction during

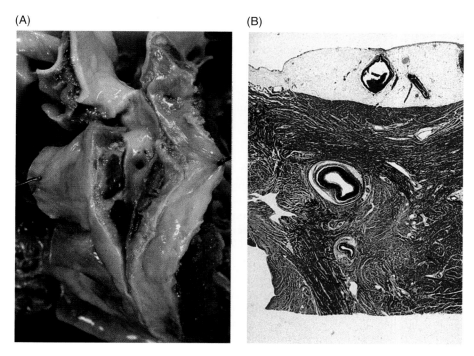

Figure 25.3 A 35-year-old competitive athlete who died suddenly on effort. (A) Gross examination showed a deep intramyocardial course (myocardial bridge) of the LAD coronary artery. (B) At histology, a thick myocardium encircled the coronary segments. Note the presence of disarray and interstitial fibrosis

systole and persistent ≥35% reduction during mid to late diastole [14]. This phenomenon can be accentuated by intracoronary nitroglycerin injection through vasodilatation of the adjacent normal coronary segment. The prevalence of this CCAA at angiography is lower than at autopsy (0.5–2.5% vs. 15–85%), since many bridges consist of thin loops of myocardium not causing haemodynamic changes [13]. Coronary bridges are quite common in hypertrophic cardiomyopathy (HCM), with a frequency of about 25% [15].

The clinical significance and pathophysiology of this CCAA are still a matter of debate. Myocardial ischaemia has been reported in patients in whom coronary angiography detected nothing but a 'milking effect' and in whom surgical debridging was revealed to be effective in relieving both signs and symptoms. Moreover, sudden death has been described in patients with myocardial bridge as the only plausible substrate accounting for sudden death (Figure 25.3) [3,5]. Maron et al. [3] have reported tunnelled coronary arteries in approximately 5% of athletic field deaths, in the absence of any other structural anomaly. Effort-induced ischaemia has been attributed to tachycardia, which increases the myocardial oxygen requirement and reduces the coronary flow during diastole.

Features such as a long (2–3 cm) and deep (2–3 mm) intramural course, with a sheath of myocardium totally encircling the coronary artery segment with disarray and fibrosis, are in keeping not only with a systolic lumen obliteration but also with persistent occlusion during diastole, when coronary blood filling occurs, due to unpaired relaxation of the myocardium surrounding the anomalous coronary segment. Clinically significant myocardial bridges can be characterised on intravascular ultrasound (IVUS) by phasic systolic vessel compression, persistent reduction in the diastolic lumen, increased blood flow velocities, retrograde systolic flow and decreased coronary flow reserve [14].

Coronary artery fistula consists of a communication of one or two coronary arteries with either a cardiac chamber or any of the great vessels [16]. The prevalence is up to 0.2% in patients who undergo selective coronary angiography. The fistula usually drains into the right ventricle, then the right atrium and the pulmonary arteries, and less commonly (<10%) into the left atrium or left ventricle. The resistance (which is determined by fistula size, tortuosity and length) and the site of drainage are the major determinants of the haemodynamic consequences of coronary artery fistulae. The blood flow from the coronary artery to a venous structure or right-sided cardiac chamber occurs throughout the cardiac cycle; with larger fistulae, a diastolic 'coronary steal' may exist, drawing blood away from the normal coronary tree, leading to symptoms and signs of myocardial ischaemia. If the fistula drains to the systemic venous circulation, a left-to-right shunt develops, with increasing pulmonary blood flow and volume overloading of both ventricles. When the drainage site is the left atrium or pulmonary vein, a left-to-left shunt and left heart volume overload occur. Small fistulae in asymptomatic children should be followed up for signs of increasing size and flow, because of their tendency to grow with age. It is recommended to close them early in both symptomatic and asymptomatic patients with large and haemodynamically significant fistulae. To the best of our knowledge, no athletic field death has been ascribed to coronary artery fistula.

In Vivo Diagnosis of CCAA Carrying a Risk of Sudden Death

In the past, CCAAs were rarely suspected or identified during life and were usually first recognised at autopsy, largely because of a lack of clinical suspicion, as well as the limits implicit in routine examination and clinical testing. With the increasing availability and use of noninvasive imaging techniques, such as echocardiography, CMR and CT, the identification of CCAA has become more frequent, even in people without symptoms or signs of myocardial ischaemia. The most studied CCAAs are wrong sinus origin and myocardial bridging.

In a series of young competitive athletes who died suddenly due to wrong sinus CCAA, sudden death was frequently the first manifestation, although premonitory cardiac symptoms commonly occurred shortly before sudden death, particularly in the setting of anomalous left main coronary artery origin, suggesting that a history of exertional syncope or chest pain requires exclusion of this anomaly [4]. Notably, all the resting 12-lead and exercise ECGs available during life were normal. Moreover, by reviewing the literature concerning exercise ECG findings in young patients with documented CCAA, only 4 out of 18 (22%), including two who were already symptomatic, showed ischaemic changes. The observation that the conventional 12-lead ECG and even the maximal exercise stress test are usually within normal limits (i.e. show no evidence of myocardial ischaemia) suggests that the latter is not always present in the clinical course of the disease. These findings have important implications for preventive strategies and in vivo identification. Therefore, ECG stress testing and even myocardial perfusion scintigraphy may provide little or no diagnostic information in patients with suspected CCAA. If the index of suspicion is sufficiently high, because of potential clinical markers such as exertional syncope or chest pain – even in the setting of a normal 12-lead and effort ECG – the origin and proximal course of the coronary artery should be established noninvasively by TTE or transoesophageal echocardiography (TOE), and if needed by more advanced imaging. Indeed, in one study, in young individuals presenting with symptoms and/or ECG changes, echocardiography provided correct identification of wrong aortic sinus origin, which was subsequently confirmed by coronary angiography [17].

Echocardiography has the potential to make the correct diagnosis, because it provides good anatomic definition of the ostium and proximal epicardial course of the coronary artery. In a series of 1360 young athletes prospectively evaluated by echocardiography, Pelliccia et al. [9] were able to visualise the ostium and proximal course of the left coronary artery in 97% and those of the right coronary artery in 80% of subjects. As a consequence, the failure to demonstrate that coronary arteries actually originate from their usual location in a young person with a history of syncope or angina suggests the need for further anatomic investigation by angiography or possibly CMR and CT angiography [4]. However, false negatives may occur when using TTE, as demonstrated by Davis et al. [8], due either to misinterpretations or to the inability to fully identify the origin of the coronary arteries as a result of poor acoustic windows.

The American Heart Association (AHA) committee on cardiovascular imaging has offered a class IIa/b recommendation that evaluation of CCAA be performed by either CT or CMR, although due to radiation concerns, CMR is preferred [18]. The European Society of Cardiology (ESC) recommends CT angiography for investigation in patients with a clinical suspicion of CCAA [19].

Functional assessment of CCAA is even more challenging than in vivo diagnosis. According to Angelini et al. [6], after a CCAA of wrong sinus origin is identified, clinical management should be based on nuclear stress, coronary angiography to evaluate for the presence of atherosclerotic disease and IVUS of the anomalous vessel. These authors suggest a grading of CCAA severity according to IVUS criteria (i.e. the amount of hypoplasia of the proximal vessel compared with the circumference of the distal vessel, and the degree of lateral compression of the proximal vessel). Combined fractional flow reserve (FFR) assessment is also recommended for a more complete assessment of the haemodynamic importance of the CCAA [14]. Both IVUS and FFR should be performed both at baseline and with dobutamine pharmacological stress.

After the imaging diagnosis of myocardial bridging by angiography ('milking effect') and/or CT (where bridges are defined as coronary segments surrounded by myocardium), the major challenge is again functional assessment to guide management decisions [14,20].

Recent developments such as stress single-photon emission CT can detect reversible myocardial perfusion defects in patients with myocardial bridging, with a correlation between the amount of ischaemia and the degree of systolic luminal narrowing.

Coronary physiological measurements across a myocardial bridge during pharmacological infusion can also be valuable. The bridged segment produces a distinctive flow velocity called the 'fingertip' phenomenon. FFR can be measured to assess haemodynamically significant stenosis, with a value <0.75 suggesting the presence of ischaemia. In the setting of abnormal but nonischaemic FFR (>0.80), intravenous administration of dobutamine can lead to higher pressure gradients with angina symptoms. However, there is a grey zone with an FFR of 0.75–0.80. Higher average peak velocity and greater pressure gradients with infusion of dobutamine compared with adenosine suggest a haemodynamically significant myocardial bridge. Finally, intracoronary acetylcholine infusion (off-label use) could provoke vasoconstriction, unmasking endothelial dysfunction or coronary vasospasm.

Adjunctive imaging by IVUS can reveal the characteristic 'half-moon' sign, an echolucent area between the bridged coronary segment and epicardial tissue that persists throughout the cardiac cycle. Moreover, IVUS can visualise noncritical atherosclerosis proximal to the bridged segment.

Both in symptomatic patients and in those with an 'incidental' finding of myocardial bridging by angiography or CT, there is no consensus on whether further diagnostic studies are needed before therapy.

Risk Stratification and Clinical Management

Timely in vivo diagnosis of CCAA raises questions about the clinical management of affected patients. The clinical challenge is to identify high-risk patients, in order to decide who should undergo medical or surgical therapy, and when.

Notably, even when dealing with a sudden death victim with CCAA, we recognise that it is important to accept that different degrees of certainty (certain, highly probable, uncertain) exist in defining the cause–effect relationship between the CCAA and the sudden death event [21]. For instance, ALCAPA is listed amongst certain causes of sudden death, the anomalous origin of the left coronary artery from the right sinus and interarterial course is listed amongst highly probable causes and all the other 'minor' CCAAs from the aorta (right coronary artery from the left sinus, left coronary artery from the right without interarterial course, high take-off from the tubular portion, left circumflex branch originating from the right sinus or right coronary artery etc.) are listed amongst uncertain causes of sudden death. In the probable and, especially, the uncertain categories, each case should be considered on its individual merits. The clinical history and the circumstances of death may influence the final determination of cause of death.

Recommendations for CCAA of ectopic arterial origin, for anomalous left coronary artery from the pulmonary artery and for coronary arteriovenous fistula have been developed within the American College of Cardiology (ACC)/AHA 2008 guidelines for the management of adults with congenital heart diseases (CHDs) [22].

The definitive treatment for ALCAPA is surgical intervention, with direct reimplantation of the anomalous coronary artery into the aortic coronary artery or coronary bypass grafting. The AHA/ACC recommendations for ALCAPA are class I, level of evidence C: (i) in patients with ALCAPA, reconstruction of a dual coronary artery supply should be performed – the surgery should be performed by surgeons with training and expertise in CHD at centres with expertise in the management of anomalous coronary artery origins; (ii) for adult survivors of ALCAPA repair, clinical evaluation with echocardiography and noninvasive stress testing are indicated every 3–5 years.

Patients with CCAA of wrong sinus type can be managed medically, surgically or even by percutaneous coronary intervention. Medical treatment consists of beta blockers and avoidance of physical exercise.

Surgical correction of CCAA with wrong aortic sinus origin may be accomplished either by coronary artery bypass grafting or by newer techniques such as reimplantation of the anomalous vessel in the proper coronary sinus or 'unroofing' of the common wall between the aorta and the anomalous coronary artery, resulting in a new orifice with a more natural take-off. According to the ACC/AHA 2008 guidelines, surgical coronary revascularisation should be performed in patients with any of the following indications:

- *Class I, level of evidence B.* (i) Anomalous left main coronary artery coursing between the aorta and pulmonary artery. (ii) Documented coronary ischaemia due to coronary compression (when coursing between the great arteries or in intramural fashion). (iii) Anomalous origin of the right coronary artery between the aorta and pulmonary artery, with evidence of ischaemia.
- *Class IIa, level of evidence C.* (i) Documented vascular wall hypoplasia, coronary compression or documented obstruction to coronary flow, regardless of the inability to document coronary ischaemia. (ii) Documented anomalous coronary artery origin from the opposite sinus.
- *Class IIb, level of evidence C.* Anomalous LAD coronary artery coursing between the aorta and the pulmonary artery.

Treatment options for coronary artery fistulae include surgical ligation, either isolated or in association with coronary artery bypass grafting, and interventional closure with occlusion coils, umbrellas, vascular plugs and covered stents [16]. The ACC/AHA 2008 recommendations indicate that:

- *Class I, level of evidence C.* (i) If a continuous murmur is present, its origin should be defined by echocardiography, CMR, CT angiography or cardiac catheterisation. (ii) A large fistula, regardless of symptomatology, should be closed via either a transcatheter or a surgical route, after delineation of its course and its potential to fully obliterate the fistula. (iii) A small to moderate fistula in the presence of documented myocardial ischaemia, arrhythmia, otherwise unexplained ventricular systolic or diastolic dysfunction or enlargement or endarteritis should be closed via either a transcatheter or a surgical approach, after delineation of its course and its potential to fully obliterate the fistula.
- *Class IIa, level of evidence C.* Clinical follow-up with echocardiography every 3–5 years can be useful for patients with small, asymptomatic fistulae, to exclude development of symptoms or arrhythmias, growth or chamber enlargement that might alter management.
- *Class III, level of evidence C.* Patients with small, asymptomatic fistulae should not undergo closure.

Finally, for myocardial bridges, the 'Schwarz classification' has been suggested as a guide to therapy, because it has been linked to clinical outcomes following pharmacological and invasive interventions [14,20]. Patients with incidental finding of myocardial bridge on angiography and no objective signs of ischaemia (Schwarz type A) need no treatment, but patients with ischaemia on stress test and objective signs of ischaemia (type B) or with altered intracoronary haemodynamics – quantitative coronary angiography/coronary flow reserve/Doppler – with or without objective signs of ischaemia (type C) show significant symptomatic improvement with beta blockers or calcium channel blockers at 5-year follow-up. Patients with Schwarz type C refractory to medical therapy may be considered for revascularisation of the myocardial bridge. To this end, myotomy, coronary artery bypass grafting and even percutaneous coronary intervention with stent implantation can be considered.

CCAA and Consensus Guidelines for Eligibility/Disqualification

In this section, we examine three official consensus guidelines for eligibility/disqualification decisions in competitive athletes with cardiovascular abnormalities which consider CCAAs: (i) the 36th Bethesda Conference, published in 2005 [23]; (ii) the Study Group of Sports Cardiology of the Working Group of Cardiac Rehabilitation and Exercise Physiology and the Working Group of Myocardial and Pericardial Diseases of the European Society of Cardiology, published in 2005 [24]; and (iii) the fourth edition of the Italian Cardiological Guidelines for Sports Eligibility, published in 2009 [25].

The *36th Bethesda Conference* recommends that all patients with *CCAA of wrong sinus with an interarterial course* be excluded from all participation in competitive sports [23]. If ischaemia is present on exercise testing, corrective surgery should be performed. Participation in all sports is permitted 3 months after successful operation for an athlete without ischaemia, ventricular arrhythmia or tachyarrhythmia or dysfunction during maximal exercise testing. In cases where there is evidence of previous myocardial infarction, the recommendations for ischaemic heart disease are the same as those reported in the pertinent subchapter of the Bethesda Conference. The management of patients with *isolated myocardial bridging* depends on objective evidence of myocardial ischaemia at rest or with exercise. In the absence of these symptoms or signs, the athlete can participate in all competitive sports. If there is evidence of ischaemia or a prior myocardial infarction, activity should be limited to low-intensity competitive sports. Athletes with surgical resection of the myocardial bridge or stenting should be restricted to low-intensity sports for at least 6 months after the procedure. Athletes who remain asymptomatic after the procedure should undergo exercise testing. If exercise tolerance is normal for age and gender and there is no evidence of exercise-induced ischaemia, the athlete may participate in all competitive sports. Special recommendations for the management of myocardial bridging in patients with HCM are reported in the cardiomyopathy chapter of the Bethesda Conference.

In the *2005 ESC recommendations* for competitive sports participation in athletes with CVD, the CCAAs are listed together with other CHDs considered not compatible with competitive sports, due to their morphologic severity/complexity and their tendency to cause serious arrhythmias [24]. However, the CCAAs are not further subdivided according to the type of anomaly, without any ad hoc recommendation (wrong sinus vs myocardial bridge vs fistulae, etc.).

Finally, the *fourth edition of the Italian Cardiological Guidelines for Sports Eligibility*, also known as COCIS, includes CCAA in the chapter on CHDs and acquired valve diseases [25]. People with a diagnosis of *CCAA from the wrong sinus*, without any further distinction, should not participate in competitive sports activities. Surgical correction is recommended in symptomatic patients. In cases that undergo surgical correction, it is recommended that evaluation for sport eligibility be conducted at referral centres with relevant experience. For *coronary artery fistulae*, asymptomatic athletes with small fistulae and without evidence of ischaemia, arrhythmias or ventricular dysfunction are eligible for all sports so long as they undergo periodic check-up. Athletes with large coronary artery fistulae, with significant shunt and/or myocardial ischaemia and/or arrhythmias and/or ventricular dysfunction, should not participate in any competitive sports activities. Surgical or interventional closure is recommended, and sport eligibility must be assessed following correction at centres with relevant experience. Finally, people with a diagnosis of a *myocardial bridge*, even in the absence of ischaemia at rest or on effort, should not participate in any competitive sports activities, with the exception of group A sports (i.e. neurogenic, characterised mainly by increases in heart rate from minimum to moderate, due to the emotional component).

Overall, there are many 'weak points' in the field of recommendations for sport activity in athletes with CCAA. First, the Italian guidelines group conditions with different 'clinical weights', such as the anomalous left coronary artery from the right sinus and the anomalous right coronary artery from the left, and give them the same level of recommendation. There is no mention of the different behaviours of CCAAs with an interarterial course and of those without in the COCIS, the ESC or the Bethesda guidelines. The anomalous origin of the left circumflex branch from the right is not separately mentioned, and as such, without a detailed analysis of this subgroup of CCAA, the current recommendations are the same as for wrong sinus CCAA. The Bethesda conference makes a clear distinction between those myocardial bridges that are symptomatic and/or have ischaemia signs and those that do not, whilst the ESC and Italian guidelines consider the myocardial bridge per se at risk.

Obviously, these consensuses emanate from largely different cultural, social and legal backgrounds. Updated recommendations for the evaluation, management and eligibility/disqualification of athletes with CCAA were recently published by the AHA/ACC [26]. Additional study, taking into account all the previous considerations and possibly incorporating prospective data from clinical registries of affected patients is needed to further refine management recommendations.

We provide our personal perspective on the management of CCAA in Figure 25.4.

	Wrong sinus LCA[a]	Wrong sinus RCA[a]	LCx from RCA or RCS	MB
Chest pain: Ischaemia/VAs /syncope	Surgery	Surgery	Surgery	Medical therapy surgery
IVUS compression/ hypoplasia	Surgery? sport restriction	Surgery? sport restriction	NA	NA
Asymptomatic	Sport restriction Surgery?	Sport restriction	Regular sport activity	Regular sport activity

Figure 25.4 Authors' perspective on the management of CCAA. [a]With an interarterial or intramural course. LCA, left coronary artery; RCA, right coronary artery; LCx, left circumflex; RCS, right coronary sinus; MB, myocardial bridge; VAs, ventricular arrhythmias; IVUS, intravascular ultrasound; NA, not applicable

Conclusion

CCAAs are a major cause of sudden death in athletes. There are many different anatomic anomalies, each with its own risk based on its precise location and morphologic features. A careful evaluation for CCAA should be made in athletes who present with exertional chest pain, syncope or ventricular arrhythmia. Existing guidelines for the management of CCAA present inconsistencies that require more research but can serve as a foundation for management. Prudent treatment of CCAA should be guided by the location and course of the anomaly, a detailed assessment of anatomic risk characteristics and the specific sporting demands of the athlete. Treatment can be assisted by expert centres.

Acknowledgement

Supported by the Registry of Cardio-Cerebro-Vascular Pathology, Veneto Region, Venice, Italy.

References

1 Roberts, W.C. Major anomalies of coronary arterial origin seen in adulthood. *Am Heart J* 1986; **111**: 941–63.

2 Frescura, C., Basso, C., Thiene, G. et al. Anomalous origin of coronary arteries and risk of sudden death: a study based on an autopsy population of congenital heart disease. *Hum Pathol* 1998; **29**: 689–95.

3 Maron, B., Doerer, J., Haas, T. et al. Sudden deaths in young competitive athletes: analysis of 1866 deaths in the United States, 1980–2006. *Circulation* 2009; **119**: 1085–92.

4 Basso, C., Maron, B.J., Corrado, D. and Thiene, G. Clinical profile of congenital coronary artery anomalies with origin from the wrong aortic sinus leading to sudden death in young competitive athletes. *J Am Coll Cardiol* 2000; **35**: 1493–501.

5 Corrado, D., Basso, C., Rizzoli, G. et al. Does sports activity enhance the risk of sudden death in adolescents and young adults? *J Am Coll Cardiol* 2003; **42**: 1959–63.

6 Angelini, P. Coronary artery anomalies: an entity in search of an identity. *Circulation* 2007; **115**: 1296–305.

7 Yau, J.M., Singh, R., Halpern, E.J. and Fischman, D. Anomalous origin of the left coronary artery from the pulmonary artery in adults: a comprehensive review of 151 adult cases and a new diagnosis in a 53-year-old woman. *Clin Cardiol* 2011; **34**: 204–10.

8 Davis, J.A., Cecchin, F., Jones, T.K. and Portman, M.A. Major coronary artery anomalies in a pediatric population: incidence and clinical importance. *J Am Coll Cardiol* 2001; **37**: 593–7.

9 Pelliccia, A., Spataro, A. and Maron, B.J. Prospective echocardiographic screening for coronary artery anomalies in 1360 elite competitive athletes. *Am J Cardiol* 1993; **72**: 978–9.

10 Page, H.L., Engel, H.J., Campbell, W.B. and Thomas, C.S. Anomalous origin of the left circumflex coronary artery: recognition, angiographic demonstration and clinical significance. *Circulation* 1974; **50**: 768–73.

11 Desmet, W., Vanhaecke, J., Vrolix, M. et al. Isolated single coronary artery: a review of 50 000 consecutive coronary angiographies. *Eur Heart J* 1992; **13**: 1637–40.

12 Zugibe, F.T., Zugibe, F.T. Jr, Costello, J.T. and Breithaupt, M.K. Hypoplastic coronary artery disease within the spectrum of sudden unexpected death in young and middle age adults. *Am J Forensic Med Pathol* 1993; **14**: 276–83.

13 Angelini, P., Trivellato, M., Donis, J. and Leachman, R.D. Myocardial bridges: a review. *Prog Cardiovasc* 1983; **26**: 75–88.

14 Corban, M.T., Hung, O.Y., Eshtehardi, P. et al. Myocardial bridging: contemporary understanding of pathophysiology with implications for diagnostic and therapeutic strategies. *J Am Coll Cardiol* 2014; **63**: 2346–55.

15 Basso, C., Thiene, G., Mackey-Bojack, S. et al. Myocardial bridging, a frequent component of the hypertrophic cardiomyopathy phenotype, lacks systematic association with sudden cardiac death. *Eur Heart J* 2009; **30**: 1627–34.

16 Mangukia, C. Coronary artery fistula. *Ann Thorac Surg* 2012; **93**: 2084–92.

17 Zeppilli, P., Dello Russo, A., Santini, C. et al. In vivo detection of coronary artery anomalies in asymptomatic athletes by echocardiographic screening. *Chest* 1998; **114**: 89–93.

18 Bluemke, D.A., Achenbach, S., Budoff, M. et al. Noninvasive coronary artery imaging: magnetic resonance angiography and multidetector computed tomography angiography: a scientific statement from the American Heart Association committee on cardiovascular imaging and intervention of the council on cardiovascular radiology and intervention, and the councils on clinical cardiology and cardiovascular disease in the young. *Circulation* 2008; **118**: 586–606.

19 Schroeder, S., Achenbach, S., Bengel, F. et al. Cardiac computed tomography: indications, applications, limitations, and training requirements: report of a Writing Group deployed by the Working Group Nuclear Cardiology and Cardiac CT of the European Society of Cardiology and the European Council of Nuclear Cardiology. *Eur Heart J* 2008; **29**: 531–56.

20 Schwarz, E.R., Gupta, R., Haager, P.K. et al. Myocardial bridging in absence of coronary artery disease: proposal of a new classification based on clinical-angiographic data and long-term follow-up. *Cardiology* 2009; **112**(1): 13–21.

21 Basso, C., Burke, M., Fornes, P. et al. Guidelines for autopsy investigation of sudden cardiac death. *Virchows Arch* 2008; **452**: 11–18.

22 Warnes, C., Williams, R.G., Bashore, T.M. et al. ACC/AHA 2008 guidelines for the management of adults with congenital heart disease: a report of the American College of Cardiology/American Heart Association Task Force on Practice Guidelines (Writing Committee to Develop Guidelines on the Management of Adults With Congenital Heart Disease). *J Am Coll Cardiol* 2008; **52**: e143–263.

23 Maron, B.J. and Zipes, D.P. 36th Bethesda Conference: eligibility recommendations for competitive athletes with cardiovascular abnormalities. *J Am Coll Cardiol* 2005; **45**: 2–64.

24 Pelliccia, A., Fagard, R., Bjørnstad, H.H. et al. Recommendations for competitive sports participation in athletes with cardiovascular disease: a consensus document from the Study Group of Sports Cardiology of the Working Group of Cardiac Rehabilitation and Exercise Physiology and the Working Group of Myocardial and Pericardial Diseases of the European Society of Cardiology. *Eur Heart J* 2005; **26**: 1422–45.

25 Cardiovascular Guidelines for Eligibility in Competitive Sports (COCIS – 4th edn). *Med Sport* 2010; **63**: 5–136.

26 Van Hare, G.F., Ackerman, M.J., Evangelista, J.A. et al. Eligibility and disqualification recommendations for competitive athletes with cardiovascular abnormalities: Task force 4: Congenital Heart Disease: A Scientific Statement From the American Heart Association and American College of Cardiology. *J Am Coll Cardiol* 2015; **66**: 2372–84.

Section 3
Ion Channelopathies, Accessory Pathways and Electrical Disease

26 Long QT Syndrome

David J. Tester and Michael J. Ackerman

Departments of Medicine, Pediatrics, and Molecular Pharmacology & Experimental Therapeutics, Divisions of Cardiovascular Diseases and Pediatric Cardiology, Windland Smith Rice Sudden Death Genomics Laboratory, Mayo Clinic, Rochester, MN, USA

Introduction

Long QT syndrome is a potentially lethal, genetically mediated ventricular arrhythmia syndrome with the hallmark electrocardiographic (ECG) feature of QT prolongation. Symptoms, if present, include syncope, seizures and aborted cardiac arrest stemming from torsades de pointes. Cut-off values that define QT prolongation (corrected for heart rate) in an asymptomatic athlete must be carefully chosen, given the wide variation of QT interval corrected for heart rate (QTc) values found in population-derived cohorts. This chapter will examine the prevalence and clinical presentation of long QT syndrome, its contribution as a cause of sudden cardiac death (SCD), the diagnostic and therapeutic approach to the athlete with suspected long QT syndrome and considerations in the context of exercise and physical activity recommendations.

Clinical Presentation of Long QT Syndrome

With an estimated incidence as high as 1 in 2000 persons, congenital long QT syndrome is a distinct group of cardiac channelopathies characterised by delayed repolarisation of the ventricular myocardium, QT prolongation (QTc >480 ms as the 50th percentile amongst long QT cohorts) and increased risk for torsadogenic syncope, seizures and SCD in an otherwise healthy young individual with a structurally normal heart [1]. The mean age of onset for symptoms is 12 years, and earlier manifestation typically associates with more severe disease [2]. Long QT individuals may or may not express QT prolongation, due to cardiac action potential duration lengthening, as seen on a resting 12-lead surface ECG [3]. In addition, lengthening of the ventricular repolarisation duration is often accompanied by distinct morphological T-wave alterations (i.e. diphasic T-waves, notches, low amplitude or very low onset), some of which may be gene-specific [3]. Although rare, macroscopic T-waves may correlate with a poor prognosis [2].

This cardiac repolarisation abnormality often has no consequence; rarely, however, the heart is caught off guard and precipitated into a potentially lethal ventricular arrhythmia following triggers associated with an adrenergic surge, such as exertion, swimming, extreme emotion, sudden auditory stimuli (e.g. an alarm clock, phone ringing, doorbell) or the postpartum period [1]. Although most events are triggered by adrenergic stress, approximately 10–15% of patients experience symptoms at rest [2]. Whilst the cardiac rhythm usually spontaneously returns to a normal rhythm, resulting only in a transient episode of syncope, about 5–10% of unsuspecting and untreated long QT individuals succumb to a fatal arrhythmia as their sentinel event. However, it is estimated that nearly half of undiagnosed patients experiencing SCD stemming from this highly treatable disorder may have displayed unrecognised 'warning signs' (e.g. exertional syncope, family history of premature sudden death) prior to their fatal event [4]. In fact, long QT syndrome may explain as much as 20% of autopsy-negative sudden unexplained death in the young (SUDY) [4]. Therefore, the clinical approach to evaluation, diagnosis and therapy is critical to the safeguarding of an individual with long QT syndrome.

IOC Manual of Sports Cardiology, First Edition. Edited by Mathew G. Wilson, Jonathan A. Drezner and Sanjay Sharma.
© 2017 International Olympic Committee. Published 2017 by John Wiley & Sons, Ltd.

Diagnostic Approach for an Athlete with Suspected Long QT Syndrome

Because of the potential enormity of the price paid by the athlete and their family when long QT syndrome is misdiagnosed and mismanaged, it is critical for the sports cardiologist to have a thoughtful and systematic diagnostic approach when evaluating someone who they suspect to have long QT syndrome. Recently, two of the world's long QT syndrome experts provided their personal systematic six-step approach to the evaluation of such patients (Figure 26.1), which takes into consideration, in sequential order, (i) the pre-test probability of long QT syndrome, (ii) the patient's personal story, (iii) family history, (iv) ECG findings, (v) provocative testing, and (vi) genetic testing results [5].

Pre-Test Probability

It must be recognised that before evaluating a patient, obtaining their personal and family history and reviewing their 12-lead ECG, the chance of their having long QT syndrome is only 1 in 2000 [5]. In contrast, the pre-test probability may be as high as 50% for a relative of someone who already has clinically established and genetically confirmed long QT syndrome.

Personal Story

Understanding the patient's storyline should be one of the strongest factors that either increases or decreases the likelihood of disease [5]. Considering that about half of all patients with long QT syndrome have manifested or will experience at least one episode of long QT syndrome-triggered syncope, seizure or cardiac arrest and that experiencing a torsadogenic episode is the leading clinical determinant for a subsequent episode, the meticulous interrogation of every spell the patient has experienced is necessary, and in each

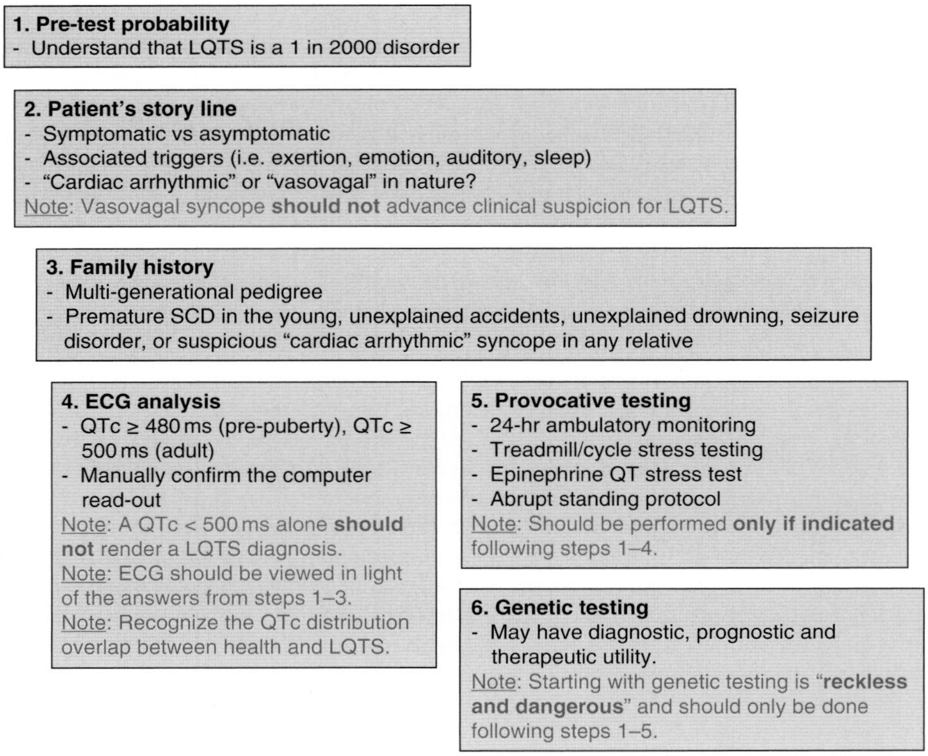

---

1. Pre-test probability
- Understand that LQTS is a 1 in 2000 disorder

2. Patient's story line
- Symptomatic vs asymptomatic
- Associated triggers (i.e. exertion, emotion, auditory, sleep)
- "Cardiac arrhythmic" or "vasovagal" in nature?
Note: Vasovagal syncope **should not** advance clinical suspicion for LQTS.

3. Family history
- Multi-generational pedigree
- Premature SCD in the young, unexplained accidents, unexplained drowning, seizure disorder, or suspicious "cardiac arrhythmic" syncope in any relative

4. ECG analysis
- QTc ≥ 480 ms (pre-puberty), QTc ≥ 500 ms (adult)
- Manually confirm the computer read-out
Note: A QTc < 500 ms alone **should not** render a LQTS diagnosis.
Note: ECG should be viewed in light of the answers from steps 1–3.
Note: Recognize the QTc distribution overlap between health and LQTS.

5. Provocative testing
- 24-hr ambulatory monitoring
- Treadmill/cycle stress testing
- Epinephrine QT stress test
- Abrupt standing protocol
Note: Should be performed **only if indicated** following steps 1–4.

6. Genetic testing
- May have diagnostic, prognostic and therapeutic utility.
Note: Starting with genetic testing is "**reckless and dangerous**" and should only be done following steps 1–5.

Figure 26.1 Six-step diagnostic approach to the evaluation of a patient suspected of having long QT syndrome (LQTS) (*Source:* Schwartz and Ackerman [5]. Reproduced with permission of OUP)

case it must be decided whether the event was triggered by a cardiac arrhythmia or was simply vasovagally mediated (neurocardiogenic) syncope [5]. It is important to note that a vasovagal faint in the athlete should not advance the clinical level of suspicion for long QT syndrome [5]. In fact, the combination of a vasovagal faint and a so-called 'borderline' prolonged QT interval has been the number one reason for an erroneous overdiagnosis of long QT syndrome [6].

Family History

A multigenerational family history and pedigree construction and analysis should be conducted in every patient evaluated for the possibility of long QT syndrome [5]. The family history should be inventoried and itemised, with an explanation for premature sudden death, unexplained accident, unexplained drowning, seizure disorder or suspicious 'cardiac arrhythmic-sounding' fainting episode in every first-, second- and third-degree relative, if possible [5]. A genetic counsellor specifically trained in cardiovascular genetics can assist greatly in obtaining such information.

ECG Findings

The diagnosis of long QT syndrome is centred significantly on the measurement of QTc using Bazett's formula ($QTc = QT/RR^{1/2}$) [3]. However, it is critically important that the 12-lead ECG be interrogated in light of the results of the aforementioned evaluations [5]. Normally, and in the majority of healthy subjects, the QTc does not exceed 440 ms in males or 460 ms in postpuberal females [2]. However, failure to recognise the overlap between the normal sex- and age-dependent distributions of QTc, including the QTc 'outliers', and patients with long QT syndrome (Figure 26.2) may result in the premature and erroneous proclamation of 'possible long QT syndrome' in a patient with a so-called 'borderline' QTc [5].

Whilst the probability of long QT syndrome in an athlete with a QTc of only 440 ms is 50% when he/she is the offspring of an adult with unequivocally diagnosed long QT syndrome, this exact same QTc identified incidentally in an athlete with no personal or family history of concern has less than a 1 in 1000 chance of indicating the presence of long QT syndrome [5]. Even when the QTc measures 481 ms in an asymptomatic female athlete without a family history, the positive predictive value (PPV) for long QT syndrome is less than 10% [5]. In fact, a diagnosis of long QT syndrome should seldom be made from the inspection of an ECG alone. Further, the sports cardiologist must keep in clear view that in an *asymptomatic athlete with no family history*, it is not until the QTc is >500 ms that the athlete is statistically more likely to have incidentally

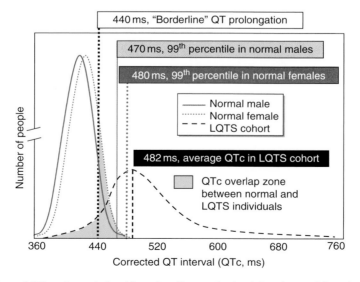

Figure 26.2 Distribution of QTc values derived from healthy postpubertal males and females [7] and from an analysis of the ECGs of all patients with genetically proven long QT syndrome evaluated in the Mayo Clinic's Long QT Syndrome Clinic (*Source:* Taggart et al. [6]. Reproduced with permission of Wolters Kluwer Health)

detected long QT syndrome than to be a normal extreme QTc outlier [5]. Nevertheless, the QTc screening cut-offs for male and female athletes have been set at 470 and 480 ms, respectively, because although an athlete with no personal symptoms and no family history is still more likely to be just a QTc outlier, the pre-test probability is increased from a 1 in 2000 population-based chance to a 1 in 10 chance, which is deemed worthy of further investigation.

When evaluating QTc, it is important that secondary causes such as drug exposure, acquired cardiac conditions, electrolyte imbalance and unbalanced diet be excluded prior to considering QT prolongation [3]. Whilst the computer QTc measurement is about 90% accurate, it must be confirmed manually, as underestimation becomes frequent when the return to baseline is slow [5]. To avoid over- or underestimation, it is suggested that measurement of the QTc be carried out on ECG traces in which the RR interval is constant for at least 10 beats [2]. In addition, given the intricate limitations of Bazett's formula, it is suggested that traces with heart rates >100 or <50 beats.min^{-1} be excluded from the evaluation [2]. This can be particularly challenging when calculating the QTc in an athlete with profound sinus bradycardia or tachycardia; Fridericia's formula ($QTc = QT/RR^{1/3}$) may be useful in such athletes [8]. However, if long QT syndrome is being invoked or refuted based on the heart rate-correction formula being used, then one should be slow to diagnose long QT syndrome. Rather than remembering different formulas, it is probably more prudent to remember that for the bradycardic athlete, Bazett's formula *underestimates* their QTc reality. In other words, if an athlete with a heart rate of 40 exhibits a Bazett's-derived QTc of 460 ms, be concerned. Consider repeating the ECG after getting his/her heart rate above 60 betas.min^{-1} and reassessing the length and look of repolarisation in that setting. Additionally, the inclusion of a physiologically normal U-wave often results in QT inflation and is a major reason for overdiagnosis of long QT syndrome (Figure 26.3) [6]. To avoid U-wave inflations, many long QT syndrome specialists recommend a method whereby the end of the T-wave is considered to be the intersection of the tangent to the steepest slope of the last limb of the T-wave and the baseline (Figure 26.4) [9]. Use of the 'teach-the-tangent' method (also referred to as 'avoid-the-tail') results in a significantly improved accuracy in the diagnosis of long QT syndrome [8]. Conversely,

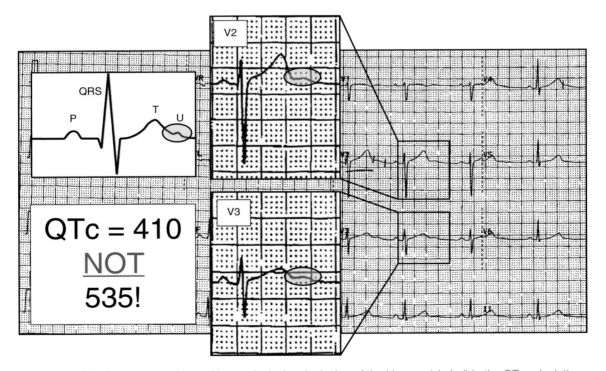

Figure 26.3 QT inflation secondary to U-wave inclusion. Inclusion of the U-wave (circled) in the QTc calculation would result in inflation of the QTc from 410 to 535 ms. This often results in QT inflation and is a major reason for overdiagnosis of long QT syndrome. This ECG comes from an athlete who was not only disqualified because of this erroneous QTc overestimate (the sin of QT inflation secondary to U-wave inclusion) but also received an implantable cardioverter-defibrillator (ICD). After his Mayo Clinic evaluation, he had his QTc measured correctly, his long QT syndrome diagnosis reversed and his ICD removed, and he was able to resume his athletic career

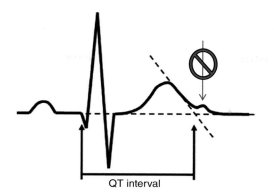

QT interval

Figure 26.4 Teach-the-tangent and avoid-the-tail. To avoid U-wave inflations, the T-wave is considered the intersection of the tangent to the steepest slope of the last limb of the T-wave and the baseline

		Points
ECG findings[a]		
QTc[b]	≥480 ms	3
	460–479 ms	2
	450–459 ms (males)	1
QTc 4th minute of recovery from exercise stress test ≥480 ms		1
Torsades de pointes[c]		2
T-wave alternans (TWA)		1
Notched T-wave in three leads		1
Low heart rate for age[d]		0.5
Clinical history		
Syncope[c]	With stress	2
	Without stress	1
Congenital deafness		0.5
Family history		
Family members with definite long QT syndrome[e]		1
Unexplained SCD at age <30 years amongst immediate family members		0.5

Table 26.1 Long QT syndrome diagnostic criteria (Schwartz score)

A cumulative score ≤1.0 gives a low probability of long QT syndrome, 1.5–3.0 gives an intermediate probability and ≥3.5 gives a high probability.

[a] In the absence of medications or disorders known to affect these features.
[b] QTc calculated by Bazett's formula (QTc = QT/RR$^{1/2}$).
[c] Mutually exclusive.
[d] Resting heart rate below the second percentile for age.
[e] The same family member cannot be counted twice.

subtle T-wave changes – specifically, notched T-waves in limb lead II or precordial leads V4–V6 – should elevate the suspicion for long QT syndrome [5].

In an effort to assist physicians in assessing the probability of long QT syndrome, a diagnostic scoring system has been established that takes into consideration the ECG findings and the clinical and family history of the patient (Table 26.1) [10]. Points are awarded for specific diagnostic criteria and tabulated to give a diagnostic ('Schwartz') score. From a clinical perspective, a score ≥3.5 is actionable and should prompt further investigation for the possibility of long QT syndrome [10]. However, this score certainly should not be taken to mandate a diagnosis of long QT syndrome [5]. Table 26.2 provides the 2013 Heart

1. Long QT syndrome is diagnosed in the presence of

- A long QT syndrome risk score >3.5 in the absence of a secondary cause for QT prolongation
- An unequivocally pathogenic mutation in one of the long QT syndrome genes
- A QT interval corrected for heart rate using Bazett's formula (QTc) ≥500 ms in repeated 12-lead ECG and in the absence of a secondary cause for QT prolongation

2. Long QT syndrome can be diagnosed in the presence of

- A QTc between 480 and 499 ms on repeated 12-lead ECGs in a patient with unexplained syncope in the absence of a secondary cause for QT prolongation and in the absence of a pathogenic mutation

Table 26.2 HRS/EHRA/APHRS expert consensus recommendations on the diagnosis of long QT syndrome

Rhythm Society (HRS)/European Heart Rhythm Association (EHRA)/Asia Pacific Heart Rhythm Society (APHRS) expert consensus recommendations on the diagnosis of long QT syndrome.

Provocative Testing

Provocative testing for QT measurements can be used in the evaluation of the patient [5]. It is important to recognise that approximately 20–25% of long QT patients with a definitive long QT syndrome gene mutation may have a QTc in the normal range [3]. Additional surveillance using 24-hour ambulatory monitoring or provocative ECG testing (e.g. treadmill/cycle stress testing, the epinephrine QT stress test, abrupt standing) may allow for the unmasking of the long QT individual with a normal resting QTc [5,11]. However, these tests should only be considered following the previous four steps, or each may erroneously advance a diagnosis of long QT syndrome [5].

For example, a night-time QTc of 500 ms in a patient with a baseline QTc <440 ms should not automatically prompt a diagnosis of long QT syndrome [5]. Rather, ambulatory monitoring offers value in identifying specific morphological alternations of the T-wave that may be associated with long QT syndrome [5]. Provocative studies are best used to confirm or unmask the presence of long QT syndrome type 1 (LQT1), where abnormal QTc values (>470 ms at 2–3 minutes of recovery) in the recovery phase of stress testing, paradoxical QT lengthening of the absolute QT interval during the Mayo Clinic epinephrine infusion protocol and paradoxical lengthening of the QTc with the Shimizu epinephrine bolus protocol all increase the likelihood of LQT1, with PPVs >70% and negative predictive values (NPVs) = 95% [5,11]. However, restraint must be used when interpreting various stress-testing results, as a positive test response by itself does not equate to a diagnosis of long QT syndrome [5]. These tests may be considered complementary and additive, as there are plenty of examples of LQT1 patients who have had a positive treadmill stress test but a negative epinephrine stress test and vice versa [5].

Genetic Testing

Genetic testing can be incorporated into the overall diagnostic evaluation for long QT syndrome. However, beginning with genetic testing is 'reckless and dangerous', and reflects a failure to understand the probabilistic nature of genetic testing and the so-called 'background genetic noise' associated with long QT syndrome [5]. When used properly, genetic testing for long QT syndrome has substantial diagnostic, prognostic and therapeutic utility. From a clinical test standpoint, genetic testing should be pursued for any athlete with a strong clinical index of suspicion for a long QT syndrome diagnosis (equivalent to a score ≥3.5) based on the clinical impression following the aforementioned steps, or for an asymptomatic athlete with an incidentally detected and unequivocally prolonged QTc (>480 ms during prepuberty, >500 ms during adulthood) in the absence of other clinical conditions [12]. If an asymptomatic athlete without a family history consistently presents with a QTc ≥470 ms on serial ECGs, genetic testing may be considered, as long as it is recognised that as the level of clinical suspicion decreases, the probability of a false-positive genetic test increases. If a definitive long QT syndrome-causing mutation is identified, then appropriate relatives should undergo mutation-specific genetic testing. It is imperative that genetic tests be understood as probabilistic tests rather than as unconditionally deterministic ones, and the genetic test results must be interpreted cautiously and incorporated into the overall diagnostic evaluation for these disorders [12,13].

Genetic Basis for Long QT Syndrome

Long QT syndrome is a genetically heterogeneous disorder typically inherited as an autosomal-dominant trait However, it is rarely inherited recessively and is typically characterised by a severe cardiac phenotype and sensorineural hearing loss. Spontaneous or sporadic germline mutations may account for nearly 10% of all cases of long QT syndrome. At present, 3 major and 11 minor long QT syndrome-susceptibility genes are known to account account for nearly 80% of the disorder, whilst 20% of patients remain genetically elusive [13]. In addition, three atypical long QT syndrome or multisystem syndromic disorders associated with either QT or QTU prolongation have been described, namely ankyrin B syndrome (formerly LQT4), Andersen–Tawil syndrome (ATS, formerly LQT7) and Timothy syndrome (TS, formerly LQT8) [13]. The focus of this chapter is on the more common 'pure' nonsyndromic long QT syndrome subtypes, and we will not address these distinct and atypical forms.

Approximately 75% of patients with a clinically certain diagnosis of long QT syndrome have mutations in one of three major long QT syndrome-susceptibility genes (Figure 26.5) that encode for ion-channel alpha subunits that critically orchestrate the cardiac action potential: *KCNQ1*-encoded I_{Ks} ($K_v7.1$) potassium channel, *KCNH2*-encoded I_{Kr} ($K_v11.1$) potassium channel or *SCN5A*-encoded I_{Na} ($Na_v1.5$) sodium channel [13]. Loss-of-function mutations in *KCNQ1* underlie about 35% of cases of long QT syndrome (LQT1),

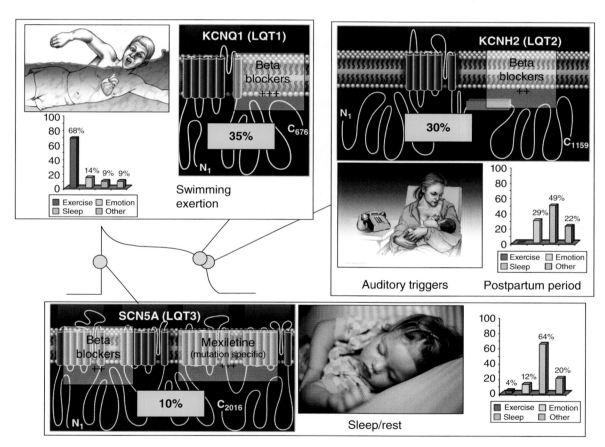

Figure 26.5 Genotype–phenotype correlations in long QT syndrome. Mutations in three genes encoding for ion channels – responsible for the cardiac action potential – underlie 75% of cases of long QT syndrome with a clinically certain diagnosis (35% *KCNQ1*, 30% *KCNH2* and 10% *SCN5A*). Observed genotype–phenotype correlations include swimming/exertion and LQT1, auditory triggers/postpartum period and LQT2 and sleep/rest and LQT3. The inset bar graphs represent data from Schwartz et al. [14]. Also illustrated is the relative gene-specific effectiveness in beta-blocker therapy, where beta blockers are extremely protective in LQT1 patients and moderately protective in LQT2 and LQT3. The sodium channel blocker Mexiletine may be protective in LQT3, but is often mutation-specific (*Source:* Tester and Ackerman [13]. Reproduced with permission of Wolters Kluwer Health)

whilst loss-of-function *KCNH2* mutations underlie ~30% (LQT2). Gain-of-function *SCN5A* mutations cause ~10% of cases (LQT3) [13]. About 5–10% of long QT patients host multiple mutations in these genes, often presenting at a younger age with a more severe phenotype. Because the 11 additional minor long QT syndrome-susceptibility genes contribute to only a minor portion of the genetic basis of long QT syndrome, only limited genotype–phenotype correlations have been generated [13]. In fact, to date, genotype-specific treatment strategies and risk stratification are based largely on the three major genotypes (LQT1, LQT2 and LQT3).

Risk Stratification in Long QT Syndrome

Relatively gene-specific triggers, ECG patterns and therapeutic responses have emerged. For example, whilst swimming- and exertion-induced cardiac events are associated strongly with LQT1, auditory triggers and events occurring during the postpartum period usually occur in patients with LQT2 and events occurring during periods of sleep/rest are most common in LQT3 (Figure 26.5) [1]. However, it is important to recognise that overlap exists between these genotype–phenotype correlations [2]. Just as a LQT1 patient may have an episode during sleep, so might an LQT3 individual have an episode during exertion.

Whilst exceptions to relatively gene-specific T-wave patterns exist, LQT1 is associated with a broad-based T-wave, LQT2 with a low-amplitude notched or biphasic T-wave and LQT3 with a long isoelectric segment followed by a narrow-based T-wave (Figure 26.6). Whilst beta blockers are extremely protective in LQT1 patients, they are only moderately protective in LQT2 and LQT3 (Figure 26.5). Female LQT2 patients may not be as fully protected by beta blockers as males [5]. Given the electrophysiological consequence of an LQT3-causing *SCN5A* mutation, late sodium current blockers, including mexiletine, flecainide and ranolazine, may represent a gene-specific therapeutic option for LQT3 [15]. However, the response to sodium channel blockers is mutation-specific, and whilst there has been clear evidence for the benefit of mexiletine in some LQT3 patients, there have been examples of failures in others [1].

In general, when the QTc is >500 ms, LQT2 females and LQT3 males are at a higher risk for a cardiac event [1]. In addition, intragenic risk stratification has been realised for LQT1 and LQT2 based upon mutation type, location and cellular function [13]. LQT1 patients with transmembrane-spanning domain-localising KCNQ1 missense mutations and patients with mutations resulting in a greater degree of $K_v7.1$ loss of function (dominant-negative) are at greater risk of a LQT1-triggered cardiac event (compared to those with C-terminal-region mutations and those with mutations that less severely damage the biology of the $K_v7.1$ channel (haplo-insufficiency), respectively). LQT2 patients with pore-region KCNH2 mutations have a longer QTc, a more severe clinical manifestation of the disorder and a greater number of arrhythmia-related cardiac events occurring at a younger age than those patients with nonpore mutations in KCNH2. In addition, LQT2 patients with transmembrane pore-region mutations have the greatest risk for cardiac events, those with frame-shift/nonsense mutations in any channel region have an intermediate risk and those with C-terminus missense mutations have the lowest risk. Despite these genotype-specific risk factors, it is advised that physicians use a multiparametric and individualised approach in their risk assessment and avoid using genotype as a generalised indicator of risk [2].

Regardless of genotype, risk of a cardiac event is high whenever QTc >500 ms and extremely high whenever QTc >600 ms [3]. Patients with a QTc of >500 ms and multiple unequivocally pathogenic mutations are at high risk, especially when symptomatic [3]. Long QT patients experiencing syncope or cardiac arrest before the age of 7 years have a greater probability of recurrence of arrhythmic events, even when on beta blockers [3]. Patients who have had syncope or cardiac arrest during the first year of life are particularly at risk for a lethal event and may not be adequately protected by traditional therapies [3]. Patients with a breakthrough event whilst on full medical therapy are at a higher risk for additional potentially lethal events [3]. Conversely, some mutation-positive patients have concealed long QT syndrome and are considered at low risk for an arrhythmic event [3]. The risk for an arrhythmic event in this group of patients is estimated to be 10% between birth and 40 years of age in the absence of therapy [3]. However, asymptomatic patients are at an increased risk whilst on drugs known to block I_{Kr} current (so-called 'HERG channel blockers') and when they have conditions that lower their plasma potassium level [5]. A list of drugs to avoid can be found at www.crediblemeds.org; this should be given to every patient, as their local family physician/medical provider may be unaware of this potentially lethal side effect.

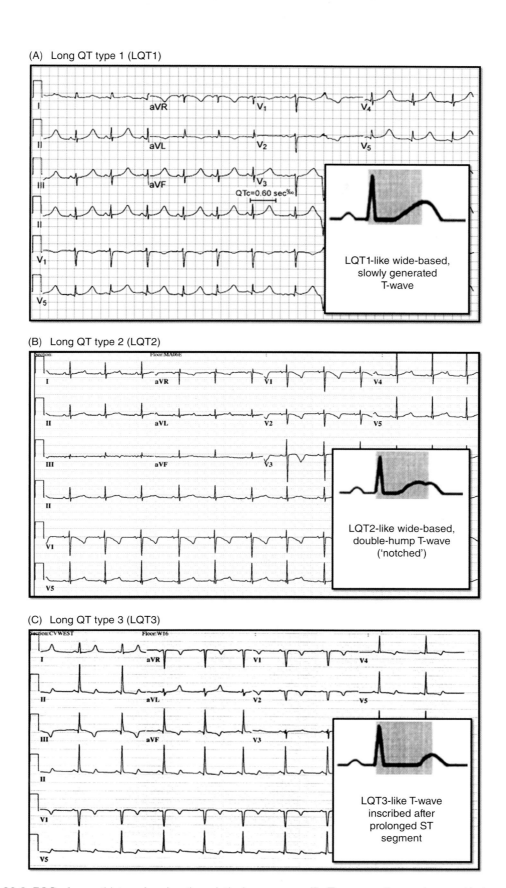

(A) Long QT type 1 (LQT1)

LQT1-like wide-based, slowly generated T-wave

QTc=0.60 sec‰

(B) Long QT type 2 (LQT2)

LQT2-like wide-based, double-hump T-wave ('notched')

(C) Long QT type 3 (LQT3)

LQT3-like T-wave inscribed after prolonged ST segment

Figure 26.6 ECGs from athletes showing the relatively gene-specific T-wave patterns observed in long QT syndrome. (A) LQT1 is associated with a broad-based T-wave. (B) LQT2 is associated with a low-amplitude notched or biphasic T-wave. (C) LQT3 is associated with a long isoelectric segment followed by a narrow-based T-wave

Disease Management in Long QT Syndrome

Besides specific lifestyle modifications, such as avoidance of swimming without supervision for LQT1 patients, reduced exposure to sudden and startling loud noises (alarm clocks, phone ringing) for patients with LQT2 and avoidance of QT-prolonging drugs in all long QT patients, the use of beta blockers, left cardiac sympathetic denervation (LCSD) and implantable cardioverter-defibrillators (ICDs) are the key therapeutic modalities for long QT patients [3,5].

Beta blockers should be considered the first line of defence in patients with long QT syndrome (including those who are genetically diagnosed but have a normal QTc) unless otherwise contraindicated, such as in the setting of active asthma [3]. Long-lasting beta blockers (e.g. propranolol, nadolol) are recommended, as they can be given once or twice daily. Propranolol is commonly used in infants and children at 2–4 mg.kg^{-1}. day^{-1} divided three times daily [5]. The longer-lasting nadolol may be used as a one-a-day administration (0.75–1.50 mg.kg^{-1}.day^{-1}) in adolescents and adults where compliance with multiple doses each day may be an issue [5]. Beta blockers have been shown to be highly effective in treating long QT patients. In fact, the mortality rate observed amongst 869 long QT patients with unknown genotype on beta-blocker therapy was 2% [16]. Specifically, beta blockers are highly effective in protecting LQT1 patients, where the mortality rate is about 0.5%. Almost all life-threatening events occurring in LQT1 patients are the result of beta-blocker therapy noncompliance or the use of QT-prolonging drugs, whilst compliance with beta-blocker therapy and avoidance of QT-prolonging drugs are associated with a 97% reduction in risk for an adverse cardiac event [5,17].

Whilst extremely effective in treating LQT1 patients, beta-blocker therapy is only moderately effective in LQT2 and LQT3 patients. About 6–7% of LQT2 and 10–15% of LQT3 patients may have life-threatening events despite beta-blocker therapy [17,18]. However, these mortality rates should not prompt intensification of therapy to an ICD solely because of an LQT2 or LQT3 genotype. Individualisation of therapy must be the cornerstone. For example, cardiac events occurring during infancy are associated with an extremely poor prognosis independent of the treatment, whereas LQT3 patients who were not symptomatic during the first year of life have a mortality rate of around 3% when on beta blockers, largely related to a QTc >600 ms [5].

As already stated, some patients with LQT3 may respond positively to a sodium-channel blocker such as mexiletine, flecainide or ranolazine. Because not all LQT3 patients will respond to these specific drugs, it is suggested that the correct clinical approach specifically for mexiletine use is to monitor its QT-shortening effect via acute oral drug testing, using one-half of the daily dose for 2 hours whilst monitoring the patient's ECG [1]. If the QTc shortens more than 40 ms without unwanted PR interval lengthening, combination therapy involving a beta blocker and mexiletine may be reasonable [1]. It must be recognised that sodium-channel blockers have the potential to negatively impact cardiac conduction, with serious consequence, and that careful ECG monitoring must be performed in the mexiletine-treated LQT3 patient [1].

For the minority of long QT patients who experience a long QT syndrome-triggered event whilst on beta-blocker therapy and for those who do not tolerate their beta-blocker therapy, LCSD (involving the resection of the lower half of the left stellate ganglion and the left-sided sympathetic chain at the level of thoracic ganglia T2–T4) can be an effective therapy. It is suitable for patients of all ages, ranging from infancy to the elderly, especially when the videoscopic approach is used [5,19]. In fact, in a cohort of 147 long QT patients with very high-risk disease (99% symptomatic, mean QTc = 563 ± 65 ms, 48% with previous cardiac arrest, 75% with recurrent syncope despite full-dose beta-blocker therapy), LCSD resulted in a 91% reduction in cardiac events over an 8-year mean follow-up period [19]. In a subgroup of five patients with reoccurring appropriate ICD shocks and electrical storms, LCSD provided a 95% decrease in the number of shocks and dramatically improved the quality of life over a 4-year follow-up period [19]. However, whilst there was a remarked reduction in the number of cardiac events, a Mayo Clinic study of 52 long QT patients undergoing LCSD illustrated that approximately 50% of high-risk patients had at least one post-LCSD breakthrough event (i.e. appropriated ICD shock, arrhythmogenic syncope, seizure or aborted cardiac arrest) [20]. Importantly, LCSD should not be considered a curative or alternative therapeutic strategy in place of an ICD for the high-risk long QT patient [5]. Rather, LCSD may provide an alternative option capable of offseting a suboptimal quality of life stemming from medication-related side effects. Current indications for LCSD include patients with appropriate ventricular fibrillation-terminating ICD shocks, patients with breakthrough cardiac events whilst on adequate drug therapy, patients who do not tolerate beta-blocker therapy side effects or who cannot take beta blockers because of asthma and high-risk young patients in whom primary drug therapy is inadequately protective, where LCSD can serve as a 'bridge' to an ICD [5].

There is overall consensus for immediate ICD implantation in a long QT patient who has experienced cardiac arrest whilst either on or off therapy, with perhaps an exception for the otherwise asymptomatic patient with a modest QT prolongation who has experienced a documented drug-induced cardiac arrest. ICD therapy should not be used as a first-line therapy in an asymptomatic long QT individual. Yet, there appears to be a large disparity in ICD usage, with some US medical centres reportedly implanting devices in ~80% of their long QT patients, compared to 3 and 15% in two of the world's largest long QT clinics [5]. Because ICD therapy has lifelong implications and complications are not infrequent, especially in the young patient, the risk/benefit ratio must be weighed carefully before initiating this invasive therapy [3].

Drs Schwartz and Ackerman suggest that implantation of an ICD should be indicated for all patients who have survived a cardiac arrest whilst being adequately treated with drug therapy; for most patients who have survived a cardiac arrest (those with a reversible/preventable cause and those with previously undiagnosed and untreated LQT1 may be exceptions); for those patients experiencing long QT syndrome-triggered syncope despite a full dose of beta blocker, especially when the use of LCSD therapy is not an option; for all patients with syncope despite full-dose beta blocker therapy and LCSD; for asymptomatic postpubertal LQT2 women with a QTc ≥550 ms; and for asymptomatic patients with a QTc >550 ms who also present with signs of high electric instability (e.g. T-wave alternans, TWA) or other evidence suggesting high risk (e.g. long sinus pauses followed by abnormal T-wave morphology) despite beta-blocker therapy and LCSD [5]. Importantly, a long QT syndrome-related death in a family member is not an automatic indication for an ICD in a surviving affected relative unless a profile of high risk for arrhythmic events has been indicated following a thorough clinical investigation of the relative [3]. Furthermore, the decision to implant an ICD should be made mutually between the physician and the patient/guardian following careful consideration has been given to the risk of sudden death and the short- and long-term risk associated with ICD implantation [3].

Considerations in the Context of Exercise and Physical Activity

The continued participation of an athlete with long QT syndrome in competitive sports is still debated amongst the experts. In 2005, Task Force 7 of the 36th Bethesda Conference provided guidelines for competitive sports recommendations for patients with long QT syndrome (Table 26.3) [21]. In the same year, the European Society of Cardiology (ESC) provided its own guidelines (Table 26.3) [22].

The North American guidelines recommend disqualification from all competitive sports except for Bethesda-permitted class IA sports (i.e. billiards, bowling, cricket, curling, golf and riflery) for all symptomatic long QT patients regardless of the QTc or underlying genotype and for asymptomatic long QT patients with baseline QT prolongation (QTc ≥470 ms in males and ≥480 ms in females). They also recommend that the restrictions can be lifted for the asymptomatic patient with genetically proven LQT3 even in the setting of manifest QT prolongation.

The ESC used a less stringent definition for long QT syndrome and recommended disqualification from all competitive sports for athletes with a QTc ≥440 ms in males and ≥460 ms in females, regardless of symptomatic status. Further, a positive genetic test alone was sufficient to prompt a comprehensive sports disqualification according to the ESC guidelines. In stark contrast, the Bethesda guidelines state that athletes who are genotype-positive yet phenotype-negative (i.e. asymptomatic with nondiagnostic QT prolongation) may be allowed to play competitive sports, except for LQT1 patients, who it is recommended refrain from competitive swimming. Both the Bethesda and the ESC guidelines recommend disqualification of all athletes with an ICD from all competitive sports (except for class IA activities per Bethesda).

These guidelines are conservative in nature and, by their own admission, base the recommendations for sports disqualification on 'expert opinion' rather than a primary evidence base. However, observation evidence has emerged that suggests that in an appropriately treated and counselled athlete with long QT syndrome, continued sports participation may not be an excessive or unacceptable risk exposure, even for the long QT athlete with an ICD [23,24]. In 2007, Basavarajaiah et al. [25] analysed the prevalence and significance of a prolonged QTc in 2000 (1260 male and 540 female) elite athletes aged between 14 and 35 years and identified 7 (6 male and 1 female; 0.35%) with a QTc ≥440 ms (males) or ≥460 ms (females), ranging from 460 to 570 ms. All 7 athletes were asymptomatic. Three athletes had a baseline QTc >500 ms, all of whom exhibited paradoxical QT prolongation during exercise and additional phenotypic manifestation of LQT1 or LQT2 or had a first-degree relative with a prolonged QTc [25]. Conversely, none of the four athletes with a QTc <500 ms (460, 474, 490 and 492 ms) had any characteristic features of long QT

2005 Bethesda Conference Guidelines

Disqualified from nearly all competitive sports (except billiards, bowling, cricket, curling, golf and riflery)

Symptomatic athlete (regardless of QTc or long QT syndrome genotype)

1   Previous out-of-hospital cardiac arrest

2   Long QT syndrome-precipitated syncope

Asymptomatic athlete with baseline QT prolongation

1   Males QTc ≥470 ms

2   Females with QTc ≥480 ms

Athletes with an ICD/pacemaker

Disqualification from competitive swimming

Genotype-positive/phenotype-negative (asymptomatic with normal QTc) patients with concealed LQT1

2005 European Society of Cardiology (ESC) Guidelines

Disqualified from all competitive sports

All athletes with baseline QT prolongation or diagnosed with long QT syndrome

1   Males QTc ≥440 ms

2   Females with QTc ≥460 ms

Genotype-positive/phenotype-negative (asymptomatic with normal QTc)

Athletes with an ICD/pacemaker

22013 HRS/EHRA/APHRS consensus statement

All long QT patients who wish to engage in competitive sports should be referred to a clinical expert for evaluation of risk

Table 26.3 Current published guidelines for competitive sports disqualification for athletes with long QT syndrome

syndrome on exercise stress testing and Holter monitoring or any family members with a prolonged QTc interval [25]. Based on their observations, the authors concluded that an athlete with a QTc ≥500 ms should be disqualified from sports. However, athletes with an isolated prolonged QTc <500 ms represent a group with low probability of long QT syndrome and should undergo close monitoring rather than immediate disqualification [25].

In 2013, Johnson and Ackerman [23] reported on 130 long QT athletes (60 females, mean age 11 ± 7 years, mean QTc = 471 ± 46 ms, mean length of follow up = 5.1 ± 2.9 years) who continued to participate in competitive sports following their diagnosis. Of the 130 athletes, 112 were treated on beta-blocker therapy, 21 had an LCSD and 20 had an ICD. The most common long QT syndrome genotype was LQT1 (57%), followed by LQT2 (32%), LQT3 (8%) and multiple mutations (3%). Despite their long QT diagnosis, these athletes continued to participate in a wide variety of competitive sports, including basketball, competitive cheerleading/dance/gymnastics, football, baseball/softball, volleyball and American football, across all levels of competition, ranging from youth city leagues to high school, college and professional [23]. Nearly 40% were participating in multiple sports. During a combined 650 athlete-year follow-up, only one athlete (0.8%) experienced two competitive sporting-related cardiac events. This previously symptomatic 9-year-old LQT1 patient with extreme QT prolongation (QTc >550 ms) and a history of aborted cardiac arrest experienced two appropriate ventricular fibrillation-terminating shocks, one during football and the other during baseball. Each of these events occurred in the setting of noncompliance with his beta-blocker therapy [23].

The Bethesda guidelines recommending disqualification for all athletes with an ICD were based on the assumed risks of the device failing to defibrillate, injury resulting from loss of control due to an arrhythmia-related shock and damage to the ICD system [21,24]. However, in the study by Johnson and Ackerman [23], none of the 20 athletes with an ICD who participated in a variety of sports had any ICD-related complications. Furthermore, over a median 31-month follow-up, Lampert et al. [24] reported that there were no occurrences of (i) disease-related mortality, (ii) shock-related injury, (iii) excessive inappropriate shocks, or (iv) excessive device malfunction or damage during sports amongst 372 athletes with an ICD participating in organised (e.g. running, basketball, football) or high-risk (e.g. skiing) sports. Overall, 77 athletes (21% of the cohort) experienced 121 ICD shock episodes (49 shocks in 37 athletes during competition/sports; 39 shocks in 29 athletes during other physical activity; 33 shocks in 24 athletes during rest) [24]. Whilst most shocks occurred during physical activity, there was no difference in the percentage of athletes who experienced shocks during competition/practice compared to those receiving shocks during other recreational or other physical activities [24].

Based in part on these emerging observational data, the latest 2013 HRS/EHRA/APHRS expert consensus statement on the diagnosis and management of inherited arrhythmia syndromes recommends that 'low-risk patients with genetically confirmed LQTS [long QT syndrome] but with borderline QTc prolongation, no history of cardiac symptoms, and no family history of multiple sudden cardiac deaths, may be allowed to participate in competitive sports in special cases after full clinical evaluation, utilization of appropriate LQTS therapy and when competitive activity is performed where automated external defibrillators are available and personnel [are] trained in basic life support' [3]. Furthermore, these guidelines indicate a possible shift towards shared decision-making, as they now stipulate as a class I indication that an athlete with long QT syndrome who desires to remain an athlete must be evaluated by an expert. These recommendations are also reflected in the 2015 joint ACC/AHA recommendations for eligibility in competitive sport [26].

For nearly 15 years, the Mayo Clinic's Long QT Syndrome/Heart Rhythm Clinic has embraced this notion regarding the importance of athlete/family autonomy and respect for the athlete's right to make a well-informed decision about continuation in competitive athletics [23]. The well-informed decision-making process begins with an initial 2–3-day long QT clinical evaluation, which includes an ECG on two consecutive days, echocardiography, 24-hour ambulatory monitoring, treadmill exercise testing, pharmacological stress testing (if indicated), genetic counselling and genetic testing (if indicated), plus additional consultations with a psychologist or psychiatrist, an ICD implant specialist and/or a surgeon specialising in LCSD [23]. The primary evaluation concludes with a 1–2 hour consultation with a long QT specialist to discuss the implications of the athlete's long QT syndrome. A treatment plan is implemented based on the perceived risk of cardiac events. Most athletes return for an annual or alternate-year 1–2 day follow-up evaluation and reassessment of their risk profile and treatment strategy [23]. In addition, they undergo extensive counselling to discuss how their present diagnosis and clinical presentation fit with the published sports participation guidelines regarding their continuation in competitive athletics. Each athlete/family is provided with a copy of the latest guidelines and has a thorough discussion about their decision to remain an athlete at each follow-up visit [23]. With regards to the paediatric athlete, they and both parents (whenever possible) must agree to allow for athletic participation. If even one family member objects over safety concerns, then the athlete is disqualified. It is required that any athlete who participates against published guidelines be protected with the best evidence-based therapy, most often beta blockers [23]. The athlete is also advised to avoid QT-prolonging drugs, to stay properly hydrated, to replenish electrolytes and to minimise elevations in core body temperature. The long QT athlete is also instructed to acquire his/her own automated external defibrillator (AED), to have as a part of his/her personal athletic safety gear. In addition, school officials, coaches and other authorities must be informed and must agree to the outlined plan for competitive sports participation [23].

References

1 Schwartz, P.J., Ackerman, M.J., George, A.L. Jr and Wilde, A.A.M. Impact of genetics on the clinical management of channelopathies. *J Am Coll Cardiol* 2013; **62**: 169–80.

2 Cerrone, M., Cummings, S., Alansari, T. and Priori, S.G. A clinical approach to inherited arrhythmias. *Circ Cardiovasc Genet* 2012; **5**: 581–90.

3 Priori, S.G., Wilde, A.A., Horie, M. et al. HRS/EHRA/APHRS expert consensus statement on the diagnosis and management of patients with inherited primary arrhythmia syndromes: document endorsed by HRS, EHRA, and APHRS in May 2013 and by ACCF, AHA, PACES, and AEPC in June 2013. *Heart Rhythm* 2013; **10**: 1932–63.

4 Tester, D.J., Medeiros-Domingo, A., Will, M.L. et al. Cardiac channel molecular autopsy: insights from 173 consecutive cases of autopsy-negative sudden unexplained death referred for postmortem genetic testing. *Mayo Clin Proc* 2012; **87**: 524–39.

5 Schwartz, P.J. and Ackerman, M.J. The long QT syndrome: a transatlantic clinical approach to diagnosis and therapy. *Eur Heart J* 2013; **34**: 3109–16.

6 Taggart, N.W., Haglund, C.M., Tester, D.J. and Ackerman, M.J. Diagnostic miscues in congenital long-QT syndrome [see comment]. *Circulation* 2007; **115**: 2613–20.

7 Mason, J.W., Ramseth, D.J., Chanter, D.O. et al. Electrocardiographic reference ranges derived from 79 743 ambulatory subjects. *J Electrocardiol* 2007; **40**: 228–34.

8 Charbit, B., Samain, E., Merckx, P. and Funck-Brentano, C. Evaluation of automatic QTc measurement and new simple method to calculate and interpret corrected QT interval. *Anesthesiology* 2006; **104**: 255–60.

9 Postema, P.G., De Jong, J.S., Van der Bilt, I.A. and Wilde, A.A. Accurate electrocardiographic assessment of the QT interval: teach the tangent. *Heart Rhythm* 2008; **5**: 1015–18.

10 Schwartz, P.J. and Crotti, L. QTc behavior during exercise and genetic testing for the long-QT syndrome. *Circulation* 2011; **124**: 2181–4.

11 Viskin, S., Postema, P.G., Bhuiyan, Z.A. et al. The response of the QT interval to the brief tachycardia provoked by standing: a bedside test for diagnosing long QT syndrome. *J Am Coll Cardiol* 2010; **55**: 1955–61.

12 Ackerman, M., Priori, S., Willems, S. et al. HRS/EHRA expert consensus statement on the state of genetic testing for the channelopathies and cardiomyopathies: this document was developed as a partnership between the Heart Rhythm Society (HRS) and the European Heart Rhythm Association (EHRA). *Heart Rhythm* 2011; **8**: 1308–39.

13 Tester, D.J. and Ackerman, M.J. Genetic testing for potentially lethal, highly treatable inherited cardiomyopathies/ channelopathies in clinical practice. *Circulation* 2011; **123**: 1021–37.

14 Schwartz, P.J., Priori, S.G., Spazzolini, C. et al. Genotype-phenotype correlation in the long-QT syndrome: gene-specific triggers for life-threatening arrhythmias. *Circulation* 2001; **103**: 89–95.

15 Moss, A.J. and Goldenberg, I. Importance of knowing the genotype and the specific mutation when managing patients with long QT syndrome [see comment]. *Circ Arrhyth Electrophysiol* 2008; **1**: 213–26, disc. 226.

16 Moss, A.J., Zareba, W., Hall, W.J. et al. Effectiveness and limitations of beta-blocker therapy in congenital long-QT syndrome. *Circulation* 2000; **101**: 616–23.

17 Vincent, G.M., Schwartz, P.J., Denjoy, I. et al. High efficacy of beta-blockers in long QT syndrome type 1: contribution of non-compliance and QT prolonging drugs to the occurrence of beta-blocker treatment 'failures'. *Circulation* 2009; **119**: 215–21.

18 Priori, S.G., Napolitano, C., Schwartz, P.J. et al. Association of long QT syndrome loci and cardiac events among patients treated with B-blockers. *JAMA* 2004; **292**: 1341–4.

19 Schwartz, P.J., Priori, S.G., Cerrone, M. et al. Left cardiac sympathetic denervation in the management of high-risk patients affected by the long-QT syndrome. *Circulation* 2004; **109**: 1826–33.

20 Bos, J.M., Bos, K.M., Johnson, J.N. et al. Left cardiac sympathetic denervation in long QT syndrome: analysis of therapeutic nonresponders. *Circ Arrhyth Electrophysiol* 2013; **6**: 705–11.

21 Zipes, D.P., Ackerman, M.J., Estes, M. et al. Task Force 7: arrhythmias. *J Am Coll Cardiol* 2005; **45**: 1354–63.

22 Pelliccia, A., Fagard, R., Bjornstad, H.H. et al. Recommendations for competitive sports participation in athletes with cardiovascular disease: a consensus document from the Study Group of Sports Cardiology of the Working Group of Cardiac Rehabilitation and Exercise Physiology and the Working Group of Myocardial and Pericardial Diseases of the European Society of Cardiology. *Eur Heart J* 2005; **26**: 1422–45.

23 Johnson, J.N. and Ackerman, M.J. Return to play? Athletes with congenital long QT syndrome. *Br J Sports Med* 2013; **47**: 28–33.

24 Lampert, R., Olshansky, B., Heidbuchel, H. et al. Safety of sports for athletes with implantable cardioverter-defibrillators: results of a prospective, multinational registry. *Circulation* 2013; **127**: 2021–30.

25 Basavarajaiah, S., Wilson, M., Whyte, G. et al. Prevalence and significance of an isolated long QT interval in elite athletes. *Eur Heart J* 2007; **28**: 2944–9.

26 Maron, B.J., Zipes, D.P. and Kovacs, R.J. Eligibility and disqualification recommendations for competitive athletes with cardiovascular abnormalities: Preamble, principles, and general considerations: A scientific statement from the American Heart Association and American College of Cardiology. *J Am Coll Cardiol* 2015; **66**(21): 2343–9.

27 Brugada Syndrome

Elena Arbelo and Josep Brugada

Department of Cardiology, Thorax Institute, Hospital Clinic Barcelona, University of Barcelona, Barcelona, Spain

Concept and Epidemiology

Over 20 years ago, eight individuals were resuscitated from sudden death caused by ventricular fibrillation; all eight showed a characteristic ST-segment elevation in the right precordial leads and a structurally normal heart [1]. Since 1996, the term 'Brugada syndrome' has been used to refer to the clinical setting characterised by 'right bundle branch block, persistent ST segment elevation and sudden death' due to polymorphic ventricular tachycardia (PVT) and/or ventricular fibrillation in the absence of structural heart disease [2]. The syndrome has attracted great interest because of its high incidence in some parts of the world and its association with sudden death in young adults and, albeit less frequently, in infants and children.

It has been estimated that Brugada syndrome is responsible for 4–12% of all sudden death and 20% of sudden death in the absence of structural heart disease. Arrhythmias in Brugada syndrome are mainly due to PVT or ventricular fibrillation.

Because the characteristic electrocardiographic (ECG) pattern of Brugada syndrome is so dynamic and often unapparent, it is difficult to determine the true prevalence of the disease in the general population. Current estimates suggest that the prevalence in Europe and the US is 1–5 in 10 000. However, it is significantly higher in Asia (especially in Thailand, the Philippines and Japan): estimated at up to 12 per 10 000. The reason for this is unknown, but it could be related to a specific sequence of the *SCN5A* promoter region. In these endemic areas, Brugada syndrome could represent the leading cause of death in individuals younger than 40 years, after accounting for accidents.

Genetic Basis

Brugada syndrome is an inherited disease with an autosomal-dominant pattern of transmission and variable penetrance. However, up to 60% of cases may be sporadic; that is, absent other relatives [3].

The first genetic mutations associated with Brugada syndrome were described in the *SCN5A* gene, which encodes the alpha subunit of the voltage-gated $Na_v1.5$ cardiac sodium channel, responsible for regulating rapid sodium current. Over the past 2 decades, more than 100 mutations have been described in the same gene, representing the most common genotype. Most mutations result in a loss of function of the transmembrane sodium current (INa), either as a result of a quantitative reduction of the expression of the sodium ion channel within cardiac myocyte cell membranes or via qualitative dysfunction of such channels.

There are other genes associated with the disease, mostly related to sodium current (*GPD-IL*, *SCN1B*, *SCN3B*), although other channels – such as calcium (*CACNA1C* and *CACNB2B*) and potassium (*Ito*) – can also be involved (Table 27.1). Functional studies have shown that in these cases, although the sodium channel is not affected, the Brugada syndrome phenotype may be explained by imbalances in the ionic currents during phase 1 of the action potential.

IOC Manual of Sports Cardiology, First Edition. Edited by Mathew G. Wilson, Jonathan A. Drezner and Sanjay Sharma.
© 2017 International Olympic Committee. Published 2017 by John Wiley & Sons, Ltd.

Channel	Inheritance	Locus	Gene
Sodium	Autosomal-dominant	3p21-p24	*SCN5A*
		3p22.3	*GPD1-L*
		19q13.1	*SCN1B*
		11q24.1	*SCN3B*
		11q23.3	*SCN2B*
		3p22.2	*SCN10A*
Sodium-associated	Autosomal-dominant	17p13.1	*RANGRF*
		3p14.3	*SLMAP*
		12p11.21	*PKP2*
Potassium		12p12.1	*ABCC9*
		11q13-q14	*KCNE3*
	Autosomal-dominant	12p12.1	*KCNJ8*
		15q24.1	*HCN4*
		1p13.2	*KCND3*
	X chromosome	Xq22.3	*KCNE5*
Calcium	Autosomal-dominant	2p13.3	*CACNA1C*
		10p12.33	*CACNB2B*
		7q21-q22	*CACNA2D1*
		19q13.33	*TRPM4*

Table 27.1 Genes associated with Brugada syndrome

Unfortunately, despite the identification of 18 genes associated with the disease, it is possible to identify a mutation in only 25–30% cases.

Importantly, even though the identification of a causal mutation may be useful in patients with suspected Brugada syndrome, the diagnosis is always based on the clinical phenotype and requires the presence of a typical ECG pattern associated with other clinical features of the disease.

Clinical Presentation

Symptoms

Most patients with Brugada syndrome are asymptomatic at the time of evaluation and remain so throughout their lives. Recognised symptoms include syncope, seizures and nocturnal agonal breathing, which may be secondary to PVT/ventricular fibrillation. It is estimated that 17–42% of Brugada syndrome patients may present with syncope or sudden death [4–7]. However, this figure probably overestimates the true incidence of events, since most asymptomatic individuals are never diagnosed. About 25% of patients who experience sudden death have already experienced syncope [5]. Events usually occur during rest or sleep, in febrile episodes or under vagal predominance, and rarely during exercise.

Brugada syndrome typically manifests in adulthood, with a mean age of presentation with sudden death of 41 ± 15 years; however, it can also occur in children and the elderly. The Brugada syndrome phenotype is 8–10 times more common in men than in women. This may be due to constitutional differences in the transmembrane ion currents between genders. Moreover, there are data suggesting hormonal influences on phenotypic differences between sexes, such as regression of ECG type 1 after castration or androgen suppression therapy for prostate cancer in men with Brugada syndrome, with higher concentrations of testosterone in Brugada syndrome men in comparison to controls [8]. Prognosis also differs between sexes, with a 4.5–5.5-fold increased risk of sudden death in men. This increased expression of Brugada syndrome in men has not been reported in children under 16.

Other manifestations, such as palpitations or dizziness, may also be present due to supraventricular arrhythmias, which predominantly consist of atrial fibrillation (up to 20% of cases) or sinus node dysfunction.

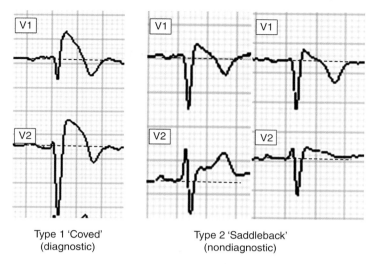

Type 1 'Coved'   Type 2 'Saddleback'
(diagnostic)   (nondiagnostic)

Figure 27.1 ECG patterns in Brugada syndrome

Rest ECG

ECG changes in Brugada syndrome can be dynamic and are occasionally concealed. Certain situations, such as fever, vagal stimulation, alcohol binging, cocaine use and electrolyte abnormalities, may expose the diagnostic ECG pattern when manifestations are not apparent at baseline.

In 2012, a new expert consensus was issued to establish accurate ECG criteria for the diagnosis of Brugada syndrome (Figure 27.1) [9]:

- The type 1 ('coved-type') Brugada ECG pattern is the only one considered diagnostic of Brugada syndrome. Its main features include:
  - ST-segment elevation ≥2 mm (0.2 mV) in one or more right precordial leads (V1–V3), followed by a concave ST segment.
  - A <4 mm reduction of the QRS–ST height from the point of maximum elevation to 40 ms later.
  - A descending ST segment crossing the isoelectric line, followed by a negative and symmetric T-wave.
- The type 2 ('saddleback-type') Brugada ECG pattern is not diagnostic but is highly suggestive of Brugada syndrome. Its main features include:
  - ST-segment elevation ≥0.5 mm (generally ≥2 mm in V2) in one or more right precordial leads (V1–V3), followed by a convex ST.
  - A slow downward slope of the r′ wave, which may or may not overlap the J-point .
  - An ST segment followed by a positive T-wave in V2 and of variable morphology in V1.

Pharmacological Tests and Other Diagnostic Tools

A diagnostic ECG pattern is observed in only 25% of baseline tracings, and most patients with a type 1 ECG at diagnosis will eventually show a normal ECG during follow-up examinations. For this reason, when there is clinical suspicion of Brugada syndrome without a spontaneous type 1 ECG pattern or during familial screening, a pharmacological challenge test with sodium-channel blocking agents should be performed in order to unmask concealed forms of Brugada syndrome.

The test is performed under continuous ECG monitoring. It is recommended to place leads V1 and V2 in the third and second intercostal spaces, respectively, at the beginning and end of the test, as this increases the sensitivity of ECG to the diagnostic pattern (Figure 27.2). The test is considered positive only if a type 1 ECG pattern is obtained, and it should be discontinued in the event of frequent ventricular extrasystoles and ventricular arrhythmias, or of widening of the QRS >130% over the baseline value. Almost 25% of drug-induced tests may result in a false-negative result, and a repeat test should be considered if the clinical suspicion of Brugada syndrome persists [10]. Table 27.2 shows drugs used, doses and routes of administration.

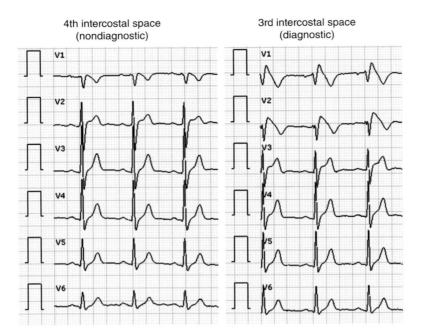

Figure 27.2 Diagnostic value of recording the ECG with higher V1–V2 leads (at the third intercostal space)

Drug	Dose	Administration	Sensibility	Specificity	Predictive positive value	Negative predictive value
Ajmaline	1 mg.kg^{-1} over 5 minutes	Intravenous	80% [1]	94.4% [1]	93.3% [1]	82.9% [1]
Flecainide	2 mg.kg^{-1} over 10 minutes 400 mg	Intravenous Oral	77% [2]	80% [2]	96% [2]	36% [2]
Procainamide	10 mg.kg^{-1} over 10 minutes	Intravenous	NA	NA	NA	NA
Pilsicainide	1 mg.kg^{-1} over 10 minutes	Intravenous	NA	NA	NA	NA

Table 27.2 Drugs used in provocation tests to unmask the ECG in Brugada syndrome

NA, not available.

Stress ECG

Heart rate during exercise testing can be considered as a parameter by which to evaluate cardiac autonomic function. Sympathetic withdrawal and parasympathetic activation occur on early recovery after exercise, and are expected to augment ST-segment elevation directly through inhibition of calcium-channel current or by decreasing heart rate.

Several cases of ST-segment augmentation during and ventricular arrhythmia induction after exercise have been reported in Brugada syndrome patients. On the other hand, experiments in right ventricular tissue preparations indicate that tachycardia aggravates ST-segment elevation in Brugada syndrome and in vitro studies using heterologous expression systems suggest that loss-of-function *SCN5A* mutations associated with Brugada syndrome have a greater impact in reducing INa at faster heart rates.

In 2009, Amin et al. [11] evaluated the ECG response to exercise in Brugada syndrome patients with *SCN5A* mutations, in Brugada syndrome patients without *SCN5A* mutations and in control subjects. They

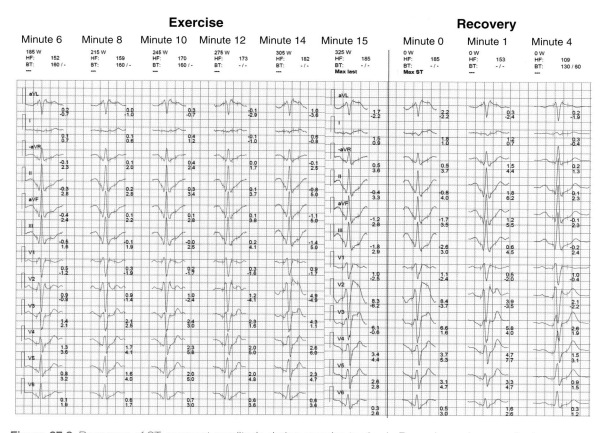

Figure 27.3 Response of ST-segment amplitude during exercise testing in Brugada syndrome patients

found that exercise aggravated the ECG phenotype in Brugada syndrome by producing an increase in peak J-point amplitude in all groups and QRS widening in Brugada syndrome patients with an *SCN5A* mutation, which was more apparent at fast heart rates. Therefore, it has been suggested that the exercise test may be a safe alternative tool for diagnosis in subjects suspected of having Brugada syndrome (Figure 27.3).

The prognostic value of exercise-related ECG changes in Brugada syndrome was explored in a Japanese population by Makimoto et al. [12]. The authors observed that the augmentation of ST-segment elevation during recovery was specific for patients with Brugada syndrome. These Brugada syndrome individuals showed a significantly larger heart rate reduction compared with patients who did not show augmentation of the ST segment, something that could be related to a higher parasympathetic activity. Moreover, ST-segment augmentation during early recovery following exercise was a significant and independent predictor of subsequent cardiac events in our study. These results suggest a possible role for stress ECG in the diagnosis and risk stratification of Brugada syndrome patients. Further studies with a larger number of Brugada syndrome patients will be required to confirm the significance of the augmentation of ST-segment elevation during exercise as a predictor of subsequent cardiac events.

Other ECG Findings

Depolarisation abnormalities, such as a prolonged P-wave, PR or QRS duration, are frequently observed, particularly in patients with Brugada syndrome secondary to *SCN5A* mutations. PR prolongation is most likely related to conduction delay at the His–Purkinje system. QRS prolongation could have prognostic value.

On the other hand, repolarisation abnormalities in the inferior and lateral leads have been reported in up to 11% of Brugada syndrome patients, seemingly related to a more severe phenotype. The QT interval is generally normal, but is occasionally slightly prolonged in the right precordial leads, possibly secondary to the greater prolongation of the action potential duration in the right ventricular epicardium. Finally, in up to 20% of cases, there may be supraventricular arrhythmias, mainly AF, although atrioventricular (AV) nodal re-entry and Wolff–Parkinson–White (WPW) have also been described. Additionally, an association between Brugada syndrome and sinus node dysfunction has been described.

Diagnostic Criteria

Until recently, in order to diagnose Brugada syndrome, it was necessary to demonstrate [13]:

1. The presence of a type 1 ECG pattern (descending ST elevation ≥2 mm in at least one right precordial lead); AND
2. The presence of one or more of the following clinical manifestations:
   a. Resuscitated sudden death.
   b. Documented PVT.
   c. A history of nonvasovagal syncope.
   d. A family history of sudden death in patients <45 years with a structurally normal heart.
   e. A type 1 ECG pattern in relatives.

However, as many individuals who have a type 1 ECG are asymptomatic, the Expert Consensus published in 2013 proposed the following definition: 'BrS [Brugada syndrome] is diagnosed when a type 1 ST elevation is observed either spontaneously or after intravenous administration of a sodium channel blocker in at least one right precordial lead (V1 and V2), placed in a standard or superior position (up to the 2nd intercostal space)' (Figure 27.4) [14]. This definition no longer requires any other evidence of malignant arrhythmias. In these asymptomatic individuals, other findings which support the diagnosis of Brugada syndrome include [14]:

- Attenuation of ST elevation during maximal exercise, with reappearance during the recovery phase. It should be noted that in selected patients, usually carrying an *SCN5A* mutation, the ST elevation may become more evident with exercise.

Ajmaline infusion

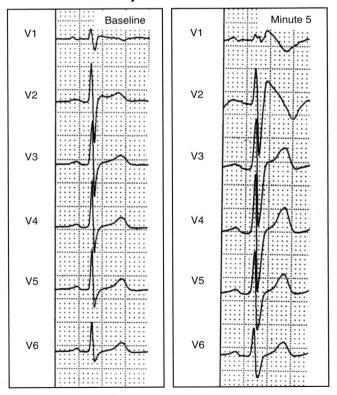

Figure 27.4 Ajmaline test to unmask the diagnostic Brugada syndrome pattern (type 1 pattern: coved-type)

A. Factors that unmask the Brugada syndrome pattern in case of genetic predisposition

Hyperkaliaemia
Hypercalcaemia
Fever
Treatment with:

1. Antiarrhythmic drugs: sodium channel blockers (class Ic, class Ia), calcium antagonists, beta blockers
2. Antianginal drugs: calcium antagonists, nitrates, potassium channel openers
3. Psychotropic drugs: tricyclic/tetracyclic antidepresssants, phenothyazines, selective serotonin reuptake inhibitors (SSRIs), lithium
4. Others: histamine H1 antagonist, alcohol intoxication, cocaine intoxication

B. Differential diagnosis

Atypical right bundle branch block (RBBB)
Left ventricular hypertrophy (LVH)
Early repolarisation (particularly in athletes)
Acute pericarditis/myocarditis
Acute myocardial ischaemia or infarction (especially of the right ventricle)
Acute pulmonary thromboembolism
Prinzmetal angina
Aortic dissecant aneurism
Disorders of the central and autonomic nervous systems
Duchenne's muscular dystrophy
Friedreich's ataxia
Arrhythmogenic right ventricular dysplasia
Mechanical compression of the right ventricular outflow tract (RVOT) (e.g. pectus excavatum, mediastinic tumour etc.)
Hemopericardium
Hypothermia

Table 27.3 Differential diagnosis of Brugada syndrome

- First-degree AV block and left-axis deviation.
- AF.
- Late potentials in high-resolution ECG (SAECG).
- Fragmentation of the QRS.
- Alternation of the ST–T segment (beat-to-beat fluctuations in the ECG ST–T segment) andspontaneous ventricular premature beats with a left bundle branch block (LBBB) pattern.
- A ventricular refractory period <200 ms and an HV interval >60 ms (obtained by an electrophysiological (EP) study).
- Absence of structural heart disease.

Importantly, other causes of ST-segment elevation should be excluded before establishing the diagnosis of Brugada syndrome; for example, psychotropic drugs and antiallergenic agents may induce a Brugada syndrome-like ECG pattern, often without a concomitant risk of arrhythmia (Table 27.3A). On the other hand, there are modulating factors that can unmask or exacerbate the typical Brugada syndrome pattern. Fever modulates the phenotype by accentuating sodium channel inactivation, unmasking the type 1 ECG pattern and triggering ventricular arrhythmias. Exposure to certain other drugs or electrolyte imbalances may also produce ST elevation suggestive of Brugada syndrome, which can be related to a possible genetic predisposition. If any of these modulating factors is present, it should be corrected (Table 27.3B). ECG changes compatible with Brugada syndrome can appear immediately after electrical cardioversion, although it is unknown whether they occur in carriers of Brugada syndrome mutations.

Risk Stratification

Accurate identification and treatment of individuals at high risk of SCD is one of the main challenges in the clinical management of Brugada syndrome patients. Sudden death is an indisputable risk factor and is recognised by all studies. These patients should be protected with an implantable cardioverter-defibrillator

(ICD) (class I indication) [14,15]. Most studies are in agreement that syncope in combination with a spontaneous type 1 ECG pattern is a strong marker of poor prognosis during follow-up.

Risk stratification in asymptomatic patients is much more complex and is a matter of debate. The incidence of major arrhythmic events varies between 0.5 and 8.2% during an average follow-up of 35 months [5–7, 16,17]. Despite these differences, it is clear that it is necessary to identify clinical variables in order to stratify risk in this subgroup of patients.

Male gender is a risk factor associated with the occurrence of cardiac events during follow-up. Moreover, risk markers differ between men and women. Indeed, poor prognostic factors described for mixed populations in the series by Brugada et al. [4,6] (which included the presence of symptoms, a spontaneous type 1 ECG pattern and inducibility in EP study) were confirmed as valid for risk stratification in men but not in women, given the low event rate in this group.

Interestingly, neither family history of sudden death nor the presence of an *SCN5A* mutation have been identified as risk factors in any of the large series reported to date. However, some mutation types, such as those resulting in a truncated protein, may have prognostic value.

Various registries agree that the inducibility of arrhythmias during an EP study is higher in symptomatic patients [5,7]; nevertheless, the utility of EP testing for risk stratification is a matter of debate. The results published by Brugada et al. [6] indicate that the EP study is an independent predictor of arrhythmic events, and Giustetto et al. [16] highlight its high negative predictive value (NPV). However, other records have not obtained the same results [5,7,17,18]. The PRELUDE (PRogrammed ELectrical stimulation preDictive valUe) registry could not confirm the high NPV [18]. Moreover, the FINGER (France, Italy, Netherlands, Germany) registry found that the inducibility of sustained ventricular arrhythmias in the EP study was significantly associated with time to first arrhythmic event in the univariate analysis, but in a subsequent multivariate analysis induction of ventricular arrhythmias during an EP study did not predict adverse events during follow-up [17].

Both the Expert Consensus and the current American College of Cardiology (ACC)/American Heart Association (AHA)/European Society of Cardiology (ESC) guidelines for the prevention of sudden death recommend performing an EP test for risk stratification in Brugada syndrome as a class IIb indication [14,15].

Management

Table 27.4 shows the Expert Consensus recommendations for the management of inherited primary arrhythmia syndromes [14].

General Measures

To date, treatment options in Brugada syndrome have been limited to ICD or drugs. However, education and lifestyle changes for the prevention of arrhythmias are critical. Patients should be informed of the various modulators and precipitating factors that can induce malignant arrhythmias (such as fever, electrolyte disturbances and drugs). Fever should be treated promptly with antipyretics and/or physical measures. Any contraindicated substance should be avoided (see www.brugadadrugs.org).

Finally, the study of first-degree relatives should always be recommended. Family genetic analysis is useful if the causal mutation in the proband is known.

Implantable Cardioverter-Defibrillator

ICD therapy is the only effective strategy for the prevention of sudden death in Brugada syndrome patients. The current indications for ICD follow the recommendations proposed by the International Consensus published in 2013 [14]. Briefly, symptomatic patients should always receive an ICD. In asymptomatic patients with a spontaneous type 1 ECG pattern, an EP study can be used to assess the need for ICD implantation [14]. In asymptomatic patients in whom a type 1 ECG pattern is documented only after the administration of sodium channel-blocking agents, regular follow-up is recommended, without the need for an EP study for risk stratification or ICD implantation [14].

Class I	1. The following lifestyle changes are recommended in all patients with a diagnosis of Brugada syndrome:
	  a. Avoidance of drugs that might induce or aggravate ST-segment elevation in right precordial leads (see www.brugadadrugs.org)
	  b. Avoidance of excessive alcohol intake
	  c. Immediate treatment of fever with antipyretic drugs
	2. ICD implantation is recommended in patients with a diagnosis of Brugada syndrome who:
	  a. Are survivors of a cardiac arrest; and/or
	  b. Have documented spontaneous sustained ventricular tachycardia with or without syncope

Class IIa	3. ICD implantation can be useful in patients with a spontaneous diagnostic type 1 ECG who have a history of syncope judged likely to be caused by ventricular arrhythmias
	4. Quinidine can be useful in patients with a diagnosis of Brugada syndrome and history of arrhythmic storms, defined as more than two episodes of ventricular tachycardia/ventricular fibrillation in 24 hours
	5. Quinidine can be useful in patients with a diagnosis of Brugada syndrome:
	  a. Who qualify for an ICD but present a contraindication to the ICD or refuse it; and/or
	  b. Have a history of documented supraventricular arrhythmias that require treatment
	6. Isoproterenol infusion can be useful in suppressing arrhythmic storms in Brugada syndrome patients

Class IIb	7. ICD implantation may be considered in patients with a diagnosis of Brugada syndrome who develop ventricular fibrillation during programmed electrical stimulation (inducible patients) 8. Quinidine may be considered in asymptomatic patients with a diagnosis of Brugada syndrome and a spontaneous type 1 ECG 9. Catheter ablation may be considered in patients with a diagnosis of Brugada syndrome and a history of arrhythmic storms or repeated appropriate ICD shocks
Class III	10. ICD implantation is not indicated in asymptomatic Brugada syndrome patients with a drug-induced type 1 ECG and on the basis of a family history of SCD alone

Table 27.4 Therapeutic recommendations in Brugada syndrome

The annual rate of appropriate ICD therapies in Brugada syndrome patients reaches up to 7% [19], although its incidence depends on the indication for ICD implantation: 6.9% in patients with sudden death, 2% in patients with a history of syncope and 1% in asymptomatic individuals. It is important to note that this rate refers to a young and otherwise healthy population, whose life expectancy can exceed 30 years. But, perhaps because it is a young, active population, there is a significant device complication rate, mainly due to inappropriate shocks and lead failure (20–36% after a 21–47-month follow-up) [19,20]. Programming a single zone of therapy (ventricular fibrillation) with a high cut-off limit (>220 beats.min^{-1}) and long sensing intervals may prevent therapy in self-limited arrhythmias. Other measures to prevent complications include the restriction of high-intensity sports, particularly those that could damage the electrode. The use of the new subcutaneous ICDs may be an effective option, as it avoids problems associated with the placement of an intravascular lead.

Exercise Considerations

Ventricular arrhythmias are rare in athletes, but by nature they may be life-threatening. Physical activity is associated with a 2.5-fold greater risk of sudden death [21]. Adrenergic stress during competitive sport is a commonly accepted trigger for arrhythmia and SCD in the presence of underlying inherited cardiac disease, such as cardiomyopathy, primary arrhythmia syndromes or vascular disease.

In the majority of Brugada syndrome patients, however, the malignant ventricular arrhythmias occur at rest and, in many cases, at night, as a consequence of an increased vagal activity and/or withdrawal of sympathetic activity. Thus, it could be hypothesised that enhanced adrenergic tone, such as that occurring during sports activity, could have an inhibitory effect and theoretically reduce the risk sudden death risk. On the other hand, increased vagal predominance as a consequence of chronic athletic conditioning may eventually enhance the propensity of athletes with Brugada syndrome to die at rest, during sleep or during recovery after exercise. Furthermore, elevation of body temperature during high-intensity efforts could potentially trigger fatal arrhythmias in these patients.

Intensity level	Points		Intensity level	Points
High			Hiking	
Basketball			• Modest	4
• Full-court	2		• Normal	4
• Half-court	2		Motorcycling	2
Body building[a]	1		Jogging	4
Ice hockey[a]	0		Sailing[b]	4
Racquetball/squash	2		Surfing[b]	1
Rock climbing[a]	1		Swimming (lap)[b]	4
Running (sprinting)	2		Tennis (doubles)	4
Skiing			Treadmill/stationary bicycle	5
• Downhill[a]	1		Weightlifting (free weights)[a,c]	1
• Cross-country	4		*Low*	
Football	2		Bowling	5
Tennis (singles)	2		Golf	5
Windsurfing	1		Horseback riding[a]	3
Moderate			Scuba diving[b]	0
Baseball/softball	4		Skating	5
Biking	5		Snorkelling[b]	4
			Weightlifting (non-free weights)	4
			Brisk walking	5

Table 27.5 Recommendations for the acceptability of recreational (noncompetitive) sports in Brugada syndrome [3]

0–1, generally not advised or strongly discouraged; 2–3, intermediate (to be assessed clinically on an individual basis); 4–5, probably permitted.

[a] These sports involve the potential for traumatic injury, which should be taken into consideration for individuals with a risk of impaired consciousness.

[b] The possibility of impaired consciousness occurring during water-related activities should be taken into account, bearing in mind the clinical profile of the individual patient.

[c] Recommendations generally differ from those for weight-training machines (non-free weights), based largely on the potential risks of traumatic injury associated with episodes of impaired consciousness during bench-press manoeuvres. Otherwise, the physiological effects of all weight-training activities are regarded as similar with respect to the present recommendations.

Unfortunately, there is a scarcity of large-scale or prospective data on the safety of sports participation in individuals suffering from Brugada syndrome, and clinical common sense should always be applied.

Based on the potential risk of lethal arrhythmias secondary to hyperthermia and to increased vagal tone and/or abrupt cessation of sympathetic activity, the Recommendations for Physical Activity and Sports Participation of the ESC [22] indicate abstinence from most competitive sporting activities, with the exception of those involving a low static and dynamic component. The joint 2015 ACC/AHA guidelines permit competitive sport in asymptomatic patients with Brugada syndrome provide adequate precautions such as avoiding dehydration, participation in endurance events associated with high core temperature and avoiding medications which may precipitate fatal arrhythmias. Competition must only occur in events where there are adequate provisions for immediate advanced cardiopulmonary resuscitation [23]. Athletes with ICDs and who have not experienced an episode of rapid ventricular arrhythmia requiring device therapy for 6 months may engage in class Ia competitive sports of low dynamic and static intensity but must avoid contact sports.

The AHA recommendations for recreational sport engagement in Brugada syndrome are given in Table 27.5 [24].

It must be noted that no association between physical exercise and sudden death has been clearly established in Brugada syndrome. For this reason, both the 2nd BrS Consensus Conference [13] and the 2013

Expert Consensus on inherited primary arrhythmia syndromes [14] and on the management of arrhythmias in the paediatric population [25] provide no guidelines regarding the limitation of sports in this pathology.

Conclusion

Since its discovery, there has been considerable progress in the understanding of various aspects of Brugada syndrome. However, there are still many controversies and unanswered questions regarding this relatively novel ion channelopathy, including issues around safety during sports participation. Future research will hopefully provide solutions and help characterise Brugada syndrome in more detail.

References

1 Brugada, P. and Brugada, J. Right bundle branch block, persistent st segment elevation and sudden cardiac death: a distinct clinical and electrocardiographic syndrome: a multicenter report. *J Am Coll Cardiol* 1992; **20**: 1391–6.

2 Miyazaki, T., Mitamura, H., Miyoshi, S. et al. Autonomic and antiarrhythmic drug modulation of st segment elevation in patients with brugada syndrome. *J Am Coll Cardiol* 1996; **27**: 1061–70.

3 Schulze-Bahr, E., Eckardt, L., Breithardt, G. et al. Sodium channel gene (SCN5A) mutations in 44 index patients with brugada syndrome: different incidences in familial and sporadic disease. *Hum Mutat* 2003; **21**: 651–2.

4 Brugada, J., Brugada, R., Antzelevitch, C. et al. Long-term follow-up of individuals with the electrocardiographic pattern of right bundle-branch block and st-segment elevation in precordial leads v1 to v3. *Circulation* 2002; **105**: 73–8.

5 Priori, S.G., Napolitano, C., Gasparini, M. et al. Natural history of brugada syndrome: insights for risk stratification and management. *Circulation* 2002; **105**: 1342–7.

6 Brugada, J., Brugada, R. and Brugada, P. Determinants of sudden cardiac death in individuals with the electrocardiographic pattern of brugada syndrome and no previous cardiac arrest. *Circulation* 2003; **108**: 3092–6.

7 Eckardt, L., Probst, V., Smits, J.P.P. et al. Long-term prognosis of individuals with right precordial st-segment–elevation brugada syndrome. *Circulation* 2005; **111**: 257–63.

8 Shimizu, W., Matsuo, K., Kokubo, Y. et al. Sex hormone and gender difference – role of testosterone on male predominance in brugada syndrome. *J Cardiovasc Electrophysiol* 2007; **18**: 415–21.

9 Bayés de Luna, A., Brugada, J., Baranchuk, A. et al. Current electrocardiographic criteria for diagnosis of brugada pattern: a consensus report. *J Electrocardiol* 2012; **45**: 433–42.

10 Meregalli, P.G., Ruijter, J.M., Hofman, N. et al. Diagnostic value of flecainide testing in unmasking SCN5A-related Brugada syndrome. *J Cardiovasc Electrophysiol* 2006; **17**: 857–64.

11 Amin, A.S., de Groot, E.A.A., Ruijter, J.M. et al. Exercise-induced ecg changes in brugada syndrome. *Circ Arrhyth Electrophysiol* 2009; **2**: 531–9.

12 Makimoto, H., Nakagawa, E., Takaki, H. et al. Augmented st-segment elevation during recovery from exercise predicts cardiac events in patients with brugada syndrome. *J Am Coll Cardiol* 2010; **56**: 1576–84.

13 Antzelevitch, C., Brugada, P., Borggrefe, M. et al. Brugada syndrome: Report of the second consensus conference: endorsed by the heart rhythm society and the european heart rhythm association. *Circulation* 2005; **111**: 659–70.

14 Priori, S.G., Wilde, A.A., Horie, M. et al. Executive summary: Hrs/ehra/aphrs expert consensus statement on the diagnosis and management of patients with inherited primary arrhythmia syndromes. *Europace* 2013; **15**: 1389–406.

15 Zipes, D.P., Camm, A.J., Borggrefe, M. et al. ACC/AHA/ESC 2006 guidelines for management of patients with ventricular arrhythmias and the prevention of sudden cardiac death – executive summary. *Eur Heart J* 2006; **27**: 2099–140.

16 Giustetto, C., Drago, S., Demarchi, P.G. et al. Risk stratification of the patients with brugada type electrocardiogram: a community-based prospective study. *Europace* 2009; **11**: 507–13.

17 Probst, V., Veltmann, C., Eckardt, L. et al. Long-term prognosis of patients diagnosed with brugada syndrome: results from the finger brugada syndrome registry. *Circulation* 2010; **121**: 635–43.

18 Priori, S.G., Gasparini, M., Napolitano, C. et al. Risk stratification in brugada syndrome: Results of the prelude (programmed electrical stimulation predictive value) registry. *J Am Coll Cardiol* 2012; **59**: 37–45.

19 Sacher, F., Probst, V., Maury, P. et al. Outcome after implantation of a cardioverter-defibrillator in patients with brugada syndrome: a multicenter study – part 2. *Circulation* 2013; **128**: 1739–47.

20 Miyazaki, S., Uchiyama, T., Komatsu, Y. et al. Long-term complications of implantable defibrillator therapy in brugada syndrome. *Am J Cardiol* 2013; **111**: 1448–51.

21 Corrado, D., Basso, C., Rizzoli, G. et al. Does sports activity enhance the risk of sudden death in adolescents and young adults? *J Am Coll Cardiol* 2003; **42**: 1959–63.

22 Pelliccia, A., Corrado, D., Bjørnstad, H.H. et al. Recommendations for participation in competitive sport and leisure-time physical activity in individuals with cardiomyopathies, myocarditis and pericarditis. *Eur J Cardiovasc Prev Rehabil* 2006; **13**: 876–85.

23 Ackerman, M.J., Zipes, D.P., Kovacs, R.J. and Maron, B.J. Eligibility and disqualification recommendations for competitive athletes with cardiovascular abnormalities: Task Force 10: The cardiac channelopathies: A scientific statement from the American Heart Association and American College of Cardiology. *J Am Coll Cardiol* 2015; **66**(21): 2424–8.

24 Maron, B.J., Chaitman, B.R., Ackerman, M.J. et al. Recommendations for physical activity and recreational sports participation for young patients with genetic cardiovascular diseases. *Circulation* 2004; **109**: 2807–16.

25 Brugada, J., Blom, N., Sarquella-Brugada, G. et al. Pharmacological and non-pharmacological therapy for arrhythmias in the pediatric population: EHRA and AEPC-arrhythmia working group joint consensus statement. *Europace* 2013; **15**(9): 1337–82.

28 Wolff–Parkinson–White Syndrome

Jack C. Salerno

University of Washington School of Medicine, Seattle Children's Hospital, Seattle, WA, USA

Introduction

Wolff–Parkinson–White (WPW) syndrome was first described in 1930 in a landmark article in the *American Heart Journal*, in which the authors reported a case series of 11 otherwise healthy patients with electrocardiogram (ECG) findings of a short PR interval and 'bundle branch block' morphology who also suffered from paroxysmal tachycardia [1]. Shortly after their discovery, electrophysiologists were able to elucidate the relationship between accessory pathways and re-entrant supraventricular tachycardia (SVT). However, it wasn't until 40 years later that rapid conduction of atrial fibrillation was discovered as the mechanism of sudden death [2].

Before reviewing the mechanism of WPW, a review of how the electrical signals normally propagate through the heart is worthwhile. In the normal heart, the atrial and ventricular myocardia are electrically insulated from one another except at the atrioventricular (AV) node and bundle of His. Impulse generation originates in the sinus node and is conducted through the atrial myocardium to the AV node. The major role of the AV node is to allow conduction of the impulse to the ventricle; equally important, however, is the inherent delay in the AV node that slows conduction from the atrium to the ventricle, allowing ventricular filling. From the AV node, there is rapid conduction via the specialised His–Purkinje system to the ventricle. There is an important conduction characteristic of the AV node whereby there is an inverse relationship of AV conduction to the atrial rate: as atrial rate accelerates, conduction within the AV node slows. This decremental property of the AV node serves as a safety net during rapid atrial rates (e.g. AF) by slowing conduction to the ventricles.

WPW is a cardiac conduction system disorder that is characterised by an abnormal electrical connection known as an accessory pathway, which bypasses the AV node and directly connects the atria to the ventricle. This condition is manifest on the surface ECG by a short PR interval and a delta wave which is the slurred upstroke of the QRS complex. These ECG findings are related to the accessory pathway bypassing the AV node, resulting in early activation of the ventricular myocardium. The accessory pathway not only creates the characteristic appearance on the ECG but may also provide the substrate for re-entrant SVT and/or allow rapid transmission of AF, with potentially life-threatening consequences.

Epidemiology

When discussing the prevalence of WPW, it is important to distinguish between the WPW pattern and WPW syndrome. The WPW pattern, also known as isolated ventricular pre-excitation, is used to describe athletes with ECG evidence of WPW without symptoms. Asymptomatic WPW pattern is much more common and has a prevalence of approximately 1 in 1000 amongst athletes [3].

Aetiology

The accessory pathways associated with WPW are thought to be an embryologic remnant resulting from failure of resorption of the ventricular syncytium during foetal development. There is evidence that over time the accessory pathway may lose conduction capabilities, with up to 30% of adults losing

IOC Manual of Sports Cardiology, First Edition. Edited by Mathew G. Wilson, Jonathan A. Drezner and Sanjay Sharma.
© 2017 International Olympic Committee. Published 2017 by John Wiley & Sons, Ltd.

ventricular pre-excitation over 5 years [4]. The loss of pre-excitation in children and adolescents over a similar period is more variable (0–26%) [5,6].

Genetics

Most cases of WPW syndrome are sporadic. However, patients with WPW have a threefold higher risk than the general population of having an affected first-degree relative with WPW [7]. The familial form is usually inherited as a Mendelian autosomal-dominant trait. There has been a long-recognised association of WPW and cardiomyopathy [8]. Mutations in the gene encoding the gamma-2 regulatory subunit of AMP-activated protein kinase (PRKAG2) and lyosomal-associated membrane protein (LAMP2) are also associated with WPW [9]. The exact mechanism explaining how this gene abnormality results in WPW is not known.

Associated Cardiac Abnormalities

The majority of athletes with WPW have normal cardiac anatomy. There is an increased prevalence of WPW in Ebstein's anomaly of the tricuspid valve. Patients with Ebstein's anomaly frequently have multiple accessory bypass tracts, mostly on the right side of the heart, near the anatomically displaced tricuspid valve. Hypertrophic cardiomyopathy (HCM) may also be associated with WPW, often in the setting of specific gene mutations (PRKAG2 and LAMP2) [8,9].

ECG Criteria for Diagnosis

The diagnosis of WPW is made by ECG. In WPW, the accessory pathway conducts the impulse generated by the sinus node in the same direction as the AV node. Because the AV node has decremental properties, the more rapidly conducting accessory pathway activates the ventricle prematurely and shortens the PR interval. Since the activation of the ventricular myocardium occurs outside of the His–Purkinje system, it results in a broad QRS. The classic ECG triad is a short PR interval (<120 ms), a slurred QRS upstroke ('delta' wave) and a prolonged QRS complex (>120 ms) with secondary ST and T-wave changes (Figure 28.1) [10].

Clinical Presentation

Asymptomatic WPW

The majority of patients with WPW are asymptomatic: approximately 65% of adolescents and 40% of those over 30 years of age [5,11]. Asymptomatic athletes are often identified after an ECG has been performed as part of a preparticipation evaluation or for other indications (chest pain). Young patients with WPW may be considered 'presymptomatic', as they have not had time to develop symptoms or a sentinel event [12].

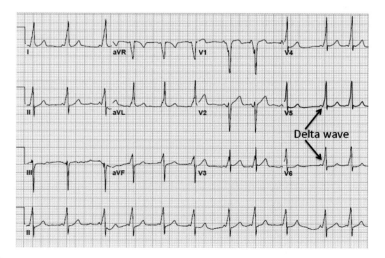

Figure 28.1 12-lead ECG showing the characteristic findings of WPW: short PR, delta wave and broad QRS

Conversely, individuals surviving to adulthood without symptoms may harbour lower risk pathways [12]. In a large community-based WPW population study, approximately one-third of individuals under 40 years of age became symptomatic with SVT or palpitations [11], whereas no patients in whom pre-excitation was first uncovered after the age of 40 years developed symptoms [13]. The athletes with WPW who are most susceptible to SCD are those with symptoms [14]. Thus, the onset of symptoms in any individual requires a heightened awareness and evaluation. Although most patients with WPW who have a sudden cardiac death (SCD) event have had prior symptoms, there are asymptomatic patients whose initial presentation is sudden death [2,14].

Symptomatic WPW

Supraventricular Tachycardia The most common presentation of symptomatic WPW related to the accessory pathway is associated with SVT. The presence of an accessory pathway with the ability to conduct retrograde from the ventricle to the atrium establishes a circuit that consists of two distinct pathways for conduction: the normal AV node and the accessory pathway (Figure 28.2). The electrical impulse during SVT usually traverses the AV node to the ventricle and then cycles back to the atrium via the accessory pathway. The overall risk of SVT developing in an asymptomatic individual is 16 per 1000 person-years of follow-up [15]. Re-entrant SVT is usually well tolerated, but it can degenerate into AF with significant consequences if there is rapid pathway conduction.

Sudden Death WPW accounts for at least 1% of deaths in a long-term registry of SCD in athletes, although it may account for a fraction of a larger percentage of cases in autopsy-negative sudden unexplained death [16]. The paediatric population has been reported to have an SCD rate of 1.9 per 1000 patient-years, in comparison with 0.9 in adults [15]. The risk of sudden death in symptomatic patients is estimated to be approximately 3–4% over a lifetime [15]. The initial presentation with sudden death is more common in younger patients and is a rare initial presentation in patients over 30 years of age. Whilst prediction of the risk of SCD by history is difficult, there are several high-risk factors: age <30 years, male gender, history of AF, prior syncope, associated congenital heart disease (CHD) and familial WPW [12].

Impact of Medications There are several medications (verapamil, digoxin) that have been associated with an increased risk of ventricular fibrillation in patients with WPW due to their ability to enhance conduction down the accessory pathway [17,18]. These medications are AV nodal blocking agents, which are occasionally used to treat SVT; they should be avoided in a patient with WPW.

Subtle Pre-excitation At times, the degree of pre-excitation is subtle and the delta wave is not obvious. This occurs when the conduction is predominantly down the AV node, with only a small influence from the accessory pathway. It is important to recognise that there is no correlation between the degree of

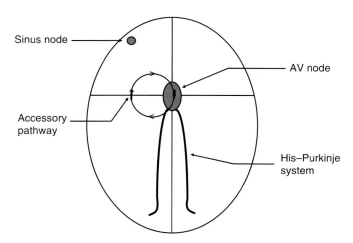

Figure 28.2 Diagram showing the 'circuit' in re-entrant SVT, wherein the impulse travels to the ventricle via the AV node and returns to the atrium via the accessory pathway

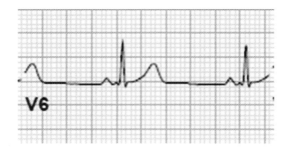

Figure 28.3 Lead V6 rhythm strip, showing subtle pre-excitation. This presentation is mostly evident from the lack of the normal Q-waves in the lateral precordial leads

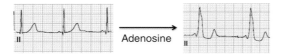

Figure 28.4 Adenosine administration during sinus rhythm in a patient with subtle pre-excitation. The diagnosis of WPW is confirmed by the increasing degree of pre-excitation. If there were no pathway, AV block would follow the adenosine administration

pre-excitation and the conduction characteristics of the accessory pathway. ECG findings associated with a subtle WPW pattern include left-axis deviation, abnormal Q-waves in leads V5 and V6 (Figure 28.3), ST-segment depression and T-wave changes [19]. Some of these findings can be difficult to distinguish from a myocardial infarction (MI) [20]. In these instances, where there is concern over subtle pre-excitation, adenosine administration can transiently inhibit conduction through the AV node without impacting conduction through the accessory pathway, thereby unmasking the pathway (Figure 28.4) [21,22].

Risk assessment of WPW

Athletes with ventricular pre-excitation are at risk for sudden death based on rapid conduction of atrial arrhythmias (particularly AF) over the accessory pathway, with resultant VF. The goal of risk stratification is to identify those athletes at risk of lethal arrhythmias. Although there are historical elements associated with increased risk, history and physical are largely inadequate for assessing the risk of sudden death. Both noninvasive and invasive electrophysiologic measures can be used to identify a pathway's ability to allow AF to degenerate into VF.

Noninvasive Evaluation

Noninvasive measures include ECG, 24-hour Holter monitoring and exercise testing. The noninvasive measure takes advantage of the fact that if the pathway cannot conduct at sinus rates achieved during exertion, it should not be able to conduct sufficiently rapidly to place the athlete at risk of sudden death.

Sudden Block during Exertion The best indicator of low risk is the sudden disappearance of pre-excitation during exercise [23]. When sudden block of the accessory pathway is reached during exercise, the patient is assumed to be at low risk of rapid conduction during AF, even during sympathetic stimulation. A recent consensus paper supported the abrupt loss of the delta wave during exercise as a sign of low risk [12]. Some caution should be applied when assessing changes in QRS during exertion. With sympathetic stimulation, there is an increased rate of conduction within the AV node, which may overcome the accessory pathway, resulting in gradual loss of conduction, as compared to abrupt loss (Figure 28.5). This situation commonly occurs with left-sided pathways, because the AV node is closer to the sinus node and therefore most of the ventricular activation occurs over the AV node, with only a small fraction occurring via the accessory pathway.

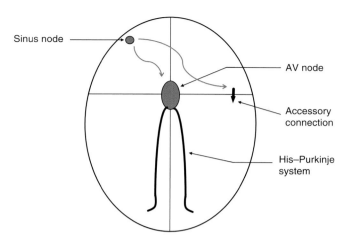

Figure 28.5 During exercise, there is an increase in AV nodal conduction. As in this example, if the AV node is closer to the sinus node than the accessory pathway, there may be a more gradual loss of pre-excitation, as the AV node accounts for a larger degree of ventricular activation. This gradual loss is not the same as abrupt change, and caution is advised when assigning low risk in this situation

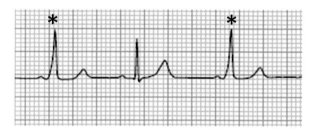

Figure 28.6 Lead II rhythm strip showing intermittent pre-excitation. The broad QRS complexes (*) are associated with accessory pathway conduction, whereas the narrow QRS represents conduction over the AV node

Intermittent Pre-excitation Intermittent pre-excitation is present when, during stable sinus rhythm, pre-excited QRS complexes are followed by normal QRS complexes showing conduction over the AV node (Figure 28.6). Intermittent loss of the delta wave during sinus rhythm relates to failure of conduction over the accessory pathway. The actual mechanism of intermittent pre-excitation is not well understood, but is likely related to a long refractory period of the accessory pathway and inability to conduct rapidly [24].

ECG during AF The ECG performed during AF provides a true assessment of the potential of the accessory pathway for rapid conduction. The shortest pre-excited RR interval (SPERRI) has been used to determine accessory pathway properties. The space between RR intervals is measured in milliseconds and can be converted to a heart rate. A short cycle length is associated with rapid conduction, whilst a longer interval between conducted beats is associated with slower conduction. A SPERRI <250 ms implies conduction across the pathway at a rate faster than 240 beats.min^{-1} (Figure 28.7). This characteristic is more commonly seen in patients with WPW who have experienced cardiac arrest. Importantly, slow conduction during AF as defined by SPERRI >250 ms has a well established negative predictive value (NPV) for sudden death [25].

Invasive Evaluation

If noninvasive testing does not provide a clear understanding of the accessory pathway conduction characteristics, invasive electrophysiology testing should be considered. This involves the placement of intracardiac or oesophageal catheters. The purpose is to define the characteristics of the pathway and identify those athletes who may be at high risk for lethal arrhythmias.

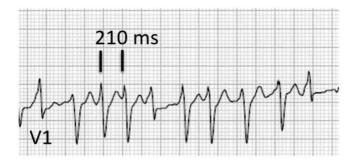

Figure 28.7 Lead V1 rhythm strip during AF with rapid conduction across the accessory pathway. The SPERRI is 210 ms, which is a rate of 285 beats.min⁻¹

During intracardiac procedures, access is obtained to the venous or arterial circulation and catheters with electrode sensors are advanced into the heart. Using various pacing manoeuvres, the electrical properties of the accessory pathway can be identified. With transoesophageal pacing, a catheter is placed in the oesophagus, enabling pacing of the left atrium via the anatomic proximity of the structures.

Several measurements are obtained during electrophysiological evaluation that can be used to assess the risk of a potentially lethal arrhythmia. The most broadly accepted high-risk feature is SPERRI during AF. A SPERRI of 250 ms during sustained induced atrial fibrillation is a very sensitive, but not specific, marker of the risk of ventricular fibrillation in WPW patients [14]. Unfortunately, because there is considerable overlap of measured variables between patients in whom life-threatening arrhythmias develop and those in whom they do not, the positive predictive value (PPV) of SPERRI remains low [15]. However, the NPV of SPERRI >250 ms is well established for risk assessment [25]. Therefore, the subgroup of athletes who have a SPERRI >250 ms has essentially no risk of SCD, which is helpful for decision-making.

In addition to SPERRI <250 ms, the following are also considered higher-risk features: multiple accessory pathways and easily inducible AF [26].

Transcatheter Ablation

Ablation therapy begins with the diagnostic electrophysiology (EP) study detailed in the previous section. During the same procedure, a specialised ablation catheter is advanced to the heart and used to perform mapping of the abnormal electrical signals until the precise location of the pathway is identified. The tip of the mapping catheter is then used to disrupt (or ablate) the tissue beneath the catheter, thus eliminating the abnormal electrical connection.

For those athletes with symptoms including palpitations, syncope or near syncope, it is mandatory to assess the functional capabilities and electrophysiologic properties of the accessory pathway [27]. Ablation is a well-established therapy for these symptomatic athletes, as the benefits outweigh the procedural risks [13,27]. In asymptomatic athletes without structural heart disease, the optimal management is less certain.

In selected asymptomatic athletes, particularly those under 25 years of age who participate in moderate- or high-level activity, it may be advisable to perform an EP study [27]. Those athletes in whom SPERRI <250 ms or who have multiple accessory pathways should undergo ablation of the accessory pathway [27].

Most of the complications of an EP study are minor and non-life-threatening. Radiofrequency (RF) ablation is associated with risks of perforation of the heart or vessel, MI, transient ischaemic attack, stroke and heart block which range from 2 to 4% in large surveys [28–30]. The procedure-related mortality reported for catheter ablation of accessory pathways ranges from 0 to 0.2% [28,30].

Catheter-based ablation therapy includes RF and cryotherapy. RF ablation causes destruction of tissue through resistive heating. The success rate of RF catheter ablation for accessory pathways is approximately 95% in most series [28–30]. After an initially successful procedure with resolution of the inflammation, there is recurrence of accessory pathway conduction in approximately 5% of patients [13].

Cryoablation is another therapeutic option that is frequently chosen for its higher safety profile. Rather than heat disruption, cryoablation technology causes tissue disruption by freezing the tissue. A significant advantage of cryoablation is that it has essentially eliminated the risk of unintentional heart block during ablation procedures. The trade-off for this higher safety profile is a lower success rate and higher recurrence rate [31]. For this reason, in most centres, cryoablation has not replaced RF ablation, but rather serves as an important adjunct technology in situations where RF energy would be deemed higher risk (e.g. near the normal conduction system).

Athletes who have had successful catheter ablation of the accessory pathway, are asymptomatic and have no inducible arrhythmia on follow-up EP study can participate in all competitive sports after several days [27]. Those without an EP study and no spontaneous recurrence of tachycardia for 2–4 weeks after ablation can participate in all competitive sports [27]. The European Society of Cardiology (ESC) postpones return to competition until 3 months after the procedure [26].

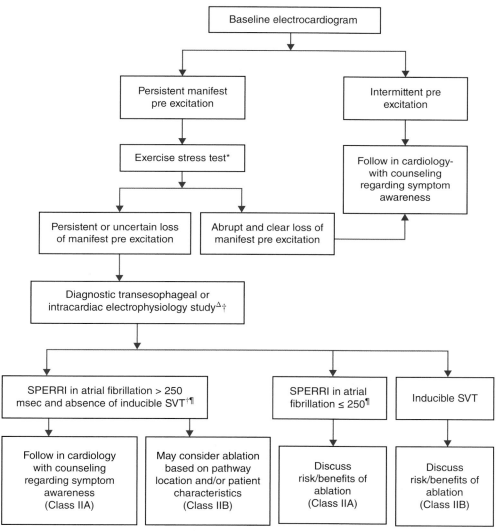

* patients unable to perform an exercise stress test should undergo risk-stratification with an EP study
Δprior to invasive testing, patients and the parents/guardians should be counseled to discuss the risks and benefits of proceeding with invasive studies, risk of observation only, and risks of medication strategy
† patients participating at moderate-hight level competitive sports should be counseled with regards to risk-benefit of ablation (Class IIA) and follow the 2016 joint ACC/AHA recommendations
¶ in the absence of inducible atrial fibrillation, the shortest pre-excited RR interval determined by rapid atrial pacing is a reasonable surrogate

Figure 28.8 Management algorithm (*Source:* Cohen et al. [12]. Reproduced with permission of Elsevier)

Management Summary

Management of athletes begins with a compete history to determine the presence of symptoms, including palpitations, near syncope and syncope. Evaluation also includes echocardiography to exclude associated structural heart disease [12].

Evaluation of the asymptomatic athlete should begin with noninvasive measures (Figure 28.8). Athletes competing in low-intensity sports who have a clear loss of pre-excitation during Holter monitoring or exercise stress test can be considered low-risk for developing a lethal arrhythmia and may be followed up periodically and counselled on symptom awareness [12]. If there is persistent pre-excitation on noninvasive testing, consultation with a cardiologist familiar with WPW risk stratification should be undertaken [12]. In addition to noninvasive testing, athletes participating in moderate- and high-intensity sports should be considered for further risk stratification via diagnostic invasive EP studies [27]. It is important to recognise that the ESC does not distinguish between intensities and mandates that all athletes with WPW undergo complete risk assessment, including EP study.

Both the 2016 joint ACC/AHA recommendations and the ESC guidelines state that athletes judged to be at increased risk on the basis of diagnostic EP study and those who are symptomatic should undergo ablation of the accessory pathway in order to retain athletic eligibility. Due to the high success rate and low incidence of complications with catheter ablation, the ESC considers ablation first-line therapy for even asymptomatic athletes [26]. For those who refuse ablation or in whom the procedure is considered high risk, competition may be allowed if the pathway meets criteria for low risk. In all other instances, it is recommended that catheter ablation be performed. The 2016 joint ACC/AHA recommendations suggest resumption of competitive sport shortly after successful ablation (4 weeks), but the ESC guidelines postpone return to competition until 3 months after the procedure.

References

1 Wolff, L., Parkinson, J. and White, P. Bundle-branch block with short PR interval in healthy young people to paroxysmal tachycardia. *Am Heart J* 1930; **V**: 685–704.

2 Dreifus, L., Haiat, R., Watanabe, Y. et al. Ventricular fibrillation. A possible mechanism of sudden death in patients and Wolff-Parkinson-White syndrome. *Circulation* 1971; **43**: 520–7.

3 Pelliccia, A., Culasso, F., Di Paolo, F.M. et al. Prevalence of abnormal electrocardiograms in a large, unselected population undergoing pre-participation cardiovascular screening. *Eur Heart J* 2007; **28**: 2006–10.

4 Klein, G.J., Yee, R. and Sharma, A.D. Longitudinal electrophysiologic assessment of asymptomatic patients with the Wolff-Parkinson-White electrocardiographic pattern. *N Engl J Med* 1989; **320**: 1229–33.

5 Deal, B.J., Keane, J.F., Gillette, P.C. and Garson, A. Jr. Wolff-Parkinson-White syndrome and supraventricular tachycardia during infancy: management and follow-up. *J Am Coll Cardiol* 1985; **5**: 130–5.

6 Santinelli, V., Radinovic, A., Manguso, F. et al. The natural history of asymptomatic ventricular pre-excitation a long-term prospective follow-up study of 184 asymptomatic children. *J Am Coll Cardiol* 2009; **53**: 275–80.

7 Vidaillet, H.J. Jr, Pressley, J.C., Henke, E. et al. Familial occurrence of accessory atrioventricular pathways (preexcitation syndrome). *N Engl J Med* 1987; **317**: 65–9.

8 Mehdirad, A.A., Fatkin, D., Dimarco, J.P. et al. Electrophysiologic characteristics of accessory atrioventricular connections in an inherited form of Wolff-Parkinson-White syndrome. *J Cardiovasc Electrophysiol* 1999; **10**: 629–35.

9 Gollob, M.H., Green, M.S., Tang, A.S. et al. Identification of a gene responsible for familial Wolff-Parkinson-White syndrome. *N Engl J Med* 2001; **344**: 1823–31.

10 Surawicz, B., Childers, R., Deal, B.J. et al. AHA/ACCF/HRS recommendations for the standardization and interpretation of the electrocardiogram: part III: intraventricular conduction disturbances: a scientific statement from the American Heart Association Electrocardiography and Arrhythmias Committee, Council on Clinical Cardiology; the American College of Cardiology Foundation; and the Heart Rhythm Society: endorsed by the International Society for Computerized Electrocardiology. *Circulation* 2009; **119**(10): e235–40.

11 Munger, T.M., Packer, D.L., Hammill, S.C. et al. A population study of the natural history of Wolff-Parkinson-White syndrome in Olmsted County, Minnesota, 1953–1989. *Circulation* 1993; **87**: 866–73.

12 Cohen, M.I., Triedman, J.K., Cannon, B.C. et al. PACES/HRS expert consensus statement on the management of the asymptomatic young patient with a Wolff-Parkinson-White (WPW, ventricular preexcitation) electrocardiographic pattern. *Heart Rhythm* 2012; **9**: 1006–24.

13 Blomstrom-Lundqvist, C., Scheinman, M.M., Aliot, E.M. et al. ACC/AHA/ESC guidelines for the management of patients with supraventricular arrhythmias – executive summary. A report of the American College of Cardiology/ American Heart Association Task Force on Practice Guidelines and the European Society of Cardiology Committee for Practice Guidelines (Writing Committee to Develop Guidelines for the Management of Patients with Supraventricular Arrhythmias) developed in collaboration with NASPE-Heart Rhythm Society. *J Am Coll Cardiol* 2003; **42**: 1493–531.

14 Klein, G.J., Bashore, T.M., Sellers, T.D. et al. Ventricular fibrillation in the Wolff-Parkinson-White syndrome. *N Engl J Med* 1979; **301**: 1080–5.

15 Obeyesekere, M.N., Leong-Sit, P., Massel, D. et al. Risk of arrhythmia and sudden death in patients with asymptomatic preexcitation: a meta-analysis. *Circulation* 2012; **125**: 2308–15.

16 Maron, B.J., Doerer, J.J., Haas, T.S. et al. Sudden deaths in young competitive athletes: analysis of 1866 deaths in the United States, 1980–2006. *Circulation* 2009; **119**: 1085–92.

17 Gulamhusein, S., Ko, P., Carruthers, S.G. and Klein, G.J. Acceleration of the ventricular response during atrial fibrillation in the Wolff-Parkinson-White syndrome after verapamil. *Circulation* 1982; **65**: 348–54.

18 Sellers, T.D. Jr, Bashore, T.M. and Gallagher, J.J. Digitalis in the pre-excitation syndrome. Analysis during atrial fibrillation. *Circulation* 1977; **56**: 260–7.

19 Perry, J.C., Giuffre, R.M. and Garson, A. Jr. Clues to the electrocardiographic diagnosis of subtle Wolff-Parkinson-White syndrome in children. *J Pediatr* 1990; **117**: 871–5.

20 Wolff, L. Diagnostic clues in the Wolff-Parkinson-White syndrome. *N Engl J Med* 1959; **261**: 637–41.

21 Grossman, A., Wand, O., Matezki, S. et al. Use of adenosine test for the exclusion of preexcitation syndrome in asymptomatic individuals. *Ann Noninvasive Electrocardiol* 2011; **16**: 180–3.

22 Garratt, C.J., Antoniou, A., Griffith, M.J. et al. Use of intravenous adenosine in sinus rhythm as a diagnostic test for latent preexcitation. *Am J Cardiol* 1990; **65**: 868–73.

23 Levy, S., Broustet, J.P., Clementy, J. et al. [Wolff-Parkinson-White syndrome. Correlation between the results of electrophysiological investigation and exercise tolerance testing on the electrical aspect of preexcitation.] *Arch Mal Coeur Vaiss* 1979; **72**: 634–40.

24 Obeyesekere, M.N. and Klein, G.J. Intermittent preexcitation and the risk of sudden death: the exception that proves the rule? *J Cardiovasc Electrophysiol* 2013; **24**: 367–9.

25 Gaita, F., Giustetto, C., Riccardi, R. et al. Stress and pharmacologic tests as methods to identify patients with Wolff-Parkinson-White syndrome at risk of sudden death. *Am J Cardiol* 1989; **64**: 487–90.

26 Pelliccia, A., Fagard, R., Bjornstad, H.H. et al. Recommendations for competitive sports participation in athletes with cardiovascular disease: a consensus document from the Study Group of Sports Cardiology of the Working Group of Cardiac Rehabilitation and Exercise Physiology and the Working Group of Myocardial and Pericardial Diseases of the European Society of Cardiology. *Eur Heart J* 2005; **26**: 1422–45.

27 Zipes, D.P., Link, M.S., Ackerman, M.J. et al. Eligibility and disqualification recommendations for competitive athletes with cardiovascular abnormalities: Task Force 9: arrhythmias and conduction defects: a scientific statement from the American Heart Association and American College of Cardiology. *J Am Coll Cardiol* 2015; **66**(21): 2412–23.

28 Calkins, H., Prystowsky, E., Berger, R.D. et al. Recurrence of conduction following radiofrequency catheter ablation procedures: relationship to ablation target and electrode temperature. The Atakr Multicenter Investigators Group. *J Cardiovasc Electrophysiol* 1996; **7**: 704–12.

29 Hindricks, G. The Multicentre European Radiofrequency Survey (MERFS): complications of radiofrequency catheter ablation of arrhythmias. The Multicentre European Radiofrequency Survey (MERFS) investigators of the Working Group on Arrhythmias of the European Society of Cardiology. *Eur Heart J* 1993; **14**: 1644–53.

30 Scheinman, M.M. NASPE survey on catheter ablation. *Pacing Clin Electrophysiol* 1995; **18**: 1474–8.

31 Lemola, K., Dubuc, M. and Khairy, P. Transcatheter cryoablation part II: clinical utility. *Pacing Clin Electrophysiol* 2008; **31**: 235–44.

29 Catecholaminergic Polymorphic Ventricular Tachycardia

Leonie C.H. Wong[1] and Elijah R. Behr[2]

[1] Cardiovascular and Cell Sciences Research Institute, St George's University of London, London, UK
[2] Cardiac Research Centre, St George's University of London, London, UK

Introduction

Catecholaminergic polymorphic ventricular tachycardia (CPVT) is an inherited arrhythmia syndrome characterised by syncope or cardiac arrest due to ventricular arrhythmias induced by adrenergic stimulation, such as exercise or acute emotion, in young individuals without underlying structural heart disease. The characteristic arrhythmia is bidirectional or polymorphic ventricular tachycardia, which may self-terminate with spontaneous recovery or degenerate into ventricular fibrillation and result in sudden cardiac death (SCD) if not resuscitated.

CPVT was first described in 1975, in a case report of a 6-year-old girl with exercise-induced bidirectional tachycardia [1]. This was followed in 1978 by a report on a series of four children with catecholamine-induced ventricular tachycardia, and in 1995 by a more comprehensive study of 21 children with CPVT [2].

There are relatively few epidemiological data on CPVT. The prevalence of the disease in the general population is estimated to be around 1 in 10 000. The mean age of symptom onset is around 8 years, although onset as late as the 4th decade of life has been reported [2,3]. Left untreated, around 30% of those affected experience at least one cardiac arrest and up to 80% experience one or more episodes of syncope. A family history of premature SCD is present in around 30% of probands with CPVT.

Genetics and Pathophysiology

A possible genetic origin for CPVT was suggested by one of the earlier studies, which found a family history of syncope or sudden death in a third of cases [2]. The disease was initially mapped to chromosome 1q42-43 through linkage analysis, prior to identification of mutations in the cardiac ryanodine receptor gene (RyR2) in 2001 [1,2]. RyR2 mutations account for around 50% of CPVT and are inherited in an autosomal-dominant manner (CPVT1). The ryanodine receptor acts as a calcium-release channel, and mutant ryanodine receptors result in increased 'leakiness' of calcium from the sarcoplasmic reticulum (SR). The penetrance of CPVT1, although incomplete, is reported to be around 80% [2].

A rarer autosomal-recessive form (CPVT2) is caused by mutations in the calsequestrin (CASQ2) gene and accounts for 2% of cases. Calsequestrin acts as a calcium buffer in the SR, and mutant calsequestrin leads to calcium overload in the SR. This too was first discovered by linkage analysis mapping the disease to chromosome 1p13-21, prior to identification of mutations in the cardiac calsequestrin gene (CASQ2) [2]. The penetrance of CPVT2 is complete, as is usually the case in homozygous disease.

Other genes involved include triadin (TRDN) and calmodulin (CALM1). Triadin forms part of the macromolecular calcium-release complex, and mutations in TRDN with an autosomal-recessive mode of inheritance have been identified in two families [2]. Genome-wide linkage analysis of a large Swedish family with autosomal-dominant CPVT mapped the disease locus to chromosome 14q31-32, and a heterozygous mutation was later identified in CALM1, which segregated with the disease phenotype [2]. Calmodulin is a

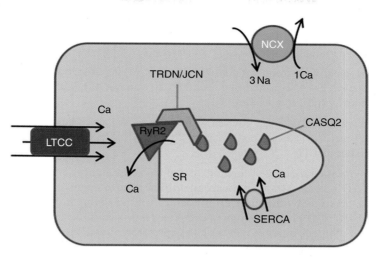

Figure 29.1 Cellular calcium haemostasis. Ryanodine receptor (RyR2), calsequestrin (CASQ2), triadin (TRDN) and junctin (JCN) form the macromolecular calcium-release complex at the SR. Calcium depolarisation activates the L-type calcium channel (LTCC) and triggers calcium release from the SR. Adrenergic stimulation leads to increased SR calcium content and spontaneous SR calcium release in diastole. The increased cytosolic calcium content activates the sodium-calcium exchanger (NCX), resulting in delayed afterdepolarisation (DAD). Na, sodium; Ca, calcium; SERCA, sarcoplasmic reticulum calcium ATPase

ubiquitous intracellular calcium sensor and acts as a calcium signal transducer. It usually binds to and inhibits *RyR2*. However, mutant calmodulin has been shown to bind to *RyR2* with high affinity and activate it [4].

Ryanodine, calsequestrin, triadin and calmodulin are all involved in the SR pathway regulating intracellular calcium fluxes and cytosolic free calcium concentration (Figure 29.1). A number of different molecular mechanisms, depending on the underlying genetic defect, have been put forward to underlie the pathophysiology of CPVT [3]. Regardless of the specific genetic defect, the resulting modification in calcium homeostasis causes increased calcium release from the SR and sets off a cellular chain reaction predisposing to arrhythmia susceptibility. Beta-adrenergic stimulation enhances SR calcium uptake through phosphorylation of *RyR2*, sarcoplasmic reticulum calcium ATPase (SERCA) and L-type calcium channels. The high SR calcium content causes *RyR2* channels to open spontaneously in diastole, generating further calcium release from the SR to the cytoplasm via neighbouring channels through the calcium-induced calcium release (CICR) mechanism. The increased intracellular calcium concentration activates the sodium-calcium exchanger (NCX) on the cell membrane, generating an inward sodium current responsible for the phenomenon of delayed afterdepolarisation (DAD), leading to triggered activity.

Contribution to SCD

One of the first epidemiological studies on sudden death in the young reported a sudden unexpected death rate of 1.3 per 100 000 person-years in children and young adults aged 1–22 years [5]. Subsequent studies have shown an SCD rate of 1.6–2.8 per 100 000 person-years in the age group 1–40 years [6,7]. The incidence of SCD in US athletes ranges from 0.3 to 1.0 per 100 000, whilst that in an Italian study is higher at 2 per 100 000 [8].

Many deaths in young individuals, including athletes, can be explained by cardiovascular abnormalities identified with macro- and microscopic examination at autopsy, such as cardiomyopathies, congenital heart defects, coronary artery anomalies and myocarditis. Amongst 1866 cases of US athletes who suffered SCD or an aborted sudden cardiac arrest (SCA), the most common cardiovascular causes of SCD were hypertrophic cardiomyopathy (36%) and coronary artery anomalies (17%), whilst 2% had structurally normal hearts at autopsy [8]. Another study in the Veneto region of Italy showed that the most common causes of SCD were arrhythmogenic right ventricular cardiomyopathy (ARVC), coronary artery disease (CAD) and myocarditis [8].

However, up to one-third of these sudden deaths in the young are unexplained following a detailed autopsy and investigations; such cases are termed 'sudden arrhythmic death syndrome' (SADS) [2,7]. This figure increases to around 40–52% in the under-19 age group [9,10]. Arrhythmia syndrome-associated SCDs, such as those due to CPVT, are initially labelled as SADS due to the absence of structural abnormalities at post mortem examination.

Several studies involving cardiological assessment of family members or targeted post mortem genetic testing, known as 'molecular autopsy', have suggested that a significant number of SADS deaths are associated with inheritable monogenic arrhythmia syndromes [7].

Familial cardiological evaluation was undertaken in 43 cases of sudden unexplained death, and CPVT was diagnosed in five (12%) [7]. However, two studies comprising 32 and 57 SADS cases respectively did not demonstrate CPVT in any of the families [7].

The first molecular autopsy of *RyR2*, targeted according to the most frequently affected exons, was undertaken in a cohort of 49 SADS cases. Mutations were identified in seven probands, representing a yield of 14% [7]. A larger follow-on study by the same group demonstrated a similar prevalence of *RyR2* mutations in 20 of 173 cases (12%) [7]. The discrepancy between results from familial evaluation and from molecular autopsy supports the possibility of incomplete expression and/or sporadic and therefore noninherited genetic disease.

Evaluation of Suspected CPVT

The initial evaluation of suspected CPVT should consist of a complete patient history, including a detailed family history for SADS or childhood and infant deaths. Investigations should include a standard 12-lead electrocardiogram (ECG), Holter monitoring and echocardiography to exclude structural heart disease. Exercise stress testing is the mainstay of CPVT diagnosis and is positive in 63–76% of clinically or genetically diagnosed CPVT patients. There is, however, less consensus on the use of epinephrine provocation as a diagnostic test due to differing results from different groups, with sensitivity ranging from 28 to 82% [3,11].

The different diagnostic yields demonstrated by different groups for exercise and epinephrine provocation testing may relate to differences in their patient populations, test indications and diagnostic end points. It has been suggested that exercise testing, although more physiological, results in a combination of sympathetic stimulation and vagal withdrawal which may be less arrhythmogenic than a pure catecholamine trigger provided by epinephrine provocation. It is likely that a combination of the two tests is most useful in the diagnosis of CPVT [12].

Following a clinical diagnosis of CPVT, genetic testing should be undertaken to identify any underlying gene mutation and so aid the screening of asymptomatic family members [13]. Immediate family should also undergo cardiological evaluation, to identify those who might be at risk [2].

Diagnostic Criteria

The resting ECG is usually normal, although a lower than normal resting heart rate and prominent U-waves have been reported [1–3]. The onset of arrhythmia with exercise testing occurs around a heart rate of 100–120 beats.min^{-1} with isolated monomorphic ventricular premature beats. These tend to worsen with increasing workload, resulting in the appearance of more complex ventricular ectopy as couplets and nonsustained ventricular tachycardia (NSVT), before the development of sustained bidirectional or polymorphic ventricular tachycardia (Figure 29.2).

The most recent diagnostic criteria were published as a Heart Rhythm Society (HRS)/European Heart Rhythm Association (EHRA)/Asia Pacific Heart Rhythm Society (APHRS) expert consensus statement in 2013 [2]:

1. CPVT is diagnosed in the presence of a structurally normal heart, normal ECG and unexplained exercise or catecholamine-induced bidirectional ventricular tachycardia, polymorphic ventricular premature beats or polymorphic ventricular tachycardia in an individual younger than 40 years.
2. CPVT is diagnosed in patients (index case or family member) who have a pathogenic mutation.
3. CPVT is diagnosed in family members of a CPVT index case with a normal heart who manifest exercise-induced premature ventricular contractions or bidirectional/polymorphic ventricular tachycardia.

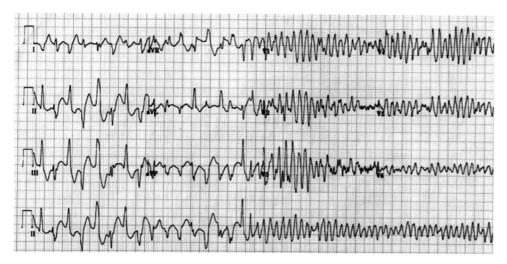

Figure 29.2 12-lead ECG showing the transition of bidirectional ventricular tachycardia to polymorphic ventricular tachycardia prior to degeneration into VF (*Source*: courtesy of Dr Jan Till, Royal Brompton Hospital)

4. CPVT can be diagnosed in the presence of a structurally normal heart and coronary arteries, normal ECG and unexplained exercise or catecholamine-induced bidirectional ventricular tachycardia or polymorphic ventricular premature beats or polymorphic ventricular tachycardia in an individual older than 40 years.

Risk Stratification

At present, risk stratification is poorly defined in CPVT. In the largest series published so far, the risk of arrhythmic events decreased with increasing age at diagnosis, whilst a prior aborted cardiac arrest was associated with future fatal or near-fatal events [2]. *RyR2*- and *CASQ2*-related CPVT appears clinically identical, although it has been suggested that *CASQ2*-related CPVT is usually more resistant to beta-blocker therapy. Mutation location may be associated with severity of phenotype, with carriers of *RyR2* mutations in the C-terminal channel-forming domain having an increased risk of NSVT [2]. Amongst asymptomatic mutation carriers identified by cascade screening, the presence of a CPVT phenotype on exercise testing has a higher risk of future cardiac events [14].

Management

Initial management on diagnosis consists of medical therapy combined with lifestyle restrictions. Interventional procedures such as an implantable cardioverter-defibrillator (ICD) or left cardiac sympathetic denervation (LCSD) are reserved for patients resistant to medical therapy.

Lifestyle and Exercise Recommendations

Exercise restriction should be implemented on diagnosis. Patients should avoid strenuous exercise or competitive sports and should limit exposure to emotionally stressful situations.

The American Heart Association (AHA), American College of Cardiology and European Society of Cardiology (ESC) have separately developed consensus statements regarding sports participation and exercise restriction in genetic cardiovascular diseases [8]. These guidelines are based on the view that physical exertion triggers potentially fatal ventricular arrhythmias in athletes with the underlying substrate of an inherited cardiovascular condition and that exercise restriction will reduce their risk profile. The recommendations are based largely on expert opinion, due to the lack of any randomised studies. The ESC has since published recommendations extending beyond competitive sports to leisure-time physical activity [15].

The general consensus is that phenotype-positive CPVT patients should avoid all competitive sports and moderate- to high-level leisure-time exercise. Low-level physical activity is allowed in patients who are symptomatically controlled with medical therapy. In genotype-positive, phenotype-negative patients ('asymptomatic or silent carriers'), there is a divergence of opinion, with the American guidelines not recommending exercise restriction but the European guidelines differentiating between phenotype-positive and -negative patients in terms of lifestyle advice. Recent evidence showing a significant proportion of asymptomatic mutation carriers developing ventricular arrhythmias on exercise lends support to the European recommendations [14,16].

It is important that physical activity recommendations do not result in a sedentary lifestyle, which may predispose to other cardiovascular morbidity. Recent findings have suggested that an individualised exercise regime can increase the threshold for developing ventricular arrhythmias in CPVT, whilst a sedentary lifestyle has the converse effect, strengthening the need to avoid a total lack of physical activity [17].

Medical Therapy

The first-line medical treatment for patients with CPVT is nonselective beta blockade [2]. The mechanism of action is thought to be inhibition of adrenergic triggered activity by heart-rate reduction and modification of calcium release from the SR. Nadolol is the beta blocker of choice, due to its long-acting properties, and has been found to be clinically effective [3]. The recommended dosage is around $1–2\,mg.kg^{-1}.day^{-1}$, with an annual rate of arrhythmic events on beta blockers of around 3–11%. If nadolol is unavailable or not tolerated, propranolol is a possible alternative, with a recommended dosage of $2–4\,mg.kg^{-1}.day^{-1}$. Exercise testing on treatment can facilitate dose titration and monitoring. However, beta blockade is not entirely effective, with 4- and 8-year breakthrough arrhythmic event rates of 18.6 and 37.2% and near-fatal event rates of 7.7 and 15.3%, respectively [2]. Strict compliance is essential, as several studies have demonstrated a ~5% rate of SCD in CPVT patients noncompliant with beta-blocker therapy [2,3].

Flecainide is included in recent CPVT management guidelines. It has been postulated to have two modes of antiarrhythmic action: directly as an *RyR2* receptor blocker, resulting in reduced amplitude of DAD, and indirectly by blocking the cardiac Na channels, increasing the threshold for triggered activity [2,18]. Flecainide has also been shown to significantly reduce the ventricular arrhythmia burden in CPVT patients. A dose of $100–300\,mg.day^{-1}$ in addition to beta-blocker therapy can be considered in patients not fully responsive to or unable to tolerate maximal beta blockade [2,18]. Propafenone, another class I antiarrhythmic, has also been shown to possess *RyR2*-blocking properties and may be considered as an alternative to flecainide [19].

Calcium-channel blockade has been shown to be effective in inhibiting ventricular arrhythmias in *CASQ2*-deficient mice, in contrast to flecainide [20]. This effect was reproduced in symptomatic *CPVT2* patients poorly controlled on beta-blocker therapy, where verapamil attenuated ventricular arrhythmias and prolonged exercise duration. Calcium-channel blockade has also been demonstrated to be effective in reducing ventricular ectopy, preventing the development of more complex and sustained ventricular arrhythmias [2].

Intervention

An ICD may be required for individuals who suffer recurrent symptoms with maximal medical therapy or who are not able to tolerate medical therapy. Medical therapy, if tolerated, should be maintained and optimised in patients implanted with an ICD to reduce the risk of an ICD shock.

Painful ICD shocks can increase sympathetic tone and act as an adrenergic trigger for further arrhythmias, leading to an electrical storm, more malignant ventricular arrhythmias and, possibly, death [21]. It has also been reported that the effectiveness of ICD shock in terminating a ventricular arrhythmia is highly dependent on the rhythm, with triggered arrhythmias such as bidirectional and polymorphic ventricular tachycardia being less likely to respond compared to ventricular fibrillation [21–23]. It is thus important that the ICD is programmed with a long delay and high cut-off rates, to avoid unnecessary and potentially ineffective shocks.

Implantation of an ICD in paediatric patients poses considerable challenges, not only from a technical standpoint, but also as a result of issues such as inappropriate shocks, the proarrhythmic potential of ICD shocks and the need for multiple interventions across the patient's lifetime.

In view of these issues, LCSD has been used to address the adrenergic trigger by altering the sympathetic supply to the heart. Several small series of LCSDs in CPVT, using either a traditional surgical or a video-assisted thoracoscopic approach, have been encouraging, with marked improvement in symptoms without significant complications [2]. LCSD could thus be considered as an add-on therapy in patients who experience recurrent symptoms or inappropriate ICD shocks whilst on maximal medical therapy. The Heart Rhythm UK position statement recommends restricting ICD implantation to CPVT patients who are unresponsive to both beta-blocker treatment and LCSD [24]. LCSD could also be considered in paediatric patients where ICD implantation is contraindicated or is not thought to be in their best interest [2].

Surveillance

Regular follow-up should be carried out every 6–12 months, using a resting 12-lead ECG, Holter monitoring and exercise testing, in order to assess the efficacy of therapy. Exercise restriction and medical therapy should then be tailored to the results of the exercise test. Regular monitoring should also be carried out in phenotype-negative mutation carriers, as many will go on to develop an overt phenotype [2].

Future Directions

A therapeutic strategy directly targeting the genetic manipulation of the underlying defect has been carried out in mice models. Denegri et al. [25] performed viral gene transfer of wild-type *CASQ2* to *CASQ2*-deficient mice and demonstrated that the phenotype is 'rescued' with normalisation of molecular ultrastructure, resulting in prevention of ventricular arrhythmias. More recently, the same group has extended its studies to evaluate gene therapy in a knock-in mouse model of the human disease. Encouragingly, it observed similar results, with *CASQ2* gene transfer not only preventing or reverting the molecular and clinical abnormalities, but also maintaining its 'curative' effects for at least a year post vector injection [25]. The potential clinical application of this finding is extremely exciting and may herald a novel approach to our treatment of CPVT, and possibly other genetic heart conditions.

References

1 Liu, N., Ruan, Y. and Priori, S.G. Catecholaminergic polymorphic ventricular tachycardia. *Prog Cardiovasc Dis* 2008; **51**(1): 23–30.

2 Priori, S.G., Wilde, A.A., Horie, M. et al. HRS/EHRA/APHRS expert consensus statement on the diagnosis and management of patients with inherited primary arrhythmia syndromes. *Heart Rhythm* 2013; **10**(12): 1932–63.

3 Venetucci, L., Denegri, M., Napolitano, C. and Priori, S.G. Inherited calcium channelopathies in the pathophysiology of arrhythmias. *Nat Rev Cardiol* 2012; **9**(10): 561–75.

4 Hwang, H.S., Nitu, F.R., Yang, Y. et al. Divergent regulation of ryanodine receptor 2 calcium release channels by arrhythmogenic human calmodulin missense mutants. *Circ Res* 2014; **114**(7): 1114–24.

5 Driscoll, D.J. and Edwards, W.D. Sudden unexpected death in children and adolescents. *J Am Coll Cardiol* 1985; **5**(6 Suppl.): 118B–21B.

6 Vaartjes, I., Hendrix, A., Hertogh, E.M. et al. Sudden death in persons younger than 40 years of age: incidence and causes. *Eur J Cardiovasc Prev Rehabil* 2009; **16**(5): 592–6.

7 Raju, H. and Behr, E.R. Unexplained sudden death, focussing on genetics and family phenotyping. *Curr Opin Cardiol* 2013; **28**(1): 19–25.

8 Vaseghi, M., Ackerman, M.J. and Mandapati, R. Restricting sports for athletes with heart disease: are we saving lives, avoiding lawsuits, or just promoting obesity and sedentary living? *Pediatr Cardiol* 2012; **33**(3): 407–16.

9 Winkel, B.G., Risgaard, B., Sadjadieh, G. et al. Sudden cardiac death in children (1–18 years): symptoms and causes of death in a nationwide setting. *Eur Heart J* 2014; **35**(13): 868–75.

10 Pilmer, C.M., Kirsh, J.A., Hildebrandt, D. et al. Sudden cardiac death in children and adolescents between 1 and 19 years of age. *Heart Rhythm* 2014; **11**(2): 239–45.

11 Sy, R.W., Gollob, M.H., Klein, G.J. et al. Arrhythmia characterization and long-term outcomes in catecholaminergic polymorphic ventricular tachycardia. *Heart Rhythm* 2011; **8**(6): 864–71.

12 Krahn, A.D., Gollob, M., Yee, R. et al. Diagnosis of unexplained cardiac arrest: role of adrenaline and procainamide infusion. *Circulation* 2005; **112**(15): 2228–34.

13 Ackerman, M.J., Priori, S.G., Willems, S. et al. HRS/EHRA expert consensus statement on the state of genetic testing for the channelopathies and cardiomyopathies. *Europace* 2011; **13**(8): 1077–109.

14 Hayashi, M., Denjoy, I., Hayashi, M. et al. The role of stress test for predicting genetic mutations and future cardiac events in asymptomatic relatives of catecholaminergic polymorphic ventricular tachycardia probands. *Europace* 2012; **14**(9): 1344–51.

15 Heidbüchel, H., Corrado, D., Biffi, A. et al. Recommendations for participation in leisure-time physical activity and competitive sports of patients with arrhythmias and potentially arrhythmogenic conditions. Part II: ventricular arrhythmias, channelopathies and implantable defibrillators. *Eur J Cardiovasc Prev Rehabil* 2006; **13**(5): 676–86.

16 Haugaa, K.H., Leren, I.S., Berge, K.E. et al. High prevalence of exercise-induced arrhythmias in catecholaminergic polymorphic ventricular tachycardia mutation-positive family members diagnosed by cascade genetic screening. *Europace* 2010; **12**(3): 417–23.

17 Manotheepan, R., Saberniak, J., Danielsen, T.K. et al. Effects of individualized exercise training in patients with catecholaminergic polymorphic ventricular tachycardia type 1. *Am J Cardiol* 2014; **113**(11): 1829–33.

18 Liu, N., Denegri, M., Ruan, Y. et al. Short communication: flecainide exerts an antiarrhythmic effect in a mouse model of catecholaminergic polymorphic ventricular tachycardia by increasing the threshold for triggered activity. *Circ Res* 2011; **109**(3): 291–5.

19 Hwang, H.S., Hasdemir, C., Laver, D. et al. Inhibition of cardiac Ca2+ release channels (RyR2) determines efficacy of class I antiarrhythmic drugs in catecholaminergic polymorphic ventricular tachycardia. *Circ Arrhythm Electrophysiol* 2011; **4**(2): 128–35.

20 Katz, G., Khoury, A., Kurtzwald, E. et al. Optimizing catecholaminergic polymorphic ventricular tachycardia therapy in calsequestrin-mutant mice. *Heart Rhythm* 2010; **7**(11): 1676–82.

21 Miyake, C.Y., Webster, G., Czosek, R.J. et al. Efficacy of implantable cardioverter defibrillators in young patients with catecholaminergic polymorphic ventricular tachycardia: success depends on substrate. *Circ Arrhythm Electrophysiol* 2013; **6**(3): 579–87.

22 Marai, I., Khoury, A., Suleiman, M. et al. Importance of ventricular tachycardia storms not terminated by implantable cardioverter defibrillators shocks in patients with CASQ2 associated catecholaminergic polymorphic ventricular tachycardia. *Am J Cardiol* 2012; **110**(1): 72–6.

23 Roses-Noguer, F., Jarman, J.W., Clague, J.R. and Till, J. Outcomes of defibrillator therapy in catecholaminergic polymorphic ventricular tachycardia. *Heart Rhythm* 2014; **11**(1): 58–66.

24 Garratt, C.J., Elliott, P., Behr, E. et al. Heart Rhythm UK position statement on clinical indications for implantable cardioverter defibrillators in adult patients with familial sudden cardiac death syndromes. *Eurospace* 2010; **12**(8): 1156–75.

25 Denegri, M., Bongianino, R., Lodola, F. et al. Single delivery of an adeno-associated viral construct to transfer the CASQ2 gene to knock-in mice affected by catecholaminergic polymorphic ventricular tachycardia is able to cure the disease from birth to advanced age. *Circulation* 2014; **129**(25): 2673–81.

30 Idiopathic Ventricular Tachycardia/Ventricular Fibrillation

André La Gerche

Baker IDI Heart and Diabetes Institute, Melbourne, Victoria, Australia

Definitions

Idiopathic ventricular tachycardia and idiopathic ventricular fibrillation refer to ventricular tachycardia and ventricular fibrillation which occur in the absence of structural heart disease. Although there is some overlap of underlying aetiologies, the two conditions are distinct, have very different prognoses and differ in their management. The exact definition of ventricular tachycardia varies slightly, but generally it refers to three or more consecutive beats arising from the ventricle at >120 beats.min^{-1}. This is identified as a regular, rapid, wide, complex tachycardia on a 12-lead electrocardiogram (ECG), although the differentiation from supraventricular tachycardias (SVTs) with aberrant conduction can be difficult. Differentiation between these two arrhythmias has been reviewed elsewhere [1] and is beyond the scope of this chapter, but all rapid, wide, complex tachycardias should be assumed to be ventricular tachycardia unless proven otherwise. Sustained ventricular tachycardia refers to ventricular tachycardia persisting beyond 30 seconds, whilst nonsustained ventricular tachycardia (NSVT) describes rhythms that revert within 30 seconds.

Ventricular fibrillation refers to very rapid and disordered electrical activity and contraction of the ventricle. It results in no meaningful contraction or cardiac output and requires immediate attention, as this rhythm is not compatible with survival without electrical reversion.

Idiopathic Ventricular Tachycardia

Amongst the general population, ventricular tachycardia is more common in older patients, reflecting the fact that ventricular tachycardia is commonly associated with underlying pathology [2]. Normally, it is associated with ischaemic heart disease or a cardiomyopathy, but in as many as 25% of cases no structural abnormalities are apparent [3]. In young athletic populations, the proportion of cases without identifiable structural heart disease may be greater, due both to the fact that ischaemic heart disease is less prevalent at younger ages and to the potential 'healthy cohort' selection bias. Idiopathic ventricular tachycardia generally carries a benign prognosis, although there are a small number of uncommon potentially serious pathologies that should be considered before providing reassurance. Table 30.1 lists the structural causes of ventricular tachycardia, as well as the causes of 'idiopathic' ventricular tachycardia. Although the term 'idiopathic' would suggest that the underlying cause is not known, in the case of idiopathic ventricular tachycardia it usually indicates the absence of structural heart disease, but a number of channelopathies represent important potentially serious causes of ventricular tachycardia in the structurally normal heart.

Inherited cardiomyopathies represent the most common causes of ventricular tachycardia and sudden cardiac death (SCD) in most contemporary studies. Hypertrophic cardiomyopathy (HCM) is an autosomal-dominant condition, most often caused by a mutation in one of the sarcomeric proteins of cardiac muscle, with a community prevalence of approximately 0.5%. It causes disarray of the cardiac myocytes, leading to abnormally thick myocardium, functional impairment and increased scar deposition, which represents a

Case Report

A 39-year-old middle-distance runner describes recurring episodes in which he feels instantly fatigued, accompanied by rapid chest palpitations. The episodes typically last 10–40 seconds and promptly resolve, and he immediately feels normal again. An exercise echocardiogram demonstrates mild dilation of all four cardiac chambers (consistent with athlete's heart) but no other structural abnormalities. During strenuous running (stage 5 of a Bruce protocol), the patient suddenly develops the same symptoms, corresponding to the onset of a wide, complex tachyarrhythmia (Figure 30.1). In the absence of structural heart disease, the wide complex tachycardia with a left bundle branch block (LBBB) appearance and inferior axis is suggestive of a right ventricular outflow tract (RVOT) tachycardia. The patient undergoes a curative ablation to a small arrhythmic focus in the RVOT and returns to competition without further symptoms.

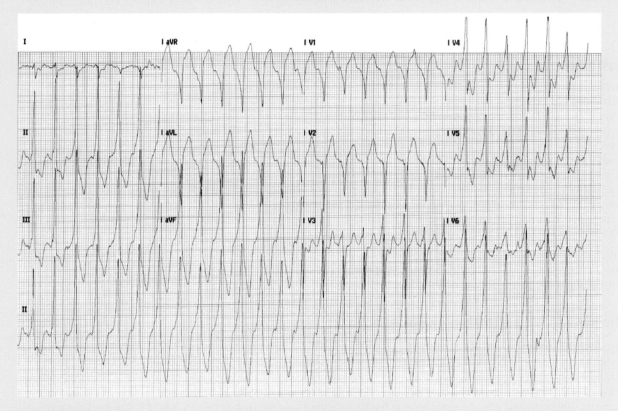

Figure 30.1 Right ventricular outflow tract (RVOT) tachycardia in a middle-distance runner. The 12-lead ECG demonstrates the onset of a wide, complex tachycardia during an exercise stimulus. The left bundle branch block (LBBB) pattern and inferior axis are consistent with RVOT tachycardia

substrate for arrhythmias and SCD. Arrhythmogenic right ventricular cardiomyopathy (ARVC) is also an autosomal-dominant condition, caused by a mutation in one of seven desmosomal genes, with a prevalence of 1 in 1000–5000 [4]. It causes fibrosis, atrophy and fatty infiltration of the myocardium, with a typical predominance in the base, apex and outflow tract region of the right ventricle, although left ventricular involvement or even left ventricular dominance can be observed. Ischaemic heart disease is most commonly observed in older populations, although is still an important cause of ventricular tachycardia and sudden death in young athletes. Dilated cardiomyopathy (DCM) is most often an acquired condition, although the underlying aetiology is frequently unknown. Myocarditis is often a presumed cause of DCM or of patches of midmyocardial fibrosis observed on cardiac magnetic resonance (CMR).

Idiopathic ventricular tachycardia is most frequently caused by triggered depolarisations from the region of the RVOT and, less commonly, the left ventricular outflow tract (LVOT) and aortic cusp. The triggered

Ventricular tachycardia associated with structural heart disease

Ischaemic heart disease (increasingly prevalent in athletes aged >30 years)

Hypertrophic cardiomyopathy (HCM)

Arrhythmogenic right ventricular cardiomyopathy (ARVC)

Dilated cardiomyopathy (DCM)

Myocarditis

Sarcoidosis

Nonatherosclerotic coronary artery disease (congenital anomalies, dissection)

Idiopathic ventricular tachycardia (no structural abnormalities)

Focal ventricular tachycardia (benign)

Right ventricular outflow tract (RVOT) tachycardia

Left ventricular outflow tract (LVOT) tachycardia

Other (fascicular, papillary muscle, etc.)

Channelopathies

Long QT syndrome

Brugada syndrome

Catecholaminergic polymorphic ventricular tachycardia (CPVT)

Short QT syndrome

Table 30.1 Causes of ventricular tachycardia

activity is believed to result from regions of myocytes that are sensitive to catecholamine-mediated increases in cyclic adenosine monophosphate (cAMP). It is typically triggered by exercise and stress, with an onset in athletes aged 30–50 years. RVOT tachycardia accounts for approximately 70% of idiopathic ventricular tachycardia cases [5] and can be identified as an LBBB QRS morphology and an inferior axis on the limb leads of a 12-lead ECG. Thus, in addition to excluding structural disease with cardiac imaging, the identification of a typical RVOT pattern on ECG is an important additional guide to a diagnosis of idiopathic ventricular tachycardia and a benign prognosis. Ventricular tachycardia arising from the LVOT accounts for an additional 10–15% of cases and shares the same inferior-axis, LBBB pattern, although the transition through the precordial leads tends to occur earlier (R-wave dominance before V3). Septal or fascicular idiopathic ventricular tachycardia is less common and is associated with a right bundle branch block (RBBB) superior-axis ventricular tachycardia. The prognosis is also benign, but it may require more intensive investigations given the less common ECG pattern.

Evaluation of the Athlete with Ventricular Tachycardia

The prognosis and treatment of ventricular tachycardia depends upon the underlying cause. Thus, the first priority is to establish whether the athlete has evidence of structural heart disease. The clinical pathway presented in Figure 30.2 suggests that the first-line investigation for athletes with ventricular tachycardia should be a transthoracic echocardiogram and 12-lead ECG. It is beyond the scope of the current chapter to detail the diagnostic features of each of the conditions associated with ventricular tachycardia. However, it is important that a comprehensive assessment of both left and right ventricular function be undertaken, as structural and functional abnormalities may suggest HCM, ARVC, DCM or coronary artery disease (CAD). Similarly, the ECG should be carefully appraised for features suggesting a channelopathy, such as a prolonged QT interval (suggesting long QT syndrome) or abnormal coved ST elevation in the anterior precordial leads (suggesting Brugada syndrome).

CMR can provide more detailed information regarding cardiac structure and function, particularly of the right ventricle, which can be difficult to assess comprehensively with echocardiography. More importantly, myocardial fibrosis can be identified as leaking of gadolinium contrast into the extracellular space, seen on gradient-echo inversion recovery imaging as a bright patch against the normal myocardium, which appears

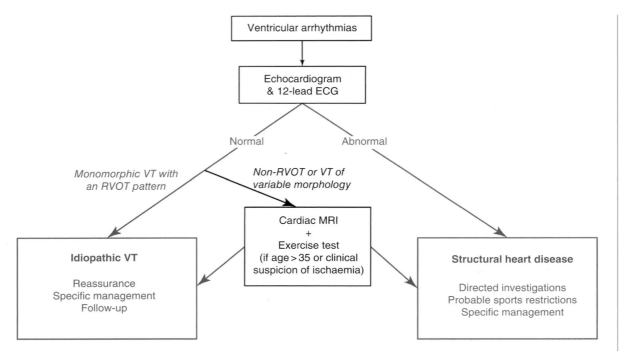

Figure 30.2 Clinical flowchart for the evaluation of ventricular tachycardia in the athlete. A combination of ECG, multimodality imaging and morphologic features of the ventricular tachycardia can be used to differentiate ventricular tachycardia due to structural abnormalities (potentially serious prognosis) from idiopathic ventricular tachycardia (usually a benign prognosis)

black. This can be a very useful means of identifying subtle abnormalities that may not be evident on echocardiography (see Figure 30.3). It should also be realised that not all cardiac pathologies will be evident with cardiac imaging performed at rest. This is especially true of ischaemic heart disease due to atherosclerotic vascular disease or congenital coronary anomalies. If these are suspected, or in athletes over 35 years of age, ischaemic heart disease should be excluded. Cardiac imaging can be performed with an exercise imaging study, such as exercise echocardiography, or with an anatomical test such as computed tomography (CT) coronary angiography or invasive coronary angiography. More detail on these modalities and their indications in athletes is provided in a review by La Gerche et al. [6].

An alternative strategy for the evaluation of patients with ventricular arrhythmias is to perform an exercise echocardiogram. This enables an assessment of the ECG, cardiac function and structure at rest, as well as of contractile reserve and inducible wall-motion abnormalities during exercise. This 'one-stop shop' can be a very useful means of determining a patient's prognosis, on the grounds that most overt structural heart disease, channelopathies and inducible arrhythmias are likely to be diagnosed during the test. In athletes, when there is any doubt, a low threshold for procedure to CMR is prudent.

Excluding Structural Heart Disease – Easier Said than Done

It can be more complex to exclude structural heart disease in athletes than in nonathletes. 'Athlete's heart' describes the structural, functional and electrical adaptations of the heart which enable athletes to generate greater cardiac outputs during exercise [7]. Distinguishing normal athletic remodelling from a DCM or ARVC can be challenging amongst endurance athletes, in whom the degree of cardiac changes can be profound. Referral for specialist assessment is recommended in any athlete in whom structural heart disease cannot be confidently excluded.

Sometimes, invasive strategies are required to determine the prognosis in ambiguous cases. It has been observed that induction of ventricular tachycardia with programmed extra stimuli during an electrophysiology

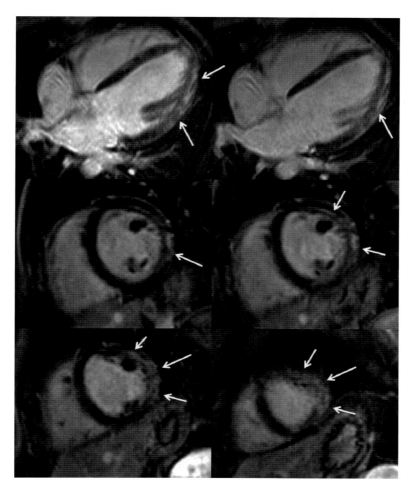

Figure 30.3 Delayed gadolinium enhancement in an elite professional cyclist with NSVT. CMR was performed in the cyclist, who was found to have asymptomatic ventricular ectopics at rest and NSVT during exercise on a Holter monitor. The atypical and varied morphology of the ventricular arrhythmias and the low–normal systolic function on echocardiogram led to performance of magnetic resonance imaging (MRI), which revealed fairly extensive gadolinium enhancement of the lateral wall of the left ventricle (white arrows). This suggests *structural* heart disease rather than *idiopathic* ventricular tachycardia and would imply a greater risk of serious arrhythmias in the future and the need for careful surveillance and possible prophylactic measures, such as insertion of an implantable cardioverter-defibrillator (ICD)

(EP) study can identify athletes at risk of subsequent serious arrhythmias [8]. From a population of 1644 screened athletes, Dello Russo et al. [9] identified 17 (1%) with frequent ventricular ectopy or NSVT but normal cardiac structure and function by conventional measures. As a means of risk stratification, electro-anatomical mapping and a guided ventricular biopsy were performed, which revealed myocardial inflammation, fibrosis and/or fatty infiltrates in 13 of the 17 athletes. In other words, these 17 athletes would have been considered to have idiopathic ventricular tachycardia by conventional measures but the majority in fact had structural heart disease.

A very recent study has suggested that exercise echocardiography and exercise CMR may identify subtle right ventricular dysfunction in some of these patients with apparently normal cardiac structure and function at rest in whom the prognosis is not as benign as typical RVOT tachycardia [10]. The take-home message for the sports clinician or cardiologist is to be rigorous in the appraisal of cardiac structure and function in the athlete with ventricular tachycardia. Even if everything appears normal, it would be prudent to review the athlete regularly and to intermittently reassess for the possibility of an evolving subclinical pathology.

Management

The discussion to date has assumed that the diagnosis of ventricular tachycardia has been made. In fact, the clinician is often faced with an athlete presenting with rapid regular palpitations or with a print-out from their heart rate monitor showing a sudden increase in heart rate above physiological levels. SVT is a more likely diagnosis in a young healthy athlete, but differentiation between SVT and ventricular tachycardia cannot be made on history. Although it may seem logical that ventricular tachycardia would be associated with more severe symptoms, this is not a reliable feature. Thus, the only means of identifying the cause of an athlete's palpitations is to obtain an ECG tracing. Patient and repeated exercise testing, Holter monitoring or, in selected cases, implantation of an implantable loop recorder may be required to make a confident diagnosis. Only then can the correct management be instituted.

The first and most important management of idiopathic ventricular tachycardia is to provide qualified reassurance to the athlete. Idiopathic ventricular tachycardia has an excellent prognosis, but, as already stated, the athlete should undergo regular assessment to ensure that it does not represent an evolving pathology. Whilst there remains some contention as to whether the athlete's heart is a completely benign entity [11], it seems prudent to remain alert, although without providing undue concern for the athlete.

Idiopathic ventricular tachycardia of RVOT origin can often be treated quite effectively with medications, but this can provide some unique issues in athletes. Usually, beta blockers are the first-line therapy, but they are often poorly tolerated by athletes. The nondihydropyridine calcium-channel blockers can also be effective and, despite their negative chronotropic effects, are often better tolerated by athletes. Low doses of class IC antiarrhythmics, such as flecainide, may be effective in suppressing arrhythmias, but they have the potential to precipitate arrhythmias in certain settings and their safety during intense sport in the remodelled athlete's heart is not completely established.

Radiofrequency (RF) catheter ablation is a safe and efficacious therapy for idiopathic ventricular tachycardia. The procedure is easier in patients with frequent ventricular ectopy, which enables the site of earliest activation to be identified as the local trigger focus and where ablation should be directed. In patients with infrequent ectopy, arrhythmias may be stimulated by medications, or pace-mapping can be used to estimate the site of origin of the ventricular tachycardia. Overall, success rates of 90–95% have been reported for catheter ablation of outflow tract ventricular tachycardia [12]. There have been some clinical observations that recurrence rates for RVOT ventricular tachycardia are higher amongst endurance athletes and that endurance training may contribute to the underlying arrhythmic substrate, however [13]. Whilst catheter ablation would seem a very appropriate early treatment, it is important to consider the role of exercise training should the ventricular tachycardia recur.

Athletes with idiopathic ventricular tachycardia do not need to be excluded from sports. The current European guidelines [14] suggest they should undergo rigorous assessment with cardiac imaging, exercise testing and electrophysiology. In the absence of structural heart disease (i.e. idiopathic ventricular tachycardia), athletes are permitted to engage in all sports, but they should be followed up every 6 months. The 2016 joint ACC/AHA guidelines [15] take a similar approach to those athletes with idiopathic ventricular tachycardia undergoing RF ablation, but are more conservative when it comes to athletes relying on medications, recommending against competitive sport for 3 months following an episode of idiopathic ventricular tachycardia and only allowing them to recommence participation if there is no recurrence, including no inducibility during exercise testing or on EP study.

Conclusion

Idiopathic ventricular tachycardia is uncommon in athletes. It is associated with a good prognosis, although frequent follow-up is recommended in athletes to ensure that structural pathology does not evolve. Although pharmacological management is efficacious, it is often poorly tolerated in athletes. RF ablation has very high rates of success and may be favoured as an early treatment to enable the athlete to compete without symptoms and complications. Although idiopathic ventricular tachycardia should not preclude athletes from competition, some recommend a period of exclusion after bouts of ventricular tachycardia.

Idiopathic Ventricular Fibrillation

VF and SCD are somewhat intertwined, because ventricular fibrillation is the most serious of all cardiac arrhythmias, leading to immediate circulatory arrest and cardiovascular collapse. Spontaneous reversion of ventricular fibrillation is rare in humans, and therefore survival is entirely dependent upon the timing and efficacy of resuscitation measures. Ventricular fibrillation is the initial rhythm recorded in approximately one-third to one-half of cardiac arrests, or in up to 80% if the rhythm is recorded within 4 minutes of arrest [16]. Unfortunately, up to 90% of patients suffering a ventricular fibrillation arrest in the absence of structural heart disease will have no preceding symptoms or risk factors for SCD [17].

Excluding Structural Heart Disease

Just as with idiopathic ventricular tachycardia, it is important to investigate for structural heart disease and channelopathies as a potential cause of idiopathic ventricular fibrillation. However, unlike with idiopathic ventricular tachycardia, those athletes who have suffered a ventricular fibrillation arrest but have no evidence of structural heart disease remain at risk of recurrent life-threatening arrhythmias and SCD. The predominant reasons for further assessment are to identify causes in which specific treatments might decrease the risk of recurrence or that might identify a familial risk, which can lead to identification of at-risk relatives.

The pathologies responsible for the majority of cases of ventricular tachycardia and ventricular fibrillation are essentially the same, although the prevalence of an ion-channel disorder as the underlying aetiology appears greater in ventricular fibrillation. In athletes of middle age and older, ischaemic heart disease must be considered likely, whilst in younger athletes the cardiomyopathies need to be excluded. Inherited heart disease may be identified in approximately 30% of patients surviving idiopathic ventricular fibrillation and their first-degree family members [18], of which long QT syndrome, Brugada syndrome and catecholaminergic polymorphic ventricular tachycardia (CPVT) make up the majority of cases, far exceeding the cardiomyopathies.

An early repolarisation pattern identified on a 12-lead ECG has recently been proposed as a risk factor for idiopathic ventricular fibrillation. Haïssaguerre et al. [19] reported an increased risk of idiopathic ventricular fibrillation associated with early repolarisation; this has since refined into benign and malignant early repolarisation, the latter comprising inferior early repolarisation with horizontal ST segments and J-waves >2 mV (see Figure 30.4). The term 'malignant' is quite misleading, given that idiopathic ventricular

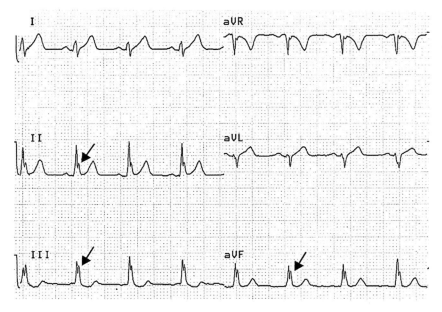

Figure 30.4 Increased-risk early repolarisation pattern in an 18-year-old male athlete. Note the large amplitude J-waves in the inferior leads (II, III and aVF), with a horizontal/descending ST segment

fibrillation is very rare and that although there may be an increase in the relative risk associated with certain early repolarisation patterns, the absolute risk remains extremely small. Early repolarisation is extremely common in young athletes and its low positive predictive value (PPV) would suggest that there is currently a very limited role for changing management or sporting recommendations based on the presence or absence of early repolarisation.

As for idiopathic ventricular tachycardia, echocardiography is recommended for the assessment of structural heart disease. In addition, exercise testing should be considered to exclude ischaemic heart disease and to assess for abnormal QT prolongation or polymorphic ventricular arrhythmias suggestive of CPVT. Finally, a CMR is prudent in all survivors of a ventricular fibrillation arrest, both given its increased sensitivity for identifying structural heart disease and because most subjects will be treated with an implantable cardioverter-defibrillator (ICD), which will largely preclude later CMR evaluation.

Management

Idiopathic ventricular fibrillation and ventricular tachycardia differ in that the former is associated with a significant risk of arrhythmias even if structural heart disease is excluded. For example, Remme et al. [20] observed that 43% of patients who had previously survived a ventricular fibrillation arrest had recurrent syncope, ventricular arrhythmias or SCD during an average of 6 years' follow-up. Thus, in most instances, treatment with an ICD is recommended. Additional management depends upon the underlying cause. There is evolving evidence of the efficacy of specific antiarrhythmic agents, such as flecainide for CPVT and quinidine for ventricular fibrillation associated with early repolarisation. In most instances, these treatments can be used as an adjunct to ICD insertion, to decrease the risk of shocks.

Conclusion

Idiopathic ventricular fibrillation is invariably fatal unless there is prompt resuscitation and defibrillation. Ion-channel disorders are an important cause of idiopathic ventricular fibrillation, and athletes should be thoroughly assessed for this possibility. Unless there is a clear reversible cause or contraindication, implantation of an ICD is recommended.

References

1 Roberts-Thomson, K.C., Lau, D.H. and Sanders, P. The diagnosis and management of ventricular arrhythmias. *Nat Rev Cardiol* 2011; **8**: 311–21.

2 Baerman, J.M., Morady, F., Dicarlo, L.A. Jr and De Buitleir, M. Differentiation of ventricular tachycardia from supraventricular tachycardia with aberration: value of the clinical history. *Ann Emerg Med* 1987; **16**: 40–3.

3 Sacher, F., Tedrow, U.B., Field, M.E. et al. Ventricular tachycardia ablation: evolution of patients and procedures over 8 years. *Circ Arrhythm Electrophysiol* 2008; **1**: 153–61.

4 Basso, C., Corrado, D., Marcus, F.I. et al. Arrhythmogenic right ventricular cardiomyopathy. *Lancet* 2009; **373**: 1289–300.

5 Hoffmayer, K.S. and Gerstenfeld, E.P. Diagnosis and management of idiopathic ventricular tachycardia. *Curr Probl Cardiol* 2013; **38**: 131–58.

6 La Gerche, A., Baggish, A.L., Knuuti, J. et al. Cardiac imaging and stress testing asymptomatic athletes to identify those at risk of sudden cardiac death. *JACC Cardiovasc Imaging* 2013; **6**: 993–1007.

7 Baggish, A.L. and Wood, M.J. Athlete's heart and cardiovascular care of the athlete: scientific and clinical update. *Circulation* 2011; **123**: 2723–35.

8 Heidbuchel, H., Hoogsteen, J., Fagard, R. et al. High prevalence of right ventricular involvement in endurance athletes with ventricular arrhythmias. Role of an electrophysiologic study in risk stratification. *Eur Heart J* 2003; **24**: 1473–80.

9 Dello Russo, A., Pieroni, M., Santangeli, P. et al. Concealed cardiomyopathies in competitive athletes with ventricular arrhythmias and an apparently normal heart: role of cardiac electroanatomical mapping and biopsy. *Heart Rhythm* 2011; **8**: 1915–22.

10 La Gerche, A., Claessen, G., Dymarkowski, S. et al. Exercise-induced right ventricular dysfunction is associated with ventricular arrhythmias in endurance athletes. *Eur Heart J* 2015; **36**(30): 1998–2010.

11 La Gerche, A. and Heidbuchel, H. Can intensive exercise harm the heart? You can get too much of a good thing. *Circulation* 2014; **130**: 992–1002.

12 Scheinman, M.M. and Huang, S. The 1998 NASPE prospective catheter ablation registry. *Pacing Clin Electrophysiol* 2000; **23**: 1020–8.

13 Heidbuchel, H., Prior, D.L. and La Gerche, A. Ventricular arrhythmias associated with long-term endurance sports: what is the evidence? *Br J Sports Med* 2012; **46**(Suppl. 1): i44–50.

14 Pelliccia, A., Fagard, R., Bjornstad, H.H. et al. Recommendations for competitive sports participation in athletes with cardiovascular disease: a consensus document from the Study Group of Sports Cardiology of the Working Group of Cardiac Rehabilitation and Exercise Physiology and the Working Group of Myocardial and Pericardial Diseases of the European Society of Cardiology. *Eur Heart J* 2005; **26**: 1422–45.

15 Zipes, D.P., Link, M.S., Ackerman, M.J., et al. Eligibility and disqualification recommendations for competitive athletes with cardiovascular abnormalities: Task Force 9: arrhythmias and conduction defects: a scientific statement from the American Heart Association and American College of Cardiology; American Heart Association Electrocardiography and Arrhythmias Committee of Council on Clinical Cardiology; Council on Cardiovascular Disease in Young; Council on Cardiovascular and Stroke Nursing; Council on Functional Genomics and Translational Biology, and American College of Cardiology. *Circulation* 2015; **132**(22): e315–25.

16 Holmberg, M., Holmberg, S. and Herlitz, J. Effect of bystander cardiopulmonary resuscitation in out-of-hospital cardiac arrest patients in Sweden. *Resuscitation* 2000; **47**: 59–70.

17 Mellor, G., Raju, H., De Noronha, S.V. et al. Clinical characteristics and circumstances of death in the sudden arrhythmic death syndrome. *Circ Arrhythm Electrophysiol* 2014; **7**: 1078–83.

18 McGorrian, C., Constant, O., Harper, N. et al. Family-based cardiac screening in relatives of victims of sudden arrhythmic death syndrome. *Europace* 2013; **15**: 1050–8.

19 Haïssaguerre, M., Derval, N., Sacher, F. et al. Sudden cardiac arrest associated with early repolarization. *N Engl J Med* 2008; **358**: 2016–23.

20 Remme, C.A., Wever, E.F., Wilde, A.A. et al. Diagnosis and long-term follow-up of the Brugada syndrome in patients with idiopathic ventricular fibrillation. *Eur Heart J* 2001; **22**: 400–9.

Section 4
Acquired Disorders

31 Commotio Cordis

Christopher Madias and Mark S. Link

Tufts Medical Center, Boston, MA, USA

Introduction

Sudden death in an athlete is tragic and usually occurs secondary to an underlying genetic or structural cardiac abnormality [1,2]; however, up to 20% of reported sudden deaths in sport occur in individuals with normal hearts who are struck in the chest by a hard object [3–5]. Sudden cardiac death (SCD) initiated by a blunt chest blow has been termed 'commotio cordis'.

Commotio cordis usually occurs in sports using firm projectiles (baseball, ice hockey, lacrosse) or involving direct chest blows (karate, judo). Sudden death occurs in the absence of any significant thoracic or cardiac trauma [6,7], such as can be seen with high-impact injuries in motor vehicle accidents and falls from extreme heights. Projectile/ball impacts in sport are not of the magnitude to produce any significant direct trauma to the underlying structures of the chest or heart. The mechanism of sudden death in commotio cordis has been determined to be arrhythmic, with a blunt chest blow inducing ventricular fibrillation. This chapter will examine the prevalence of commotio cordis as a cause of SCD and will review diagnostic criteria, including findings on electrocardiography (ECG) and cardiac imaging. The evaluation and management of suspected commotio cordis will be discussed, including risk stratification and considerations for exercise and physical activity recommendations.

Prevalence

Reports of commotio cordis can be found as early as 1763 [7]. In the 19th century, sudden death after falls or industrial accidents prompted experimental work with rabbits in an attempt to explain the pathophysiology [8]. In the early decades of the 20th century, however, commotio cordis was largely forgotten, represented in medical literature only by sporadic case reports, and its prevalence was thus thought to be rare. The first fully documented case of commotio cordis in the US occurred in 1978, during a T-ball game [9]. In 1995, a series of 25 cases of sudden death from blunt chest impact in sport was reported, forming the foundation of the commotio cordis registry [3]. It has become clear that commotio cordis is not such a rare phenomenon, with up to 20 cases a year reported in the US alone. A 2003 review of sudden deaths in young athletes revealed commotio cordis to be the second leading cause of death, behind only hypertrophic cardiomyopathy [2]. Since the creation of the National Commotio Cordis Registry in 1996, more than 220 cases of sudden death from chest impact have been accrued [4]. Cases have now been described across the globe. Interestingly, the increased recognition of commotio cordis has led to the discovery of a US registry of deaths during baseball games in the early 1900s. This registry describes 19 deaths from the years 1900 to 1910 that were due to commotio cordis [10].

Clinical Profile

Approximately 75% of commotio occurs in the setting of sports activity: 50% during competitive sporting events and 25% during recreational sport. Victims are typically struck by projectiles normally used in the game, such as balls and pucks. The majority of cases occur in sports in which a small projectile with a dense

IOC Manual of Sports Cardiology, First Edition. Edited by Mathew G. Wilson, Jonathan A. Drezner and Sanjay Sharma.
© 2017 International Olympic Committee. Published 2017 by John Wiley & Sons, Ltd.

core is propelled at a high velocity, such as baseball, lacrosse and hockey. A baseball is the most common triggering event. All impacts occur over the left precordium, directly over the cardiac silhouette.

Most subjects in the registry collapsed instantaneously, but 20% experienced brief lightheadedness before losing consciousness. The initial rhythm seen in the majority of patients where resuscitation was attempted was ventricular fibrillation (VF), but in those undergoing prolonged resuscitation, asystole has also been reported [11]. VF is immediate and carries a grim prognosis unless resuscitation and defibrillation are rapidly performed [3,12]. Whilst commotio cordis was once thought to be universally fatal, successful resuscitation is now observed in up to 60% of cases [12].

Commotio cordis is most commonly seen in the young, with a peak incidence between the ages of 13 and 18 years (median age 14 years). The predominance of young subjects in the registry likely relates to the high level of participation in youth sports in American culture. Furthermore, young individuals might also be at higher risk for commotio cordis due to an increased compliance of the chest wall compared with adults. Males account for 95% of cases for unclear reasons – theories have included a disproportionate participation in implicated sports. Caucasians account for 78% of the patients in the commotio cordis registry [4].

Physical findings in commotio are confined to anterior chest wall bruising. In an initial series of 25 commotio victims [3], 12 had bruises over the cardiac silhouette. ECG findings in commotio consist of anterior ST elevation, similar to that seen in myocardial infarctions. Thus, it is not uncommon for commotio victims to undergo cardiac catheterisation. Echocardiography is by definition normal, but it serves to rule out other cardiac pathophysiology associated with SCD, such as hypertrophic cardiomyopathy. Increasingly, cardiac magnetic resonance (CMR) is performed in order to rule out subtle structural abnormalities. Electrophysiology (EP) studies are rarely needed, but provocative drug testing for Brugada and long QT syndrome may be warranted if other causes of sudden death are suspected.

Experimental Model

A reliable, contemporary experimental model of commotio cordis was first described in 1998 [13]. In this model, anesthetised juvenile swine are placed prone in a sling. Projectiles impact the precordium and can be timed to strike throughout the cardiac cycle. Intracardiac pressures are monitored during all chest impacts. Projectile speed can be adjusted from 20 to 70 miles per hour (mph), and impacts are aimed directly over the cardiac silhouette by transthoracic echocardiographic guidance. Using this model, VF is consistently and reproducibly induced by chest wall impact if a confluence of several factors is achieved (Figure 31.1) [5].

Important Variables in the Initiation of Ventricular Fibrillation

Timing Initial experiments revealed that timing of impact is amongst the most crucial of variables for induction of VF [13]. Impacts that triggered VF occurred in a narrow window of vulnerability during cardiac repolarisation (10–30 ms prior to the peak of the T-wave). Impacts at other points in the cardiac cycle, such as during the QRS complex or ST segment, did not result in VF, but were noted to cause other arrhythmic events, such as premature ventricular contractions, heart block, ST elevation and bundle branch block.

Velocity Impact velocity has also proven to be an important variable for induction of commotio cordis. In the swine model, faster, higher-energy impacts more consistently resulted in VF than did low-velocity impacts. In animals weighing between 10 and 25 kg, chest impacts induced VF over 50% of the time at speeds between 40 and 50 mph [14]. These data are of particular relevance for youth baseball, in which ball velocity is typically between 30 and 50 mph. At impacts faster than 50 mph, an increased incidence of direct thoracic and myocardial damage was observed; at these velocities, the model becomes more consistent with one of cardiac contusion.

Location of Impact Consistent with the clinical profile of commotio cordis in humans, impact location directly over the heart is necessary for induction of VF in the swine model. Examination of impact location from base to apex using echocardiography revealed that impacts over the centre of the left ventricle most frequently induced VF [15]. Impacts at the base or apex of the heart were less likely to result in VF. Impacts that occurred outside the borders of the cardiac silhouette never resulted in induction of VF.

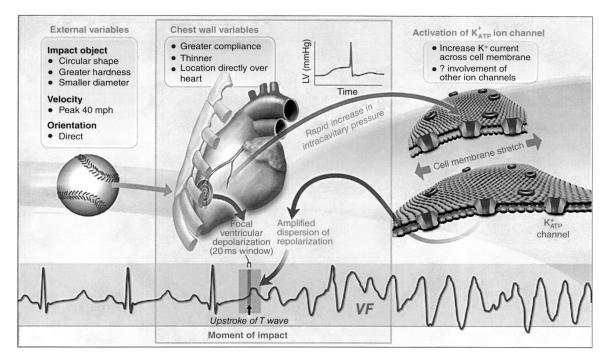

Figure 31.1 Confluence of variables necessary to cause commotio cordis (*Source*: Link [5]. Reproduced with permission of Wolters Kluwer Health)

Hardness and Shape of Object Object hardness and shape proved to be other important variables for induction of VF. Softer projectiles were associated with a lower incidence of VF [13,16]. In a series of experiments, a dense wooden object, similar in size to but harder than a regulation baseball, was noted to result in the highest incidence of VF. The lowest incidence was seen with a safety baseball, commonly known as a 'T-ball.' Smaller, more compact objects, such as those shaped like a golf ball, produced VF more frequently than objects with a larger surface, which distributed the energy of impact over a wider area [17].

Animal Size and Weight Larger animals are less susceptible to VF with ball impact. Data assessing chest impacts in 128 swine ranging in weight from 5 to 54 kg were examined. The swine were divided into five groups by weight and received 624 impacts during the vulnerable window of the cardiac cycle. VF occurred in 29.2% of impacts in the 5.0–13.9 kg group (the smallest group), compared to 34.3% in the 14.0–23.9 kg group, 26.9% in the 24.0–33.9 kg group, 29.8% in the 34–43 kg group and 15.1% in the 44–54 kg group. The highest weight group was associated with a significantly lower incidence of VF compared to other weights (p = 0.002) [18].

Individual Susceptibility Data suggest that there might be an underlying individual susceptibility to commotio cordis. In the experimental model, only a small percentage of animals appeared uniquely susceptible to VF with chest impact (a great majority of appropriately timed chest impacts resulted in VF), whilst a higher number were resistant to chest wall-impact VF [19]. Underlying cardiac repolarisation abnormalities may contribute to individual susceptibility.

Left Ventricular Pressure The variables of velocity, hardness, shape and location all likely relate to the creation of a critical threshold pressure in the heart necessary for induction of VF. It is theorised that the clinical manifestations of commotio cordis are a result of the instantaneous rise in peak left ventricular pressure seen with chest wall impact. In the experimental swine model, impact velocity correlated with the peak left ventricular pressure created by chest impacts. Furthermore, higher peak left ventricular pressures were more likely to result in induction of VF.

Prevention

Of 125 events that occurred during competitive sport noted in the National Commotio Cordis Registry, 32% involved individuals who were wearing some sort of chest protection at the time of impact [4,20]. Despite the use of chest protectors, sudden death was not prevented in these individuals. In some cases, it appears the chest protector moved during play and was not overlying the cardiac silhouette at the time of impact; however, in other cases, impact occurred directly upon the chest protector and commotio cordis was not prevented. In the experimental swine model, seven commercially available lacrosse chest protectors (circa 2003) and nine baseball chest protectors (circa 2003) proved ineffective at preventing induction of VF (Figure 31.2) [21]. These findings support the need for further research in the development of adequate chest protectors designed for the prevention of commotio cordis in youth sports.

The use of age-appropriate safety baseballs may also decrease the risk of commotio cordis. In the swine model, safety baseballs significantly reduced the frequency of induction of VF by chest impacts (Figure 31.3) [13,16]. Data from this model and other clinical data from the US Consumer Product Safety Commission (CPSC) have led to calls for the utilisation of age-appropriate safety baseballs in sports [22]. Safety baseballs are similar in weight and feel to standard ones but with more cushioned construction and represent an inexpensive and effective preventive measure.

Treatment

Reported outcomes of commotio cordis events were initially quite poor, with an overall survival of <5% in [3,12]. Impacts that result in commotio cordis can at first appear relatively benign, and it was believed that low survival was largely due to poor recognition of the severity of events and thus delayed resuscitation. More recent data from the commotio cordis registry have shown that survival is increasing and now approaches 60% (Figure 31.4) [12]. It is clear that early resuscitation from commotio cordis is the key to survival. Improved awareness of commotio, along with increased distribution of automated external defibrillators (AEDs) at many sport facilities, has correlated with this improved survival [12].

Three aspects are key to survival: (i) recognition that a collapse after chest wall impact is a cardiac arrest; (ii) excellent cardiopulmonary resuscitation (CPR); and (iii) timely use of an AED. Distinguishing 'getting the wind knocked out of you' and cardiac arrest is crucial. Unresponsiveness after collapse should be assumed a cardiac arrest. Excellent CPR prolongs the time for which the brain and vital organs survive whilst awaiting defibrillation. Finally, defibrillation at the scene of the arrest is critical to improving survival.

Coaches and athletic trainers involved in youth athletics should be made aware of the clinical scenario of commotio cordis and should become familiar with CPR and the use of AEDs. Commotio cordis should be suspected if an athlete collapses suddenly (or after several seconds) following a chest impact and remains unarousable. Emergency medical services should be contacted immediately and an AED should be placed on the victim as soon as possible. CPR should be performed as guided by standard out-of-hospital cardiac arrest algorithms.

Survivors of commotio cordis in the absence of structural heart disease might consider a return to competitive sports [23]. There are limited data to guide clinical decision-making in this regard. Guidelines state that return to training and competition may be considered if no underlying cardiac abnormality is identified, and should be based on individual cases and clinical judgment [24]. However, as already mentioned, recent data from the swine model of commotio cordis suggest that individual susceptibility may play a role in this phenomenon [19]. Survivors should have a thorough cardiac evaluation. After review of clinical data and careful assessment of the risks and benefits of sports participation, a return to play should be an individual decision made between the survivor, their family and their clinician.

Conclusion

Commotio cordis is a relatively rare, tragic event that typically occurs in adolescent boys in the setting of organised sport. Through the development of a comprehensive registry and the creation of a reliable animal model, our understanding of the clinical profile and of the underlying pathophysiology of commotio cordis has evolved considerably over the last 10–15 years. Whereas the earliest experimental and observational findings pointed to the basic physiologic requirements for induction of VF from chest impact, more recent

(A)

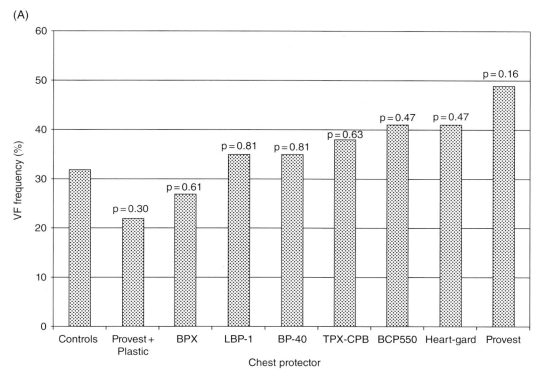

(B)

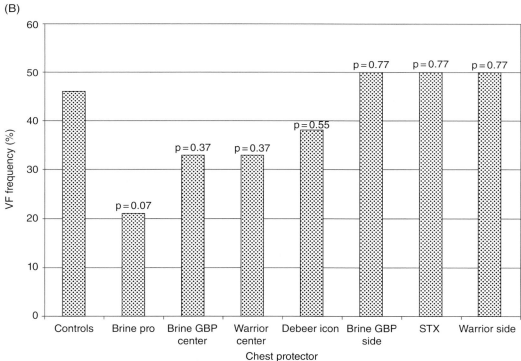

Figure 31.2 Commercial chest protectors did not prevent induction of ventricular fibrillation (VF) by lacrosse balls in an experimental swine model of commotio cordis. (A) Bar graph of the incidence of VF with baseball impacts at 40 mph in swine wearing commercially available baseball chest wall protectors. (B) Bar graph of the incidence of VF with lacrosse ball impacts at 40 mph in swine wearing lacrosse chest wall protectors (*Source*: Weinstock et al. [21]. Reproduced with permission of American Academy of Pediatrics)

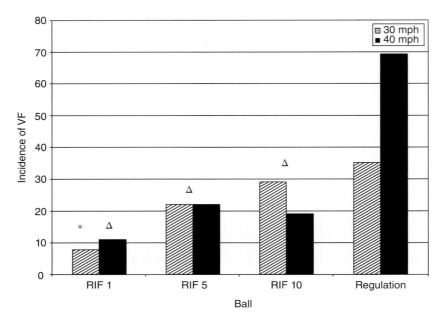

Figure 31.3 Softer-than-standard safety baseballs are available in different hardness grades. The softer balls are less likely to cause experimental VF than are standard baseballs. RIF, reduced injury factor (*Source*: Link et al. [13]. Reproduced with permission of Massachusetts Medical Society)

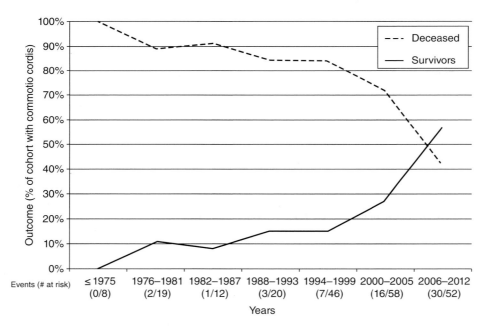

Figure 31.4 Outcomes in commotio cordis victims over the last 4 decades. Higher survival rates are likely due to improved recognition of commotio, improved cardiopulmonary resuscitation (CPR) and increased availability of automated external defibrillators (AEDs) (*Source*: Maron et al. [12]. Reproduced with permission of Elsevier)

work has been directed at more specific scenarios and parameters, such as the possibility of individual susceptibility to commotio cordis. Research in the areas of chest wall protection and the use of safety baseballs is directed at prevention. The safety of young athletes would be further advanced by increased awareness of commotio cordis and by more widespread access to AEDs at youth sporting events.

References

1 Link, M.S. and Estes, N.A. Athletes and arrhythmias. *J Cardiovasc Electrophysiol* 2010; **21**: 1184–9.

2 Maron, B.J. Sudden death in young athletes. *N Engl J Med* 2003; **349**: 1064–75.

3 Maron, B.J., Poliac, L.C., Kaplan, J.A. and Mueller, F.O. Blunt impact to the chest leading to sudden death from cardiac arrest during sports activities. *N Engl J Med* 1995; **333**: 337–42.

4 Maron, B.J. and Estes, N.A. 3rd. Commotio cordis. *N Engl J Med.* 2010; **362**: 917–27.

5 Link, M.S. Commotio cordis: ventricular fibrillation triggered by chest impact-induced abnormalities in repolarization. *Circ Arrhythm Electrophysiol* 2012; **5**: 425–32.

6 Geddes, L.A. and Roeder, R.A. Evolution of our knowledge of sudden death due to commotio cordis. *Am J Emerg Med* 2005; **23**: 67–75.

7 Nesbitt, A.D., Cooper, P.J. and Kohl, P. Rediscovering commotio cordis. *Lancet* 2001; **357**: 1195–7.

8 Meola, F. La commozione toracica. *Gior Internaz Sci Med* 1879; **1**: 923–37.

9 Dickman, G.L., Hassan, A. and Luckstead, E.F. Ventricular fibrillation following baseball injury. *Phys Sports Med* 1978; **6**: 85–6.

10 Maron, B.J., Boren, S.D., Estes, N.A. 3rd. Early descriptions of sudden cardiac death due to commotio cordis occurring in baseball. *Heart Rhythm* 2010; 7: 992–3.

11 Maron, B.J., Gohman, T.E., Kyle, S.B. et al. Clinical profile and spectrum of commotio cordis. *JAMA* 2002; **287**: 1142–6.

12 Maron, B.J., Haas, T.S., Ahluwalia, A. et al. Increasing survival rate from commotio cordis. *Heart Rhythm* 2013; **10**: 219–23.

13 Link, M.S., Wang, P.J., Pandian, N.G. et al. An experimental model of sudden death due to low-energy chest-wall impact (commotio cordis). *N Engl J Med* 1998; **338**: 1805–11.

14 Link, M.S., Maron, B.J., Wang, P.J. et al. Upper and lower limits of vulnerability to sudden arrhythmic death with chest-wall impact (commotio cordis). *J Am Coll Cardiol* 2003; **41**: 99–104.

15 Link, M.S., Maron, B.J., VanderBrink, B.A. et al. Impact directly over the cardiac silhouette is necessary to produce ventricular fibrillation in an experimental model of commotio cordis. *J Am Coll Cardiol* 2001; **37**: 649–54.

16 Link, M.S., Maron, B.J., Wang, P.J. et al. Reduced risk of sudden death from chest wall blows (commotio cordis) with safety baseballs. *Pediatrics* 2002; **109**: 873–7.

17 Kalin, J., Madias, C., Alsheikh-Ali, A.A. and Link, M.S. Reduced diameter spheres increases the risk of chest blow-induced ventricular fibrillation (commotio cordis). *Heart Rhythm* 2011; **8**: 1578–81.

18 Madias, C., Dau, N., Bir, C. et al. Mechanism of increased susceptibility of youth to sudden death with chest wall impact (commotio cordis). *Circulation* 2007; Abstracts of the Annual Scientific Sessions.

19 Alsheikh-Ali, A.A., Madias, C., Supran, S. and Link, M.S. Marked variability in susceptibility to ventricular fibrillation in an experimental commotio cordis model. *Circulation* 2010; **122**: 2499–504.

20 Drewniak, E.I., Spenciner, D.B. and Crisco, J.J. Mechanical properties of chest protectors and the likelihood of ventricular fibrillation due to commotio cordis. *J Appl Biomech* 2007; **23**: 282–8.

21 Weinstock, J., Maron, B.J., Song, C. et al. Failure of commercially available chest wall protectors to prevent sudden cardiac death induced by chest wall blows in an experimental model of commotio cordis. *Pediatrics* 2006; **117**: e656–62.

22 Kyle, S.B. *Youth Baseball Protective Equipment Project Final Report.* Washington, DC: United States Consumer Product Safety Commission, 1996.

23 Link, M.S. Prevention of sudden cardiac death: return to sport considerations in athletes with identified cardiovascular abnormalities. *Br J Sports Med* 2009; **43**: 685–9.

24 Link, M.S., Estes, N.A. 3rd and Maron, B.J. Eligibility and disqualification recommendations for competitive athletes With cardiovascular abnormalities: Task force 13: Commotio cordis: A scientific statement from the American heart association and American college of cardiology. *J Am Coll Cardiol* 2015; **66**: 2439–43.

32 Myocarditis

Jeffrey A. Towbin

The Heart Institute, University of Tennessee Health Science Center, Le Bonheur Children's Hospital and St Jude Children's Research Hospital, Memphis, TN, USA

Introduction

Myocarditis is an inflammatory disease of the myocardium that causes necrosis and/or degeneration of adjacent myocytes not typical of the ischaemic damage associated with coronary artery disease (CAD) [1]. This definition does not take into account the underlying causative mechanism of disease. The disease may be acute or chronic and is characterised by inflammatory cell infiltrates, myocyte necrosis or myocyte degeneration, with or without fibrosis. It may be caused by infectious, connective-tissue, granulomatous, toxic or idiopathic processes. There may be associated systemic manifestations of the disease, and on occasion the endocardium or pericardium is involved. Patients may be asymptomatic, have nonspecific prodromal symptoms or present with overt congestive heart failure, compromising arrhythmias or sudden death. It is thought that viral infections are the most common aetiology, especially in children, teenagers and young adults, although myocardial toxins, drug exposures, hypersensitivity reactions and immune disorders may also be responsible disease triggers.

Aetiology and Epidemiology

Cases that are definitively diagnosed as myocarditis are most commonly a result of a viral infection, which in the current era is diagnosed by the molecular biologic amplification method known as polymerase chain reaction (PCR), performed on endomyocardial biopsy samples, with or without positive viral culture or viral serology [2]. Major causes of myocarditis are listed in Table 32.1, but, importantly, most viral causes are transmitted through the air and therefore are easily transferrable.

Many cases of myocarditis in athletes remain unrecognised because they have a nonspecific or benign presentation, leaving the true incidence of myocarditis unknown. It is an underdiagnosed entity, but estimates of its incidence can be made by review of autopsy results. In the large multicentre Myocarditis Treatment Trial, there was a reported incidence of 9% in adult patients [3]. In a review of all autopsies in children (n = 1516) at a single centre over a 10-year period, only 1.8% of post mortem exams were consistent with myocarditis. Of the positive cases, 57% had presented with sudden cardiac death (SCD) [2]. Viral myocarditis appears to be a major cause of unexpected death in person less than 40 years of age, particularly in athletes and others doing moderate exercise, and may progress to chronic dilated cardiomyopathy (DCM).

IOC Manual of Sports Cardiology, First Edition. Edited by Mathew G. Wilson, Jonathan A. Drezner and Sanjay Sharma.
© 2017 International Olympic Committee. Published 2017 by John Wiley & Sons, Ltd.

Infectious causes			
Viral	*Bacterial*	*Spirochetal*	*Protozoal*
Coxsackie B virus	Diphtheria	Syphilis	Chagas' disease (South
Echovirus	Tuberculosis	Leptospirosis	American trypanosomiasis)
Epstein–Barr virus (EBV)	Salmonella	Relapsing fever	Sleeping sickness (African
Cytomegalovirus (CMV)	Staphylococcus	Lyme's disease	trypanosomiasis)
Influenza A and B	Gonococcus		Toxoplasmosis
Adenovirus	Clostridium	*Mycotic*	Malaria
Rubeola	Brucellosis	Candidiasis	Leishmaniasis
Rubella	Pisttacosis	Histoplasmosis	Amoebiasis
Varicella	Tetanus	Sporotrichosis	
Herpes virus	Tularaemia	Coccidiomycosis	*Helminthic*
Mumps	Streptococcus	Aspergillosis	Trichinosis
Hepatitis virus	Legionnaire's disease	Blastomycosis	Echinococcosis
Poliomyelitis	Meningococcus	Cryptococcosis	Schistosomiasis
Human immunodeficiency virus			Ascariasis
(HIV) (?)		*Rickettsial*	Filariasis
Variola		Typhus	Parasonimiasis
Rabies		Q fever	Strongyloidiasis
Arborvirus		Rocky Mountain	
Mycoplasma pneumoniae		spotted fever	

Noninfectious causes		
Cardiotoxins	*Hypersensitivity*	*Systemic disorders*
Catecholamines	*reactions*	Collagen – vascular
Anthracyclines	Antibiotics	diseases
Cocaine	Diuretics	Sarcoidosis
	Lithium	Kawasaki disease
	Tetanus toxoid	Hypereosinophilia
	Clozapine	

Table 32.1 Major causes of myocarditis, including infectious and noninfectious causes

Clinical Manifestations

Clinical Presentation

Adolescents and adults commonly have a recent history of viral disease 10–14 days prior to presentation, with initial symptoms that include lethargy, low-grade fever, pallor, decreased appetite, vomiting and episodic abdominal pain, diaphoresis, palpitations, rashes, exercise intolerance and general malaise. Later in the course of illness, respiratory symptoms become predominant; syncope or sudden death may occur as a result of cardiac collapse. Physical examination findings are usually consistent with heart failure [4]. Jugular venous distention and pulmonary rales may be identified, and resting tachycardia may be prominent. Occasional ectopy and arrhythmias may occur, including atrial fibrillation, supraventricular tachycardia (SVT), ventricular tachycardia and atrioventricular (AV) block [5].

Diagnostic Tests

The diagnosis of myocarditis is often difficult to establish, but it should be suspected in any individual who presents with unexplained new-onset heart failure or arrhythmia, especially ventricular tachycardia or complete heart block.

Electrocardiography Sinus tachycardia with low-voltage QRS complexes with or without low-voltage or inverted T-waves are classically described (Figures 32.1B and 32.2A,B). A pattern of myocardial injury or infarction may be seen with ST-segment changes (Figures 32.1B and 32.2B). These changes may be diffuse

(A)

(B)

(C)

(D)

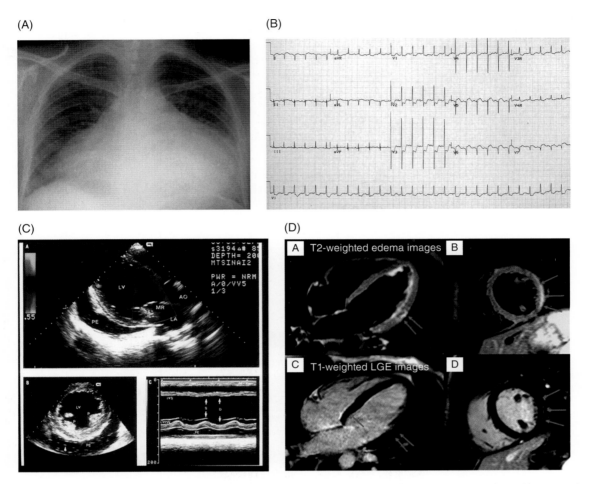

Figure 32.1 Diagnostic testing in myocarditis. (A) Chest radiograph demonstrating cardiomegaly and increased vascular markings. (B) Electrocardiogram (ECG) with sinus tachycardia, low-voltage QRS complexes, ST-segment abnormalities and Q-waves in leads I and aVL. (C) Echocardiographic features of myocarditis: two-dimensional parasternal long-axis view demonstrating left ventricular dilation and a pericardial effusion (PE) – colour Doppler interrogation provides evidence of mitral regurgitation (Panel A); parasternal short-axis view demonstrating left ventricular dilation and normal papillary muscles (P) (Panel B); and M-mode demonstrating systolic dysfunction with flattened interventricular septal motion (IVS), fair left ventricular posterior wall excursion (LVPW), left ventricular dilation with increased left ventricular end-diastolic dimension (D) and reduced systolic function (S) and PE (Panel C). Ao, aorta; LA, left atrium; MR, mitral regurgitation. (D) Cardiac magnetic resonance (CMR) images in a patient with acute myocarditis. Top panels show long-axis (Panel A) and short-axis (Panel B) T2-weighted oedema images demonstrating focal myocardial oedema in the subepicardium of the left midventricular lateral wall (red arrows). Lower panels show corresponding long-axis (Panel C) and short-axis (Panel D) T1-weighted late gadolinium enhancement (LGE) images demonstrating the presence of typical LGE in the subepicardium of the left midventricular lateral wall and the basal septum (red arrows) (*Source*: with permission from Kindermann et al. [6])

or may occur in a defined coronary distribution pattern. With sufficient time and myocardial damage, Q-waves may also be seen. Pericarditis may accompany the clinical picture, with resultant diffuse ST-segment elevation. Conduction-system disease (including AV block; Figure 32.3A) and ventricular arrhythmias (including ventricular tachycardia (Figure 32.3B) and ventricular fibrillation, SVT, atrial fibrillation and atrial flutter) may occur in some patients, and may even be the presenting complaint.

Noninvasive Imaging Echocardiography is widely used in the assessment of suspected myocarditis, due to its ready availability (Figure 32.1C). Assessment of chamber size, ventricular thickness and systolic function has been classically pursued as part of the evaluation, as has evaluation for pericardial effusion. In addition,

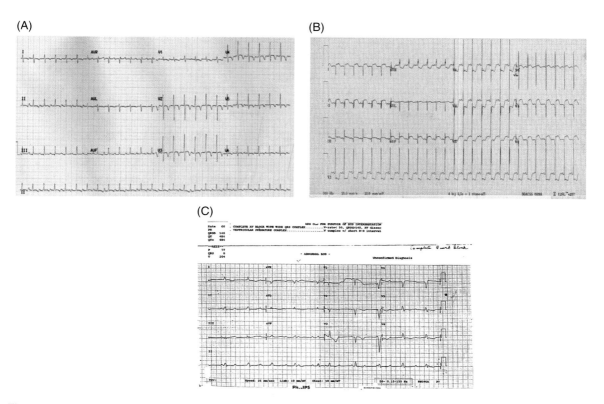

Figure 32.2 Electrocardiogram in myocarditis. (A) Tachycardia and low-voltage complexes. Additionally, there is T-wave inversion in leads V1–V6. (B) ST depression in the right precordial leads and aVR and ST elevation in leads I and II. (C) Complete AV block

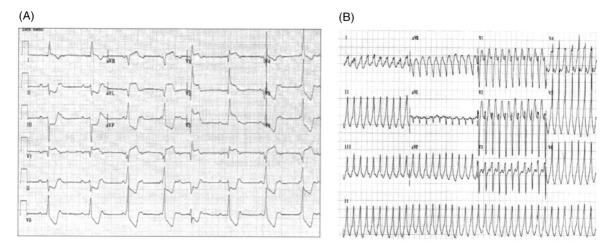

Figure 32.3 Arrhythmias in myocarditis. (A) Complete AV block. (B) Ventricular tachycardia

assessment for segmental wall-motion abnormalities is advocated, as there may be regional dysfunction in the setting of a normal ejection fraction (EF). Newer echocardiographic modalities have greatly enhanced the ability to assess diastolic function and should also be evaluated. A dilated and dysfunctional left ventricle consistent with DCM is often seen on two-dimensional (2D) (Figure 32.1C) and M-mode (Figure 32.1C) echocardiography [7]. Segmental wall-motion abnormalities are relatively common, but global hypokinesis is usually predominant. Pericardial effusion frequently occurs. Doppler and colour Doppler commonly demonstrate mitral regurgitation, which may be associated with a dilated left atrium (Figure 32.1C). Newer strategies that assess regional myocardial deformation, such as strain and strain-rate imaging, are also utilised and may offer opportunities to detect myocardial inflammation prior to overt changes in regional or global systolic function [8].

Cardiovascular magnetic resonance (CMR) is a noninvasive strategy that provides reproducible volumetric and functional data and has the unique ability to localise areas of myocardial inflammation and oedema (Figure 32.1D). Specific techniques for myocardial characterisation have been developed, including T-2-weighted imaging (to localise myocardial oedema) and T-1-weighted contrast-enhanced fast-spin echo imaging (for hyperaemic responses) (Figure 32.1D). The use of gadolinium enhancement techniques has been valuable, with late gadolinium enhancement (LGE) being able to localise areas of irreversible myocardial injury (necrosis and fibrosis) and inflammation. In a report on 203 consecutive adult patients with biopsy-proven myocarditis who also underwent CMR on presentation and during clinical follow-up, the presence of LGE resulted in hazard ratios of 8.4 and 12.8 for all-cause mortality and cardiac mortality, respectively. This was a more robust predictor than the echocardiographic markers typically assessed, including EF and left ventricular end-diastolic volume. Furthermore, SCD was not seen in any subject without LGE [9]. CMR also offers a unique modality to follow patients with myocarditis longitudinally for ongoing assessment for reversible/irreversible myocardial injury, myocardial viability, favorable remodelling and scar burden [10]. All of these findings may have an impact on clinical decision-making, including response to therapy and the need for advanced interventions (such as implantable cardioverter-defibrillators, ICDs) and cardiac transplantation.

Serologic Testing The use of serologic markers in cardiovascular disease (CVD) is common; they may identify ongoing myocardial damage and offer insight into future prognosis. However, the currently available biomarkers lack specificity, and there are none that clearly differentiate myocarditis from other causes of acute myocardial dysfunction, such as that caused by ischaemia. Traditional markers of myocardial cell lysis, such as the creatine kinase myocardial band (CK-MB) and troponins, may be elevated in acute myocarditis. These are readily available tests that help to identify the affected organ system. In patients with acute myocarditis, serum concentrations of troponin I and T are elevated more frequently than the CK-MB fraction, and higher levels of troponin T have been shown to be of prognostic value. However, troponin measurements may only be elevated in 35–45% of biopsy-proven myocarditis cases [11]. Nonspecific serum markers of inflammation, including leukocytes and C-reactive protein (CRP), can be elevated in acute myocarditis, but normal values do not exclude an acute myocardial inflammatory process.

Cardiac Catheterisation and Endomyocardial Biopsy The gold standard for identification of the underlying cause of acute and chronic myocarditis remains the analyses performed on tissue obtained by endomyocardial biopsy (Figure 32.4A). These tests include routine histologic examination (Figure 32.4B) and targeted immunohistochemical analysis. In addition, viral PCR analysis is performed on all endomyocardial biopsy samples due to the inherent limitations of the existing histopathological criteria used for diagnosis [12]. Cardiac catheterisation typically reveals low cardiac output and elevated ventricular end-diastolic pressures in patients with significant myocardial involvement. The endomyocardial biopsy (Figure 32.4A), usually obtained from the right ventricle, is microscopically evaluated for inflammation (Figure 32.4B). The inflammatory infiltrate is normally patchy and scattered in the ventricular myocardium. A mononuclear cell infiltrate is diagnostic of myocarditis, although this does not delineate cause. Myocardial biopsy has been reported to be diagnostically sensitive in 3–63% of cases [13], but because of the risks associated with biopsy, particularly in young children and those with ventricular wall thinning and/or active inflammation or malignant arrhythmias, many centres have abandoned this procedure.

It should be noted that foci of inflammation may be seen in all forms of cardiomyopathy, irrespective of aetiology, due to the disruption of cardiomyocytes as part of the pathophysiology and cellular biology of the disease. These are not cases of myocarditis in the usual sense. The Dallas criteria have been used as the gold standard for microscopic diagnosis of myocarditis; they define myocarditis as 'a process characterized by an inflammatory infiltrate of the myocardium with necrosis and/or degeneration of adjacent myocytes not typical of ischaemic damage' owing to coronary artery or other disease [15]. At the time of initial biopsy, a specimen may be classified as active myocarditis, borderline myocarditis or no myocarditis, depending on whether an inflammatory infiltrate occurs in association with myocyte degeneration or necrosis (active), too sparse an infiltrate or no myocyte degeneration (borderline). Repeat endomyocardial biopsy may be appropriate in cases where strong suspicion of myocarditis exists clinically; on repeat endomyocardial biopsy, histology may be classified as ongoing myocarditis, resolving myocarditis or resolved myocarditis. However,

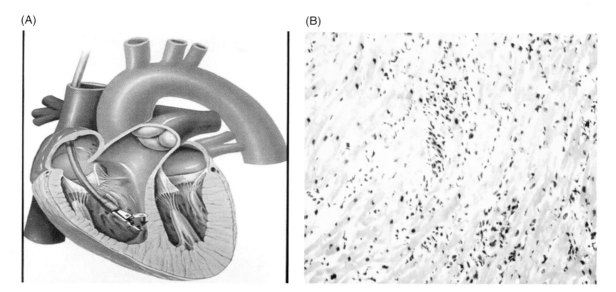

Figure 32.4 Endomyocardial biopsy and histopathology in myocarditis. (A) Endomyocardial biopsy technique. The bioptome is advanced via the superior vena cava in the neck into the right atrium, across the tricuspid valve and into the right ventricle, and finally situated against the interventricular septum, where the biopsy is performed. The bioptome can be advanced via the inferior vena cava with similar results. (B) Endomyocardial biopsy histology demonstrates lymphocytic infiltrates, myocardial oedema and necrosis (*Source*: Towbin [14]. Reproduced with permission of Elsevier)

increasing evidence has led to more extensive studies on endomyocardial biopsy samples, including histopathology, immunohistochemistry, viral PCR and cardiac antibody testing, in order to better make the diagnosis of myocarditis.

Viral Studies A positive viral culture from the myocardium used to be considered the diagnostic standard but it is rarely identified, even in patients with other classic features of the disease. Viral culture of peripheral specimens, such as blood, stool or urine, is commonly performed but is unreliable in identifying the actual causative infection of the heart. Viral antibody serologic titres have also been used for aetiologic diagnosis. A fourfold increase in viral antibody titre reportedly correlates with infection. However, these studies are nonspecific because prior infection with the causative virus is commonplace and the results take a significant amount of time to complete. Nonetheless, PCR analysis may identify the viral genome in the heart in approximately 45–50% of suspected cases [16].

Pathophysiology

Viral infection triggers interstitial inflammation and myocardial injury, resulting in cardiac enlargement and an increase in the ventricular end-diastolic volume [17]. Normally, this increase in volume results in an increased force of contraction, improved EF and improved cardiac output, as described by the Starling mechanism. In myocarditis, the myocardium is unable to respond to these stimuli, resulting in a reduction in stroke volume. A 'domino effect' of various changes occurs, resulting in pathophysiologic responses in patients with myocarditis, including:

1. Interactions with the sympathetic nervous system, preserving vital systemic blood flow via vasoconstriction. However, this increases afterload on the failing myocardium. This sympathetic nervous system input initially results in preserved blood pressure, tachycardia and diaphoresis.
2. Acute decompensated heart failure with disease progression. The progressive increase in ventricular end-diastolic volume and pressure results in increased left atrial pressure, which is transmitted into the pulmonary venous system. This causes increasing hydrostatic forces, which overcome the colloid osmotic pressure that normally prevents transudation of fluid across the capillary membranes; this results in pulmonary oedema.

3. Dilation of all cardiac chambers, particularly the left ventricle. In addition to causing poor ventricular function, this dilation creates worsening pulmonary oedema and leads to stretching of the mitral annulus and resultant mitral regurgitation, further increasing left atrial volume and pressure.

4. Replacement of normal myofibres by fibroblasts during the healing stages of myocarditis, resulting in scar formation. Reduced elasticity and ventricular performance can produce persistent heart failure. In addition, ventricular arrhythmias or AV block may accompany fibrosis.

Gross and Microscopic Pathology

Pathologic findings are nonspecific, with similar gross and microscopic changes noted irrespective of the causative agent [18]. The heart weight is increased and all four chambers are affected. The muscle is flabby and pale, with petechial haemorrhages often seen on the epicardial surfaces. A pericardial effusion may also be seen, relating to the often combined finding of pericarditis (e.g. myopericarditis). The ventricular wall is frequently thin, although hypertrophy may be found as well. The valves and endocardium are usually not involved. In cases of chronic myocarditis, the valves may be glistening white, consistent with endocardial fibroelastosis (EFE), suggesting that the findings may be the result of longstanding inflammation [19]. Mural thrombi may occur in the left ventricle, and small emboli are often found in the coronary and cerebral vessels.

Extensive necrosis of the myocardium, with loss of cross-striation in the muscle fibres and oedema, is seen in severe infections, especially with coxsackievirus. Mild to moderate inflammation with moderate to severe fibrosis is common in cases of adenoviral myocarditis, whilst coronary insufficiency is common with PVB19. Diphtheria myocarditis is frequently complicated by arrhythmias and complete AV block [20]. Diphtheria exotoxin attaches to conduction tissue and interferes with protein synthesis by inhibiting a translocating enzyme in the delivery of amino acids. Bacterial myocarditis produces microabscesses and patchy focal suppurative changes. A combined perimyocarditis is also frequently encountered.

Myocarditis and Athletics

Physical activity should be restricted during the acute phase of myocarditis, until the disease has completely resolved. Athletes should be temporarily excluded from competitive and amateur leisure-time sport activity, regardless of age, gender, severity of symptoms or therapeutic regimen. After resolution of the clinical presentation (at least 6 months after the onset of the disease), clinical reassessment is indicated before the athlete can resume competitive sport. Pre-participation screening should be performed every 6 months during the follow-up, including 12-lead electrocardiogram (ECG), exercise echocardiography, 24-hour Holter and, importantly, CMR with LGE. Asymptomatic athletes with normal ventricular function and absence of complex ventricular arrhythmias during an exercise test or Holter monitor may resume competition in all sports. Athletes who fulfill these requirements but who have persistent LGE on the CMR 6 months after initial presentation should continue to remain under annular cardiac surveillance while competing.

Long-Term Sequelae

Many patients with myocarditis survive the critical phase of the illness. It is increasingly recognised that they will present with myocardial dysfunction and evidence of heart failure at some later point in their lives [21]. It remains unclear what the underlying cause of these long-term sequelae could be, but viral persistence and autoimmunity have been widely considered.

Treatment

Care for pateints with suspected or proven myocarditis must be individualised, given the wide range of viral aetiologies and presenting symptoms, which may vary from being relatively asymptomatic to undergoing cardiogenic shock. Continual reassessment of patients with myocarditis is recommended, as their clinical picture can change dramatically in a very short period of time. Many patients present with relatively mild disease, with minimal or no respiratory compromise and only mild signs of congestive heart failure. These patients require close haemodynamic and electrocardiographic monitoring to assess whether the disease will progress to worsening heart failure and they will need more intensive medical care. Murine models of myocarditis suggest that exercise may result in increased viral replication, as well as myocardial inflammation and necrosis [22]. Thus, it appears prudent to place all athletes under this restriction at the time of diagnosis. Normal arterial blood oxygen levels should be maintained for any patient with compromised haemodynamics resulting in hypoxaemia.

Medical Management

The appropriate medical management of patients with myocarditis is dependent on their clinical presentation. Patients presenting with mild symptoms of heart failure and preserved cardiac output should be continually evaluated, as they may progress to a more decompesated state. Diuretics may be used judiciously to treat symptoms of shortness of breath or peripheral oedema. There are convincing data to show that long-term oral therapies may be of benefit. Angiotensin-converting enzyme (ACE) inhibitors or angiotensin receptor blockers (ARBs) should be considered in patients with evidence of depressed left ventricular systolic function and/or dilation of the left ventricle, to assist in favorable remodelling [23]. ACE inhibitors have been shown to reduce inflammatory infiltrates and calcification, and the ARB candesartan was shown to enhance survival and decrease inflammatory mediators in murine models of myocarditis. The use of beta blockade in patients with myocarditis has also showed success. Murine models treated with beta blockade have demonstrated decreased inflammation [24], and human studies clearly report the lack of beta blocker use as an independent predictor of poor prognosis [25].

Arrhythmias should be treated appropriately and aggressively [5]. Supraventricular and ventricular tachyarrhtyhmias may be seen and should be treated quickly. Chronic arrhythmias may persist long after the acute disease has passed, especially in the setting of myocardial fibrosis. Thus, athletes who recover from myocarditis, regardless of cause, should be followed indefinitely with appropriate arrhythmia surveillance. Our practice has been to perform ambulatory Holter monitoring annually at a minimum, with more frequent assessment or alternative strategies (such as event recoders) in patients with symptoms or with risk of ongoing arrhythmia. Finally, the use of immunosuppressive and immunomodulatory agents in suspected or proven cases of viral myocarditis has remained controversial and is not recommended.

Conclusion

Myocarditis should be suspected in athletes with unexplained cardiac arrhythmias and dysfunction, especially if preceded by a flu-like syndrome. An early diagnosis is desirable, in order to avoid fatal consequences, since physical activity can exacerbate the inflammatory process. Treatment is often difficult for highly competitive athletes to comprehend, as initial treatment for athletes with myocarditis should be complete absence from all physical activity for at least 6 months. Athletes should only resume training when ventricular function and cardiac dimensions return to normal and the clinically relevant arrhythmias disappear. Adherence to such guidelines should be strongly advocated, to reduce the potential of life-threatening arrhythmias or rapidly progressive cardiac dysfunction and the need for the introduction of antiviral or immunosuppressive treatment [26].

References

1 Jefferies, J.L. and Towbin, J.A. Dilated cardiomyopathy. *Lancet* 2010; **375**: 752–62.
2 Weber, M.A., Ashworth, M.T., Risdon, R.A. et al. Clinicopathological features of paediatric deaths due to myocarditis: an autopsy series. *Arch Dis Child* 2008; **93**: 594–8.
3 Mason, J.W., O'Connell, J.B., Herskowitz, A. et al. A clinical trial of immunosuppressive therapy for myocarditis. The Myocarditis Treatment Trial Investigators. *N Engl J Med* 1995; **333**: 269–75.
4 Bowles, N.E. and Towbin, J.A. Molecular aspects of myocarditis. *Curr Opin Cardiol* 1998; **13**: 179–84.
5 Friedman, R.A., Kearney, D.L., Moak, J.P. et al. Persistence of ventricular arrhythmia after resolution of occult myocarditis in children and young adults. *J Am Coll Cardiol* 1994; **24**: 780–3.
6 Kindermann, I., Barth, C., Mahfoud, F. et al. Update on myocarditis. *J Am Coll Cardiol* 2012; **59**: 779–92.
7 Felker, G.M., Boehmer, J.P., Hruban, R.H. et al. Echocardiographic findings in fulminant and acute myocarditis. *J Am Coll Cardiol* 2000; **36**: 227–32.
8 Di Bella, G., Gaeta, M., Pingitore, A. et al. Myocardial deformation in acute myocarditis with normal left ventricular wall motion – a cardiac magnetic resonance and 2-dimensional strain echocardiographic study. *Circ J* 2010; **74**: 1205–13.

9 Grün, S., Schumm, J., Greulich, S. et al. Long-term follow-up of biopsy-proven viral myocarditis: Predictors of mortality and incomplete recovery. *J Am Coll Cardiol* 2012; **59**: 1604–15.

10 Zagrosek, A., Abdel-Aty, H., Boye, P. et al. Cardiac magnetic resonance monitors reversible and irreversible myocardial injury in myocarditis. *JACC Cardiovasc Imaging* 2009; **2**: 131–8.

11 Lauer, B., Niederau, C., Kuhl, U. et al. Cardiac troponin T in patients with clinically suspected myocarditis. *J Am Coll Cardiol* 1997; **30**: 1354–9.

12 Baughman, K.L. Diagnosis of myocarditis: death of Dallas criteria. *Circulation*; 2006; **113**: 593–5.

13 Grogan, M., Redfield, M.M., Bailey, K.R. et al. Long-term outcome of patients with biopsy-proved myocarditis: comparison with idiopathic dilated cardiomyopathy. *J Am Coll Cardiol* 1995; **26**: 80–4.

14 Towbin, J.A. Molecular genetic aspects of cardiomyopathy. *Biochem Med Metab Biol* 1993; **49**: 285–320.

15 Aretz, H.T. Myocarditis: the Dallas criteria. *Hum Pathol* 1987; **18**: 619–24.

16 Bowles, N.E., Bowles, K.R. and Towbin, J.A. Viral genomic detection and outcome in myocarditis. *Heart Fail Clin* 2005; **1**: 407–17.

17 Sole, M.J. and Liu, P. Viral myocarditis: a paradigm for understanding the pathogenesis and treatment of dilated cardiomyopathy. *J Am Coll Cardiol* 1993; **22**: 99A–105A.

18 Dec, G.W. Jr, Palacios, I.F., Fallon, J.T. et al. Active myocarditis in the spectrum of acute dilated cardiomyopathies. Clinical features, histologic correlates, and clinical outcome. *N Engl J Med* 1985; **312**: 885–90.

19 Hutchins, G.M. and Vie, S.A. The progression of interstitial myocarditis to idiopathic endocardial fibroelastosis. *Am J Pathol* 1972; **66**: 483–96.

20 Burch, G.E., Sun, S.C., Sohal, R.S. et al. Diphtheritic myocarditis. A histochemical and electron microscopic study. *Am J Cardiol* 1968; **21**: 261–8.

21 McCarthy, R.E. 3rd, Boehmer, J.P., Hruban, R.H. et al. Long-term outcome of fulminant myocarditis as compared with acute (nonfulminant) myocarditis. *N Engl J Med* 2000; **342**: 690–5.

22 Kiel, R.J., Smith, F.E., Chason, J. et al. Coxsackievirus B3 myocarditis in C3H/HeJ mice: description of an inbred model and the effect of exercise on virulence. *Eur J Epidemiol* 1989; **5**: 348–50.

23 Jessup, M., Abraham, W.T., Casey, D.E. et al. 2009 focused update: ACCF/AHA Guidelines for the Diagnosis and Management of Heart Failure in Adults: a report of the American College of Cardiology Foundation/American Heart Association Task Force on Practice Guidelines: developed in collaboration with the International Society for Heart and Lung Transplantation. *Circulation* 2009; **119**: 1977–2016.

24 Pauschinger, M., Rutschow, S., Chandrasekharan, K. et al. Carvedilol improves left ventricular function in murine coxsackievirus-induced acute myocarditis association with reduced myocardial interleukin-1beta and MMP-8 expression and a modulated immune response. *Eur J Heart Fail* 2005; **7**: 444–52.

25 Kindermann, I., Kindermann, M., Kandolf, R. et al. Predictors of outcome in patients with suspected myocarditis. *Circulation* 2008; **118**: 639–48.

26 Chimenti, C., Pieroni, M. and Frustaci, A. Myocarditis: when to suspect and how to diagnose it in athletes. *J Cardiovasc Med (Hagerstown)* 2006; **7**: 301–6.

Section 5
Other Causes of Sudden Death

33 Alternative Noncardiac Medical Causes of Sudden Death: Sickle-Cell Trait, Exertional Heatstroke, Exercise Rhabdomyolysis, Asthma and Extreme Environmental Conditions

Juan Manuel Alonso and Paul Dijkstra

Department of Sports Medicine, ASPETAR, Qatar Orthopaedic and Sports Medicine Hospital, Doha, Qatar

Introduction

The majority of published papers on sudden death in athletes focus on acute cardiovascular events. However, other causes of sudden death during sport are relevant to the sports medicine and cardiology physician, especially when providing on-field care to a collapsed athlete. The more common noncardiac causes of medical sudden death are sickle-cell trait (SCT) (2–6%) and exertional heatstroke (EHS) (1–2%) [1,2]. Asthma, brain aneurysm, drug overdose, exertional hyponatraemia, exertional rhabdomyolysis, high altitude disorders, hypothermia, infections and pulmonary embolism represent other potential causes of sudden death in athletes, but taken together make up less than a quarter of all medical causes [1,2]. This chapter focuses on the noncardiac medical causes of sudden death in athletes.

Sickle-Cell Trait

SCT is a genetic condition resulting from the inheritance of an A-S gene (single mutant beta globin allele) for sickle haemoglobin (HbS) from one parent and an A-A gene for normal haemoglobin (HbA) from the other, allowing both HbS and HbA to be produced in every red blood cell (RBC). Patients with SCT always have more HbA (typically 60%) than HbS. In contrast, those with sickle-cell disease inherit the A-S gene from both parents and produce no HbA in their RBCs. The sickle gene is common in regions endemic with

IOC Manual of Sports Cardiology, First Edition. Edited by Mathew G. Wilson, Jonathan A. Drezner and Sanjay Sharma.

malaria, because SCT protects against early death from plasmodium infection. Approximately 300 million people worldwide and nearly 9% of African Americans (roughly 3 million individuals), 0.5% of Hispanic individuals and 0.2% of white individuals have SCT. The coexistence of alpha-thalassaemia trait, occurring in about one-third of black individuals, lowers the amount of HbS in each RBC and may reduce the risk of exertional sickling [3,4]. Exertional sickling blocks the microvasculature of working muscles by altered sickle RBCs, resulting in ischaemic rhabdomyolysis and profound metabolic disturbances, which can eventually lead to death.

SCT carriage can be confirmed by either (i) Hb separation and quantification or (ii) analysis of alpha-globin genes. The presence of HbA and HbS in RBCs in a person who has not received a RBC transfusion in 3 or more months indicates SCT [4].

Epidemiology of SCT-Associated Sudden Death

The 31-year Unites States Sudden Death in Athletes registry includes 23 SCT-related deaths (0.9%) amongst 2462 registered athlete deaths, all in African Americans [5]. Over the 10-year period 2002–2011, 11 SCT-associated deaths were registered, all in African American male athletes [2]. A recent publication by Harmon et al. [6] found 273 deaths in a total of 1 969 663 athlete-participant-years within a series of all cases of sudden death in National Collegiate Athletic Association (NCAA) student athletes from January 2004 to December 2008. Of these sudden death cases, 5 (2%) were associated with SCT, all occurring in black Division I American football athletes. Harmon et al. [6] estimated a 37-times higher risk of sudden death for Division I American football athletes with, versus without, SCT. In a subsequent interpretation of the Harmon data by Stovitz and Shrier [7], further analysis reduced the risk in black athlete SCT carriers to 22-fold, as SCT was not found to be an associated risk factor for death in white athletes. Nevertheless, it can be concluded that SCT is a major risk factor for sudden death in black collegiate athletes [6,9]. Exertional deaths associated with SCT have also been reported in other sports (basketball and track and field), although the vast majority occur in African American athletes playing American football [2,8].

Athletic Performance and SCT

Epidemiological studies on athletic performance have shown that SCT can contribute to success in brief and explosive track-and-field events involving alactic energy metabolism. As such, SCT carriers may have a greater ability to excel in short-distance, intense running. In contrast, the ability of SCT carriers to perform repeated, short bouts of predominantly anaerobic exercise with limited recovery may be lower than non-SCT carriers [4].

Pathophysiology of SCT-Associated Sudden Death

The key clinical consideration for athletes with SCT is exertional sickling, as this 'sudden collapse' syndrome can be fatal. The typical exercise stimulus for a sickling collapse is maximal exertion for at least a few minutes, which can include repeated bouts of high intensity conditioning with inadequate rest periods. Other challenging scenarios can include an abrupt increase in training intensity, mainly on the first day of fitness conditioning, such as when athletes return from holiday. These factors may trigger the 'perfect storm' from undue exercise intensity, sustained for at least a few minutes, and a 'heroic effort' beyond the athlete's limits (see case report) [3].

A complex cascade of pathophysiological changes is presumed to lead to exertional sickling and subsequent collapse. Maximal exertion (running or cycling) can induce hypoxaemia and metabolic acidosis within 2–5 minutes, alongside possible RBC dehydration and hyperthermia amid a milieu of hyperosmotic working muscles [3].

These adverse forces – hypoxaemia and acidosis, hyperthermia in working muscles, hyperosmolarity and RBC dehydration (which concentrates HbS), and a sharp rise in circulating levels of epinephrine (which makes SCT red cells sticky) – promote exertional sickling in the microcirculation [3,10,11]. Sickle cells have a propensity to block small blood vessels and thus the blood supply to working muscles. This causes further

Case Report: Exertional Sickling

A 19-year-old African American college football player in Texas collapsed after a conditioning run on a 'mild' day in September. He ran 16 successive sprints of 100 yards each, lagged behind his teammates on the final sprints, and collapsed of shortness of breath and leg pain. He was initially alert, but became lethargic after a few minutes. Too weak to stand, he was transported to the athletic training room, where despite supportive therapy and intravenous fluids, he lost consciousness within 15 minutes. He was rushed to the hospital, where he was noted to have profound lactic acidosis and fulminant rhabdomyolysis. He developed acute renal failure and disseminated intravascular coagulation, remained unresponsive, and died about 15 hours after collapse, from hyperkalaemia and pulseless electrical activity leading to asystole [3].

Source: Eichner [3]. Reproduced with permission of Elsevier

Sickling	Cardiac	Heatstroke	Asthma
Weakness > pain	No cramping	Confusion	Usually occurs in a known asthmatic
Athlete slumps to ground	Sudden collapse	Bizarre behaviour	Prior episodes, poor control
Athlete can talk at first	Unconsciousness	Incoherence	Athlete breathless, may or may not wheeze
Muscles 'normal'	Limpness or seizure	Athlete can be in coma	Athlete gasping, panicky on hands/knees
Temperature often <39 °C (103 °F)	Temperature irrelevant	Temperature >40 °C (104 °F)	Auscultate – reduced air movement
Can occur early in training session	No warning	Usually occurs late in training session	Usually occurs after sprinting

Table 33.1 Features of common nontraumatic causes of on-field collapse (*Source*: Eichner [8]. Reproduced with permission of Wolters Kluwer Health)

exertional sickling and ischaemic rhabdomyolysis, which can be explosive. The result is a metabolic storm (profound lactic acidosis, hyperkalaemia, and falling calcium), with may lead to a fatal arrhythmia or pulseless electrical activity in an otherwise normal heart [3,10].

Exercise Collapse Associated with Sickle-Cell Trait

This clinical presentation in athletes with SCT has recently been named 'exercise collapse associated with sickle-cell trait' (ECAST). It includes a spectrum from severe muscle pain to fulminant collapse. American football conditioning accounts for the majority of ECAST events. The trigger is short-duration, high-intensity exercise, typical in athletes near maximal exertion during repeated bouts of conditioning. ECAST can occur after the end of an hour-long, fast-tempo station drill, or early, after the athlete has been on-field for only a short time (e.g. near-maximal sprinting for only 2–5 minutes) [3,4,8]. Sustained maximal intensity is a trigger in all cases of ECAST [10].

All in an apparently healthy athlete during exercise collapses on-field with no apparent trauma should be considered cardiac in origin until proven otherwise; then, EHS, asthma, or exertional sickling should be considered. Sudden cardiac arrest presents with an abrupt collapse and a non-responsive athlete. Exertional sickling should be suspected in an athlete who appears to be struggling during conditioning exercise and then collapses without loss of consciousness. Not all sickling collapses are identical, but they differ from other causes of nontraumatic collapse (see Table 33.1). Pain, weakness and flaccid or soft muscles are common in ECAST, as opposed to the painful, hard, contracted muscles present in exercise-associated muscle cramps [4].

Some athletes report that symptoms begin with leg and/or low back pain. Some call it 'cramps that spread up my body'. Athletes may stop with disabling low back pain or may instead complain of weakness more than pain. Other presenting symptoms include chest 'tightness' and complaints of 'I can't catch my breath' or 'I just don't feel right' within the context of high intensity conditioning. The athlete may initially be on their hands and knees and may be very anxious. Athletes with a sickle crisis may engage in very rapid breathing (not asthma) to try to offset the metabolic acidosis. Some stoic players will just stop (e.g. after 700 m of a planned 800 m sprint) and sit or lie down, saying, 'I can't go on', or, 'my legs won't go'. The instinctive decision to stop activity or exercise has possibly saved the lives of many players with SCT [3,8].

Risk Factors

SCT carriers may have interacting factors, such as impaired blood rheology in the microcirculation, a pro-inflammatory vascular environment with abnormal adherent sickle cells, neutrophils and monocytes or coagulation abnormalities and endothelial dysfunction [4,8]. SCT carriers may be at greater risk during or after certain conditions of microcirculatory alteration that can lead to acute ischaemic episodes in skeletal muscle cells [4].

Several contributing factors have been proposed to increase the risk of adverse effects in SCT carriers: (i) exercise in the heat and/or high humidity; (ii) dehydration; (iii) exercise at altitude; and (iv) poor conditioning. Other factors hypothetically contributing to initiate adverse effects include exercise-induced asthma, pre-exercise fatigue due to illness (i.e. viral infection) or lack of sleep, high-intensity exercise and the use of dietary supplements containing stimulants [4].

Some authors have found greater oxidative stress responses in sedentary rather than in physically trained SCT carriers. In other words, for athletes with SCT being physically fit may reduce the risk of developing ECAST by decreasing endothelial dysfunction and subsequent vascular impairment through improvements in both nitric oxide and antioxidant availability [12].

A polygenetic pathogenesis is postulated for sudden death in SCT carriers, and a variety of candidate genes may be implicated. Environmental factors (exercise intensity, altitude, hydration status and the presence of concurrent illness) may interact with genetic variations to influence risk. These variations can influence microvascular flow and potassium efflux, modulating the risk of sudden death [11].

Prevention: To Screen or Not To Screen?

It is important to implement strategies to prevent complications and sudden death in athletes with SCT. However, restriction from sports participation is not recommended [6]. All newborns in the US are screened for SCT as there is strong evidence that early intervention in those who are HbS homozygous can reduce mortality and morbidity [4,6]. The NCAA adopted legislation in April 2010 mandating screening in all Division I athletes (a haemoglobin solubility as a minimum, with a positive result followed by additional testing) without known SCT status at birth [6,13]. As of January 2013, similar policies have been extended to NCAA Divisions II and III [13].

However, the American Society of Hematology (ASH) denounced the NCAA position in January 2012 [9], based on a lack of scientific evidence and the belief the recommended solubility test may give misleading results. ASH has expressed several concerns, including the potential disclosure of protected health information and the loss of privacy, stigmatisation and discrimination associated with mandatory screening [9,13]. ASH recommends the approach taken by the US Army: undertaking universal interventions (e.g. monitoring of heat acclimatisation), adjusting work to the environment, implementing guidelines for hydration and keeping staff prepared for early detection and rapid appropriate treatment of heat illness [9].

Nevertheless, appropriate sharing of medical information with coaches, managers and medical staff can be necessary in elite sport [14], and many experts in the field believe that the 'NCAA way' can reduce ECAST deaths through proper counseling and awareness that the army approach may not be as effective [10]. The significance of SCT identification and targeted training modifications to decrease mortality has not been verified, and further research is needed [6].

Management of Exertional Sickling

Targeted education and preventive interventions are recommended for athletes with known SCT (see Table 33.2). Pre-season testing for SCT status in high-risk athletes (i.e. American football players) allows appropriate counselling and provides valuable information to the medical staff in case of an

- Targeted screening of high-risk groups
- Educational interventions for athletes with SCT and their supervisors (managers, sports coaches, strength and conditioning coaches and medical staff)
- Allotment of appropriate time for and access to hydration
- Gradual acclimatisation to heat
- Modification of activity in the heat and at altitude
- Appropriate strength and conditioning programmes developed by qualified coaches
- Prohibition of punitive exercise
- Early recognition of and immediate rest for athletes who are struggling; athletes must not be pushed past the physiological limit
- Adequate emergency planning for all individuals responsible for athletes during training

Table 33.2 SCT prevention measures (*Source:* Harmon et al. [9]. Reproduced with permission of BMJ)

exertional collapse. Athletes with SCT should be educated regarding the signs, symptoms and associated risk factors of exertional sickling.

If an athlete with SCT begins to experience symptoms with high-intensity training, they should immediately stop their activity and seek medical attention. Rest, supplementary oxygen and, in some cases, cooling and intravenous fluid administration can reverse initial symptoms. For minor episodes, athletes may return to play when symptoms have fully resolved. More extreme cases of exertional sickling, associated with athlete collapse or unconsciousness, are medical emergencies and should be treated with supplementary oxygen, intravenous fluids, cooling and rapid transport to an emergency facility. An automated external defibrillator (AED) should be available in cases of exertional sickling with collapse, in case of rapid deterioration to cardiopulmonary arrest. In-hospital assessment for laboratory abnormalities (specifically hyperkalaemia and rhabdomyolysis) and monitoring for potential adverse sequelae (e.g. renal dysfunction, cardiac arrhythmias) is necessary [9].

Exertional Heatstroke

The metabolic rate is a function of running speed and body mass, with the highest rectal temperatures in the fastest runners competing in events of 8–21 km. Rectal temperatures may increase to 40.5 °C in such runners without symptoms or evidence of heat-related illness. Heat-related illness predominantly affects athletes during high-intensity exercise, but also in exercise of longer duration, resulting in withdrawal from activity or collapse during or soon after activity [15]. EHS is defined as a rectal temperature >40 °C accompanied by symptoms or signs of organ system failure – most frequently, central nervous system (CNS) dysfunction (unconsciousness, reduced level of consciousness, confusion, agitation or convulsions). When the metabolic heat produced by the exercising muscles during activity is greater than the body heat transfer to the surroundings, the core temperature rises to levels that can disrupt organ function. Almost all EHS patients exhibit sweat-soaked and pale skin at the time of collapse, as opposed to the dry, hot and flushed skin that is described in the presentation of non-exertion-related (classic) heatstroke [16].

Early recognition and rapid cooling can reduce both the morbidity and the mortality associated with EHS. Clinical changes can be subtle and easy to miss if coaches, medical personnel and athletes do not maintain a high level of awareness and monitor at-risk athletes closely. Fatigue and exhaustion during exercise occur more rapidly as heat stress increases, and are the most common causes of withdrawal from activity in hot conditions. When athletes collapse from exhaustion in hot conditions (but without confusion or other CNS changes), the term 'heat exhaustion' is often applied. This term can be confusing, and in some cases, rectal temperature >40 °C is the only discernible difference between heat exhaustion and EHS during on-site evaluations [15]. While EHS occurs most frequently in hot, humid conditions, it is important to remember it can also occur in cool conditions, during intense or prolonged exercise in susceptible individuals, especially when excessive or warm clothing is worn [16].

Predisposing Factors

Individual susceptibility (as opposed to environmental conditions) plays a more important role in the development of EHS than was previously thought [15]. Although strenuous exercise in a hot, humid environment, lack of heat acclimatisation and poor physical fitness are widely accepted as the primary factors leading to

- Low physical fitness
- Sleep deprivation
- Improper acclimatisation
- Heat load corresponding to wet bulb globe temperature (WBGT) green flag or above
- High solar radiation
- Physical effort unmatched to physical fitness
- Improper work/rest cycles
- Absence of proper medical triage
- Training at hottest hours
- Improper treatment

Table 33.3 Risk factors frequently present in EHS fatal cases (*Source:* Casa et al. [17]. Reproduced with permission of Wolters Kluwer Health)

EHS, even highly trained and heat-acclimatised athletes can develop EHS whilst exercising at a high intensity if heat dissipation is inadequate relative to metabolic heat production. The greatest risk of EHS exists when the wet bulb globe temperature (WBGT) exceeds 28 °C (82 °F) during high-intensity exercise (>75% VO_{2max}) and/or strenuous exercise that lasts longer than 1 hour. Inadequate physical fitness, incomplete heat acclimatisation, viral illness, medications and genetic predisposition may account for EHS at lower temperatures. The risk factors most frequently found in fatal cases are listed in Table 33.3 [17].

Epidemiology of EHS-Associated Sudden Death

EHS accounts for 1–3% of all exertional sudden death, and may rise to the primary cause of sudden death during the summer months [18]. Amongst organised sports in the US, the frequency of EHS-related deaths is highest in American football, with a large proportion (up to 90%) occurring during practice. In most cases, fatal EHS is a rare event. It is more likely during the initial 4 days of pre-season conditioning in American football, where the incidence of fatal EHS was about 1 in 350 000 participants between 1995 and 2002 [16]. The number of sports-related EHS deaths in the US has doubled since 1975, and more deaths were reported between 2005 and 2009 than during any 5-year period of the preceding 30 years [19]. In the period 2002–2011, Maron et al. [2] found 5 (2.7%) EHS-associated deaths amongst a total of 182 cases from the US National Registry of Sudden Death in Athletes. Harmon et al. [6] showed two exertional deaths (0.7% of total, 15% of exertional) associated with EHS amongst NCAA student athletes from January 2004 through December 2008.

Yankelson et al. [20] showed that EHS-associated sudden death was the only cause of death noticed in 23 serious adverse events resulting in hospitalisation in a series of 137 580 runners who participated in Tel Aviv races from March 2007 to November 2013. They found 10 serious and 5 life-threatening/fatal events due to EHS for every serious cardiac event, highlighting that EHS can be more common during long-distance races (up to 10 km) in warm climates and have potential fatal consequences.

Pathophysiology

The fundamental pathophysiology of EHS occurs when internal-organ tissue temperatures rise above critical levels for a substantial amount of time, when cell membranes are damaged and when cell energy systems are disrupted. The extent of multisystem tissue dysfunction and the mortality rate are directly related to the duration of temperature elevation [16]. Cardiac tissue hyperthermia suppresses cardiac function and compromises the vascular transport of heat from deep tissues to the skin. As core temperature increases, the cardiovascular system becomes further challenged as a result of blood flow diversion from the viscera to the skin and vital organs, producing intestinal ischaemia [16,19]. Rhabdomyolysis, the breakdown of muscle fibres, occurs as muscle tissue exceeds the critical temperature threshold for cell membranes (~41 °C). The release of myoglobin from damaged muscle cells may cause renal tubular toxicity and obstruction if renal blood flow is inadequate. Intracellular potassium is also released, increasing serum potassium levels and potentially inducing cardiac arrhythmias. Heating renal tissue above its critical threshold can directly suppress renal function and induce acute renal failure, which is worsened by sustained hypotension, crystallisation of myoglobin and disseminated intravascular coagulation [16]. A systemic inflammatory response syndrome (SIRS) may develop, leading to vascular endothelial damage and a consumptive coagulopathy [19].

Recognition and Management of EHS

Prompt recognition of EHS is imperative to survival. The two main criteria for diagnosis of EHS are (i) core body temperature >40.0 °C (104 °F), taken with a rectal thermometer and (ii) CNS dysfunction [18]. The degree and duration of hyperthermia determine the presence of signs and symptoms, which are often nonspecific and can include disorientation, clumsiness, headache, nausea, dizziness, apathy, confusion, impairment of consciousness, irrational or unusual behaviour, inappropriate comments, irritability, inability to walk, loss of balance and muscle function resulting in collapse, profound fatigue, hyperventilation, vomiting, diarrhoea, delirium, seizures and coma. Any significant change of personality or performance should trigger immediate assessment for EHS, especially in hot, humid conditions or long-distance events [16,19].

It is essential to measure body core temperature in order to make the definitive diagnosis of EHS. Rectal and gastrointestinal temperature (if available) are the preferred methods for accurate core temperature measurement in a patient with EHS [18]. Ear (i.e. aural), oral, skin, temporal and axillary temperature measurements are less reliable and should not be used to diagnose or distinguish EHS from other causes of collapse [15,16].

EHS is a life-threatening medical emergency that requires immediate whole-body cooling. In treating EHS, the adage 'cool first, transport second' should guide immediate care when qualified medical staff are on site (i.e. athletic trainer, physiotherapist or team physician). Cooling should be initiated until the rectal temperature reaches 39 °C (102 °F) and, if there are no other life-threatening complications, completed on-site prior to evacuation to the hospital emergency department. Athletes who rapidly become lucid during cooling have the best prognosis. The gold standard for rapid body cooling is cold-water and ice-water immersion therapy (water temperature 2–15 °C), preferably initiated within 10 minutes; this results in a survival rate of nearly 100%. When water immersion is unavailable, a reasonable alternative is an aggressive combination of rapidly rotating ice water-soaked towels to the head, trunk and extremities and ice packs to the neck, axillae and groin [16,19,21].

In addition to rapid body cooling, normal saline infusion should be considered to assist in preserving intravascular volume and to improve renal blood flow, thereby protecting the kidney from rhabdomyolysis, increasing organ tissue perfusion and facilitating heat exchange, oxygenation and the removal of waste products. In-hospital assessment should monitor for rhabdomyolysis, renal dysfunction, cardiac arrhythmias and other end-organ damage [16,19,21].

Prevention

It is essential to adjust exercise intensity and breaks when environmental conditions are dangerous. Extreme environmental conditions should be approached with caution, and practices should be altered and events cancelled as appropriate [18]. Athletes should be allowed to acclimatise to the heat before being subjected to stressful conditions, such as full equipment, multiple practices, performance trials or major events. Appropriate hydration can help reduce heart rate, fatigue and core body temperature. Safeguards should be put in place to ensure that athletes arrive at practice and competition well hydrated and that they rehydrate according to thirst in order to replace fluid loss during practice [18].

Other, Less Frequent Causes of Noncardiac Sudden Death

Exercise Rhabdomyolysis

Exercise rhabdomyolysis (ER) is an acute syndrome of major muscle breakdown provoked by physical trauma, muscle hypoxia, genetic defects, infections, elevations in body temperature, metabolic and electrolyte disturbances and excessive unaccustomed physical exercise [19]. It is a relatively uncommon condition, but can have very serious consequences, including muscle ischaemia, cardiac arrhythmia and death [22]. Muscle breakdown products, electrolytes, myoglobin and other proteins leak into the blood stream, and serum creatine kinase (s-CK) levels typically rise dramatically [19]. ER presents clinically with muscle pain, soreness, stiffness and swelling, with progression to loss of mobility and weakness. It is associated with hyper- and hypothermia, SCT (and other ischaemic conditions), exertion, crush syndromes, certain medications (statins, stimulants and nonsteroidal anti-inflammatory drugs (NSAIDs)), and pre-existing illness or infection [22]. Prior history of EHS (7–11 times increased risk), male gender and African American ethnicity are risk factors for ER.

Accurate diagnosis relies on the history (including risk factors) and examination findings, which may include marked tenderness of the affected muscle groups, signs of altered mental status, reduced systolic blood pressure and increased heart rate. The characteristic laboratory findings are significantly elevated s-CK levels ($>10\,000\,IU.l^{-1}$) and myoglobin in the urine with a positive dipstick test. Appropriate management is hospitalisation with aggressive fluid replacement, forced diuresis and careful urine alkalinisation [23]. Unexpectedly severe EHS and ER should prompt clinicians to look for susceptibility to malignant hyperthermia.

Asthma

Sudden fatal asthma attacks are rare occurrences in both competitive and recreational athletes, but can be precipitated by sporting activity. Although it is possible that a patient with mild asthma will suddenly die, asthmatic deaths usually occur in severely affected or poorly compliant individuals and in those with recent hospital admittances due to severe crisis. Becker et al. [24] recently described a series of 61 deaths resulting from asthma crisis between July 1993 and December 2000, the majority (81%) of which occurred under the age of 21. Basketball and track-and-field athletics were most frequently associated with these fatal events. Preventive measures for asthmatic athletes might include a structured warm-up protocol before exercise or sport activity to decrease reliance on medications and minimise asthmatic symptoms and exacerbations. The sports medicine staff should educate asthmatic athletes about the use of medications as prophylaxis before exercise, asthma triggers, recognition of signs and symptoms and compliance with prescribed medication [18].

Extreme Environmental Conditions

Mortality during high-altitude mountaineering can be in the order of 1–40 per 1000 persons above Everest base camp, for both expedition members and high-altitude porters. On high (8000 m) peaks, the mortality during descent from the summit can reach 134 in 1000 summiteers [25]. High-altitude pulmonary oedema (HAPO) and high-altitude cerebral oedema (HACO) are thought to be responsible for the majority of non-traumatic deaths that occur at altitude. An ascent to altitude results in a fall in barometric pressure and a subsequent reduction in the partial pressure of inspired oxygen. In order to cope with this change, the human body undergoes a process of acclimatisation. In those who ascend rapidly, this can be incomplete, resulting in the development of life-threatening conditions such as HAPO and HACO. The incidence of these conditions also increases with higher altitude. In a number of cases, HAPO and HACO coexist. It is possible that HAPO and HACO also contribute in some part to those deaths attributed to trauma or hypothermia. In the early stages of HACO, changes in consciousness, abnormalities in motor function and visual disturbances can occur, whilst in HAPO, lethargy, malaise and breathlessness are commonly seen.

Since ambient temperature falls by approximately 5.5 °C for every 1000 m of altitude, the cold environment can contribute to a number of deaths in the mountains. Deaths caused by hypothermia tend to occur as a result of an unexpected event, such as a musculoskeletal injury or an episode of high-altitude illness [26].

References

1 Harmon, K.G., Asif, I.M., Klossner, D. and Drezner, J.A. Incidence of sudden cardiac death in National Collegiate Athletic Association Athletes. *Circulation* 2011; **123**: 1594–600.

2 Maron, B.J., Haas, T.S., Murphy, C.J. et al. Incidence and causes of sudden death in US college athletes. *J Am Coll Cardiol* 2014; **63**: 1636–43.

3 Eichner, E.R. Sickle cell considerations in athletes. *Clin Sports Med* 2011; **30**: 537–49.

4 O'Connor, F.G., Bergeron, M.F., Cantrell, J. et al. ACSM and CHAMP summit on sickle cell trait: mitigating risks for warfighters and athletes. *Med Sci Sports Exerc* 2012; **44**: 2045–56.

5 Harris, K.M., Haas, T.S., Eichner, E.R. and Maron, B.J. Sickle Cell trait associated with sudden death in competitive athletes. *Am J Cardiol* 2012; **110**: 1185–8.

6 Harmon, K.G., Drezner, J.A., Klossner, D. and Asif, I.M. Sickle cell trait associated with a RR of death of 37 times in national collegiate athletic association football athletes: a database with 2 million athlete-years as the denominator. *Br J Sports Med* 2012; **46**: 325–30.

7 Stovitz, S.D. and Shrier, I. Sickle cell trait, exertion-related death and confounded estimates. *Br J Sports Med* 2014; **48**: 285–6.

8 Eichner, E.R. Sickle cell trait in sports. *Curr Sports Med Rep* 2010; **9**: 347–51.

9 Harmon, K.G., Drezner, J.A. and Casa, D.J. To screen or not to screen for sickle cell trait in American football? *Br J Sports Med* 2012; **46**: 158.

10 Eichner, E.R. Preventing exertional sickling deaths: the right way, the wrong way, and the army way. *Curr Sports Med Rep* 2013; **12**: 352–3.

11 Loosemore, M., Walsh, S.B., Morris, E. et al. Sudden exertional death in sickle cell trait. *Br J Sports Med* 2012; **46**; 312–14.

12 Chirico, E.N., Martin, C., Faes, C. et al. Exercise training blunts oxidative stress in sickle cell trait carriers. *J Appl Physiol* 2012; **112**: 1445–53.

13 Thompson, A.A. Sickle cell trait testing and athletic participation: a solution in search of a problem? *Hematology Am Soc Hematol Educ Program* 2013; **2013**: 632–37.

14 Dijkstra, H.P., Pollock, N., Chakraverty, R. and Alonso, J.M. Managing the health of the elite athlete: a new integrated performance health management and coaching model. *Br J Sports Med* 2014; **48**: 523–31.

15 Noakes, T. Exercise in the heat. In: Khan, K. and Brukner, P. (eds) *Clinical Sports Medicine*. North Ryde, NSW: McGraw-Hill, 2012. pp. 1132–43.

16 American College of Sports Medicine, Armstrong, L.E., Casa, D.J. et al. American College of Sports Medicine position stand. Exertional heat illness during training and competition. *Med Sci Sports Exerc* 2007; **39**: 556–72.

17 Casa, D.J., Armstrong, L.E., Ganio, M.S. and Yeargin, S.W. Exertional heat stroke in competitive athletes. *Curr Sports Med Rep* 2005; **4**: 309–17.

18 Casa, D.J., Guskiewicz, K.M., Anderson, S.A. et al. National athletic trainers' association position statement: preventing sudden death in sports. *J Athl Train* 2012; **47**: 96.

19 Nichols, A.W. Heat-related illness in sports and exercise. *Curr Rev Musculoskelet Med* 2014; **7**: 355–65.

20 Yankelson, L., Sadeh, B., Gershovitz, L. et al. Life-threatening events during endurance sports. *J Am Coll Cardiol* 2014; **64**: 463–9.

21 Casa, D.J., McDermott, B.P., Lee, E.C. et al. Cold water immersion: the gold standard for exertional heatstroke treatment. *Exerc Sport Sci Rev* 2007; **35**: 141–9.

22 Tietze, D.C. and Borchers, J. Exertional rhabdomyolysy in the athlete: a clinical review. *Sports Health* 2014; **6**: 336–9.

23 Milne, C. Renal symptoms during exercise. In: Khan, K. and Brukner, P. (eds) *Clinical Sports Medicine*. North Ryde, NSW: McGraw-Hill, 2012. pp. 1063–7.

24 Becker, J.M., Rogers, J., Rossini, G. et al. Asthma deaths during sports: report of a 7-year experience. *J Allergy Clin Immunol* 2004; **113**: 264–7.

25 Weinbruch, S. and Nordby, K.C. Fatalities in high altitude mountaineering: a review of quantitative risk estimates. *High Alt Med Biol* 2013; **14**(4): 346–59.

26 Windsor, J.S., Firth, P.G., Grocott, M.P. et al. Mountain mortality: a review of deaths that occur during recreational activities in the mountains. *Postgrad Med J* 2009; **85**: 316–21.

Part 4
Cardiovascular Management

34 Guidelines for Sports Practice in Athletes with Cardiovascular Disease

Andrew D'Silva[1] and Sanjay Sharma[2]

[1]St George's University Hospital Foundation NHS Trust, St George's University of London, London, UK
[2]Department of Cardiovascular Sciences, St George's University of London, London, UK

It is a widely accepted clinical perception, occasionally substantiated by scientific evidence, that athletes with underlying cardiovascular disease (CVD) have an increased risk of sudden cardiac death (SCD) or clinical deterioration when compared with relatively sedentary individuals, by virtue of the demands placed on the CV system during regular intensive exercise regimes and sports participation [1]. Therefore, an expert consensus document is required to guide physicians and cardiologists in the evaluation of athletes with CV abnormalities and to recommend sports activities that can be safely performed. Two such documents currently exist, namely the American Heart Association/American College of Cardiology (AHA/ACC) guidelines, from the United States [2], and the European Society of Cardiology (ESC) Consensus Recommendations [1], from Europe. Both were originally published in 2005. Since then, the US guidelines have been updated and the European guidelines are in the process of being updated. Whilst most recommendations in the two documents are similar, it is important to appreciate that they draw from largely different cultural, social and legal backgrounds and, therefore, in some instances present different approaches to disqualification decisions and implications for clinical practice. It must be emphasised that both sets of recommendations are based on published scientific evidence where available, but given the scarcity and inconsistency of scientific investigations concerning the effect of regular sporting activities on the pathophysiology and clinical course of several CVDs [1], they are largely reliant on circumstantial evidence and the expert opinion of the respective consensus panels. Given that risk of clinical deterioration or SCD is difficult to predict, both guidelines are conservative in principle, in an attempt to encompass all preventable deaths, and acknowledge that many athletes who may never suffer such events will be unnecessarily restricted. Over the last 10 years, few studies have been conducted that would challenge the current recommendations, but efforts should be made wherever possible to tailor precise advice to the individual.

Competitive athletes are defined as individuals of young and adult age, either amateur or professional, who are engaged in exercise training on a regular basis and who participate in official sports competition [1].

This chapter will address each group of CVDs in turn, compare the US and European recommendations and explain the underlying rationale behind them. It includes relevant evidence that has come to light since their original publications.

Reference will be made to the Mitchell classification (Figure 34.1), which divides various sports activities into two main categories (dynamic and static) and according to intensity (low, moderate and high) [3]. The classification is intended to provide a schematic indication of the CV demand associated with different sports and to identify those disciplines associated with increased risk of bodily collision or syncope, which should be avoided in certain cardiac patients [1].

IOC Manual of Sports Cardiology, First Edition. Edited by Mathew G. Wilson, Jonathan A. Drezner and Sanjay Sharma.
© 2017 International Olympic Committee. Published 2017 by John Wiley & Sons, Ltd.

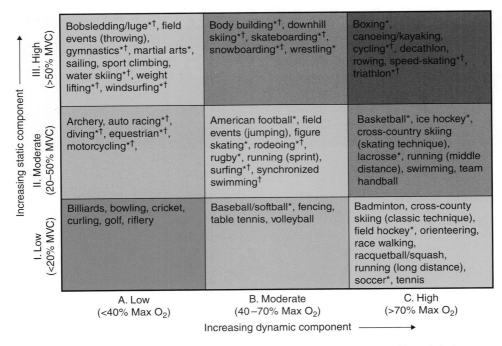

Figure 34.1 Sports classification based on peak static and dynamic components achieved during competition. The lowest total CV demands (cardiac output and blood pressure, BP) are shown in green, and the highest in red. Max O₂, maximal oxygen uptake; MVC, maximal voluntary contraction. *Danger of bodily collision. †Increased risk if syncope occurs (*Source*: Mitchell et al. [3]. Reproduced with permission of Elsevier)

Cardiomyopathies, Myocarditis and Pericarditis

The ESC and AHA/ACC recommendations for competitive athletes with cardiomyopathies, myocarditis or pericarditis are summarised in Table 34.1.

Hypertrophic Cardiomyopathy

Hypertrophic cardiomyopathy (HCM) is a relatively common genetically transmitted primary myocardial disease, with a prevalence of 1 in 500 in the general population and is the most common cause of unexpected SCD in young people, including competitive athletes [4]. Mutations in the genes encoding sarcomeric contractile proteins are responsible in 50–60% of cases. The condition is characterised by unexplained left ventricular hypertrophy (LVH) and a predilection to fatal ventricular arrhythmias, but is highly heterogeneous with respect to cardiac morphology, clinical penetrance and natural history. Although most individuals with HCM are unable to augment stroke volumes sufficiently long to compete in sports at an elite level, due to a small LV cavity size, impaired diastolic function, dynamic LV outflow tract (LVOT) obstruction, microvascular ischaemia or a combination of these factors, some are completely asymptomatic and may be able to demonstrate excellence in sports disciplines with an explosive start–stop component, such as basketball, football and American football. Unfortunately, their index presentation may be SCD, during or immediately after exercise.

The ESC guidelines restrict any individual with HCM and cardiac symptoms or risk factors for SCD from all competitive sports. Risk factors for SCD include prior cardiac arrest, ventricular tachycardia (VT), a family history of SCD, syncope, an LV wall thickness ≥30 mm and an abnormal BP response to exercise. HCM individuals without symptoms or risk factors are restricted to low-dynamic, low-static (class IA) sports, with annual follow-up.

The ACC guidelines restrict all HCM individuals to low-intensity (class IA) sports. Given that most class IA sports are relatively sedentary, the authors believe that all patients with HCM should be permitted to participate in class I sport irrespective of risk factors.

Condition	ESC	AHA/ACC
HCM with symptoms or high risk	No competitive sports	Low-dynamic, low-static sports (IA)
HCM low risk	Low-dynamic, low-static sports (IA)	Low-dynamic, low-static sports (IA)
HCM G+/P−	No competitive sports, only recreational sports[a]	All competitive sports
ARVC	No competitive sports	Possibly low-dynamic, low-static sports (IA)
ARVC G+/P−	No competitive sports	Low-dynamic, low-static sports (IA)
DCM with symptoms or high risk	No competitive sports	Possibly low-dynamic, low-static sports (IA)
DCM low risk	Low–moderate-dynamic and low-static sports (IA, IB)	Possibly low dynamic low static sports (IA)
Myocarditis and pericarditis	No competitive sports for 6 months, then all competitive sports upon satisfactory evaluation	No competitive sports for 6 months, then all competitive sports upon satisfactory evaluation

Table 34.1 Summary of selected differences between ESC and AHA/ACC recommendations for competitive athletes with cardiomyopathies, myocarditis or pericarditis

[a] Revised recommendations will permit such individuals from competing in all sports.

HCM, hypertrophic cardiomyopathy; ARVC, arrhythmogenic right ventricular cardiomyopathy; DCM, dilated cardiomyopathy.

Genotype-Positive/Phenotype-Negative Individuals

The natural history of genotype-positive/phenotype-negative (G+/P−) individuals is not fully understood. Previous reports suggest that such individuals exhibit a high concentration of serum biomarkers of collagen synthesis, late gadolinium enhancement on cardiac MRI [5], expanded extracellular volume detectable by T1 mapping [6] and subtle impairment of diastolic dysfunction [7]. The impact of exercise on the development of the overt phenotype or the arrhythmogenic substrate is unclear, so the ESC recommendations adopt a cautious view and advise that competition be confined to class IA sports in affected athletes. However, over the past few years emerging studies have shown that G+/P− individuals have a benign clinical course, with low penetrance and absence of symptoms or adverse events [8, 9]. Based on these considerations, it is recommended that all G+/P− individuals be assessed comprehensively with a cardiac MRI, exercise test and Holter monitor to exclude the broader phenotypic features of HCM. In the absence of abnormal investigations, the athlete may compete in all sports, but they should be kept under annual surveillance as follow-up studies in this cohort are relatively short.

According to the AHA/ACC guidelines, G+/P− individuals can participate in all competitive sports, provided that they are asymptomatic and do not have a family history of SCD [10]. In the light of new evidence, future ESC guidelines are likely to become more liberal and take the same view.

Athletes with Marked Repolarisation Changes but a Structurally Normal Heart

On occasion, and particularly among athletes of African or Afro-Caribbean origin, the presence of deep T-wave inversion on the electrocardiogram (ECG) may raise the possibility of HCM. In such circumstances, if the echocardiogram cannot confirm the diagnosis, comprehensive assessment with cardiac MRI, exercise stress test and a 24-hour Holter monitor is necessarily to exclude the broader phenotypic features of HCM. In the absence of a diagnosis, both sets of recommendations permit competition in all sports, but both suggest that the athlete should be evaluated annually whilst competing, since such repolarisation changes may reflect the onset of cardiomyopathy in the future [1, 10].

Arrhythomogenic Right Ventricular Cardiomyopathy

Arrhythmogenic right ventricular cardiomyopathy (ARVC) is a primary myocardial disease characterised histologically by fibro-fatty replacement of the RV myocardium and clinically by life-threatening ventricular tachyarrhythmias in young individuals. ARVC represents the commonest cause of SCD in young athletes in Italy [1]. The ESC guidelines restrict athletes with a definite diagnosis of ARVC from all competitive sports [1].

The ACC guidelines state that all individuals with a definite or probable diagnosis of ARVC should be excluded from most competitive sports, with the possible exception of low-intensity (class IA) sports [10]. The authors believe that the American guidelines are more pragmatic and that there is no evidence to disqualify affected athletes from class IA sports.

G+/P− Individuals

Data from animal studies show that plakophilin-deficient mice develop the ARVC phenotype with intensive exercise [11]. Recently, a plethora of publications have shown that asymptomatic gene-positive family members of first-degree relatives with overt ARVC who exercise regularly are more likely to go on to develop overt disease, potentially fatal arrhythmias and heart failure, as compared to sedentary gene-positive family members [12-15]. The AHA/ACC guidelines permit low-intensity (class IA) sports [10]. By virtue of the recommendations for G+/P− HCM individuals, the authors assume that the ESC guidelines restrict G+/P− athletes with ARVC from all competitive sports [1].

Dilated Cardiomyopathy

Dilated cardiomyopathy (DCM) is a myocardial disease characterised by LV dilatation and impaired systolic function. DCM includes disorders that are familial/genetic in origin; that are secondary to infection or inflammation, exposure to toxic substances or metabolic disorders; or that are of idiopathic origin. Although not frequent, DCM can cause SCD in athletes [1].

The ESC guidelines restrict athletes with DCM and symptoms or risk factors for SCD from all competitive sports. Risk factors for SCD with DCM include an ejection fraction (EF) <40%, complex ventricular arrhythmias and an abnormal BP response to exercise. Athletes with DCM but no symptoms or risk factors are permitted to participate in low–moderate-dynamic and low-static (class IA and IB) sports, with annual follow-up [1].

AHA/ACC guidelines acknowledge that whilst little information is available regarding DCM and other myocardial diseases, it is prudent to exclude athletes with DCM from most competitive sports, with the possible exception of low-intensity (class IA) sports in selected cases [10]. The authors consider the AHA/ACC recommendations to be more pragmatic.

Left Ventricular Noncompaction

Left ventricular noncompaction (LVNC) is a relatively novel yet unclassified cardiomyopathy that is characterised by prominent trabeculation within the LV myocardium, separated by deep recesses. The disease is characterised by progressive systolic heart failure, and a predisposition to serious ventricular arrhythmias and systemic thromboembolism. The diagnosis of LVNC can be difficult in athletes because LV trabeculations are common in sports players (see Chapter 21). Based on the available literature, we would not consider an asymptomatic athlete with incidental features of LVNC to necessarily harbour a cardiomyopathy in the absence of symptoms, family history, abnormal ECG patterns and impaired LV function. In athletes with impaired LV function and T-wave inversion, we propose abstinence from competitive sports involving medium- or high-intensity exercise, as for all other cardiomyopathies.

Myocarditis

Myocarditis is defined as an inflammatory process of the myocardium, with histological evidence of myocyte degeneration and necrosis of nonischaemic origin, associated with inflammatory infiltration [1].

The ESC guidelines state that athletes with active myocarditis should be restricted from competitive sports for a convalescence period of 6 months following the onset of clinical manifestations. Athletes may then return to all competitive sports, provided there are no remaining symptoms, LV function has returned to normal and there are no arrhythmias as evaluated by ECG, echocardiography and exercise testing [1]. The AHA/ACC guidelines are almost identical in this respect, but they add that serum markers of inflammation and heart failure must normalise before the athlete returns to training and competitive sport [10].

The convalescence period of 6 months is based purely on consensus advice and is not supported by any clinical evidence. It may be possible for athletes to return to competitive sport as early as 3 months after the onset of symptoms, if LV function is completely normal and there are no resting or exercise-induced arrhythmias. Both recommendations have also relied on the echocardiogram, whereas the gold standard imaging test for myocarditis is cardiac MRI, which has the advantage of detecting the extent of myocardial inflammation and fibrosis. In this regard, there are no data relating to the management of an athlete with preserved LV size and function who is free of arrhythmias but is rendered with permanent myocardial scarring. Further studies in this field, particularly relating to the quantity of scar burden, are prudent to inform future recommendations, but the authors would advise that all athletes with scarring should be assessed annually with an echocardiogram and an exercise stress test.

Pericarditis

Pericarditis is an inflammatory process of the pericardium which may also affect the subepicardial layers of the myocardium.

The ESC guidelines for athletes with pericarditis are the same as those for myocarditis: restriction for 6 months, with return to all competitive sports upon normalisation of ECG, echocardiography and exercise testing [1]. The AHA/ACC guidelines add a requirement for normalisation of serum markers of inflammation before the athletes return to play. Also, the presence of chronic pericardial disease resulting in constriction disqualifies athletes from all competitive sports [10].

As with myocarditis, the authors believe that a convalescence period of 3 months may suffice in some athletes.

Primary Electrical Disease

The ESC and AHA/ACC recommendations for competitive athletes with primary electrical disease are summarised in Table 34.2.

Congenital Long QT Syndrome

Congenital long QT syndrome (LQTS) can be a difficult clinical diagnosis to secure definitively, and a diagnostic algorithm, such as the Priori–Schwarz score, is best employed for this purpose (see Chapter 26) [16]. An increasing proportion of asymptomatic individuals with genetically proven LQTS are found to

Condition	ESC	AHA/ACC
Long QT syndrome	No competitive sports	No competitive sports until asymptomatic on treatment for 3 months and precautionary measures taken
		Then all sports except swimming/diving for LQT1
Long QT syndrome G+/P−	No competitive sports	All sports, except swimming/diving
Brugada syndrome	No competitive sports	All sports with precautionary measures taken
CPVT	No competitive sports (as for malignant VT)	Possibly low-dynamic, low-static sports (IA)
WPW	All competitive sports 3 months after successful catheter ablation	Low-risk accessory pathway: all competitive
		High-risk pathway: all competitive sports 4 weeks after catheter ablation
ICD patients	No competitive sports	Possibly low-dynamic, low-static sports (IA)

Table 34.2 Summary of selected differences between ESC and AHA/ACC recommendations for competitive athletes with primary electrical disease

LQT1, type 1 long QT syndrome; CPVT, catecholaminergic polymorphic ventricular tachycardia; WPW, Wolff–Parkinson–White syndrome; ICD, implantable cardioverter-defibrillator.

have normal resting ECGs with a heart rate–corrected QT interval (QTc) by Bazette's formula of <460 ms (G+/P− LQTS). To add complexity, a QTc of 440 ms, used in the past as an upper limit of normal, is found far too frequently in normal individuals (>25%) [17]. In general, a QTc of >470 ms in males or >480 ms in females requires further investigation as to whether a congenital or acquired cause of QT prolongation is present. Exercise testing and 24-hour Holter monitoring can be useful in making a diagnosis. Gene testing for responsible cardiac ion channel mutations can identify an abnormality in 75% of LQTS sufferers [17]. All affected individuals should receive treatment with a nonselective beta blocker, and this in itself may result in disqualification from particular sports.

According to the ESC, competitive sports are contraindicated in all athletes with LQTS, including those who are G+/P− [1]. The AHA/ACC guidelines restrict only athletes with symptomatic or electrocardio-graphically manifest LQTS from competitive sports. However, once rendered asymptomatic on therapy for 3 months, competitive sports participation can be considered provided precautionary measures are taken, including avoidance of QT-prolonging drugs, electrolyte and hydration replenishment, avoidance of hyper-thermia, acquisition of a personal automated external defibrillator as part of the athlete's personal safety gear and establishment of an emergency action plan [18]. Asymptomatic G+/P− athletes are allowed to participate in all competitive sports with the appropriate precautionary measures listed in the text. It is acknowledged that although the risk of SCD may be higher than baseline, there are insufficient compelling data to justify excluding these individuals from competitive sports [17]. However, due to a strong association between SCD in sports involving swimming/diving and type 1 LQTS (LQT1), athletes with G+/P− LQT1 should refrain from competitive sports with swimming/diving.

Brugada Syndrome

Brugada syndrome is a genetic condition characterised by a typical ECG pattern in anterior precordial leads V1–V3, with a 'coved-type' ST segment elevation >2 mm. It may be spontaneous or induced by pharmaco-logical sodium channel blockade. It is associated with arrhythmia-related syncope or cardiac arrest. Up to 20% of affected individuals carry a gene mutation in the sodium channel gene, *SCN5A* [19]. Most events occur at rest, and often at night, when sympathetic activity is withdrawn and vagal tone increased. High temperature is known to increase ST segment elevation and is associated with event risk. However, no clear relationship between exercise and arrhythmia has been found (see Chapter 27).

Despite this, the ESC guidelines restrict all athletes affected with Brugada syndrome from competitive sports [1]. The AHA/ACC guidelines acknowledge the lack of association between exercise and SCD and permit competitive sports participation provided appropriate precautionary measures and disease-specific treatments are in place and that the athlete has been asymptomatic on treatment for at least 3 months [18].

It is difficult to justify restrictions based on currently available evidence. In the future, ESC recommenda-tions may be liberalised, allowing more competitive sports (taking into account dehydration and sporting environments that might precipitate hyperthermia). Individuals who develop a type 1 Brugada ECG pattern on exercise testing may be an exception. At present, it is difficult to justify any restriction on individuals who harbour an SCN5A mutation but do not have any evidence of the Brugada ECG pattern.

Catecholaminergic Polymorphic Ventricular Tachycardia

Catecholaminergic polymorphic VT (CPVT) is characterised by exercise-induced PVT (often with a 'bidi-rectional pattern'), which can degenerate into ventricular fibrillation. This condition has been linked to mutations of the ryanodine receptor and calsequestrin genes, which result in abnormal calcium release from the sarcoplasmic reticulum (SR). CPVT does not manifest any abnormalities on the resting ECG, but it requires exercise testing or epinephrine provocation to establish the diagnosis. All affected individuals require treatment with a nonselective beta blocker and consideration of an implantable cardioverter-defi-brillator (ICD).

The ESC guidelines restrict all athletes with CPVT from all competitive sports, on the basis that they have a permanent substrate for malignant VT [1]. The AHA/ACC guidelines restrict all athletes from competitive sports, with the possible exception of minimal contact, class IA activities. It is also advised that affected individuals are restricted from competitive sports involving swimming. Asymptomatic sufferers, identified on family screening, should be treated the same way if exercise-induced or pharmacological provocation-induced VT is present. A less restrictive approach may be suitable for the G+/P− (asymptomatic, no inducible VT) athletes [18].

Wolff–Parkinson–White Syndrome

Wolff–Parkinson–White (WPW) syndrome is defined as the presence of paroxysmal arrhythmias in a patient with overt ventricular pre-excitation. The tachyarrhythmias related to WPW syndrome include atrioventricular (AV) re-entry tachycardia (either orthodromic or antidromic), atrial fibrillation and, rarely, ventricular fibrillation.

Both ESC and AHA/ACC guidelines are in agreement that symptomatic athletes with ventricular pre-excitation and atrial fibrillation or flutter should undergo catheter ablation [1, 20]. For those who are asymptomatic, a low but definite risk of SCD exists, and for this reason the ESC guidelines recommend that catheter ablation is the first-choice treatment, due to its high success rate and low risk of complications [1]. For athletes who refuse or in whom the procedure is associated with higher risks, competitive sport participation is allowed if invasive electrophysiological (EP) study demonstrates a low-risk accessory pathway with a long refractory period [1]. The AHA/ACC guidelines advocate exercise stress testing assessment of the EP properties of the accessory pathway. Specifically, abrupt and complete loss of pre-excitation during exercise denotes a low-risk pathway with a long refractory period. Those with a low-risk accessory pathway can participate in all competitive sports. If an athlete cannot be ascertained as being at low risk by stress testing, then an EP study is advocated. Those with high-risk features of the accessory pathway, with an effective refractory period ≤250 ms, should undergo catheter ablation and are then permitted to participate after 4 weeks, if follow-up EP study is satisfactory [20].

Athletes with Implantable Cardioverter-Defibrillators

Athletes with ICDs are generally considered to have cardiac diseases that are life-threatening and, therefore, represent a contraindication for competitive sports. Furthermore, rapid lunging movements of the upper limbs and bodily collision risk lead to fracture and damage to the generator box, respectively. Both ESC and AHA/ACC guidelines recommend restriction from competitive sports, although the American guidelines allow class IA sports if free from arrhythmia requiring device therapy for 3 months [1, 20]. The AHA/ACC guidelines also allow scope for participation in sports with higher peak static and dynamic components based on an individualised approach in stable athletes. Similar concerns exist in athletes with pacemakers, due to the risks of damage to a device or lead; sports with physical contact are contraindicated in ESC guidelines and cautioned in AHA/ACC guidelines [1, 20].

A new registry tracking athletes with normal LV EFs and transvenous ICDs who choose to continue participation in sports of higher classifications than IA shows low rates of cardiac events and no increased risk of device/lead malfunction [21]. These observations may provide justification in the future for more liberal recommendations for some athletes with ICDs and pacemakers. Ultimately, the underlying cardiac condition will remain the most significant factor influencing the appropriateness of sports participation.

Aortopathies, Coronary Artery Disease and Hypertension

The ESC and AHA/ACC recommendations for competitive athletes with aortopathies, coronary artery disease or hypertension are summarised in Table 34.3.

Marfan Syndrome

Marfan syndrome is an autosomal-dominant connective-tissue disorder caused by fibrillin 1 (*FBN1*) gene defects and by mutation of transforming growth factor beta receptor 2 (TGFBR2). Penetrance is complete, but there is large phenotypic heterogeneity, with variable involvement of different organs/tissues, including osteoskeletal, CV, ocular, skin, pulmonary and nervous system. The primary cause of mortality in athletes is aortic root dilatation, dissection and rupture.

Condition	ESC	AHA/ACC
Marfan syndrome	Full phenotype or positive genetic test: no competitive sports	Aortic root dilatation, moderate-to-severe mitral regurgitation, left ventricular (LV) systolic dysfunction (EF < 40%) or family history of aortic dissection: no competitive sports
	Incomplete phenotype, no family history, no gene mutation or family history alone: all competitive sports with annual follow-up	None of the above: low dynamic, low–moderate-static sports (IA, IIA)
Ischaemic heart disease	High probability of events: no competitive sports	Unstable IHD: no competitive sports
	Low probability of events: low–moderate-dynamic and low-static sports (IA, IB)	Stable, clinically manifest IHD: low-dynamic and low–moderate-static sports (IA, IIA)
		Clinically concealed IHD with low probability of events: all competitive sports
Anomalous coronary artery origins	–	No competitive sports with possible exception of low-dynamic, low-static class IA sports
		Postsurgical correction: all competitive sports, upon satisfactory evaluation after 3 months
Hypertension	Low risk: all competitive sports with annual follow-up	Mild hypertension with no target organ damage: all competitive sports
	Moderate risk: all sports except high-static, high-dynamic sports (IIIC), with annual follow-up	Moderate hypertension without target organ damage: all sports except high-static sports (IIIA–C), until hypertension controlled
	High risk: all sports with exclusion from high-static sports (IIIA–C) with annual follow-up	
	Very high risk: only low–moderate-dynamic, low-static sports (IA, IB), with 6-monthly follow-up	With any associated clinical condition: dependent on type and severity of condition
	With any associated clinical condition: no competitive sports	

Table 34.3 Summary of selected differences between ESC and AHA/ACC recommendations for competitive athletes with aortopathies, coronary artery disease or hypertension

The ESC guidelines recommend that athletes with the full Marfan syndrome phenotype, as well as those with an incomplete phenotype but positive family history, should refrain from all competitive sports. Athletes with an incomplete phenotype, no FBN1 mutation and no family history are allowed to continue sports participation with annual follow-up. The same recommendations apply to athletes with a family history of Marfan syndrome, negative phenotype and no FBN1 mutation [1].

The AHA/ACC recommendations are based largely on aortic root dimensions, with 6–12 monthly monitoring by echocardiography or magnetic resonance angiography. Athletes with Marfan syndrome who do not have ≥1 of aortic root dilatation (transverse dimension ≥40 mm in men or ≥36 mm in women, or >2 standard deviations from the mean for body surface area in children); moderate-to-severe mitral regurgitation; LV systolic dysfunction (EF < 40%); or a family history of aortic dissection at an aortic diameter <50 mm are restricted to low–moderate-static, low-dynamic (class IA, IIA) competitive sports [22]. Otherwise, athletes with Marfan syndrome at higher risk of aortic dissection are restricted from competitive sports. The authors concur with the AHA/ACC recommendations.

Ischaemic Heart Disease

Ischaemic heart disease (IHD) is the leading cause of SCD in athletes over the age of 35 years. Younger athletes with familial hypercholesterolaemia are prone to premature atherosclerosis and are at risk of SCD and acute coronary syndromes. These events may occur in asymptomatic individuals without any prior symptoms of ischaemia.

The ESC guidelines recommend assessing all athletes who have a definite diagnosis of IHD (which includes angina, acute coronary syndromes and previous revascularisation) for the probability of future cardiac events. The assessment includes exercise-induced ischaemia, symptoms of complex ventricular arrhythmias significant coronary stenosis (70% of major coronary artery or >50% of left main stem) and reduced LV EF (<50%). Any of these signs indicates a higher probability of future cardiac events and results in disqualification from all competitive sports. In their absence, the probability of cardiac events is deemed low, and low–moderate-dynamic, low-static (class IA, IB) sports are permitted, with annual follow-up [1].

The AHA/ACC guidelines recommend a similar assessment of risk for future cardiac events. Athletes deemed at higher risk (exercise-induced ischaemia, impaired LV function or haemodynamically significant coronary artery stenosis) are restricted from competitive sports participation, though once stabilised may return to sports with low-dynamic and low-to-moderate static demands, classes IA and IIA. Athletes with clinically manifest IHD who are asymptomatic and athletes with clinically concealed IHD can participate in all competitive sports provided they have no inducible ischaemia or electrical instability and a resting LV EF >50%. Aggressive risk factor modification with high-intensity statin therapy is also advocated to reduce the chance of plaque disruption [23].

Anomalous Coronary Artery Origins

Anomalous coronary artery origins deserve special mention as an important cause of SCD in athletes in a large US registry [4]. The AHA/ACC guidelines recommend exclusion from all competitive sports with the possible exception of class IA sports. In order to be eligible to compete, an athlete with this condition must undergo surgical correction, with re-evaluation for ischaemia, arrhythmia and dysfunction on maximal exercise testing after 3 months. Any athletes presenting with a myocardial infarction (MI) should be risk-assessed in the same way as someone with IHD [24].

Hypertension

Hypertension is the most common CV condition observed in competitive athletes [25]. It is defined as a systolic BP ≥140 mmHg and/or diastolic BP ≥90 mmHg. Although hypertension may be associated with an increased level of risk for complex ventricular arrhythmias and sudden death, it has not directly been implicated as a cause of SCD in young competitive athletes. Athletes with hypertension should be treated according to the general guidelines for the management of hypertension. However, in endurance athletes, diuretics and beta blockers may impair exercise performance or cause electrolyte and fluid disturbances, and they may be prohibited by certain athletic training bodies. Therefore, calcium channel blockers and blockers of the renin–angiotensin system are the medications of choice for hypertensive endurance athletes [1].

The ESC guidelines recommend that athletes are risk-stratified according to the presence of risk factors, 10-year CV risk scores, target organ damage and/or associated clinical conditions. Athletes with well-controlled, mild (grade 1) hypertension, with no risk factors, a 10-year CV risk of <20% and no end organ damage, can participate in all competitive sports, with annual follow-up. Athletes with well-controlled mild-to-moderate hypertension (grade 1–2) with one or two risk factors but no end organ damage should not participate in high-dynamic, high-static (class IIIC) sports and be followed up yearly. Athletes with well-controlled mild-to-moderate (grade 1–2) hypertension with three or more risk factors, diabetes or target-organ damage should be excluded from all high-static (class IIIA–IIIC) sports, with annual follow-up. The same recommendation applies to athletes with well-controlled severe (grade 3) hypertension and no other risk factors. Athletes with treated severe (grade 3) hypertension and any risk factors, including those with target organ damage, should be restricted to low–moderate-dynamic, low-static (class IA, IB) sports, with 6-monthly follow-up. Any athlete with well-controlled hypertension who has an associated clinical condition of cerebrovascular disease, IHD, peripheral vascular disease (PVD), established nephropathy or retinopathy should be restricted from all competitive sports [1].

The AHA/ACC guidelines are simpler: athletes with mild (stage 1) hypertension without target organ damage or concomitant heart disease are eligible for all sports. Athletes with moderate (stage 2) hypertension

Condition	ESC	AHA/ACC
Mitral stenosis (MS)	Mild MS, sinus rhythm: all competitive sports, excluding high-dynamic, high-static (IIIC)	Mild MS, sinus rhythm, normal pulmonary artery pressure: all competitive sports
	Mild MS and atrial fibrillation: non-contact, low–moderate-dynamic, low–moderate-static (IA, IB, IIA, IIB)	Severe MS or elevated pulmonary artery pressures: low-intensity sports (IA)
	Moderate and severe MS: non-contact, low-dynamic, low-static (IA)	Anticoagulation for atrial fibrillation: no contact sports
Mitral regurgitation (MR)	Mild-to-moderate MR, sinus rhythm, normal LV size/function and normal exercise testing: all sports	Mild-to-moderate MR, sinus rhythm, normal LV size/function and normal pulmonary artery pressures: all competitive sports
	On anticoagulation for atrial fibrillation: no contact sports	Mild-to-moderate MR and only mild LV dilatation, compatible with athletic training (EDV < 60 mm): all competitive sports
	Mild-to-moderate MR, mild LV dilatation (ESV < 55 ml.m^{-2}): Low–moderate-dynamic, low–moderate-static sports (IA, IB, IIA, IIB)	
	Severe MR or mild-to-moderate MR with marked LV dilatation (ESV > 55 ml.m^{-2}) or LV dysfunction (EF < 50%): no competitive sports	Severe MR, sinus rhythm and only mild LV dilatation: low-intensity and some moderate-intensity sports (IA, IIA, IB)
		Severe MR, definite LV enlargement (EDV ≥ 60 ml.m^{-2}), pulmonary hypertension or any degree of LV systolic dysfunction: low-intensity sports (IA)
		On anticoagulation for atrial fibrillation: no contact sports
Aortic stenosis (AS)	Asymptomatic mild AS, normal LV size/function, no significant arrhythmia: low–moderate-dynamic, low–moderate-static sports (IA, IB, IIA, IIB)	Mild AS: all competitive sports if normal maximal exercise response, with annual re-evaluation
		Moderate AS and satisfactory exercise tolerance test: low–moderate-static, low–moderate dynamic sports (IA, IIA, IB)
	Moderate AS or frequent/complex arrhythmias: low-dynamic, low-static sports (IA)	Asymptomatic severe AS: low-intensity competitive sports (IA)
	Severe AS or moderate AS with symptoms or LV dysfunction: no competitive sports	Symptomatic severe AS: no competitive sports
Aortic regurgitation (AR)	Mild-to-moderate AR, normal LV size/function, normal exercise testing and no arrhythmia: all competitive sports, with annual follow-up	Mild-to-moderate AR
		+ only mild LV enlargement and satisfactory exercise test: all competitive sports
	Mild-to-moderate AR with progressive LV dilatation: low-dynamic and low-static sports only (IA)	+ moderate LV enlargement (ESV < 50 mm in men and < 40 mm in women) and satisfactory exercise test: all competitive sports
	Severe AR, or mild-to-moderate AR with dilatation of the ascending aorta or ventricular arrhythmias: no competitive sports	Severe AR, moderate enlargement and EF >50%: all competitive sports if satisfactory exercise test
		Symptomatic severe AR, EF <50% and more than moderate LV enlargement: no competitive sports
Prosthetic heart valves	Valve function and LV function normal: low–moderate-dynamic, low–moderate-static sports (IA, IB, IIA, IIB)	Valve function and LV function normal: low–moderate-dynamic, low–moderate-static sports (IA, IB, IC, IIA)
	Anticoagulation required: no contact sports	Anticoagulation required: sports with low likelihood of bodily contact

Table 34.4 Summary of selected differences between ESC and AHA/ACC recommendations for competitive athletes with valvular heart disease (VHD)

ESV, end systolic volume; EDV, end diastolic volume.

without evidence of target organ damage should be restricted from high-static (class IIIA–IIIC) sports, until hypertension is controlled. Eligibility for competitive sport participation in athletes with coexistent CVD is usually based on the type and severity of the associated condition [25].

Valvular Heart Disease

Valvular heart disease (VHD) encompasses any stenotic or regurgitant lesion of any or multiple cardiac valves, as well as patients with prosthetic heart valves. In general, valvular regurgitation is better tolerated than valvular stenosis and exercise recommendations for these individuals are more liberal. The general recommendations are summarised in Table 34.4, and a detailed account can be found in Chapter 23.

Congenital Heart Disease

Congenital heart disease (CHD) encompasses a broad range of different cardiac abnormalities, varying from simple to highly complex lesions. The available literature regarding exercise and sports participation with CHD is sparse, and some conditions are not compatible with the haemodynamic changes required in exercise due to the morphological severity/complexity or the tendency to compromising arrhythmias. However, the haemodynamic balance in patients with CHD varies considerably, even amongst patients with the same lesions. This makes it impossible to state recommendations that are valid in all cases, and highlights the importance of cardiologists with expertise in CHD tailoring recommendation to the individual patient. As a general principle, only those patients with CHD who are likely to deteriorate as a consequence of regular physical exercise should be restricted from sports participation [1].

Otherwise, summarised simply, the ESC guidelines allow sports competition for athletes with atrial septal defects, small ventricular septal defects, AV septal defects with competent valvular function, anomalous pulmonary venous connection and patent ductus arteriosus, provided that they are asymptomatic and have normal ventricular function, normal pulmonary artery pressures, a normal BP response to exercise and no significant arrhythmias [1]. More complex lesions are covered in greater detail in both the ESC and AHA/ACC guidelines [1, 24]; this falls beyond the scope of this chapter.

This chapter comprehensively summarises the current guidelines pertaining to CV conditions associated with SCD in athletes or which one might commonly expect to face in an athletic population. In general, it is prudent to advise any individual with a CV condition to avoid sudden explosive exertions, such as sprinting. Graded increases in workload are better tolerated by the heart. They should also avoid exercising in extreme adverse environmental conditions (hot, humid or very cold), as this may precipitate cardiac events in predisposed individuals. Finally, it may be considered safe and conservative practice to advise athletes with certain CV conditions to maintain their heart rate at ≤80% of maximum or at the level for the anaerobic threshold, if this is known.

In summary, whilst it is appreciated that exercise can trigger significant cardiac events in individuals with underlying CV conditions, it is difficult to predict the risk of a future cardiac event and what impact regular physical activity and competitive sports participation might have on this risk. Current guidelines are predominantly based on the interpretation of circumstantial evidence by a consensus group and are conservative in nature in an attempt to encompass all preventable deaths. Nevertheless, some athletes may choose not to follow the recommendations of their physicians and although they place themselves at perceived risk, they should be followed up and included in registries to add to the currently limited evidence base.

References

1 Pelliccia, A., Fagard, R., Bjornstad, H.H. et al. Recommendations for competitive sports participation in athletes with cardiovascular disease: a consensus document from the Study Group of Sports Cardiology of the Working Group of Cardiac Rehabilitation and Exercise Physiology and the Working Group of Myocardial and Pericardial Diseases of the European Society of Cardiology. *Eur Heart J* 2005; 26(14): 1422–45.
2 Maron, B.J., Zipes, D.P. and Kovacs, R.J. Eligibility and Disqualification Recommendations for Competitive Athletes With Cardiovascular Abnormalities: Preamble, Principles, and General Considerations: A Scientific Statement From the American Heart Association and American College of Cardiology. *J Am Coll Cardiol* 2015; 66(21): 2343–9.
3 Mitchell, J.H., Haskell, W., Snell, P. and Van Camp, S.P. Task Force 8: classification of sports. *J Am Coll Cardiol* 2005; 45(8): 1364–7.
4 Maron, B.J., Doerer, J.J., Haas, T.S. et al. Sudden deaths in young competitive athletes: analysis of 1866 deaths in the United States, 1980–2006. *Circulation* 2009; 119(8): 1085–92.

5   Ho, C.Y., López, B., Coelho-Filho, O.R. et al. Myocardial fibrosis as an early manifestation of hypertrophic cardio-myopathy. *N Engl J Med* 2010; 363(6): 552–63.

6   Ho, C.Y., Abbasi, S.A., Neilan, T.G. et al. T1 measurements identify extracellular volume expansion in hypertrophic cardiomyopathy sarcomere mutation carriers with and without left ventricular hypertrophy. *Circ Cardiovasc Imaging* 2013; 6(3): 415–22.

7   Ho, C.Y., Sweitzer, N.K., McDonough, B. et al. Assessment of diastolic function with Doppler tissue imaging to predict genotype in preclinical hypertrophic cardiomyopathy. *Circulation* 2002; 105(25): 2992–7.

8   Gray, B., Ingles, J. and Semsarian, C. Natural history of genotype positive-phenotype negative patients with hyper-trophic cardiomyopathy. *Int J Cardiol* 2011; 152(2): 258–9.

9   Jensen, M.K., Havndrup, O., Christiansen, M. et al. Penetrance of hypertrophic cardiomyopathy in children and adolescents: a 12-year follow-up study of clinical screening and predictive genetic testing. *Circulation* 2013; 127(1): 48–54.

10   Maron, B.J., Udelson, J.E., Bonow, R.O. et al. Eligibility and Disqualification Recommendations for Competitive Athletes With Cardiovascular Abnormalities: Task Force 3: Hypertrophic Cardiomyopathy, Arrhythmogenic Right Ventricular Cardiomyopathy and Other Cardiomyopathies, and Myocarditis: A Scientific Statement From the American Heart Association and American College of Cardiology. *J Am Coll Cardiol* 2015; 66(21): 2362–71.

11   Kirchhof, P., Fabritz, L., Zwiener, M. et al. Age- and training-dependent development of arrhythmogenic right ven-tricular cardiomyopathy in heterozygous plakoglobin-deficient mice. *Circulation* 2006; 114(17): 1799–806.

12   James, C.A., Bhonsale, A., Tichnell, C. et al. Exercise increases age-related penetrance and arrhythmic risk in arrhythmogenic right ventricular dysplasia/cardiomyopathy-associated desmosomal mutation carriers. *J Am Coll Cardiol* 2013; 62(14): 1290–7.

13   Sawant, A.C., Bhonsale, A., te Riele, A.S. et al. Exercise has a disproportionate role in the pathogenesis of arrhythmo-genic right ventricular dysplasia/cardiomyopathy in patients without desmosomal mutations. *J Am Heart Assoc* 2014; 3(6): e001471.

14   Saberniak, J., Hasselberg, N.E., Borgquist, R. et al. Vigorous physical activity impairs myocardial function in patients with arrhythmogenic right ventricular cardiomyopathy and in mutation positive family members. *Eur J Heart Fail* 2014; 16(12): 1337–44.

15.   Ruwald, A.C., Marcus, F., Estes, N.A. et al. Association of competitive and recreational sport participation with cardiac events in patients with arrhythmogenic right ventricular cardiomyopathy: results from the North American multidisciplinary study of arrhythmogenic right ventricular cardiomyopathy. *Eur Heart J* 2015; 36(27): 1735–43.

16   Priori, S.G., Schwartz, P.J., Napolitano, C. et al. Risk stratification in the long-QT syndrome. *N Engl J Med* 2003; 348(19): 1866–74.

17   Zipes, D.P., Ackerman, M.J., Estes, N.A. et al. Task Force 7: arrhythmias. *J Am Coll Cardiol* 2005; 45(8): 1354–63.

18   Ackerman, M.J., Zipes, D.P., Kovacs, R.J. and Maron, B.J. Eligibility and Disqualification Recommendations for Competitive Athletes With Cardiovascular Abnormalities: Task Force 10: The Cardiac Channelopathies: A Scientific Statement From the American Heart Association and American College of Cardiology. *J Am Coll Cardiol* 2015; 66(21): 2424–8.

19   Probst, V., Wilde, A.A., Barc, J. et al. SCN5A mutations and the role of genetic background in the pathophysiology of Brugada syndrome. *Circ Cardiovasc Genet* 2009; 2(6): 552–7.

20   Zipes, D.P., Link, M.S., Ackerman, M.J. et al. Eligibility and Disqualification Recommendations for Competitive Athletes With Cardiovascular Abnormalities: Task Force 9: Arrhythmias and Conduction Defects: A Scientific Statement From the American Heart Association and American College of Cardiology. *J Am Coll Cardiol* 2015; 66(21): 2412–23.

21   Lampert, R., Olshansky, B., Heidbuchel, H. et al. Safety of sports for athletes with implantable cardioverter-defibril-lators: results of a prospective, multinational registry. *Circulation* 2013; 127(20): 2021–30.

22   Braverman, A.C., Harris, K.M., Kovacs, R.J. and Maron, B.J. Eligibility and Disqualification Recommendations for Competitive Athletes With Cardiovascular Abnormalities: Task Force 7: Aortic Diseases, Including Marfan Syndrome: A Scientific Statement From the American Heart Association and American College of Cardiology. *J Am Coll Cardiol* 2015; 66(21): 2398–405.

23   Thompson, P.D., Myerburg, R.J., Levine, B.D. et al. Eligibility and Disqualification Recommendations for Competitive Athletes With Cardiovascular Abnormalities: Task Force 8: Coronary Artery Disease: A Scientific Statement from the American Heart Association and American College of Cardiology. *J Am Coll Cardiol* 2015; 66(21): 2406–11.

24   Van Hare, G.F., Ackerman, M.J., Evangelista, J.A. et al. Eligibility and Disqualification Recommendations for Competitive Athletes With Cardiovascular Abnormalities: Task Force 4: Congenital Heart Disease: A Scientific Statement From the American Heart Association and American College of Cardiology. *J Am Coll Cardiol* 2015; 66(21): 2372–84.

25   Black, H.R., Sica, D., Ferdinand, K. and White, W.B. Eligibility and Disqualification Recommendations for Competitive Athletes With Cardiovascular Abnormalities: Task Force 6: Hypertension: A Scientific Statement from the American Heart Association and the American College of Cardiology. *J Am Coll Cardiol* 2015; 66(21): 2393–7.

35 Management of the Symptomatic Athlete

Meagan M. Wasfy and Aaron L. Baggish

Cardiovascular Performance Program, Massachusetts General Hospital, Boston, MA, USA

Introduction

Whilst routine physical exercise is one cornerstone of a healthy lifestyle, athletes and physically active patients are not immune to cardiovascular disease (CVD). With the rising popularity of both competitive and recreational sports across the full age spectrum from youth to masters athletes, athletic patients are increasingly common in clinical practice. Athletes seeking medical evaluation often present with complaints suggestive of underlying CVD, including exertional chest pain, dyspnoea, palpitations and syncope. These symptoms, particularly when provoked by the stress of exercise, may be the first manifestation of occult, life-threatening cardiac disease. In the majority of cases, however, exertional symptoms do not ultimately reflect malignant cardiovascular pathology and athletes are successfully returned to competition following evaluation. Differentiating malignant heart disease from benign symptoms is amongst the principal responsibilities of clinicians charged with the care of athletic patients. This chapter is designed to provide a clinical framework for the evaluation of the athlete with symptoms suggestive of underlying heart disease.

General Considerations

Whilst the general fundamentals of patient care apply to athletes with cardiovascular symptoms, athletic patients are a unique clinical population. From the initial ascertainment of the medical history and performance of the physical examination through to the ordering and interpretation of diagnostic testing, it is essential that clinicians be familiar with key attributes of the athletic patient, including age, gender, ethnicity, antecedent medical history, exercise training and competition regimen, possible exposure to performance-enhancing agents (PEAs), and athlete-specific normative findings on all available forms of diagnostic testing.

The comprehensive medical history should begin with a focused assessment of the presenting symptom, with careful consideration of numerous issues, including symptom severity, duration, exacerbating and ameliorating factors and association with exercise. Additional items meriting consideration include changes in training regimens and competition outcomes, dietary intake and medication/supplement use that correlates with the development of symptoms. Questions focused on the use of PEAs are crucial. Anabolic steroids, the most widely used PEAs, have been shown to have numerous deleterious cardiovascular side effects, including exaggerated blood pressure response and myocardial dysfunction [1,2]. The use of erythropoietin Zanalogues, whilst most commonly associated with central nervous system (CNS) vascular dysfunction, can precipitate microvascular coronary artery infarction due to excessive red cell mass. A family history of sudden cardiac death (SCD) is a major risk factor for the presence of a heritable and potentially dangerous cause of cardiovascular symptoms. Therefore, a detailed family history focused on sudden or unexplained accidents or death, unexplained syncope, athletic restriction and/or placement of an implantable intracardiac device (e.g. pacemaker or implantable cardioverter–defibrillator (ICD)) is an essential element of the medical history. A comprehensive history guides a focused physical exam, which often includes specific provocative manoeuvres as detailed later in this chapter.

When the history and physical are not sufficient to establish or exclude underlying disease, subsequent testing should be customised to maximise diagnostic yield. All athletes with exertional symptoms should undergo maximal-effort or symptom-limited exercise testing with the goal of provoking the presenting symptom. Exercise testing in athletes is ideally performed with an emphasis on simulating the demands of training and competition by using sport-specific exercise modalities and customised testing protocols. Many symptomatic athletes will also require some form of noninvasive cardiac imaging (e.g. echocardiography, cardiac magnetic resonance (CMR)) and/or ambulatory rhythm monitoring. The results of all testing must be interpreted in the context of athlete-specific ranges of normality, when supplied by the available literature – and in its absence, by provider expertise.

Traditionally, cardiovascular specialists have not been considered core members of the sports medicine team. This historical approach fosters numerous limitations to optimal care. Consequently, there is increasing recognition that athletes with suspected CVD are best cared for by a team of experts that includes a dedicated sports cardiologist. This approach holds the most potential to provide a comprehensive and cost-effective evaluation and treatment plan. In this chapter, we expand upon these general recommendations and present suggestions for the evaluation of specific common cardiovascular symptoms.

Syncope

Syncope and pre-syncope are common amongst athletes. Syncope is defined as a transient loss of consciousness accompanied by loss of postural tone with spontaneous recovery. Pre-syncope refers to alteration without complete loss of consciousness, and may be characterised by a myriad of nonspecific symptoms, including lightheadedness, 'faintness' and darkening of vision. A differential diagnosis for the most common and clinically relevant causes of syncope and pre-syncope in the athlete is shown in Table 35.1.

The history and physical examination are the most important parts of the syncope evaluation and can identify the aetiology in about 45% of cases in which a cause is found [3]. History-taking in syncope can be difficult, because the patient often has some degree of amnesia for the event; when possible, it is useful to refer to witness accounts or video documentation of the event. The most important aspect of the athlete's history is the association of syncope with exertion. Syncope that truly occurs during exercise is relatively rare compared to syncope that occurs immediately following termination of exercise or syncope that is unrelated to exercise. Importantly, syncope during exercise should raise a high level of concern for an underlying and potentially dangerous cardiovascular cause (Table 35.1) [4,5].

The vast majority of syncope in athletes, particularly post-exertional syncope, is caused by neurally mediated cerebral hypoperfusion [4]. During exercise, peripheral vascular resistance falls but venous return to the heart is augmented by peripheral muscle activity, which acts like a 'muscle pump'. Sudden cessation of exercise leads to loss of this muscle pump and can result in a rapid reduction in central venous return. Sudden reduction in central venous return coupled with post-exertional reductions in heart rate and blood pressure results in a diminished cerebral blood flow, which may ultimately lead to syncope. In our experience, post-exertional syncope is more common amongst women than men, and reduced or low normal body mass may be an additional risk factor. Similar physiology and resultant syncope may occur in the absence of exertion in the settings of prolonged standing, sudden changes in position from supine to standing or emotional perturbation [6]. A careful history and basic evaluation may be all that is required if the clinical scenario is classic for neurally mediated cerebral hypoperfusion. Patients with this form of syncope are often successfully managed with conservative measures, including improved hydration, increase in dietary sodium intake, use of a commercially available compression stocking and education about avoidance tactics.

Syncope that occurs during and not following exertion must be considered a manifestation of underlying CVD until proven otherwise. Athletes who experience syncope or develop near-syncopal symptoms during exercise therefore require a more in-depth evaluation, designed to look for the presence of underlying cardiac conditions that are associated with SCD (Table 35.1). Salient historical features of an exertional syncopal episode include the presence of prodromal symptoms (e.g. palpitations, sustained subjective tachycardia, chest pain), inciting factors (including changes in exercise intensity), the activity being undertaken at the time of the episode, duration of loss of consciousness, the presence of involuntary muscular movements or bowel/bladder incontinence during loss of consciousness, and post-syncopal symptoms (e.g. confusion) [7,8]. Particular attention should be paid to a prior personal history of syncope or pre-syncope or a family history of sudden death. Important factors in the physical examination of the athlete with syncope are complete vital signs, including orthostatic vital signs, and careful cardiac auscultation, including positional

Cause	History and physical exam	Resting ECG findings	Additional diagnostic testing
Primary arrhythmia: ventricular tachycardia	Prior palpitations Prodromal symptoms may be brief or absent, in which case there may be significant resultant injury	See below	See below
Long or short QT syndrome	Specific exposures (exercise, cold water, sudden startle) Family history of SCD or deafness	Long or short QTc Abnormal T-wave morphology	Exercise testing Genetic testing
Brugada syndrome	Non-exertional syncope More common in Asian men Family history of SCD	Abnormal J-point elevation, ST elevation and T-wave inversion in leads V1–V3	Procainamide challenge Genetic testing
Catecholaminergic polymorphic ventricular tachycardia (CPVT)	Associated with exertion or emotion Family history of SCD	Normal	Exercise testing or ambulatory rhythm monitoring
Primary arrhythmia: supraventricular tachycardia (SVT)[a]	Exertional or non-exertional Prodrome of palpitations and lightheadedness	Delta wave (in WPW syndrome only)	Exercise testing or ambulatory rhythm monitoring
Structural cardiac disease	May cause syncope via tachyarrhythmia and/or failure of adequate cardiac output; with the latter, a prodrome of lightheadedness, chest pain or SOB may precede LOC	See below	See below
Hypertrophic cardiomyopathy (HCM)	Exertional syncope and/or palpitations Associated chest pain, SOB or performance decline Family history of SCD Physical examination: systolic murmur that augments with Valsalva manoeuvre, prominent apical impulse	Prominent voltage *plus* left atrial enlargement, intraventricular conduction delay, abnormal repolarisation, T-wave inversions or Q-waves	TTE CMR Genetic testing
Coronary artery anomalies/coronary artery disease (CAD)	Exertional syncope Associated chest pain, SOB or performance decline	Usually normal	Exercise testing TTE Cardiac CTA
Arrhythmogenic right ventricular cardiomyopathy (ARVC)	Exertional syncope and/or palpitations Family history of SCD Mediterranean descent	Abnormal RBBB, epsilon wave, right precordial T-wave inversions	Exercise testing TTE CMR
Myocarditis	Viral prodrome Associated chest pain and palpitations	Diffuse ST-segment elevation and PR depression	TTE CMR Cardiac biomarkers
Other cardiomyopathy (dilated, noncompaction, restrictive), congenital or valvular heart disease	Exertional or non-exertional syncope and/or palpitations Possible family history Associated performance decline Physical examination: abnormal precordial impulses, cardiac murmurs	Bundle branch blocks, right or left ventricular hypertrophy, abnormal Q-waves, T-wave inversions	TTE CMR
Other			
Cerebrovascular disease	Associated vertigo or focal neurologic signs (vertebrobasilar insufficiency), arm exercise (subclavian steal) or head/neck movement (carotid body hypersensitivity): vascular bruits on physical examination	Normal	Vascular imaging

Table 35.1 Differential diagnosis of syncope in the athlete

Cause	History and physical exam	Resting ECG findings	Additional diagnostic testing
Seizure	Prodromal 'aura' Tonic–clonic movements prolonged during or prior to LOC Tongue biting and loss of continence Prolonged post-ictal confusion	Normal	EEG
Neurally mediated cerebral hypoperfusion	Post-exertional or independent of exertion[b] (prolonged or sudden standing, emotional stimulus, warm or crowded room, micturition or coughing, postprandial) Prodrome of lightheadedness or warmth Bracing for fall and lack of significant injury Brief tonic–clonic movements after LOC	Normal	None required
Exertional heat stroke or hyponatremia	Post-exertional, specifically after prolonged endurance exercise Prodrome of mental status changes May cause exercise-associated collapse without actual LOC	Normal	Immediate core body temperature and electrolyte measurement

Table 35.1 (Continued)

ECG, electrocardiogram; SCD, sudden cardiac death; QTc, corrected QT; WPW, Wolff–Parkinson–White; SOB, shortness of breath; LOC, loss of consciousness; TTE, transthoracic echocardiogram; CMR, cardiac magnetic resonance; CTA, computed tomography angiogram; RBBB, right bundle branch block; EEG, electroencephalogram.

[a] Bradycardia, although a common cause of syncope in the elderly, is not a common cause of syncope in otherwise healthy young athletes.

[b] Neurally mediated cerebral hypoperfusion may rarely manifest as exertional syncope. Diagnostic findings in this scenario include an inappropriate blood pressure response to exercise (i.e. a blunted rise or any fall in systolic blood pressure) that is clearly associated with reproduction of presenting symptoms in the setting of a structurally normal heart and absence of arrhythmia.

manoeuvres such as the Valsalva manoeuvre or standing from squatting to elicit dynamic murmurs (such as that heard in outflow tract obstruction in hypertrophic cardiomyopathy (HCM)).

In the vast majority of cases, evaluation of athletes with syncope should include a 12-lead electrocardiogram (ECG). Many findings that are considered abnormal in the general population are commonly observed in trained athletes due to exercise-induced cardiac adaptations, and as such several helpful sets of guidelines have been developed to distinguish between normal 'training-related' and abnormal pathologic findings in the interpretation of the athlete's ECG [9,10]. See Chapter 10 for normal ECG findings in athletes. Salient pathologic ECG findings that may suggest a dangerous cardiovascular cause for syncope are included in Table 35.1.

Unless the initial evaluation is entirely consistent with neurally mediated cerebral hypoperfusion, clinicians should have a low threshold for obtaining a transthoracic echocardiogram (TTE) to exclude structural and valvular diseases. As discussed later, TTE is useful for excluding or confirming numerous causes of SCD in young athletes (<35 years old), including HCM, anomalous coronary arteries, myocarditis and arrhythmogenic right ventricular cardiomyopathy (ARVC), as these may first present with syncope, amongst other symptoms [11]. In contemporary practice, TTE represents the most logical first-line imaging test, but it is often followed by adjunct, more diseases-specific imaging modalities, including cardiac computed tomography (CT) and CMR. Exertional syncope should also prompt customised exercise testing that simulates the specific training or competition conditions which provoked the presenting episode of syncope or pre-syncopal symptoms. If comprehensive exercise testing fails to reproduce the presenting symptoms and arrhythmia exists on the differential diagnosis, ambulatory ECG monitoring is indicated. The choice of an ambulatory rhythm monitoring device for an athlete with syncope must be individualised and should be made in conjunction with a cardiovascular specialist with the requisite expertise. Additional diagnostic testing modalities, including tilt-table testing and electrophysiology (EP) study, may be considered in isolated cases, but they have a limited role in the evaluation of unexplained syncope in athletes due to their poor sensitivity and specificity. Tilt-table testing, in particular, is prone to high false-positive rates and low reproducibility amongst athletes, and therefore is not routinely recommended.

Determining a definitive cause of syncope is not possible in up to ~35% of cases [3]. In cases in which diagnostic uncertainty persists following a comprehensive evaluation, decisions about return to play must rely upon the remaining suspicion for a dangerous cardiovascular cause, based upon the history, physical examination and diagnostic testing data. For example, if syncope and/or its prodromal symptoms have been captured on an exercise test or ambulatory rhythm monitoring and shown not to be associated with a malignant arrhythmia, then return to play may be reasonable even in the absence of a clear diagnosis. Sporting activities during which recurrent syncope may prove life-threatening even in the absence of established disease (e.g. open-water swimming, rock climbing, scuba diving) should prompt a more conservative approach.

Palpitations

Palpitations – the awareness of forceful, rapid or irregular heartbeats – are common amongst trained athletes. Whilst the majority of palpitations originate from benign causes, they may also represent clinically relevant arrhythmia or be indicative of underlying structural heart disease (Table 35.1). The differential diagnosis of palpitations in athletes is broad (Table 35.2), but may be appropriately narrowed by careful history-taking. The timing of palpitations relative to exertion is crucial and, along with the frequency and nature of symptoms, will help guide the choice of subsequent diagnostic testing. Palpitations that trigger concomitant symptoms (including pre-syncope/syncope) and palpitations in a previously healthy athlete with a family history of sudden death or heritable CVD suggest a higher likelihood of malignant tachyarrhythmia. A history of stimulant use via prescription medications, such as methylphenidate, as well as over-the-counter use of caffeine or herbal stimulants, should also be specifically questioned.

Arrhythmia	History	Diagnostic testing/prognosis
Premature atrial or ventricular contractions	'Skipped' or irregular beats; may diminish with exercise or with detraining	No structural heart disease and suppression of ectopy with exercise: benign prognosis. Complex PVCs during exercise or frequent PVCs (>2000 in 24 hours): further evaluation for structural heart disease or arrhythmia syndromes (Table 35.1)
Supraventricular tachycardia (SVT)		
Atrioventricular (AV) nodal re-entrant tachycardia, atrial tachycardia, atrial flutter	Sudden start/stop (especially for re-entry), regular palpitations	Benign prognosis in the absence of structural heart disease
Pre-excitation (i.e. bypass tract), including WPW syndrome, AVRT	May be asymptomatic. AVRT: sudden start/stop, regular palpitations	Higher incidence of atrial fibrillation, which can lead to ventricular fibrillation: risk stratification with exercise testing (low risk if delta wave disappears at high heart rate) or EP study
Atrial fibrillation	Irregular palpitations. May occur at rest or be provoked by exertion. Long-time endurance athletes may have higher incidence	Exercise testing and history are useful in establishing a mechanism (increased sympathetic activity during exercise versus augmentation of vagal tone, facilitating atrial re-entry at rest) and management strategies. Risk of cardioembolic events in the setting of structural heart disease or hypertension
Ventricular tachycardia	Regular palpitations; may be of short duration (i.e. NSVT) or prolonged and associated with pre-syncope or syncope	Especially in sustained ventricular tachycardia, a thorough evaluation for structural cardiac disease (i.e. TTE, CMR), inheritable arrhythmia syndrome (see Table 35.1) or offending medications (e.g. stimulants, QTc-prolonging drugs) is mandatory

Table 35.2 Common causes of palpitations in athletes

PVC, premature ventricular contraction; WPW, Wolff–Parkinson–White; AVRT, atrioventricular re-entry tachycardia; EP, electrophysiological; NSVT, nonsustained ventricular tachycardia; TTE, transthoracic echocardiogram; CMR, cardiac magnetic resonance; QTc, corrected QT.

Monitor	Description	Pros	Cons
Holter monitor	Leads attached to a pager-sized device 24–48 hours of continuous monitoring	High-fidelity tracings Continuous tracings good for symptoms that are short in duration	Insufficient to capture infrequent symptoms Leads cumbersome in most sports, so it is difficult to capture exertional symptoms
Traditional nonimplantable loop monitor	Leads attached to a pager-sized device Up to 1 month of continuous monitoring	Same as Holter monitor, but can be kept longer for infrequent symptoms	Leads cumbersome in most sports
Patch loop monitor	Device approximate size of a matchbook affixed to chest with a sticky patch 1–2 weeks of continuous monitoring	Continuous tracings are good for symptoms that are short in duration Low-profile device is usable during almost all sports, including swimming	Insufficient to capture infrequent symptoms
Implantable loop monitor	Device approximate size of a key implanted subcutaneously over upper chest Battery life up to 3 years	Best for infrequent symptoms that are short in duration/ without prodrome	Invasive Requires a short recovery prior to resuming contact sports
Event monitor	Device approximate size of a deck of cards placed on chest at time of symptom onset (no leads)	Can be kept for prolonged periods Good for symptoms that are long in duration but sporadic	Must be kept nearby Not useful for symptoms that are short in duration Not practical for exertional symptoms in many sports

Table 35.3 Types of ambulatory rhythm monitor

Diagnostic evaluation of the athlete with symptomatic palpitations should follow the dual goals of excluding underlying causative medical conditions or cardiac structural abnormalities and documenting the cardiac rhythm that is associated with symptoms (on ECG). Basic laboratory testing should include measurement of electrolytes, thyroid function, iron indices and blood counts. The presence of structural heart disease greatly influences the prognosis of common arrhythmias, and therefore a TTE is recommend to evaluate for cardiac structural abnormalities. There are several options for ECG documentation of cardiac rhythm associated with palpitations, including exercise testing customised to the conditions that previously triggered symptoms and/or some form of out-patient ambulatory rhythm monitoring (Table 35.3).

Therapeutic options for the athlete with palpitations are determined by the underlying cause. They include simple conservative observation and reassurance, pharmacotherapy and intracardiac ablation. In the absence of an established diagnosis for palpitations, return to play with the use of an ambulatory rhythm monitor may be reasonable based on the a priori likelihood of a malignant arrhythmia. Consensus opinions regarding return to play for various arrhythmias have been published [12].

Chest Pain

Although cardiac causes of chest pain (Table 35.4) are relatively uncommon (<6%) in athletes less than 35 years old, underlying causal conditions include potentially life-threatening diseases such as coronary artery anomalies and HCM [13]. Older athletes with exertional chest discomfort must be assumed to have atherosclerotic coronary disease until proven otherwise. Noncardiac medical and musculoskeletal causes of exertional chest pain (Table 35.5) are relevant and common across the age spectrum of athletes.

The medical history for the athletic patient with chest pain should focus on whether pain is exertional or non-exertional, and on the presence of specific provocative factors (e.g. movement, diet and climate). Associated symptoms may further guide narrowing of the differential diagnosis to a specific organ system (Tables 35.4 and 35.5). Ischaemic chest pain can result from a number of cardiac conditions, including coronary pathologies (i.e. coronary anomalies, atherosclerotic coronary disease) that limit myocardial

Disease	Chest pain features
Coronary artery disorders	*Ischaemic pain from reduced coronary blood supply*
Atherosclerosis	Effort-dependent 'warm-up angina' during first minutes of exercise
Anomalous origin of coronary artery	Infrequent/sporadic ischaemic chest pain at high level of exercise intensity
Coronary artery dissection	Acute-onset ischaemic pain without resolution at rest
Coronary artery vasospasm	More often non-exertional
Myocardial disorders	
Hypertrophic cardiomyopathy (HCM)	Exertional ischaemic pain from increased myocardial demand
Myocarditis/pericarditis	Positional sharp substernal pain
Other	
Aortic dissection	Acute onset, often during isometric activity; tearing pain in back and chest
Arrhythmia	Tracks with palpitation onset/offset
Valvular and congenital heart disease (CHD)	Exertional ischaemic pain from increased myocardial demand

Table 35.4 Cardiac causes of chest pain in athletes

blood flow, and from non-coronary conditions (i.e. cardiomyopathy and valvular heart disease) that increase myocardial demand. Regardless of the aetiology, chest discomfort caused by myocardial ischaemia is most often: (i) triggered by effort; (ii) relieved by rest within several minutes; and (iii) located in the substernal and/or left chest area. It often has an aching, pressure or tightness quality and may radiate to the jaw, neck and/or arm. Chest pain that is caused by myocardial ischaemia is typically reproducible at a given workload. However, athletes with an anomalous coronary artery may experience unpredictable and irregular episodes of ischaemic exertional chest discomfort. It is important to have a high index of suspicion for congenital coronary artery anomalies because, although rare in the general population (detected in <1% of individuals at coronary angiography), they have been shown to account for 15–20% of sudden death events in athletes [11].

Syncope or lightheadedness that occurs with exertional chest discomfort is a *clinical red flag* for a potentially life-threatening condition. The combination of chest discomfort and near syncope suggests a transient impairment of cardiac function that reduces delivery of blood to the brain. Athletes with this symptom constellation should refrain from exercise until the clinical investigation is completed.

As part of the initial diagnostic evaluation in athletes presenting with chest pain, an ECG should be obtained, and if pain is exertional, the athlete should undergo customised exercise testing in an attempt to reproduce pain and evaluate for ischaemic ECG changes and/or arrhythmia. Further diagnostic evaluation of suspected cardiac chest pain after initial history, examination, ECG and exercise ECG testing may require additional cardiac diagnostic imaging. As some of the characteristic ECG findings in athletes (e.g. left ventricular hypertrophy, LVH) can lead to uninterpretable results during exercise ECG testing, the addition of an imaging modality (i.e. stress echocardiography or nuclear scintigraphy) or the use of metabolic gas-exchange testing may be considered [14]. Alternatively, or in series, suspected anatomical coronary pathology (i.e. coronary artery disease (CAD) or anomalous coronary origin) may be directly evaluated via cardiac CT, CMR or invasive coronary angiography.

The initial evaluation for structural cardiac disease (i.e. HCM, valvular and congenital disease) is typically accomplished with TTE. TTE is also useful for ruling out anomalous coronary origin, although if coronary origin is not clearly identified, angiography may still be necessary. TTE and other imaging test results must be interpreted in the context of expected exercise-induced cardiac remodelling, which is specific to both the athlete's sport and their training load. Marked left ventricular dilation (left ventricular end diastolic diameter >60 mm) is relatively common (~15%), particularly in endurance athletes [15], and thus absolute ventricular size measurements in isolation are not useful for differentiating athletic remodelling from disease. In contrast, markedly thickened left ventricular walls (>13–15 mm, based on gender) are uncommon (<2%) [16] and should prompt a high index of suspicion for pathologic hypertrophy. Athletes with larger body size and greater exercise intensity and/or volume who are of Afro-Caribbean descent may demonstrate the greatest degree of adaptive LVH [17,18]. Sport type is also an

Diagnosis	History and physical examination	Diagnostic testing
Pulmonary causes		
Asthma	Exertional chest tightness, SOB, cough, wheezing Starts minutes after beginning of exercise or in recovery Allergens or climate extremes may be triggers May persist despite rest Physical examination: wheeze with rapid forced expiration	Spirometry
Pneumothorax	Spontaneous (tall, thin habitus) or post-trauma Sharp pain, worse with deep breath Physical examination: absent breath sounds	AP inspiratory chest film, expiratory film if not seen
Pulmonary embolus	Acute chest pain, new wheeze, pleuritic pain, haemoptysis, dyspnoea Risk after immobisation or with oral contraceptive use Physical examination: tachypnoea, leg swelling	Chest CTA
Pneumonia	Focal pain, pleuritic or achy in nature Cough, fever Physical examination: focal crackles and reduced breath sounds	PA and lateral chest films
Pleurisy	Sharp pain, worse with deep breath May occur after respiratory infections or pneumonia Physical examination: pleural friction rub	–
Gastrointestinal causes		
Gastroesophageal reflux disease (GERD)	Burning chest or epigastric pain Associated belching, nausea, vomiting Temporally associated with eating around exercise May persist despite rest Risk factors: hiatal hernia, NSAIDs, protein supplements Physical examination: bowel sounds in chest (if hernia)	History usually sufficient Endoscopy or exercise test if needed
Musculoskeletal causes		
Rib fracture	If acute: direct trauma with pleuritic pain Stress fractures cause vague pain that progresses to point tenderness, higher risk in rowers and weightlifters/throwers Physical examination: point tenderness, bruising.	Rib X-rays, bone scan
Costochondritis	Focal sharp pain at the junction of rib and sternum, provoked by movement Onset after new chest exercise or frequent coughing Physical examination: pain with direct pressure over costochondral junction	–
Rib subluxation	Pleuritic posterior chest pain Caused by to rib slipping off of transverse process Physical examination: point tenderness	Rib X-rays
Slipping rib syndrome	Sharp pleuritic pain for seconds, followed by aching pain for days Caused by increased mobility of anterior ribs 8–10 and irritation of intercostal nerve Physical examination: point tenderness, improvement with 'hooking manoeuvre' (fingers hooked under ribs at costal margin and ribs pulled forward)	–

Table 35.5 Noncardiac causes of chest pain in athletes

SOB, shortness of breath; AP, posterior–anterior; CTA, computed tomography angiography; NSAIDs, nonsteroidal anti-inflammatory drugs.

important consideration when looking at the geometry of cardiac enlargement in athletes. Isometric exercise as performed in strength-based sports (e.g. weightlifting, throwing events, American football linemen) places an increased pressure load on the heart and typically leads to mild forms of concentric LVH (i.e. increased left ventricular wall thickness without an increase in left ventricular chamber size) [19]. In contrast, isotonic exercise as performed in endurance sports (e.g. distance running, cycling, swimming) places an increased volume load on the heart and typically leads to eccentric LVH or left ventricular remodelling (i.e. balanced increase in left ventricular chamber size and mass), with concomitant right ventricular enlargement [19,20]. Advanced TTE techniques that evaluate left ventricular systolic and diastolic function may also help differentiate pathologic from adaptive cardiac enlargement [21]. Cases for which diagnostic uncertainty remains after TTE with regards to the presence of pathologic structural cardiac disease may benefit from the addition of CMR, which provides more detailed assessment of cardiac structure. CMR is particularly useful in the diagnosis of HCM with focal hypertrophy, ARVC and myocarditis [22].

Exertional Fatigue and Performance Decline

Exertional fatigue and/or performance decline in the athlete often presents a considerable diagnostic challenge. These symptoms are notoriously difficult for the athlete to describe and may be caused by dysfunction in any of the organ systems required to support the increased metabolic demands of exercise. Furthermore, the underlying cause of exertional fatigue and performance decline may range from completely benign (e.g. relative detraining) to life-threatening (e.g. CVD). In the athlete presenting with exertional fatigue or performance decline, the primary goal of the medical history is to clarify the specific limiting symptoms. Excessive shortness of breath is commonly associated with exertional fatigue, and may not be a specific sign of pulmonary pathology. However, noisy breathing or audible wheeze, especially with specific climate or allergic triggers, may suggest exertional bronchospasm or vocal cord dysfunction. Shortness of breath in the absence of other symptoms may be the cardinal manifestation of CVD, pulmonary vascular disease or nonvascular medical conditions such as anaemia. Historical data, non-exertional symptoms and physical examination signs often provide important clues regarding the aetiology of exertional fatigue caused by medical conditions such as occult infection, autoimmune disorder or endocrine disease.

Unless the patient history is able to clearly narrow the differential diagnosis, the diagnostic evaluation of exertional fatigue and shortness of breath is often necessarily broad. Guided by the history, comprehensive laboratory evaluation can rule out common medical issues in athletes, including anaemia (blood counts, iron studies), thyroid disease (thyroid-stimulating hormone, TSH), autoimmune disease (antinuclear antibodies, inflammatory markers), infection (heterospot for mononucleosis) and pregnancy (human chorionic gonadotropin).

A resting ECG serves as the initial evaluation for CVD amongst athletes with exertional fatigue or performance decline. Comprehensive and customised exercise stress testing is often the most useful next step in narrowing the differential diagnosis. Exercise testing in athletes should be performed to maximal exercise capacity and not terminated prematurely due to heart rate. Whilst the Bruce protocol is easily performed, well tolerated and commonly used, athletes who experience symptoms only during their particular activity may need specialised exercise testing designed to simulate their primary sporting activity and the specific scenarios during which they experience symptoms (e.g. intensity, duration, climate, sudden starts/stops). Exercise testing can be accompanied by a number of physiologic monitors. ECG monitoring may document ischaemia, arrhythmia or an inappropriate heart rate response to exercise. Intermittent evaluation of blood pressure via a noninvasive cuff may identify an excessive hypertensive response or blunted blood pressure response to exercise. Pulse oximetry may reveal exercise-induced desaturation, which may suggest primary pulmonary disease or an exercise-induced cardiac shunt. The addition of pre- and post-exercise spirometry is useful to identify exercise-induced asthma or vocal cord dysfunction. Finally, the addition of continuous metabolic gas exchange (i.e. cardiopulmonary exercise testing) allows for the quantification of exercise capacity (peak VO_2) and exercise effort (respiratory exchange ration), as well as identification of patterns suggestive of abnormal pulmonary or cardiac limits to exercise [23]. Exercise testing may capture abnormalities that either suggest or secure a diagnosis for exertional symptoms, and in cases in which further clarification is required can help guide the choice of additional testing.

Conclusion

The evaluation of symptoms suggestive of underlying CVD is a crucial aspect of the care of the athletic patient, and requires a customised and careful stepwise approach to differentiate dangerous and potentially life-threatening cardiovascular pathology from benign entities. Such evaluation is best accomplished by a sports medicine team that includes a cardiologist with expertise in the disease processes, diagnostic options and management challenges that may be unique to the athletic patient.

References

1 Baggish, A.L., Weiner, R.B., Kanayama, G. et al. Long-term anabolic-androgenic steroid use is associated with left ventricular dysfunction. *Circ Heart Fail* 2010; **3**(4): 472–6.

2 Riebe, D., Fernhall, B. and Thompson, P.D. The blood pressure response to exercise in anabolic steroid users. *Med Sci Sports Exerc* 1992; **24**(6): 633–7.

3 Linzer, M., Yang, E.H., Estes, N.A. et al. Diagnosing syncope. Part 1: Value of history, physical examination, and electrocardiography. Clinical Efficacy Assessment Project of the American College of Physicians. *Ann Intern Med* 1997; **126**(12): 989–96.

4 Colivicchi, F., Ammirati, F. and Santini, M. Epidemiology and prognostic implications of syncope in young competing athletes. *Eur Heart J* 2004; **25**(19): 1749–53.

5 Hastings, J.L. and Levine, B.D. Syncope in the athletic patient. *Prog Cardiovasc Dis* 2012; **54**(5): 438–44.

6 Freeman, R. Clinical practice. Neurogenic orthostatic hypotension. *N Engl J Med* 2008; **358**(6): 615–24.

7 Calkins, H., Shyr, Y., Frumin, H. et al. The value of the clinical history in the differentiation of syncope due to ventricular tachycardia, atrioventricular block, and neurocardiogenic syncope. *Am J Med* 1995; **98**(4): 365–73.

8 Sheldon, R., Rose, S., Ritchie, D. et al. Historical criteria that distinguish syncope from seizures. *J Am Coll Cardiol* 2002; **40**(1): 142–8.

9 Corrado, D., Pelliccia, A., Heidbuchel, H. et al. Recommendations for interpretation of 12-lead electrocardiogram in the athlete. *Eur Heart J* 2010; **31**(2): 243–59.

10 Drezner, J.A., Ackerman, M.J., Anderson, J. et al. Electrocardiographic interpretation in athletes: the 'Seattle criteria'. *Br J Sports Med* 2013; **47**(3): 122–4.

11 Maron, B.J., Doerer, J.J., Haas, T.S. et al. Sudden deaths in young competitive athletes: analysis of 1866 deaths in the United States, 1980–2006. *Circulation* 2009; **119**(8): 1085–92.

12 Zipes, D.P., Ackerman, M.J., Estes, N.A.M. et al. Task Force 7: arrhythmias. *J Am Coll Cardiol* 2005; **45**(8): 1354–63.

13 Perron, A.D. Chest pain in athletes. *Clin Sports Med* 2003; **22**(1): 37–50.

14 Gibbons, R.J., Balady, G.J., Bricker, J.T. et al. ACC/AHA 2002 guideline update for exercise testing: summary article. A report of the American College of Cardiology/American Heart Association Task Force on Practice Guidelines (Committee to Update the 1997 Exercise Testing Guidelines). *J Am Coll Cardiol* 2002; **40**(8): 1531–40.

15 Pelliccia, A., Culasso, F., Di Paolo, F.M. and Maron, B.J. Physiologic left ventricular cavity dilatation in elite athletes. *Ann Intern Med* 1999; **130**(1): 23–31.

16 Pelliccia, A., Maron, B.J., Spataro, A. et al. The upper limit of physiologic cardiac hypertrophy in highly trained elite athletes. *N Engl J Med* 1991; **324**(5): 295–301.

17 Sharma, S. Athlete's heart – effect of age, sex, ethnicity and sporting discipline. *Exp Physiol* 2003; **88**(5): 665–9.

18 Baggish, A.L., Yared, K., Weiner, R.B. et al. Differences in cardiac parameters among elite rowers and subelite rowers. *Med Sci Sports Exerc* 2010; **42**(6): 1215–20.

19 Baggish, A.L., Wang, F., Weiner, R.B. et al. Training-specific changes in cardiac structure and function: a prospective and longitudinal assessment of competitive athletes. *J Appl Physiol (1985)* 2008; **104**(4): 1121–8.

20 Oxborough, D., Sharma, S., Shave, R. et al. The right ventricle of the endurance athlete: the relationship between morphology and deformation. *J Am Soc Echocardiogr* 2012; **25**(3): 263–71.

21 Rawlins, J., Bhan, A. and Sharma, S. Left ventricular hypertrophy in athletes. *Eur J Echocardiogr* 2009; **10**(3): 350–6.

22 Prakken, N.H., Velthuis, B.K., Cramer, M.J. and Mosterd, A. Advances in cardiac imaging: the role of magnetic resonance imaging and computed tomography in identifying athletes at risk. *Br J Sports Med* 2009; **43**(9): 677–84.

23 Ross, R.M. ATS/ACCP statement on cardiopulmonary exercise testing. *Am J Respir Crit Care Med* 2003; **167**(2): 211–77.

36 Management of Abnormal Physical Examination Findings in Athletes

Victoria Watt[1], Mats Börjesson[2] and Mikael Dellborg[3]

[1]Department of Sports Medicine, ASPETAR, Qatar Orthopaedic and Sports Medicine Hospital, Doha, Qatar
[2]Åstrand Laboratory, Swedish School of Sport and Exercise Sciences (GIH) and Department of Cardiology, Karolinska University Hospital, Stockholm, Sweden
[3]Department of Molecular and Clinical Medicine/Östra, Institute of Medicine, Sahlgrenska Academy, University of Gothenburg and Adult Congenital Heart Unit, Sahlgrenska University Hospital/Östra, Gothenburg, Sweden

Introduction

Pre-participation cardiovascular screening of athletes includes a thorough examination of the cardiovascular system. The aim of the physical examination is to uncover signs suggestive of underlying cardiac disease that may be associated with an increased risk of sudden cardiac death (SCD), particularly with continued sports participation [1]. In addition, sports medicine physicians may be called upon to perform pre-participation evaluations (PPEs) in previously sedentary people, of a variety of ages, about to embark on an exercise programme. This should be borne in mind when reading this chapter.

The complete cardiovascular physical examination begins with a general inspection of the patient, followed by a systematic examination to detect signs of cardiac disease. In many parts of the world, physicians have easy access to a number of cardiac investigative tools, including the 12-lead electrocardiogram (ECG) and echocardiography. In addition, athletes and nonathletes have access to integrated health care services, allowing early detection and intervention if there is any suspicion of cardiac disease. It can be argued that, in this context, a discussion of the clinical signs found in established, untreated cardiac structural disease is anachronistic and, perhaps, no longer necessary.

However, screening for structural cardiac abnormalities remains less than perfect. In addition, participation in sport is a global pursuit. Sports medicine physicians may, at times, be required to practice medicine without immediate access to ECG and echocardiography. Furthermore, with increasing movement of people from their country of origin, it is not uncommon for physicians to evaluate patients and athletes who may not have had prior access to health care services and who may originate from populations with a different spectrum of diseases to those usually seen. It is important, therefore, to retain the skills required to carry out a complete cardiovascular examination, as outlined in this chapter.

General Inspection

Examination of the cardiovascular system begins with general inspection. This can provide useful information about the overall health status of the athlete. The athlete should be recumbent, reclined at approximately 45°, in a well-lit room and free from distraction. The physician can assess whether the athlete appears fit, has an appropriate body mass index (BMI), is breathing comfortably and is free from discolouration or abnormal signs suggestive of a possible congenital cardiac syndrome.

The athlete should have a normal resting respiratory rate. A mild tachypnoea is likely to be secondary to the anxiety often experienced when athletes attend for PPE. However, if the athlete appears to be breathless at rest, particularly if they have experienced a decline in their athletic performance or normal functional status or have additional cardiac or respiratory symptoms, then this should raise the index of suspicion for an underlying cause. The clinician should exclude a primary respiratory or cardiac abnormality through further examination and investigations (including ECG and echocardiography).

A simple inspection of the athlete's general appearance can offer a great deal of useful information, particularly in weight-categorised sports. Eating disorders are more prevalent in elite athletes compared to non-athletes and are more common in females, often occurring as part of the female athlete triad. Eating disorders are more often seen in sports where low body weight can have a positive impact on performance, for example endurance running, road cycling and aesthetic disciplines. Severe eating disorders are associated with a number of cardiac complications, including reduced myocardial mass, hypotension and arrhythmias related to electrolyte abnormalities and prolongation of the QT interval. Individuals with physical examination findings suggestive of an inappropriately low BMI and a possible eating disorder should be referred to competent specialists, capable of dealing with the challenging medical and psychological consequences of these conditions.

If a previously sedentary individual presents for PPE prior to embarking on an exercise programme, they may have an elevated BMI. In such cases, a careful estimation of cardiovascular risk should be made and the physician should examine carefully for hypertension and signs of cardiac and peripheral vascular disease (PVD), as discussed later in this chapter.

Examination of the athlete's stature should be part of the general inspection. Short stature may be familial and, whilst not usually associated with disease, can be a sign of skeletal dysplasia or endocrine disorders such as growth hormone deficiency or hypothyroidism. Congenital diseases such as Noonan's and Turner's syndromes are frequently associated with short stature and have a significant prevalence of cardiac disease: pulmonary stenosis, septal defects and myocardial hypertrophy in the former; aortic valve disease, coarctation, aortic dilatation and dissection in the latter.

Athletes presenting with unusually tall stature, particularly in sports where increased height may confer an advantage, such as basketball, may prompt the clinician to consider the possibility of Marfan syndrome. This is a connective-tissue disorder, inherited in an autosomal-dominant pattern or arising as a result of spontaneous mutation. Marfan syndrome affects the cardiac, skeletal, ocular and neurological systems and carries a reduced life expectancy. Cardiac complications include dilatation of the aorta, aortic dissection and mitral valve prolapse (MVP). If the clinician suspects Marfan syndrome then a further, detailed assessment of the musculoskeletal system is indicated, along with a transthoracic echo. See Chapter 22 and the Revised Ghent Nosology for further details on the diagnostic criteria for Marfan syndrome [2]. Inherited connective-tissue disorders and their findings on clinical examination are discussed further later in this chapter.

Examination of the Hands

Traditionally, inspection of the hands and skin comprises an important part of the cardiovascular system examination. However, many of the signs that can be found in the peripheries are unlikely to be seen in competitive athletes (e.g. peripheral cyanosis and fingernail clubbing seen in cyanotic congenital heart disease (CHD)). These are conditions which, by their very nature, significantly limit an individual's ability to exercise. A patient with a right-to-left cardiac shunt and therefore significant pulmonary hypertension is unlikely to present as an athlete for pre-participation screening. However, the hand and skin signs seen in familial hyperlipidaemia (tendon xanthomata) and connective-tissue diseases (joint hypermobility, arachnodactyly and skin striae) may be detected and are of relevance to the athlete and the cardiovascular system.

Examination of the Radial Pulse

Examination of the radial pulse is, of course, a central part of the cardiovascular examination. The pulse should always be palpated by the physician and never ignored, even if the heart rate has been provided by an automated measurement. The 'normal' resting heart rate is traditionally defined as being between

60 and 100 beats.min^{-1}, with bradycardia and tachycardia occurring at heart rates below and above these thresholds, respectively. The resting heart rate is inversely related to physical fitness, and an elevated resting heart rate is an independent risk factor for mortality, regardless of fitness, level of activity and other major cardiovascular risk factors [3]. However, the resting heart rate should always be interpreted in the context of the athlete's age and overall fitness.

The resting heart rate of an athlete is usually lower than 60 beats.min^{-1}, and the finding of a resting brady-cardia of *greater than* 30 beats.min^{-1} in a young, *well-trained* athlete, with confirmation of sinus bradycardia on 12-lead ECG, is of no concern. Of course, this is not the case in an older individual taking part in low-level, recreational activity or presenting for assessment prior to embarking on a physical activity programme. In these cases, a 12-lead ECG is imperative to determine the underlying rhythm and exclude underlying conduction disease. A medication history should be taken and further tests performed where indicated, including Holter monitoring, exercise testing to assess the heart-rate response to exercise, thyroid function and electrolyte studies.

The commonest cause of an irregular pulse in young athletes is sinus arrhythmia: a physiological variation in heart rate occurring with respiration. However, an ECG should be performed to exclude other causes of an irregular pulse, including supraventricular or ventricular ectopy and atrial fibrillation. The physician may choose to examine for radioradial and radiofemoral delay at this point: signs which may be found in coarctation of the aorta.

Assessment of Resting Blood Pressure

Measurement of the blood pressure is an essential component of the cardiovascular examination in the athlete. Hypertension is the commonest cardiovascular condition found in athletes, and carries a significant morbidity and mortality if left untreated over the long term. Assessment of the athlete's blood pressure should be performed in a standardised manner and in accordance with current guidelines. See Chapter 39 and the current European Society of Cardiology (ESC) and American Heart Association (AHA) advisory documents for further detail [4,5]. The athlete should be seated, at rest, and should not have recently participated in exercise. Avoidance of caffeine prior to the measurement is also recommended.

The blood pressure should be measured in both arms, with the higher reading taken as the reference. If the auscultatory method is used, phase I and V Korotkoff sounds should be used to identify systolic and dias-tolic values. An appropriately sized bladder should be fitted to the upper arm, with the cuff placed at the level of the heart. Office readings are usually higher than ambulatory and home blood pressure measurements. Hypertension is currently defined as a resting blood pressure ≥140/90 mmHg (office measurement), ≥130/80 mmHg (24-hour average ambulatory measurement) or ≥135/85 mmHg (home measurement). Chapter 39 describes the management of confirmed hypertension in athletes. However, as part of the current chapter, it is important to discuss the initial assessment of a newly discovered abnormal blood pressure measurement.

Low Resting Blood Pressure

It is well known that regular aerobic training has a favourable effect on blood pressure, through a reduction in vascular resistance, mediated by a number of mechanisms, including effects on the sympathetic, parasym-pathetic and renin–angiotensin systems. Athletes commonly present with blood pressure readings towards the lower end of the normal range, and this can be seen as a training effect, similar to resting bradycardia. In certain circumstances, such as dehydration, febrile illness or after sudden cessation of exercise, the blood pressure decrease can become more pronounced, leading to hypotensive symptoms.

Orthostatic symptoms should prompt blood pressure measurement in both the sitting and the standing positions. A systolic blood pressure decrease of more than 10 mmHg upon standing, without an increase in diastolic blood pressure, is defined as an orthostatic blood pressure response. This finding should be evaluated in the presence of symptoms. If possible, any underlying cause or exacerbating factors should be identified and corrective measures taken (e.g. advice regarding appropriate hydration strategies and post-exercise management techniques).

Increased Blood Pressure at Rest

The initial management of a single elevated blood pressure recording involves considering the circumstances in which the measurement was taken. The athlete should be in a sufficiently rested state, should not have recently participated in exercise and, ideally, should have avoided caffeine prior to the measurement. The diagnosis of hypertension should not be made after a single, elevated office recording. Office blood pressure measurements are known to be higher than ambulatory recordings or measurements taken at home. Therefore, if, on a second reading, the blood pressure remains elevated, the athlete should be referred for an ambulatory blood pressure recording, or, if this is not available, for further readings at home or in the primary care setting. The diagnosis of hypertension is made either with the result of an ambulatory monitor or after two or more readings taken after at least two separate office visits.

Normal blood pressure is defined as <120/80 mmHg. Hypertension is currently defined as a resting blood pressure >140/90 mmHg. Prehypertension is classified as a blood pressure between 120 and 130 mmHg systolic and 80 and 90 mmHg diastolic. Individuals with prehypertension are at risk of progressing to hypertension, and current guidelines (already referenced) recommend lifestyle advice for this cohort.

Hypertension may be primary or secondary. Primary hypertension arises in the absence of an identifiable cause and may be due to a number of environmental and genetic factors. Over 90% of cases of hypertension in adults fall into this category. Nevertheless, the diagnosis of hypertension in an athlete should prompt a series of further investigations to exclude a secondary cause, most commonly vascular, renal and endocrine disorders. As part of the initial assessment, and during the clinical examination, signs of coarctation should be sought (as discussed later), along with auscultation of the renal arteries. In addition, it is important to elicit signs of end-organ damage, including peripheral oedema (seen in cardiac or renal impairment) and hypertensive retinopathy (found through fundoscopy).

It is worth mentioning that a number of drugs often used by athletes have been implicated in the aetiology of hypertension, including the oral contraceptive pill, nonsteroidal anti-inflammatory drugs (NSAIDs), corticosteroids and decongestants, such as ephedrine. Therefore, the examining physician should ensure that a thorough medication history is taken for any athlete found to be hypertensive. Simple office investigations, including urinalysis and renal function tests, should be carried out without delay, whilst a more extensive series of investigations can be arranged subsequently. A resting 12-lead ECG, echocardiography and stress ECG to assess the athlete's blood pressure response to exercise are imperative, as the results will help determine the athlete's eligibility to continue participation in sport [6,7].

Coarctation of the Aorta

Coarctation of the aorta commonly presents in the first year of life, but can present at any stage in childhood and early adulthood. Patients are often asymptomatic, and the condition is only detected after an incidental finding of hypertension. The examining physician should be aware that aortic coarctation often coexists with a bicuspid aortic valve (BAV). Therefore, if the physician suspects a coarctation, the aortic valve should be carefully examined. In addition, patients who have undergone intervention or surgical repair of a coarctation may remain hypertensive or may develop hypertension afterwards. Therefore, blood pressure measurement should be carried out in any patient with a history of coarctation (whether repaired or not).

In addition, an assessment of the blood pressure in the lower limbs should be performed the first time an athlete presents for evaluation. Blood pressure in the lower limbs is usually around 10% *higher* than brachial artery pressure. A pressure drop of at least 20 mmHg from the upper to the lower limbs, when supine, may indicate an underlying coarctation. An examination of the peripheral pulses is essential – radiofemoral delay is the hallmark sign of a coarctation, but depending on the position of the stenosis in relation to the origin of the left subclavian artery, radioradial delay may also be found.

If the physician suspects a coarctation, a 12-lead ECG and echocardiography should be arranged. Transthoracic echo allows good visualisation of the aortic valve, aortic root, arch and proximal ascending and descending segments of the aorta. Increased flow velocities in the descending aorta are present in coarctation, and there may be segments of pre- or poststenotic dilatation. However, it is not possible to image the entire thoracic aorta by transthoracic echo. Therefore, in suspicious cases, it is essential to arrange more definitive imaging of the thoracic aorta in its entirety, using magnetic resonance imaging (MRI) or computed tomography angiography (CTA). In confirmed cases, or if doubt remains, the athlete should be referred to the appropriate adult CHD specialist for further evaluation. Furthermore, athletes who have previously undergone a coarctation repair should remain under long-term follow-up with a specialist in adult CHD. Lifelong blood pressure surveillance and follow-up imaging of the repair site are indicated in these individuals.

Examination of the Face and Neck

Facial signs can be associated with underlying cardiac abnormalities in some inherited and congenital syndromes. A cleft of the lip or palate is associated with CHD in approximately 25% of cases [8]. Characteristic facial signs may be seen in a number of congenital syndromes associated with cardiac disease, most notably Down's, Noonan's and Turner's syndromes. These conditions are well described in the medical literature and are associated with a significant prevalence of cardiac malformations.

Signs of possible underlying cardiac disease can also be seen in and around the eyes. Xanthalesmata and corneal arcus may be seen in young athletes with familial hypercholesterolaemia, which is associated with an increased risk of atheromatous disease. There are a number of connective-tissue disorders associated with ectopia lentis (lens dislocation), including Marfan's and Ehlers–Danlos syndromes (both associated with aortic aneurysms and dissection, MVP and regurgitation) and homocysteinuria (associated with an increased risk of atheromatous disease). Exophthalmos may be indicative of underlying thyroid disease and the associated cardiac complications of hyperthyroidism, including tachyarrhythmias, atrial fibrillation and high-output cardiac failure.

Detection of these signs should prompt further investigation, including echocardiography, thyroid function, thyroid antibody testing and lipid profile analysis. A brief inspection should also be made of the oral cavity. Central cyanosis is unlikely to be found in any athlete presenting for evaluation, and so, whilst an important sign to elicit in cyanotic CHD, is of less relevance to this chapter.

Examination of the neck should be performed with the patient reclined at 45°. Carotid bruits may indicate underlying vascular disease in the older athlete, or may represent radiation of a cardiac murmur (e.g. in a stenosed BAV in the younger athlete). Assessment of the central venous pressure can be performed through an examination of the internal jugular vein. This runs along the anterior border of the sternal head of the sternocleidomastoid muscle, and enables an estimation of the right atrial pressure. The venous waveform can be difficult to detect: the neck should be relaxed and well-illuminated, and the head should be turned slightly to the left (if examining the right internal jugular vein). If the venous pressure is low, the waveform may not be apparent at all.

If the jugular venous pressure (JVP) is found to be elevated beyond 3 cm vertical height above the manubriosternal junction, a thorough examination of the cardiovascular system and an assessment of the volume status of the athlete should be performed, looking in particular for signs of valvular heart disease and cardiac failure. This should be followed with a 12-lead ECG and echocardiography. Finally, before leaving the neck, it is worth ensuring that there is no obvious goitre, since a significantly underactive or hyperactive thyroid gland can cause cardiovascular complications.

Examination of the Thorax

The thorax should be examined for scars, including thoracotomy scars, which are sometimes located in a very lateral position and may not be apparent on first inspection. A left thoracotomy scar may be found in previous coarctation repair or ligation of a patent ductus arteriosus, and a right thoracotomy scar may result from surgical closure of an atrial septal defect (ASD). In addition, minimal-access valve surgery is increasingly being used. The physician should be aware of the variety of scars that can be found as a result of this intervention. Typically, there may be three or four small scars over the right anterior chest wall and a further scar in the right or left groin, indicating the site of femoral artery cannulation. There may also be smaller, subcostal scars, indicative of chest or mediastinal drain insertion. A central sternotomy scar generally indicates more complex cardiac surgery. The athlete may not be able to recall the exact nature of any surgery performed, particularly if it was carried out at a young age.

A general inspection of the thorax also provides useful information about the shape of the thoracic cage. Chest-wall abnormalities, kyphosis and kyphoscoliosis can affect cardiorespiratory performance and may be indicative of an underlying syndrome (e.g. pectus carinatum is associated with Noonan's and Turner's syndromes).

Inherited Connective-Tissue Disorders

Scoliosis, kyphosis and chest-wall abnormalities (pectus excavatum and carinatum) are also found in inherited disorders of connective tissue and feature in the current diagnostic criteria for Marfan syndrome. However, these signs may occur in other inherited disorders of connective tissue, including Ehler–Danlos syndrome, the vascular subtype of which carries a significant risk of cardiovascular complications, including valvular abnormalities and aneurysms of small- and medium-sized arteries, the aorta and, sometimes, the coronary arteries.

If the examining physician elicits signs suggestive of a possible inherited connective-tissue disorder, a systematic clinical approach should follow. Attention must be paid to the family history, including questions regarding joint and skin laxity, easy bruising, acute severe medical or surgical events (such as chest pain or an acute abdomen) and a family history of sudden death due to a ruptured aneurysm. A more detailed examination of the musculoskeletal system is also indicated, including specific tests for joint hypermobility and measurements of vertical height and arm span. See Chapter 22 for further details on the clinical signs that can be elicited in Marfan syndrome.

If a connective-tissue disorder is suspected, the athlete may also be referred for a formal ophthalmology review to assess for myopia, corneal flattening and lens subluxation. An echocardiogram should be arranged to detect valvular abnormalities and to assess the size of the thoracic aorta. More detailed imaging of the aorta may be indicated if further clarification is needed. Most importantly, if there is a suspicion of an inherited connective-tissue disorder, the sports medicine physician should refer the athlete to a specialist for further assessment and possible genetic testing. The diagnosis of an inherited connective-tissue disorder has implications for the athlete, their eligibility to participate in sport and their family members.

Examination of the Heart

A systematic examination of the heart is an essential component of the physical examination of athletes. The unexpected death of an athlete due to previously undiagnosed cardiac disease is a catastrophe for all concerned. Whilst many of the causes of SCD, such as the ion channelopathies, are not associated with any physical signs for the clinician to detect, signs of congenital, valvular and heart muscle diseases can be found on careful physical examination. It is important to elicit these signs in any PPE of the athlete, or of the sedentary person about to embark upon an exercise programme.

An inspection should first be made for any visible pulsations, including the apex beat, having already examined the thorax for scars. The apex beat should then be palpated; this is normally located in the fifth intercostal space in the midclavicular line. Significant displacement of the apex beat may be indicative of an underlying cardiac pathology. The physician should palpate for thrills (palpable murmurs) at the apex, the left sternal edge and over the aortic valve. In addition, a right ventricular heave may be palpable at the left sternal edge. Following this, cardiac auscultation should be performed with a stethoscope of sufficient quality and in quiet surroundings. Each valve should be auscultated in turn, often beginning at the apex (mitral valve), then the lower and upper left sternal edge (tricuspid and pulmonary valves respectively) and finally the aortic valve (right upper sternal edge, second intercostal space).

Cardiac Auscultation

When listening to the heart, the physician should begin with auscultation of the first and second heart sounds, timing the heart sounds with the pulse. The first heart sound is created by closure of the mitral and tricuspid valves, marking the onset of systole. The second heart sound is generated by the closure of the aortic and pulmonary valves, signifying the end of systole. The timing of the pulse falls between the first and second heart sounds (i.e. during systole). Once the heart sounds have been correctly identified, any murmur present can then be classified as being systolic or diastolic.

A murmur is the noise created by turbulent blood flow and can be identified as the absence of silence between the heart sounds. This can occur in a structurally normal heart, often termed an 'innocent' or physiological flow murmur, and is a common finding in young people and healthy athletes. Flow murmurs are typically short, systolic murmurs, often heard at the upper or lower left sternal edge. They may vary with position and can become louder in febrile states, or with an increased resting cardiac output, as seen in well-trained endurance athletes and during pregnancy. The physician may seek reassurance from a lack of symptoms and a normal ECG. However, if there is any doubt as to the nature of the murmur, echocardiography should be arranged.

If a murmur is heard, then attention should be paid to the following features:

- *Timing:* Is the murmur systolic (occurring with the pulse) or diastolic?
- *Location:* Where is the murmur heard the loudest? Note, this may be a poor guide to the underlying causative pathology.
- *Radiation:* Does the murmur radiate elsewhere? Typically, the murmur of mitral regurgitation radiates to the axilla, whilst the murmur of aortic stenosis can often be heard in the carotid arteries.
- *Loudness:* Different grading schemes exist for scoring the intensity of murmurs. It is also important to note the duration; for example, a pansystolic murmur begins *with* the first heart sound and is of constant intensity throughout, whereas an ejection systolic murmur begins *after* the first heart sound, with a crescendo–decrescendo pattern.
- *Provocative manoeuvres:* Murmurs arising as a result of valvular pathology on the right side of the heart may increase in intensity on held inspiration (as blood flow to the right side of the heart increases). Similarly, left-sided heart murmurs may increase in intensity on held expiration (increasing flow to the left side of the heart). The murmur of aortic regurgitation is often best heard at the lower left sternal edge, with the patient leaning forward and in held expiration. The early diastolic rumble of mitral stenosis is most easily auscultated with the patient lying in the left lateral position and the stethoscope placed directly over the apex beat.

Table 36.1 lists some common causes of pathology giving rise to murmurs. If a murmur is identified by the examining sports medicine physician, a careful examination for signs of heart failure should be made and a 12-lead ECG and echo study arranged without delay. Onward formal cardiology referral can then be made,

Systolic murmurs (frequently benign, associated with increased stroke volume)	Diastolic murmurs (always pathological)
Mitral regurgitation: High-pitched, pansystolic murmur, usually loudest at the apex and radiating to the axilla	*Mitral stenosis*: Usually caused by rheumatic mitral valve disease and rare in athletes from the developed world. This is a low-pitched, diastolic rumble, most easily heard with the athlete in the left lateral position and with the stethoscope directly over the apex
Mitral valve prolapse (MVP): Classically causes a mid/late systolic click (the leaflet prolapsing), which may or may not be followed by a mid/late high-pitched systolic murmur of MR, loudest at the apex	
Tricuspid regurgitation: Lower-pitched systolic murmur, loudest at the lower left sternal edge and on held inspiration	*Tricuspid stenosis*: Rare. Most often caused by rheumatic valve disease and usually coexistent with TR
Aortic stenosis: Ejection systolic murmur over the aortic valve. May radiate to the carotids. If heard in an athlete, suspect BAV and listen specifically for aortic regurgitation	*Aortic regurgitation*: In athletes, most likely a result of a BAV. An early diastolic 'whooshing' murmur, best heard at the lower left sternal edge, with the patient leaning forwards and in held expiration
Pulmonary stenosis: Ejection systolic murmur, loudest at the upper left sternal edge. Common in Noonan's syndrome	*Pulmonary regurgitation*: Significant pulmonary regurgitation may be heard as a low-pitched diastolic murmur over the pulmonary valve
Atrial septal defect (ASD): Depending on the nature and location of the defect, can cause the murmurs of TR and MR. Commonly, due to increased flow through the right side of the heart, a systolic flow murmur across the pulmonary valve is the only audible feature	*Atrial septal defect (ASD)*: A large ASD may give rise to a diastolic rumble at the lower left sternal edge, caused by increased flow across the tricuspid valve
Ventricular septal defect (VSD): A large VSD will present in childhood, prohibiting vigorous exercise and requiring surgical repair. However, small, 'restrictive' VSDs can be followed up, often without need for surgery. They cause a loud, high-pitched, pansystolic murmur, loudest at the left sternal edge, and may be a dramatic finding in a healthy athlete	

Table 36.1 Common causes of pathology giving rise to murmurs

MR, mitral regurgitation; TR, tricuspid regurgitation; BAV, bicuspid aortic valve; ASD, atrial septal defect; VSD, ventricular septal defect.

depending on the findings. Continuous murmurs, audible throughout systole and diastole, are extremely uncommon, and are caused by a communication between the high-pressure arterial system and the low-pressure venous system. Causes include patent ductus arteriosus (which can rarely present in adulthood), pulmonary arteriovenous fistulae, ruptured sinus of Valsalva aneurysms and aortic coarctation with significant collateralisation. Referral to a CHD specialist is recommended in such cases, as the diagnosis may not be readily apparent on a standard transthoracic echo.

Hypertrophic Cardiomyopathy

Hypertrophic cardiomyopathy (HCM) is one of the commonest causes of SCD in athletes. Indeed, the unheralded collapse of an athlete on the field of play may be the first presentation of this potentially lethal condition. HCM causes characteristic changes on the ECG and cardiac echo. It is extensively described in Chapter 19. The sports medicine physician should be aware that HCM can cause a number of clinical signs which should be sought during the cardiovascular examination.

The apical impulse may be laterally displaced and abnormally forceful. A double apical impulse may be palpated, caused by vigorous left atrial contraction against a noncompliant ventricle. This same mechanism can give rise to a fourth heart sound. Involvement of the mitral valve apparatus in HCM is common, and the murmur of mitral regurgitation may be present.

If there is a significant gradient in the left ventricular outflow tract (LVOT), an ejection systolic murmur at the left sternal edge may be heard. This is similar to the murmur of aortic stenosis, with a crescendo–decrescendo pattern, but typically does not radiate to the carotids. Importantly, the murmur caused by an increased LVOT gradient is affected by preload and afterload. An increase in preload (e.g. squatting) or afterload (e.g. handgrip) will reduce the gradient and hence the intensity of the murmur. The converse applies, and a reduction in preload (standing or the valsalva manoeuvre) will increase the LVOT gradient and the intensity of the murmur. More advanced HCM may present with signs of heart failure and atrial arrhythmias, but individuals with these signs are unlikely to be participating in sport.

If the physician suspects the possibility of HCM, then, after a thorough family and personal history to elicit symptoms and a careful clinical examination, the next step is to carry out a 12-lead ECG. Further imaging with echocardiography is indicated. Cardiac magnetic resonance (CMR) should be performed if doubt remains. A normal echo does *not* exclude the disease, particularly if the athlete is symptomatic, the ECG is abnormal or the hypertrophy selectively affects the apex of the heart – an area that may not be clearly visualised on transthoracic echo.

The diagnosis of HCM can be difficult to make, especially in well-trained athletes with athletic cardiac remodelling. Furthermore, in younger patients, ECG changes may manifest before structural changes can be identified on imaging. This is a genetic, often inherited cardiomyopathy and, in addition to the important implications of a diagnosis for the athlete's eligibility to participate in sport, there are significant implications for the athlete's family members. Referral to a cardiologist with expertise in HCM is essential if the physician has any suspicion of this condition.

Added Heart Sounds

In a normal resting heart, only two heart sounds should be heard: the first and second heart sounds (S_1 and S_2), as previously described. S_1 has mitral and tricuspid components, S_2 aortic (A_2) and pulmonary (P_2) components. The separate components of the first heart sound can be heard individually in S_1 splitting: the mitral valve usually closes just before the tricuspid valve, but this difference is not often appreciable. A fixed, wide split of the second heart sound is characteristic of ASDs, but is not always audible. A_2 and P_2 may be unusually loud in systemic and pulmonary hypertension, respectively. In addition to the first and second heart sounds, two extra sounds (S_3 and S_4) occur in diastole, caused by rapid early and late ventricular filling, respectively. In well-trained athletes with high stroke volumes, a third heart sound may be heard. However, the presence of an added heart sound is not always normal in the athletic population and may be indicative of underlying cardiac disease.

In summary, systolic murmurs are common findings and are often benign. Diastolic murmurs are more difficult to detect and should never be dismissed as physiological flow murmurs, as they are always pathological.

If a murmur is auscultated, a thorough examination of the heart must be carried out, followed by a 12-lead ECG and echocardiography. If a *physiological* or *functional* ejection systolic murmur is suspected, conditions associated with increased stroke volume (and therefore increased flow across the aortic and pulmonary valves) should be excluded, including thyrotoxicosis, anaemia, pregnancy and fever.

Examination of the Lungs

A thorough examination of the cardiovascular system should include an examination of the lungs. The athlete who presents with chest pain, breathlessness, wheeze, cough, fatigue or a decline in athletic performance may have an underlying cardiac or respiratory condition, since all these symptoms can occur with disorders of either system. Therefore, any athlete presenting with such symptoms requires a thorough examination of both the respiratory and the cardiovascular systems. In addition, significant heart disease often leads to pulmonary sequelae. Cardiac conditions with increased flow to the lungs cause an increase in pulmonary artery pressure and eventual pulmonary hypertension. Similarly, left-sided heart disease leads to an increase in left atrial pressure and subsequent pulmonary oedema. The likelihood of pulmonary complications increases with the severity of the underlying cardiac condition and, perhaps not surprisingly, there is a corresponding decrease in the likelihood of these individuals presenting to the sports medicine physician.

The physician will already have inspected the patient for an increased respiratory rate and any chest-wall deformities and scars. Chest-wall expansion can be assessed and the athlete should then be sat forwards in order to examine the posterior chest wall. A further inspection for scars should be made; lateral thoracotomy scars can be easily missed if only the anterior chest wall is examined. In addition, the physician can examine for kyphoscoliosis (if not already done). The lungs should be percussed and then auscultated. For this, the athlete should be asked to breathe in and out, slowly, through an open mouth. All areas of the lungs should be examined. For the purposes of a cardiac examination, the bases of the lungs hold the most interest for cardiologists, sometimes revealing a dull percussion note and reduced breath sounds, with the bilateral pleural effusions occurring in right heart failure or the inspiratory crepitations found in left heart failure. Some cardiac murmurs can be heard over the posterior chest wall, including the murmurs of aortic coarctation, patent ductus arteriosus and, sometimes, severe mitral regurgitation.

The differential diagnosis of an athlete presenting with breathlessness, fatigue and a decline in athletic performance includes cardiac disease, but asthma should also be considered. Asthma typically causes breathlessness with an *expiratory* wheeze on examination and may be induced or exacerbated by exercise. This is in contrast to another condition, common in athletes and often misdiagnosed as asthma: vocal cord dysfunction. This condition is characterised by a difficulty *breathing in* and is associated with stridor (inspiratory noise) rather than wheeze (expiratory noise), as well as throat tightness and changes in the voice or difficulty speaking. This difference is diagnostically important and should be readily apparent with careful history-taking and examination. Any athlete complaining of breathlessness merits a full cardiac and respiratory evaluation. If the heart is found to be normal in structure and function, then the athlete should be referred to a respiratory specialist for further evaluation and lung function studies.

Examination of the Abdomen

For the cardiologist, palpation and auscultation of the abdomen is an important part of the cardiovascular system examination. However, most of the clinical signs in the abdomen are unlikely to be found in the competitive athlete. Congestive cardiac failure leads to hepatic congestion and hepatomegaly, severe tricuspid regurgitation can cause a pulsatile liver and infective endocarditis may lead to hepatosplenomegaly. For the sports medicine physician, any athlete with hypertension should undergo auscultation of the renal arteries to examine for renal artery bruits, noting that the absence of a bruit does not exclude a haemodynamically significant stenosis.

Examination of the Lower Limbs

As previously discussed, when considering the possibility of coarctation of the aorta, the femoral pulses should be palpated, with simultaneous palpation of the radial pulse, and a blood pressure measurement of the lower limb should be taken. The young, competitive, nonsmoking athlete is unlikely to have PVD and, unless complaining of claudicant symptoms, does not warrant further examination of the peripheral pulses. However, if an older recreational athlete presents with claudicant symptoms, atherosclerosis is the most likely cause. In this case, all peripheral pulses should be examined and ankle brachial pressure indices (ABPIs) arranged, along with a cholesterol profile, glucose measurement and lifestyle advice, where indicated. Onward referral to a vascular surgeon may be considered.

Iliac Artery Insufficiency

If a competitive athlete is complaining of claudication or weakness of the lower limbs during exercise, particularly if they are a cyclist, then they should be examined for signs of iliac artery insufficiency. This condition is principally found in competitive cyclists, but has been described in other sports, including long-distance running and speed skating. In contrast to conventional peripheral (atheromatous) vascular disease, the underlying pathology is usually endofibrosis and can be associated with abnormal vessel kinking during hip-flexion activity. The athlete usually presents with exertional lower limb pain, affecting the thigh and sometimes also the calf and buttock. The pain is claudicant in nature and is often described as a feeling of 'lactic acid in the muscles', typically associated with loss of power. Symptoms resolve quickly with rest and are predictable, occurring at a particular exercise intensity. Important differential diagnoses include piriformis syndrome and lumbar radiculopathy.

If an athlete presents with these symptoms, the sports medicine physician should examine carefully for a femoral bruit. The patient should be supine, with the hip in a neutral position. Such a finding is highly specific for endofibrosis in the appropriate clinical context. The femoral bruit typically becomes significantly louder as the hip is moved into flexion, but a femoral bruit that is *only* audible in hip flexion is a far less specific finding. However, the examination can be normal even in the presence of significant symptoms. If an athlete presents with symptoms – with or without signs – suggestive of this condition, post-exercise ABPIs should be arranged and the athlete should be referred on to a vascular surgeon with expertise in this field for further evaluation.

Popliteal artery entrapment is an uncommon condition that presents with claudication symptoms in a young or athletic population. In contrast to iliac artery insufficiency, symptoms are usually isolated to the calf. The reader is referred to recent reviews for further information [9]. Finally, a routine check for pedal oedema should be made; this is a classic sign of right heart failure, but is also found in renal disease (which may occur as a cause or consequence of hypertension). Peripheral oedema is more likely to be positional in a healthy athlete, particularly if it disappears with exercise.

Conclusion

A careful examination of the cardiovascular system is essential in the PPE of competitive athletes and in the assessment of the athlete presenting with symptoms of chest pain, breathlessness, syncope, fatigue or a decline in athletic performance. It is perhaps even more relevant to the previously sedentary individual presenting for evaluation prior to participation in an exercise programme.

Any assessment of the cardiovascular system should begin with a careful personal and family history, with an overall assessment of cardiovascular risk where clinically indicated, followed by a systematic approach to the clinical examination. The assessment should be completed by a 12-lead ECG, which, when performed on a well-trained athlete, should be interpreted in accordance with current international guidelines. Further imaging can be arranged where necessary. Finally, if cardiac disease is suspected or identified, the athlete should be referred to the appropriate specialist for expert assessment, management, advice on eligibility to continue participation in sport and long-term follow-up.

References

1 Corrado, D., Pellicia, A., Bjornstad, H.H. et al. Cardiovascular pre-participation screening of young competitive athletes for prevention of sudden death: proposal for a common European protocol. Consensus statement of the Study Group of Sports Cardiology of the Working Group of Cardiac Rehabilitation and Exercise Physiology and the Working Group of Myocardial and Pericardial diseses of the European Society of Cardiology. *Eur Heart J* 2005; **26**: 516–24.

2 Loeys, B.L., Dietz, H.C., Braverman, A.C. et al. The revised Ghent nosology for the Marfan syndrome. *J Med Genet* 2010; **47**(7): 476–85.

3 Jensen, M.T., Suadicani, P., Hein, H.O. and Gyntelberg, F. Elevated resting heart rate, physical fitness and all-cause mortality: a 16 year follow-up in the Copenhagen Male Study. *Heart* 2013; **99**: 882–7.

4 Mancia, G., Fagard, R., Narkiewicz, K. et al. ESH/ESC Task Force for the Management of Arterial Hypertension. 2013 Practice guidelines for the management of arterial hypertension of the European Society of Hypertension (ESH) and the European Society of Cardiology (ESC): ESH/ESC Task Force for the Management of Arterial Hypertension. *J Hypertens* 2013; **31**(10): 1925–38.

5 James, P.A., Oparil, S., Carter, B.L. et al. 2014 Evidence-based guideline for the management of high blood pressure in adults: report from the Panel Members Appointed to the Eighth Joint National Committee (JNC 8). *JAMA* 2014; **311**(5): 507–20.

6 Maron, B.J. and Zipes, D.P. 36th Bethesda Conference eligibility recommendations for competitive athletes with cardiovascular abnormalities. *J Am Coll Cardiol* 2005; **45**: 1311–75.

7 Pelliccia, A., Fagard, R., Bjørnstad, H.H. et al. Recommendations for competitive sports participation in athletes with cardiovascular disease. A consensus document from the Study Group of Sports Cardiology of the Working Group of Cardiac Rehabilitation and Exercise Physiology and the Working Group of Myocardial and Pericardial Diseases of the European Society of Cardiology. *Eur Heart J* 2005; **26**: 1422–45.

8 Bonow, R., Mann, D., Zipes, D. et al. *Braunwald's Heart Disease*. Philadelphia, PA: Elsevier, 2012.

9 Hislop, M., Kennedy, D., Cramp, B. and Dhuphelia, S. Functional popliteal artery entrapment syndrome: poorly understood and frequently missed? A review of clinical features, appropriate investigations, and treatment options. *J Sports Med* 2014; **2014**: 105953.

37 Management of Atrial Fibrillation in Athletes

Eduard Guasch[1] and Lluis Mont[2]

[1]Unitat de Fibril·lació Auricular, Hospital Clinic, University of Barcelona, Barcelona, Catalonia, Spain
[2]Institut d'Investigacions Biomèdiques August Pi i Sunyer (IDIBAPS), Barcelona, Catalonia, Spain

Introduction

Atrial fibrillation is the most frequent sustained arrhythmia in clinical practice and affects as many as 33.5 million individuals worldwide. The arrhythmia exhibits an age-related prevalence, which rises from 1.5% in the 5th decade of life to approximately 20% in those aged >85 years. Given the prevailing demographic, life-expectancy and heart-disease burden trends, the number of patients with atrial fibrillation could double by 2060 if the age- and sex-specific prevalence remains stable.

A diagnosis of atrial fibrillation is associated with a fivefold increase in the risk of ischaemic stroke. Long-term and severe disabling symptoms are more frequent after stroke in patients with atrial fibrillation compared to those with sinus rhythm. Additionally, patients with atrial fibrillation have a twofold increase in all-cause mortality, and the arrhythmia is associated with a substantial increase in health care costs. The national cost of atrial fibrillation is estimated at $6–26 billion in the US and approximately £450 million in the UK. In 2000, costs relating to the management of atrial fibrillation accounted for 1% of total National Health Service (NHS) budget in the UK.

Hypertension and structural heart disease are the most common causes of atrial fibrillation. Nevertheless, in up to one-third of cases, atrial fibrillation cannot be explained by hypertension or structural disease; this is frequently referred to as 'idiopathic atrial fibrillation'. An increasing number of newly recognised aetiologies for atrial fibrillation, such as obstructive sleep apnoea, obesity and tall stature, were formerly considered idiopathic atrial fibrillation.

Recent evidence suggests that lifelong exercise may be implicated as an aetiologic factor for atrial fibrillation. An association between endurance training and atrial fibrillation was first suggested in veteran Finnish orienteers [1], who were found to have a higher than expected incidence of atrial fibrillation in the absence of structural heart disease. In parallel, our group confirmed this association in a case–control study and demonstrated a higher proportion of athletes in a cohort of 'lone atrial fibrillation' patients than in the age- and sex-matched Catalan population [2]. We subsequently demonstrated a high risk of atrial fibrillation in trained athletes in a prospective study which included marathon runners. Athletes who had run the 1992 Barcelona Marathon had an 8.8-fold higher risk of being diagnosed with atrial fibrillation after an 11-year follow-up in comparison to a sedentary cohort reporting <300 kcal.day^{-1} of physical activity [3]. Further small studies from our group and others confirmed this association in elite cyclists [4], skiers [5], handball players [6] and other athletes. Overall, these reports show that top-level athletes have a three- to eightfold increased risk of atrial fibrillation.

IOC Manual of Sports Cardiology, First Edition. Edited by Mathew G. Wilson, Jonathan A. Drezner and Sanjay Sharma.
© 2017 International Olympic Committee. Published 2017 by John Wiley & Sons, Ltd.

The association between endurance exercise and atrial fibrillation was highly debated in the scientific community until the publication of large epidemiological studies involving thousands of individuals, which have consistently demonstrated a higher atrial fibrillation incidence in the group with the highest load of physical activity [7–10]. Aizer et al. [7] first found a progressive increase in comorbidity-adjusted atrial fibrillation risk with increasingly higher amounts of daily jogging. Andersen et al. [8] confirmed a dose–risk response within a highly trained athlete cohort. Those who competed at a higher level and reached higher performance were at twice the risk of developing atrial fibrillation as those who engaged in lower physical activity levels. The largest published study analysed over 300 000 middle-aged Norwegian men and women included in a large nationwide health screening programme. Those men who self-reported practising intensive exercise had a 3.1 hazard risk of being prescribed flecainide, a surrogate marker for the diagnosis of atrial fibrillation [10].

The association between atrial fibrillation and exercise appears to exhibit a U-shaped curve [11]. The risk of atrial fibrillation seems to be confined to high-intensity physical activity. Conversely, regular, moderate exercise may protect against atrial fibrillation by impacting positively on the risk of ischaemic heart disease and hypertension. Recent data suggest that the most active elderly individuals are protected from atrial fibrillation [12] in a dose-dependent manner. In the elderly, the benefits of exercise with respect to preventing heart disease probably outweigh the direct atrial fibrillation-promoting mechanisms. A healthy-individual bias may be involved, however, as older individuals suffering comorbidities such as atrial fibrillation are less prone to exercise. This protective effect is supported by a large body of evidence, including meta-analyses [13].

Epidemiology and Relevance

The prevalence of atrial fibrillation amongst exercising individuals is not evenly distributed but appears to be concentrated in specific subgroups, characteristically middle-aged individuals. The average age at presentation of atrial fibrillation ranges from the 4th to the 6th decade of life in most studies in athletes (Figure 37.1) [2,4,7,8,14]. A former history of high-intensity exercise for a variable time, generally endurance training for more than 10 years, is a common finding. Atrial fibrillation may be diagnosed many years after finishing high-intensity training [2,9]. Conversely, atrial fibrillation is uncommon in young athletes [15], suggesting that regular high-intensity exercise slowly promotes an atrial proarrhythmogenic substrate over >10 years of intensive training. Experimental data in an animal model of high-intensity running are consistent with this hypothesis. Exercise only promoted an arrhythmogenic substrate after 16 weeks of running (roughly equivalent to 10 years in human), but not at the 4 or 8 weeks' training time-points [16]. Whilst high-intensity exercise has been estimated to convey a two- to eightfold increase in atrial fibrillation risk, the contribution of high-intensity exercise to atrial fibrillation prevalence in the general population remains unknown. Large registries focusing on this issue have not been constructed. Moreover, exercise-induced atrial fibrillation has no definite, strict diagnostic criteria. A large variety of definitions of high-intensity exercise-induced atrial fibrillation have been used, but standardised diagnostic criteria are required to obtain robust prevalence data. However, rough estimations can be obtained from small studies.

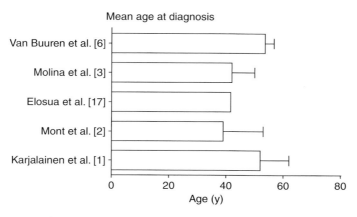

Figure 37.1 Publications reporting mean age at diagnosis of exercise-induced atrial fibrillation

In a cohort of patients with atrial fibrillation without structural heart disease or hypertension, we found a long-lasting endurance exercise history in roughly 30–40% of cases [2,11]. The increase in the number of amateur endurance runners is paving the way for a future rise in the incidence of exercise-induced atrial fibrillation. The number of runners in the US who have completed a marathon has increased 20-fold in the last 30 years, and similar values are probably valid for Europe. If a similar trend is maintained, and considering that the atrial arrhythmogenic substrate slowly progresses throughout 10 or more years of high-intensity exercise, the prevalence of exercise-induced atrial fibrillation is likely to increase exponentially in the future.

Clinical Presentation

Clinical manifestations of atrial fibrillation in athletes range from being asymptomatic to severe disabling hypotension and syncope. Palpitations and fatigue are the most common symptoms. Atrial fibrillation is amongst the most frequent causes of longstanding palpitations in young elite athletes [18]. Fatigue and decreased maximal exercise performance are common complaints in individuals engaged in competitive sports. Half of all sufferers report reducing their physical activity as a consequence of arrhythmia symptoms, eventually leading to discontinuation of exercise [14]. Atrial contraction contributes up to 40% of left ventricle filling volume during exercise. Consequently, loss of atrial contraction during atrial fibrillation rhythm may lead to a significantly reduced cardiac output during exercise and physical performance. In this regard, successful cardioversion of patients with atrial fibrillation associates to a 30% increase in maximal exercise capacity.

A minority of athletes with atrial fibrillation report being asymptomatic [14]. However, in a cohort of patients with allegedly 'asymptomatic' persistent atrial fibrillation, those who remained in sinus rhythm after an ablation procedure showed a roughly 20% increase in objective markers of exercise capacity [19].

The most widely accepted classification of atrial fibrillation is based on the clinical evolution pattern. Atrial fibrillation may present as a self-limiting (<7 days) arrhythmia (*paroxysmal atrial fibrillation*) or a sustained arrhythmia that requires therapeutic intervention to return to sinus rhythm (*persistent atrial fibrillation*). Patients in whom attempts to restore sinus rhythm have been abandoned are said to have *permanent atrial fibrillation*. The autonomic tone balance plays a critical role in triggering atrial fibrillation episodes, and both sympathetic and parasympathetic tone enhancements may initiate bouts of atrial fibrillation. Onset of atrial fibrillation in situations in which the parasympathetic tone is dominant, such as during sleep or after meals, is a common presentation in athletes [2,18,20]. Sympathetic-triggered episodes during intense exercise or other predominantly adrenergic situations are also frequently reported by affected athletes.

Stroke is the most serious complication of atrial fibrillation. Most athletes with atrial fibrillation will be classified into low-risk groups based on the absence of structural heart disease and young age. It is noteworthy that exhausting exercise, such as marathon-running, promotes a transient prothrombotic status in which the ischaemic heart rate is increased. At the present time, however, we do not have data on a specific thromboembolic risk status for athletes.

Pathology

The mechanisms by which exercise promotes the development of an atrial arrhythmogenic substrate have yet to be studied in detail. Some mechanisms have been proposed, but the level of evidence is low and their contribution to exercise-induced atrial fibrillation pathology is still speculative.

Some authors suggest that exercise-induced atrial fibrillation is supported by an extreme, yet physiological, form of cardiac adaptation to exercise (so called 'athlete's heart'). Nevertheless, recent data suggest that an additive, pathological substrate might develop after extremely high sustained hemodynamic loads of exercise [16].

Some of the characteristics encompassed in the physiological remodelling of the athlete's heart have been shown to potentially promote atrial fibrillation. For instance, dilated atria and bradycardia increase cardiac output reserve and exercise capacity in athletes. Dilated atria increase the atrial muscle mass, thereby increasing the substrate in which atrial fibrillation can be established. Nevertheless, atrial dilation beyond normal range is common in highly trained athletes in the absence of clinical arrhythmic events [18], suggesting that atrial dilation may contribute to the atrial arrhythmogenic substrate but needs additional factors to sustain atrial fibrillation. On the other hand, parasympathetic tone enhancement occurs early after initiating regular physical activity. Increased parasympathetic tone shortens atrial action potential and effective refractory period, facilitating re-entry formation and atrial fibrillation. A recent experimental report highlighted parasympathetic enhancement as a critical factor in exercise-induced atrial fibrillation instauration [16].

Extreme forms of exercise may induce distinct, pathological remodelling. Atrial fibrosis is a cornerstone of atrial fibrillation substrate, inducing slower, heterogeneous electrical conduction throughout the atria, and hence facilitating re-entry formation and atrial fibrillation. A recent study in an animal model showed the development of atrial interstitial fibrosis as a consequence of high-intensity exercise [16]. After 16 weeks of endurance training in a treadmill, rats developed increased susceptibility to inducible atrial fibrillation. Trained rats showed larger atria and enhanced parasympathetic tone – but also increased atrial interstitial fibrosis – in comparison to sedentary rats. Scarring after high-intensity exercise clearly denotes pathologic adaptation. These results are still to be reproduced in humans, but are supported by recent data in highly trained athletes. P-wave duration, a surrogate for total atrial conduction time, is specifically prolonged in the most physically active athletes [21]. P-wave duration has been shown to correlate to atrial fibrosis in atrial surgical samples. Plasma PICP-I, CITP-I and TIMP-1 [22] are profibrotic markers that have been reported to be increased in veteran and top-level athletes. Unfortunately, a cardiac origin for these biomarkers has not been demonstrated, and further research is warranted.

Very high-intensity bouts of exercise promote transient, intensity-dependent proinflammatory and immuno-suppressive systemic effects. Some authors have speculated about the role of repetitive inflammatory insults in the development of an atrial arrhythmogenic substrate. Indeed, inflammatory infiltrates have been detected in atrial specimens from patients with atrial fibrillation and no structural heart disease, but not yet in specimens from athletes. On the other hand, it has been suggested that silent, limited myocarditis may occur after transient immunosuppression following exhausting endurance exercise.

Therapeutic Approach

General Approach and Therapeutic Aims

The therapeutic objectives and strategies in athletes with atrial fibrillation are as per general clinical guidelines for all patients with atrial fibrillation [23]. However, the nature of individuals affected with exercise-induced atrial fibrillation merits specific consideration. Particular details concerning the long-term management of atrial fibrillation in athletes are summarised in Figure 37.2.

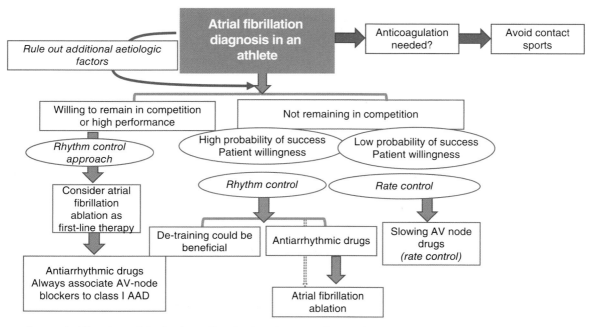

Figure 37.2 Therapeutic approach to patients with exercise-induced atrial fibrillation

Atrial fibrillation is diagnosed by obtaining an ECG, which will typically record absence of P-waves, irregular baseline f-waves and irregular RR cycles. The diagnosis of atrial fibrillation in young or middle-aged individuals should prompt a detailed clinical examination, even when the clinical suspicion of exercise-induced atrial fibrillation is high. Exercise-induced atrial fibrillation usually presents in individuals without structural heart disease, adopting an idiopathic atrial fibrillation-like phenotype. Nevertheless, concomitant, alternative causes of atrial fibrillation should be pursued. Treatable diseases such as obstructive sleep apnoea, undetected hypertension and thyrotoxicosis, or nonreversible ones such as a strong genetic component, need to be assessed before establishing high-intensity exercise as the sole cause of atrial fibrillation. Echocardiography should be performed in all affected individuals in order to assess left atrial size, but also to rule out acquired or congenital underlying structural heart disease. If symptoms appear during exercise, an exercise test or long-term recording during physical activity may provide a diagnosis. An exercise stress test is also useful for assessing ventricular rate during exercise in active individuals who opt out of rate control.

The therapeutic approach should involve two main considerations: therapy for the arrhythmia itself and reduction of the risk of systemic thromboembolism.

Arrhythmia Therapy

A patient with atrial fibrillation can be approached through a *rhythm-control* or a *rate-control* strategy. Whilst a rhythm-control approach pursues restoration and maintenance of sinus rhythm, rate control accepts atrial fibrillation as baseline rhythm and aims to achieve a heart rate within a physiological range. At this point in time, there is no consistent evidence supporting a rhythm- or rate-control strategy in terms of survival or prevention of complications, but ongoing trials (EAST -NCT01288352- and CABANA -NCT00911508-) will provide further data and refine criteria for an objective decision scheme selection.

In this scenario, the therapeutic approach should aim to relieve symptoms and improve quality of life. The decision between rhythm- and rate-control therapy (Figure 37.2) should be individualised, and the participation of the patient in the therapeutic decision should be encouraged. As previously stated, atrial fibrillation will likely impair physical fitness in most individuals and will steer therapy towards a rhythm-control regimen in those willing to maintain a high physical activity performance. On the other hand, rate control might be acceptable in those who remain asymptomatic and are not in need of high physical activity performance. Clinical and imaging data may provide objective arguments in certain circumstances. For example, long-lasting persistent atrial fibrillation (>1 year with continuous atrial fibrillation) or very dilated atria (left atrial anteroposterior diameter >50 mm in transthoracic echocardiography) substantially increase atrial fibrillation recurrence rate and may make sinus rhythm restoration and long-term maintenance unlikely in some patients.

Lifestyle Modification From a theoretical point of view, a certain disease might stabilise or even regress if the exposure to its aetiologic factor is reduced or avoided. If true for exercise-induced atrial fibrillation, this would strongly advocate for discontinuation of high-intensity exercise in affected individuals. Unfortunately, studies addressing this issue are lacking, and concrete evidence underlying a recommendation for exercise discontinuation is still required. Only experimental research and a study in the clinical setting suggest a benefit from stopping high-intensity exercise in secondary atrial fibrillation prevention. The role of deconditioning was studied in an animal model of atrial fibrillation induced by high-intensity endurance training. Rats were more prone to atrial fibrillation inducibility in an electrophysiology (EP) study after running in a treadmill for 16 weeks, but regressed to control values a little after 4 weeks of deconditioning [16]. These results in the experimental setting are supported by a clinical observational study. In athletes undergoing atrial flutter ablation, Heidbuchel et al. [24] showed that those who continued to practise physical activity were more likely to develop subsequent atrial fibrillation. Conversely, the risk of atrial fibrillation in those who stopped training was similar to that in the nonathletic population.

Atrial dilation and fibrosis, parasympathetic enhancement and proinflammatory bouts are potential contributors to atrial fibrillation arrhythmogenic substrate. Their complete or partial regression after stopping regular exercise may provide surrogate indicators for a benefit of physical activity deconditioning in the therapy of atrial fibrillation. Atrial dilatation regresses, although incompletely, after deconditioning, and similar results have been found for atrial fibrosis in an experimental animal model [16]. Parasympathetic enhancement regresses shortly after finishing regular intense physical activity.

Even if a benefit were demonstrated for high-intensity exercise discontinuation, important barriers to its implementation should be considered. Professional athletes are unwilling to decondition due to financial losses. Up to 40% of athletes exhibit negative addiction to exercise (NAEx) symptoms. Affected athletes continue to run despite serious physical injuries and social isolation, eventually developing anxiety and depressive symptoms when training cannot be completed. In these athletes, the diagnosis of atrial fibrillation may have little impact on their will to retire. In either case, athletes would likely desire a definitive therapy aimed at 'curing' atrial fibrillation and permitting sport participation.

The usefulness of exercise discontinuation is subject to an early diagnosis. Once atrial fibrillation episodes occur, fibrillatory activity promotes self-perpetuating mechanisms (*atrial fibrillation begets atrial fibrillation*) that eventually lead to a deep atrial remodelling and structural disorganisation. Exercise discontinuation at this stage is likely futile. However, adherence to moderate doses of physical activity is to be encouraged, in order to prevent acquired risk factors for coronary disease.

Pharmacological Therapy Antiarrhythmic agents are first line in both rate and rhythm control strategies for atrial fibrillation. It is worth noting that the efficacy and side effects of antiarrhythmic drugs have not been specifically tested in athletes. Drugs aimed at restoring or maintaining sinus rhythm include class I antiarrhythmics such as flecainide and propafenone and class III agents such as amiodarone, dronedarone and sotalol. Beta blockers, calcium antagonists and digoxin are commonly used in a rate-control strategy due to their atrioventricular (AV) node slowing conduction properties.

Some antiarrhythmic drugs exert deleterious haemodynamic effects that may impact on exercise performance. The negative inotropic effects of flecainide and propafenone are recognised. Flecainide significantly blunts chronotropic response and prolongs QRS duration during exercise [25]. Propafenone provides a mild vagolytic effect that can yield additional benefits in the parasympathetic enhancement found in patients with atrial fibrillation induced by exercise. Type I antiarrhythmics should be prescribed in conjunction with AV nodal blocking drugs (such as beta blockers) to reduce the risk of 1 : 1 AV conduction in the event of atrial flutter, which can degenerate to ventricular fibrillation and sudden death. Amiodarone is not associated with deleterious haemodynamic effects during exercise, but the side-effect profile of the drug makes it undesirable for chronic use in young patients.

In athletes with infrequent, symptomatic atrial fibrillation relapses, a *pill-in-the-pocket* approach may serve to limit the negative inotropic and chronotropic effects of type I antiarrhythmic drugs. Self-administered flecainide or propafenone shortly after beginning arrhythmia symptoms might safely restore sinus rhythm in those patients in whom heart disease has been ruled out. Nevertheless, sinus bradycardia in athletes prompts an initial test in a monitored environment in order to exclude adverse arrhythmic events.

Beta blockers are frequently used to reduce heart rate during episodes of atrial fibrillation, but they reduce exercise tolerance in individuals without structural heart disease [26] by reducing both the chorontropic and inotropic effects of catecholeamines and possibly decreasing hyperventilation during exercise. Nondihydro-piridinic calcium-channel blockers also possess negative chronotropic and inotropic properties, but a recent randomised study showed their superiority in terms of exercise tolerance in comparison to beta blockers [27]. Nevertheless, sinus bradycardia and Wenckebach-type AV block in athletes may limit the use of beta blockers and nondihydropiridinic calcium-channel blockers in these patients. Digoxin is rarely used due to its low AV node-slowing efficacy during exercise and reports showing increased mortality from its use.

It is important to discuss with competitive athletes the fact that some antiarrhythmic drugs are prohibited by the World Anti-Doping Agency (WADA). At present, beta blockers are the only antiarrhythmic drugs prohibited in a few sports, such as shooting, darts, billiards and golf.

Whilst classic antiarrhythmic drugs aim to prevent atrial fibrillation episodes by acting on basic electrophysiological properties at the ion-channel level and promoting membrane stabilisation, upstream therapies target the development of the atrial structural substrate sustaining atrial fibrillation. Prevention or regression of atrial arrhythmogenic substrate is particularly desirable in those athletes not willing to stop exercising, in whom remodelling will continue. Experiments in trained rats demonstrate that the angiotensin II receptor blocker (ARB) losartan prevents exercise-induced right ventricular fibrosis, and suggest a similar effect in the atria [28]. Confirmatory results have not been published in humans.

Nonpharmacological Therapy Nonpharmacological strategies, particularly atrial fibrillation ablation, have evolved as a cornerstone of atrial fibrillation therapy. Pulmonary vein isolation was first shown to reduce atrial fibrillation burden in patients with paroxysmal atrial fibrillation. Substrate modification with linear lesions and a variety of novel techniques have since been proposed for patients with a more advanced substrate. Both catheter and surgical ablation techniques have proved effective and yield a better antiarrhythmic effect than any other drug in patients with either paroxysmal or persistent atrial fibrillation. Due to a higher complication rate, atrial fibrillation ablation is commonly reserved for patients who remain symptomatic after being on at least one antiarrhythmic drug.

Whether atrial fibrillation ablation is as effective in athletes as in other patients with atrial fibrillation was first addressed by our group [29]. We demonstrated that atrial fibrillation ablation yields a similar success rate in athletes and sedentary patients without structural heart disease. Later studies confirmed our results and suggested that non-endurance athletes were more likely to revert back to atrial fibrillation than were endurance athletes [30]. Overall, atrial fibrillation ablation may enable competitive athletes to resume training and return to regular competition [31], and it appears an attractive approach for those athletes keen to remain active in whom antiarrhythmic drugs might impair their competitive status. Atrial fibrillation ablation may be considered as a first-line therapy in competitive athletes after the risks and benefits have been explained by the treating physician and considered by the patient. Indeed, a role for atrial fibrillation ablation in athletes is endorsed in the recently published atrial fibrillation clinical guidelines [23].

Prevention of Thromboembolic Complications

Prevention of thromboembolic complications is a critical aspect of atrial fibrillation management in all patients, including athletes. Current guidelines support the use of the CHA_2DS_2-VASc (**C**ongestive heart failure; **H**ypertension; **A**ge >75 – **2 points**; **D**iabetes; **S**troke – **2 points**; **V**ascular disease; **A**ge 65–75; **S**ex category female) scheme for decision-taking. Chronic anticoagulation is mandatory in those individuals with a score >1. The decision for patients with 1 point should be individualised. On the basis of low comorbidity and young age, anticoagulation will not usually be required in the long-term management of athletes. Nevertheless, anticoagulation may be needed for short periods of time in low-risk athletes undergoing cardioversion (if the epsiode of atrial fibrillation lasted for more than 48 hours) or atrial fibrillation ablation procedures. Whilst receiving anticoagulant drugs, atrial fibrillation patients should avoid collision sports.

Prevention

The main aim when considering atrial fibrillation in athletes is to prevent the development of the arrhythmia, rather than to treat it. Whilst an exercise dose–atrial fibrillation risk relationship has been suggested, there are no consistent data showing the existence of a risk threshold. Some reports demonstrate that atrial fibrillation risk increases after 1500 hours of lifetime cumulated intensive exercise [3]. Epidemiological studies have reported an increased risk after competing in 1 hour of exercise per day [9] or >5 hours of jogging per week [7]. However, it is likely that the dose–response curve is continuous. Overall, we do not believe that current evidence is strong enough to provide physical activity limits as a general measure for the primary prevention of atrial fibrillation.

Conclusion

Although the benefits of exercise are well recognised, there is evidence from small cohorts and large epidemiological studies that longstanding endurance exercise is associated with an increased prevalence of atrial fibrillation in middle-aged and older athletes. Atrial dilation and fibrosis, parasympathetic tone enhancement and inflammatory insults have been suggested to mediate this association.

The therapeutic approach is largely driven by patient decision, symptoms and the patient's desire to continue to engage in competitive sport. A strong evidence-based recommendation for discontinuation of high-intensity exercise is lacking, with the guidelines based on small studies and surrogate markers. Most antiarrhythmic drugs impair performance, so there is a move towards more invasive yet potentially curative approaches, such as atrial fibrillation ablation. The need for anticoagulation should be assessed on the basis of the CHA_2DS_2VASc scheme, and contact sports are forbidden in athletes who are anticoagulated.

References

1 Karjalainen, J., Kujala, U.M., Kaprio, J. et al. Lone atrial fibrillation in vigorously exercising middle aged men: case-control study. *BMJ* 1998; **316**(7147): 1784–5.

2 Mont, L., Sambola, A., Brugada, J. et al. Long-lasting sport practice and lone atrial fibrillation. *Eur Heart J* 2002; **23**(6): 477–82.

3 Molina, L., Mont, L., Marrugat, J. et al. Long-term endurance sport practice increases the incidence of lone atrial fibrillation in men: a follow-up study. *Europace* 2008; **10**(5): 618–23.

4 Baldesberger, S., Bauersfeld, U., Candinas, R. et al. Sinus node disease and arrhythmias in the long-term follow-up of former professional cyclists. *Eur Heart J* 2008; **29**(1): 71–8.

5 Grimsmo, J., Grundvold, I., Maehlum, S. and Arnesen, H. High prevalence of atrial fibrillation in long-term endurance cross-country skiers: echocardiographic findings and possible predictors – a 28–30 years follow-up study. *Eur J Cardiovasc Prev Rehabil* 2010; **17**(1): 100–5.

6 van Buuren, F., Mellwig, K.P., Faber, L. et al. The occurrence of atrial fibrillation in former top-level handball players above the age of 50. *Acta Cardiol* 2012; **67**(2): 213–20.

7 Aizer, A., Gaziano, J.M., Cook, N.R. et al. Relation of vigorous exercise to risk of atrial fibrillation. *Am J Cardiol* 2009; **103**(11): 1572–7.

8 Andersen, K., Farahmand, B., Ahlbom, A. et al. Risk of arrhythmias in 52 755 long-distance cross-country skiers: a cohort study. *Eur Heart J* 2013; **34**(47): 3624–31.

9 Drca, N., Wolk, A., Jensen-Urstad, M. and Larsson, S.C. Atrial fibrillation is associated with different levels of physical activity levels at different ages in men. *Heart* 2014; **100**(13): 1037–42.

10 Thelle, D.S., Selmer, R., Gjesdal, K. et al. Resting heart rate and physical activity as risk factors for lone atrial fibrillation: a prospective study of 309 540 men and women. *Heart* 2013; **99**(23): 1755–60.

11 Calvo, N., Ramos, P., Montserrat, S. et al. Emerging risk factors and the dose.response relationship between physical activity and lone atrial fibrillation: a prospective case.control study. *Europace* 2016; **18**(1): 57–63.

12 Mozaffarian, D., Furberg, C.D., Psaty, B.M. and Siscovick, D. Physical activity and incidence of atrial fibrillation in older adults: the cardiovascular health study. *Circulation* 2008; **118**(8): 800–7.

13 Ofman, P., Khawaja, O., Rahilly-Tierney, C.R. et al. Regular physical activity and risk of atrial fibrillation: a systematic review and meta-analysis. *Circ Arrhythm Electrophysiol* 2013; **6**(2): 252–6.

14 Hoogsteen, J., Schep, G., Van Hemel, N.M. and Van Der Wall, E.E. Paroxysmal atrial fibrillation in male endurance athletes. A 9-year follow up. *Europace* 2004; **6**(3): 222–8.

15 Pelliccia, A., Maron, B.J., Di Paolo, F.M. et al. Prevalence and clinical significance of left atrial remodeling in competitive athletes. *J Am. Coll. Cardiol* 2005; **46**(4): 690–6.

16 Guasch, E., Benito, B., Qi, X.Y. et al. Atrial fibrillation promotion by endurance exercise: demonstration and mechanistic exploration in an animal model. *J Am Coll Cardiol* 2013; **62**(1): 68–77.

17 Elosua, R., Arquer, A., Mont, L. et al. Sport practice and the risk of lone atrial fibrillation: a case-control study. *Int J Cardiol* 2006; **108**(3): 332–7.

18 Furlanello, F., Bertoldi, A., Dallago, M. et al. Atrial fibrillation in elite athletes. *J Cardiovasc Electrophysiol* 1998; **9**(8 Suppl.): S63–8.

19 Mohanty, S., Santangeli, P., Mohanty, P. et al. Catheter ablation of asymptomatic longstanding persistent atrial fibrillation: impact on quality of life, exercise performance, arrhythmia perception, and arrhythmia-free survival. *J Cardiovasc Electrophysiol* 2014; **25**(10): 1057–64.

20 Mont, L., Tamborero, D., Elosua, R. et al. Physical activity, height, and left atrial size are independent risk factors for lone atrial fibrillation in middle-aged healthy individuals. *Europace* 2008; **10**(1): 15–20.

21 Wilhelm, M., Roten, L., Tanner, H. et al. Atrial remodeling, autonomic tone, and lifetime training hours in nonelite athletes. *Am J Cardiol* 2011; **108**(4): 580–5.

22 Lindsay, M.M. and Dunn, F.G. Biochemical evidence of myocardial fibrosis in veteran endurance athletes. *Br J Sports Med* 2007; **41**(7): 447–52.

23 January, C.T., Wann, L.S., Alpert, J.S. et al. 2014 AHA/ACC/HRS guideline for the management of patients with atrial fibrillation: a report of the American College of Cardiology/American Heart Association Task Force on Practice Guidelines and the Heart Rhythm Society. *J Am Coll Cardiol* 2014; **64**(21): e1–76.

24 Heidbuchel, H., Anne, W., Willems, R. et al. Endurance sports is a risk factor for atrial fibrillation after ablation for atrial flutter. *Int J Cardiol* 2006; **107**(1): 67–72.

25 Ranger, S., Talajic, M., Lemery, R. et al. Amplification of flecainide-induced ventricular conduction slowing by exercise. A potentially significant clinical consequence of use-dependent sodium channel blockade. *Circulation* 1989; **79**(5): 1000–6.

26 Atwood, J.E., Sullivan, M., Forbes, S. et al. Effect of beta-adrenergic blockade on exercise performance in patients with chronic atrial fibrillation. *J Am Coll Cardiol* 1987; **10**(2): 314–20.

27 Ulimoen, S.R., Enger, S., Pripp, A.H. et al. Calcium channel blockers improve exercise capacity and reduce N-terminal Pro-B-type natriuretic peptide levels compared with beta-blockers in patients with permanent atrial fibrillation. *Eur Heart J* 2014; **35**(8): 517–24.

28 Gay-Jordi, G., Guash, E., Benito, B. et al. Losartan prevents heart fibrosis induced by long-term intensive exercise in an animal model. *PLoS ONE* 2013; **8**(2): e55427.

413

29 Calvo, N., Mont, L., Tamborero, D. et al. Efficacy of circumferential pulmonary vein ablation of atrial fibrillation in endurance athletes. *Europace* 2010; **12**(1): 30–6.

30 Koopman, P., Nuyens, D., Garweg, C. et al. Efficacy of radiofrequency catheter ablation in athletes with atrial fibrillation. *Europace* 2011; **13**(10): 1386–93.

31 Furlanello, F., Lupo, P., Pittalis, M. et al. Radiofrequency catheter ablation of atrial fibrillation in athletes referred for disabling symptoms preventing usual training schedule and sport competition. *J Cardiovasc Electrophysiol* 2008; **19**(5): 457–62.

38 Implantable Cardioverter-Defibrillators in Athletes

Victoria Watt

Department of Sports Medicine, ASPETAR, Qatar Orthopaedic and Sports Medicine Hospital, Doha, Qatar

Introduction

International guidelines on sports participation for athletes with cardiovascular conditions recommend that people with implantable cardioverter-defibrillators (ICDs) should not take part in most competitive sports, at either amateur or professional level [1,2]. These guidelines were published 10 years ago, and since then, ICD implantation rates in the developed world have increased year on year. The safety and performance of ICDs have not been tested under conditions of strenuous activity. Perceived risks to sports participants include exercise-induced arrhythmia, ICD failure in high adrenergic states, damage to the system from physical stress or trauma, inappropriate therapies due to high heart rates and risk to the athlete of syncope during sports such as swimming, climbing and cycling. Recent data have challenged these guidelines, and surveys have indicated that most athletes with an ICD continue to take part in some form of sporting activity [3]. Indeed, a number of professional footballers have made a successful return to play following ICD implantation. There are multiple factors to take into account before a decision can be made regarding sports participation. These include the underlying diagnosis, the sport involved, the support network available to the athlete and medicolegal issues. This chapter will outline the basic principles of ICD therapy and how to safely manage an athlete with an ICD.

ICD Structure and Function

An ICD is implanted in patients who are at risk of, or have suffered from, an aborted sudden cardiac death (SCD) due to a ventricular arrhythmia. The ICD is not able to prevent arrhythmia onset, it can only detect and treat the arrhythmia as it occurs. The device consists of a titanium pulse generator (the 'box' or 'can') and a defibrillator lead, implanted into the right ventricle via a transvenous route (Figures 38.1 and 38.2). In recent years, a new, entirely subcutaneous system has been developed, which avoids the complications associated with a transvenous system, but this can only be used in a subset of patients and is not yet in widespread use.

The pulse generator houses the lithium battery, a capacitor to store and deliver the charge and the hardware used to programme the device. This is implanted beneath the skin, usually on the left side of the chest, in the same location as a standard pacemaker. The battery lasts from 5 to 10 years, depending on manufacturer, type and number of therapies delivered. When the battery life is low, the entire box has to be changed. Therefore, a patient who has a device implanted in early adulthood can expect to undergo multiple box changes over their lifetime.

IOC Manual of Sports Cardiology, First Edition. Edited by Mathew G. Wilson, Jonathan A. Drezner and Sanjay Sharma.
© 2017 International Olympic Committee. Published 2017 by John Wiley & Sons, Ltd.

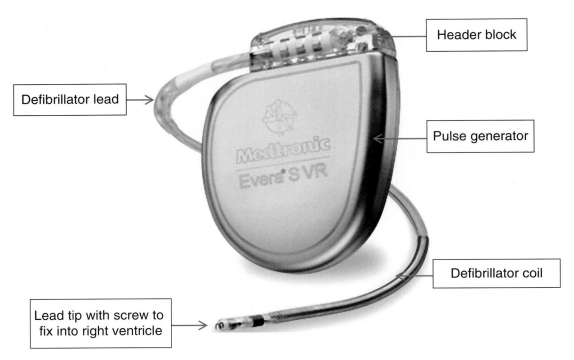

Header block

Defibrillator lead

Pulse generator

Defibrillator coil

Lead tip with screw to fix into right ventricle

Figure 38.1 Standard single-chamber ICD (Medtronic)

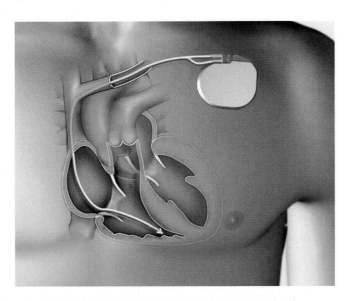

Figure 38.2 Standard location of the ICD pulse generator and transvenous lead

The defibrillator lead is implanted via the cephalic, axillary or subclavian vein into the right ventricle. The lead senses intrinsic ventricular electrical activity, enabling continuous monitoring of heart rate and ventricular complex morphology through the detection of intracardiac electrograms. Pacing impulses are transmitted along the lead conductor to the right ventricle to stimulate depolarisation if the intrinsic heart rate is too slow (standard bradycardia pacing). The device can also deliver rapid pacing in the event of a ventricular tachyarrhythmia (antitachycardia pacing, ATP). This form of 'overdrive pacing' will often successfully terminate ventricular tachycardia, avoiding the need for a shock. Defibrillation is delivered to the myocardium from the defibrillator coil(s), located at the distal segment of the lead in the right ventricle (single-coil lead) and sometimes in the superior vena cava (dual-coil lead). Other pacing leads may also be implanted, depending on the underlying cardiac condition (Table 38.1). All leads are radiopaque, and a defibrillator lead is easily identifiable on chest X-ray (Figure 38.3).

ICD type	Lead position	Pacing	ATP	When to use
Single-chamber	RV	RV	Yes	Standard ICD indication
Dual-chamber	RV, RA	RV, RA	Yes	Standard ICD indication and need for bradycardia pacing
Biventricular (CRT-D)	RV, LV (via epicardial vein) +/− RA	RV, LV +/− RA	Yes	Standard ICD indication and heart failure requiring CRT
S-ICD	Subcutaneous	Post-shock pacing only	No	ICD indication No pace-terminable ventricular tachycardia required No bradycardia pacing required No CRT required

Table 38.1 Types of ICD

RV, right ventricle; RA, right atrium; LV, left ventricle; CRT-D, cardiac resynchronisation therapy defibrillator; ICD, implantable cardioverter-defibrillator; CRT, cardiac resynchronisation therapy; S-ICD, subcutaneous implantable cardioverter-defibrillator.

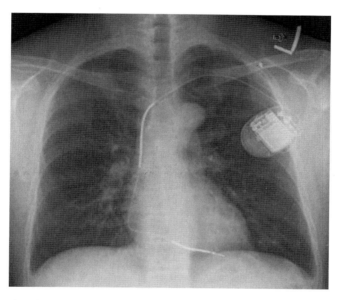

Figure 38.3 Chest X-ray showing a single-chamber ICD with defibrillator coils in the superior vena cava and the right ventricle (dual-coil lead)

Data from arrhythmia and therapy episodes are stored by the device, along with information about lead performance and integrity, battery longevity and some physiological indices. The device is interrogated and programmed noninvasively in the device clinic. In addition, most devices have 'home monitoring', allowing data to be sent to the hospital every night whilst the patient is asleep.

The function of an ICD depends entirely upon how it is programmed. Device programming can and should be tailored to the individual patient [4]. The device is programmed according to 'zones' determined by heart rate, with therapy delivered only when the heart rate reaches the designated zone. The device uses discriminators (heart rate, complex morphology, arrhythmia onset and stability of the RR interval) to optimise supraventricular tachycardia (SVT)/ventricular tachycardia discrimination, and makes use of complex algorithms in arrhythmia detection and therapy delivery. Young patients with a high-normal sinus rate when exercising (e.g. up to 200 beats.min⁻¹) will require a therapeutic zone higher than this in order to avoid an inappropriate shock. Up to three therapeutic zones can be programmed, and the device can deliver both types of therapy within each zone.

Therapies are delivered according to individualised programming. ATP has been shown to be effective in terminating even very rapid ventricular arrythmias, so most algorithms start with ATP, which can be delivered whilst the device is charging [5]. If ATP fails to terminate the tachycardia, a shock is delivered (energy up to 40 J, charge time around 10 s). Following the shock, if the patient remains in ventricular tachycardia/ventricular fibrillation, the device will immediately recharge. However, it will not continue to shock indefinitely: for each episode, a maximum number of shocks will be delivered (usually up to eight).

Subcutaneous ICDs

Lead-related complications are the most common cause of failure of a transvenous ICD system and can render the ICD ineffective or cause inappropriate device therapy. In addition, patients can outlive the lead's longevity and need to undergo revision or replacement procedures over the lifetime of their device. In an attempt to address these issues, an entirely subcutaneous ICD (S-ICD) has been developed [6]. The S-ICD comprises a box positioned over the left lateral ribs and a lead tunnelled beneath the skin, which detects surface electrograms (Figure 38.4). There are no endovascular components. This device is not able to pace the heart (apart from transient post-shock pacing), or deliver ATP. It is therefore not suitable for patients with a pacing indication or for patients with pace-terminable ventricular tachycardia.

S-ICDs are of particular interest in paediatric patients, as they do not physically impact on the anatomy of the heart or vasculature. They have been used successfully in children and in individuals with hypertrophic cardiomyopathy (HCM) and ion channelopathies [7]. Current international guidelines for ICD implantation do not include specific recommendations for the subcutaneous system, and there are particular concerns that need to be taken into account for the athletic population. Protective clothing is advised if there is a risk of trauma, and contact sports should be avoided. Early data have demonstrated a higher incidence of inappropriate shocks compared to transvenous systems, due to issues with T-wave over-sensing [6]. This may be important during vigorous physical activity and times of increased heart rate, which could be detected as a malignant tachyarrhythmia. Data from large prospective comparative trials are required to characterise S-ICD performance compared to the transvenous system, and, as yet, there are no published data on the use of the S-ICD in athletes.

ICDs in Athletes: Underlying Diagnosis

The current international guidelines for ICD implantation are based on underlying aetiology and are the same for both athletes and nonathletes [8–10]. The causes of cardiac arrest in athletes include HCM, coronary artery anomalies, arrhythmogenic right ventricular cardiomyopathy (ARVC), myocarditis and ion channelopathies. HCM, ARVC and the ion channelopathies are genetic conditions that cannot be cured and carry a high risk of sustained ventricular tachycardia/ventricular fibrillation, usually without impairment of

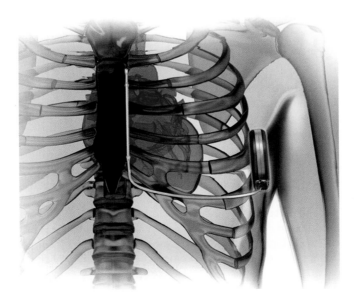

Figure 38.4 Subcutaneous ICD (Boston Scientific). Note the position of the pulse generator over the left lateral ribs and the subcutaneous lead

cardiac function. They are the most frequent indications for ICD implantation amongst the athletic population. Advice regarding fitness to participate in sport for athletes with an ICD depends upon the limitations of their underlying condition. Even moderate physical activity in patients with ICDs has been shown to be associated with an increased number of ventricular arrythmias requiring therapy [11], and the potential impact of this on disease progression must be considered.

Hypertrophic Cardiomyopathy

HCM accounts for more cases of SCD in athletes than any other cardiac disease. It is characterised by left ventricular hypertrophy (LVH) of various distributions and by histological evidence of myocardial disarray and fibrosis. SCD is caused by ventricular tachyarrhythmias, which are unpredictable and occur most commonly in asymptomatic individuals. ICDs are effective in preventing SCD in patients with HCM; aborted sudden death and sustained ventricular tachycardia are class I indications for implantation. In other cases, risk stratification is advised, and according to the American guidelines, an ICD should be considered if there is an immediate family history of SCD, recent unexplained syncope or left ventricular wall thickness ≥30 mm. Recently, the European Society of Cardiology (ESC) HCM outcome investigators recommended a 5-year risk calculator derived from a model equation incorporating seven parameters (age, family history of SCD, maximal left ventricular wall thickness, left atrial diameter, maximal left ventricular outflow obstruction, nonsustained ventricular tachycardia (NSVT) and unexplained syncope) to calculate the 5-year risk of SCD. A cut-off value of ≥6% SCD risk in 5 years is recommended for consideration of an ICD implant in primary prevention. Risk stratification should be performed annually. The recent American Heart Association (AHA) and ESC guidelines for the management of HCM advise against moderate- and high-intensity competitive sports [12,13].

For more information on HCM, see Chapter 19.

Arrhythmogenic Right Ventricular Cardiomyopathy

ARVC is characterised by fibro-fatty infiltration of the myocardium, with right ventricular dilatation, regional hypokinesis and aneurysm formation. Disruption of the cellular architecture causes electrical instability, manifesting as electrocardiogram (ECG) abnormalities and ventricular arrhythmias. It is an important cause of SCD, with considerable differences in regional prevalence. ARVC is progressive and can involve both ventricles. A number of causative genetic mutations have been identified, affecting cell-adhesion proteins. Inheritance is usually autosomal-dominant, but the penetrance and resultant phenotype are highly variable and the diagnosis is made with reference to task-force criteria [14].

ARVC often presents with sustained ventricular tachycardia and cardiac arrest associated with exertion [15]. There is a risk of catecholamine-induced ventricular tachycardia during exercise, and regular physical activity has been shown to worsen fibro-fatty infiltration [16]. It is widely accepted that athletes with ARVC should be excluded from most competitive sports, except those of low intensity. ARVC patients with ICDs have been shown to have a low incidence of arrhythmic death and a high frequency of appropriate device therapies. An ICD is indicated if there is a history of sustained ventricular tachycardia or an aborted SCD. Risk stratification for primary-prevention cases is more difficult, and decisions are made on a case-by-case basis.

For more information on ARVC, see Chapter 20.

Long QT Syndrome

Long QT syndrome is an inherited cardiac ion channelopathy characterised by repolarisation abnormalities, prolongation of the QT interval and risk of ventricular arrhythmias. To date more than 10 types have been described, each with a specific genetic mutation; the most common are LQT1, 2 and 3. Presence of the mutation does not automatically confer disease (genotype-positive, phenotype-negative), and guidelines differ for this patient group [17]. Long QT patients are at higher risk of ventricular arrhythmias during states of excitement, including exercise and intense emotion. Swimming is known to trigger events in

LQT1 and sudden noise (e.g. alarm clocks, starter pistols) in LQT2. Both the Bethesda and the ESC guidelines advise disqualification of individuals with long QT syndrome from all competitive sports, other than low-intensity activities.

Despite current recommendations, athletes with long QT syndrome, including some with ICDs, have continued to compete. Over a 5-year follow-up period, Johnson and Ackerman [18] observed a group of 130 such individuals, participating in sports from Mitchell classification IA to IIIB, to have a low rate of cardiac events. Only one athlete had a sporting-related event that triggered an ICD therapy (this individual was noncompliant with beta-blocker therapy at the time). These findings led the authors to suggest that the current recommendations for participation in competitive sports for athletes with long QT syndrome may be excessive.

Beta blockers are highly effective in LQT1 and are the treatment of choice. ICDs are recommended for selected patients with syncope despite beta-blocker treatment, sustained ventricular arrhythmia or a history of aborted SCD. In athletes with long QT syndrome and an ICD, careful counselling, risk stratification and medical management are mandatory before return to play can be allowed. It is essential to ensure strict compliance with beta-blocker therapy and avoidance of all QT-prolonging drugs. Swimming should be avoided in patients with LQT1. Hypokalaemia should also be avoided; appropriate measures must be taken if the athlete has significant vomiting or diarrhoea.

For more information on long QT syndrome, see Chapter 26.

Brugada Syndrome

Brugada syndrome is an ion channelopathy caused by mutations in the SCN5A sodium-channel gene, leading to repolarisation abnormalities, ECG changes and a risk of lethal ventricular arrhythmias. Inheritance is autosomal–dominant, and the syndrome is more common in Asian populations and males. The ECG changes may be absent at rest but can be unmasked with pharmacological testing. Arrhythmias occur without warning, and are more likely during a febrile illness. There is no effective treatment and ICD implantation is indicated for patients with a history of aborted SCD or syncope with inducible significant ventricular tachycardia on electrophysiology testing (class I indications) [19]. Unlike ARVC, there is no clear demonstrable relationship between exercise and arrhythmic events. However, given the lack of warning symptoms, sporting activity which might be dangerous in the event of transient loss of consciousness should be avoided. In addition, the athlete should not exercise if febrile or at risk of hyperthermia (e.g. in the heat). It is recommended that patients be disqualified from all competitive sports, with the exception of class IA activities. Guidelines differ for genotype-positive, phenotype-negative patients [17].

For more information on Brugada syndrome, see Chapter 27.

Catecholaminergic Polymorphic Ventricular Tachycardia

Catecholaminergic polymorphic ventricular tachycardia (CPVT) is a rare arrhythmogenic disorder that affects genes involved in calcium transport within the sarcomere. Ventricular arrhythmias are triggered by exercise or stress. Beta blockers and avoidance of triggers are effective treatments. An ICD is indicated if the patient has had an aborted SCD, or if they have had breakthrough arrhythmias whilst on treatment. Implantation of an ICD does not reduce the risk of an arrhythmia occurring, and therefore does not permit the athlete to return to competition. Given the clear relationship between exercise and arrhythmias in this condition, participation in sport is not advised, despite recent data suggesting that it is possible for CPVT patients to exercise safely following a careful period of retraining and if they stay below a 'threshold' heart rate [20].

For more information on CPVT, see Chapter 29.

Short QT Syndrome

This extremely rare disorder is characterised by a short resting QT interval (males <330 ms, females <340 ms) [21], which typically does not change with heart rate. Mutations in genes encoding for potassium and calcium channels lead to shortening – and increased dispersion – of the cardiac action potential repolarisation time. This results in a short QT interval and shortened atrial and ventricular refractory periods, with a consequent increased risk of both atrial and ventricular fibrillation. There are no clear triggers for arrhythmia onset, there is no proven drug treatment and presentation is usually with cardiac arrest. ICD implantation is indicated for patients with a history of aborted SCD, but due to the small number of cases, risk stratification for asymptomatic individuals has not been clearly defined. Only low-intensity (class IA) activities are advised, and individuals should avoid activities where they might be a risk of injury in the event of syncope [22].

ICDs in Athletes: Implications for Return to Play

Nature of the Sport

Consideration must be given to the dynamic nature of the sporting activity, including intensity, risk of collision and trauma to the device pocket, risk of damage to the lead and risk to the athlete in the event of syncope (e.g. swimming, climbing, cycling, motor racing). Sports with obligatory body contact (e.g. rugby, ice hockey, American football, martial arts, boxing) should be avoided. There is no evidence that participation in sports involving significant arm movements (e.g. swimming, golf, racquet sports) leads to an increased incidence of lead failure [3], but appropriate guidance regarding timing of return to play following ICD implantation should be given by the implanting physician. The physical risk of an episode of syncope occurring during certain activities (e.g. swimming, cycling, motor sports, climbing) also needs to be considered, and appropriate measures must be taken to mitigate it (including cessation of the activity, if necessary). There may be particular issues with regard to the sport involved and the underlying cardiac condition (e.g. swimming and LQT1).

Ethical and Medicolegal Considerations

Most individuals with an ICD wish to continue their sporting activities, but the decision-making process regarding return to play is fraught with difficulties. Implantation of an ICD may lead to the misconception that all is well and the athlete can continue to participate in sport without concern for the disease, the consequences of ICD therapies or the medical support that they will require. In professional athletes, the desire to return to play may be influenced by financial considerations. The economic, emotional and psychological impact on an athlete if they are unable to resume their sport should not be underestimated. Any decision regarding return to play can only be made after consideration of all these issues and after discussion with all parties concerned.

However, if an athlete returns to play with an ICD, the question arises over who is liable if an adverse event occurs. Does the athlete have a right to participate in sport regardless of risk, if they are willing to assume responsibility for that risk? Does this assumption of liability mean that the athlete's club or organisation will not be held liable in the future? Are there medicolegal implications for the cardiologist or team doctor involved in the athlete's care?

Recognised guidelines should be used in the decision-making process, but adherence is not mandatory. Decisions should be made on an individual basis. The Bethesda guidelines state that 'a clinician has the flexibility to deviate from the recommendations if he or she believes it is in the best interests of a patient-athlete to reach an alternative decision' [2]. Compliance with international guidelines may be taken as supportive evidence that an appropriate decision has been reached. The physician must ensure that any advice given is in line with 'good medical practice', however that may be defined in their jurisdiction, and is protective of the athlete's health. These factors could be used to negate accusations of malpractice, even if the advice given were contrary to published recommendations.

Complications of ICDs and Implications for Athletes

When an ICD is implanted into a young patient, they can expect to undergo further procedures over the course of their lifetime in order to maintain device function. These include mandatory pulse generator replacements and sometimes lead revision procedures. Every time the device pocket is opened either for a routine box change or to deal with a complication, there is a risk of infection [23]. Device infection is a very serious condition that usually mandates extraction of the device (a high-risk procedure) and reimplantation on the contralateral side. It is therefore of the utmost importance that measures be taken to avoid device complications, including giving appropriate advice to an athlete considering participation in sport.

Pocket Complications

Pocket complications include infection, skin erosion and haematoma, all of which may occur following direct trauma to the device. A submuscular pocket is sometimes used for a better cosmetic result, but it also provides greater protection to the device, so is often used if the overlying skin is very thin or if the patient wishes to participate in activities involving a risk of contact. Protective clothing can be worn to minimise the risk of device trauma (Figure 38.5). If the athlete sustains direct trauma to the pocket or if there is any evidence of erythema, swelling or infection, they should be referred without delay to the local device clinic for ICD interrogation and wound evaluation.

Lead Failure

Lead failure can occur secondary to lead displacement or damage to any component of the lead, particularly a breach in insulation or a conductor fracture. Symptoms may not be immediately apparent, but early signs of lead failure can be detected from changes in lead performance parameters – information that is stored in the device and analysed during device interrogation. Lead displacement occurs most frequently during the first month post-implantation. Excessive movement of the ipsilateral arm can cause traction on the lead and subsequent displacement. Patients are advised to limit arm movement for the first 6 weeks post-implantation. This recommendation may be extended to several months for individuals who wish to participate in certain sports perceived to pose an increased risk, such as golf, but currently there are no evidence-based guidelines and advice is given on a case-by-case basis.

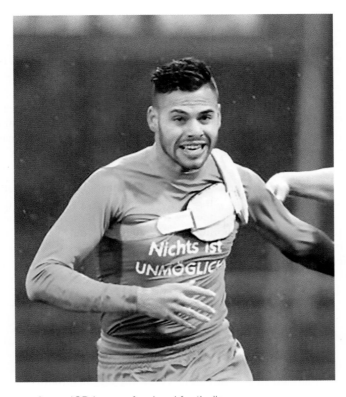

Figure 38.5 Protective cover for an ICD in a professional footballer

A second cause of lead failure is subclavian crush injury. This can occur if the lead is implanted into the sub-clavian vein and, over time, is crushed as it traverses the costoclavicular ligament. The risk of lead damage is theoretically increased in activities involving extremes of arm movement. There have been case reports of pacemaker lead fracture caused by subclavian crush injury during weightlifting. However, an international registry of athletes with ICDs has shown that, over a 30-month follow-up period, participation in contact sports, sports with intense arm activity (e.g. swimming) or weightlifting was not predictive of lead failure [3].

Inappropriate Shocks

An inappropriate shock occurs when the device delivers a therapy for sinus or SVT, or for 'noise' detected if there is damage to the lead. If this occurs, then the device must be reprogrammed to prevent further episodes. ICD shocks, whether appropriate or inappropriate, are not a benign entity. They are responsible for much of the morbidity associated with ICDs, reducing quality of life through significant psychological distress, and, rarely, can cause further arrhythmias. Additionally, ICD shocks have been reported to be asso-ciated with excess mortality [24]. In recent years, changes have been made to device programming in an attempt to reduce the incidence of inappropriate shocks. These include improved algorithms and discrimi-nators, longer detection times to avoid shocks for self-terminating ventricular tachycardia and individualised programming; this latter change is especially important for younger patients and athletes who can reach high sinus rates during exercise [25,26]. In addition, a single cycle of ATP, delivered whilst the device is charging, will often successfully terminate very fast ventricular tachycardia, thereby reducing the number of shocks delivered and improving quality of life [5].

If an athlete receives a therapy from a device, this should not be seen as a harmless event but as an aborted sudden death episode with an immediate risk of further arrhythmias. The athlete should be transferred to hospital for urgent evaluation and device interrogation. It is not advisable for the athlete to resume their activities until this review has taken place.

How to Care for an Athlete with an ICD: Practical Considerations

Following ICD implantation, advice on when and if the athlete can resume training and competition should be given by the athlete's cardiologist, in conjunction with the team physician. Once the decision has been made, there are a number of issues that the team physician and supporting staff need to consider in order to minimise potential adverse events:

- There must be a clear understanding of the underlying cardiac pathology and the specific risks involved.
- A copy of the athlete's ICD identification card should be kept on record, along with their medication his-tory and a note of any contraindicated drugs (e.g. long QT syndrome).
- There must be regular follow-up with the athlete's cardiologist and device clinics.
- An automated external defibrillator (AED) should be available at all times (and individuals should be trained in its use), with an emergency response plan.
- If the athlete receives a therapy from the device, there should be immediate transfer to hospital for device interrogation and cardiology review.
- The athlete should be referred to the device clinic without delay in the event of trauma to the device pocket or signs of inflammation, infection or swelling.

Medical Equipment that may Interfere with an ICD

Automated External Defibrillator

On very rare occasions, the ICD may fail to recognise an episode of ventricular tachycardia or ventricular fibrillation, or the ICD therapy may be ineffective, in which case an AED must be used. AEDs can be used safely in patients with ICDs, but there is a risk of damage to the device and to the myocardium at the lead–tissue interface. In order to minimise this risk, defibrillator pad placement should be as far away from the pulse generator as possible – at least 10 cm from the edge of the ICD. Usually, the anteroposterior, posterolateral or biaxillary positions are used [27].

There have been case reports of rescuers receiving mild shocks from ICDs when in contact with patients during cardiopulmonary resuscitation (CPR). It is important to wear gloves when giving CPR to someone with an ICD, but they are not designed to insulate against electrical current and may not provide total protection. However, it should be noted that the maximum energy delivered from an ICD is less than 40 J, so the risk to the rescuer is very small and delivery of effective CPR should not be delayed.

Magnetic Resonance Imaging

Some ICDs are 'magnetic resonance imaging (MRI) compatible', but this depends on the exact generator and lead type, and there is still an exclusion zone of at least the thorax, which cannot be imaged. If an MRI scan is required, the device clinic must be informed beforehand. Precise details will be checked to ensure MRI compatibility and arrangements will be made for a device technician to be present at the time of the study for device interrogation and programming.

Other Medical Interventions

Extracorporeal shockwave lithotripsy (ESWL) should be avoided in patients with ICDs. Diathermy, therapeutic radiation and transcutaneous electrical nerve stimulation (TENS) are all possible, although specific precautions are required.

Nonmedical Equipment

Security and antitheft systems are safe to walk through, but individuals with an ICD should not stay near or lean on them. For airport travel, the athlete should carry their ICD identification card and inform security personnel that they have a device. It is safe to pass through metal detectors. Handheld metal detectors should not be placed over the device for any longer than necessary, and, ideally, an alternative form of inspection should be used.

Mobile phones should be used on the ear opposite to the ICD and not kept in an overlying pocket. MP3 players are safe, but most headphones contain a magnetic substance that can cause interference if placed too close to the ICD, so they should be kept at least 15 cm away and not placed in a chest pocket or draped over the ICD site. Power-generating and arc-welding equipment carry a risk of pulse generator inhibition and should not be used. Magnets can deactivate the ICD (and are sometimes used in hospital to 'turn off' therapies in an emergency situation). Close and prolonged contact with magnets should be avoided; this includes magnetic items such as bracelets and necklaces. Equipment containing powerful magnets should not be used.

Conclusion

A growing number of sportsmen and women are choosing to continue their sporting activities after ICD implantation. There is an increasing body of evidence to suggest that it may be possible for an athlete to participate in activities with a higher dynamic component than the class IA sports permitted in the current Bethesda guidelines. The decision to return to play is complex, fraught with difficulties and can only be made after appropriate counselling with the athlete, team management and team physician. Until more evidence becomes available, decisions must be made on a case-by-case basis, with issues surrounding liability for the club and doctor remaining uncertain. If the athlete is allowed to return to their sport, the team physician must have a clear understanding of the implications for the athlete and of what to do if the device delivers a therapy or there is a suspected device complication. It is essential that the athlete has regular follow-up and is compliant with medication and medical advice in order to minimise further risk. Finally, eligibility for the athlete to continue participation in competitive sport should be reviewed by the team physician and cardiologist on an annual basis.

References

1 Pelliccia, A., Fagard, R., Bjørnstad, H.H. et al. Recommendations for competitive sports participation in athletes with cardiovascular disease. A consensus document from the Study Group of Sports Cardiology of the Working Group of Cardiac Rehabilitation and Exercise Physiology and the Working Group of Myocardial and Pericardial Diseases of the European Society of Cardiology. *Eur Heart J* 2005; **26**: 1422–45.

2 Maron, B.J. and Zipes, D.P. 36th Bethesda Conference Eligibility Recommendations for competitive athletes with cardiovascular abnormalities. *J Am Coll Cardiol* 2005; **45**:1311–75.

3 Lampert, R., Olshansky, B., Heidbuchel, H. et al. Safety of sports for athletes with implantable cardioverter-defibrillators: results of a prospective, multinational registry. *Circulation* 2013; **127**: 2021–30.

4 Koneru, J.N., Swerdlow, C.D., Wood, M.A. and Ellenbogen, K.A. Minimizing inappropriate or 'unnecessary' implantable cardioverter-defibrillator shocks. Appropriate programming. *Circ Arrhyth Electrophysiol* 2011; **4**: 778–90.

5 Wathen, M.S., DeGroot, P.J., Sweeney, M.O. et al. Prospective randomized multicenter trial of empirical antitachy-cardia pacing versus shocks for spontaneous rapid ventricular tachycardia in patients with implantable cardioverter-defibrillators. Pacing Fast Ventricular Tachycardia Reduces Shock Therapies (PainFREE Rx II) Trial Results. *Circulation* 2004; **110**: 2591–6.

6 Weiss, R., Knight, B.P., Gold, M.R. et al. Safety and efficacy of a totally subcutaneous implantable-cardioverter defibrillator. *Circulation* 2013; **128**: 944–53.

7 Lambiase, P.D., Barr, C., Theuns, D.A.M.J. et al. Worldwide experience with a totally subcutaneous implantable defibrillator: early results from the EFFORTLESS S-ICD Registry. *Eur Heart J* 2014; **35**: 1657–65.

8 Zipes, D.P., Camm, A.J., Borggrefe, M. et al. ACC/AHA/ESC 2006 guidelines for management of patients with ventricular arrhythmias and the prevention of sudden cardiac death executive summary: a report of the American College of Cardiology/American Heart Association Task Force and the European Society of Cardiology Committee for Practice Guidelines (Writing Committee to Develop Guidelines for Management of Patients with Ventricular Arrhythmias and the Prevention of Sudden Cardiac Death). *Eur Heart J* 2006; **27**: 2099–140.

9 Russo, A.M., Stainback, R.F., Bailey, S.R. et al. ACCF/HRS/AHA/ASE/HFSA/SCAI/SCCT/SCMR 2013 appropri-ate use criteria for implantable cardioverter-defibrillators and cardiac resynchronization therapy. A report of the American College of Cardiology Foundation Appropriate Use Criteria Task Force, Heart Rhythm Society, American Heart Association, American Society of Echocardiography, Heart Failure Society of America, Society for Cardiovascular Angiography and Interventions, Society of Cardiovascular Computed Tomography, and Society for Cardiovascular Magnetic Resonance. *J Am Coll Cardiol* 2013; **61**: 1318–68.

10 Tracy, C.M., Epstein, A.E., Darbar, D. et al. 2012 ACCF/AHA/HRS focused update incorporated into the ACCF/AHA/HRS 2008 guidelines for device-based therapy of cardiac rhythm abnormalities. A report of the American College of Cardiology Foundation/American Heart Association Task Force on Practice Guidelines and the Heart Rhythm Society. *J Am Coll Cardiol* 2013; **61**: e6–75.

11 Lampert, R., Joska, T., Burg, M. et al. Emotional and physical precipitants of ventricular arrhythmia. *Circulation* 2002; **106**: 1800–5.

12 Gersh, B.J., Maron, B.J., Bonow, R.O. et al. ACCF/AHA guideline for the diagnosis and treatment of hypertrophic cardiomyopathy. A report of the American College of Cardiology Foundation/American Heart Association Task Force on Practice Guidelines Developed in Collaboration With the American Association for Thoracic Surgery, American Society of Echocardiography, American Society of Nuclear Cardiology, Heart Failure Society of America, Heart Rhythm Society, Society for Cardiovascular Angiography and Interventions, and Society of Thoracic Surgeons. *Circulation* 2011; **124**: e783–831.

13 Elliott, P.M., Anastasakis, A., Borger, M.A. et al. 2014 ESC guidelines on diagnosis and management of hypertrophic cardiomyopathy: the Task Force for the Diagnosis and Management of Hypertrophic Cardiomyopathy of the European Society of Cardiology (ESC). *Eur Heart J* 2014; **35**: 2733–79.

14 Marcus, F.I., McKenna, W.J., Sherrill, D. et al. Diagnosis of arrhythmogenic right ventricular cardiomyopathy/dys-plasia. Proposed modification of the task force criteria. *Circulation* 2010; **121**: 1533–41.

15 Sadjadieh, G., Jabbari, R., Risgaard, B. et al. Nationwide (Denmark) study of symptoms preceding sudden death due to arrhythmogenic right ventricular cardiomyopathy. *Am J Cardiol* 2014; **113**: 1250–4.

16 Maron, B.J., Chaitman, B.R., Ackerman, M.J. et al. Recommendations for physical activity and recreational sports participation for young patients with genetic cardiovascular diseases. *Circulation* 2004; **109**: 2807–16.

17 Pelliccia, A., Zipes, D.P. and Maron, B.J. Bethesda Conference #36 and the European Society of Cardiology Consensus Recommendations Revisited. A comparison of US and European criteria for eligibility and disqualifica-tion of competitive athletes with cardiovascular abnormalities. *J Am Coll Cardiol* 2008; **52**: 1990–6.

18 Johnson, J.N. and Ackerman, M.J. Return to play? Athletes with congenital long QT syndrome. *Br J Sports Med* 2013; **47**: 28–33.

19 Epstein, A.E., DiMarco, J.P., Ellenbogen, K.A., et al. 2012 ACCF/AHA/HRS focused update incorporated into the ACCF/AHA/HRS 2008 guidelines for device-based therapy of cardiac rhythm abnormalities: a report of the American College of Cardiology Foundation/American Heart Association Task Force on Practice Guidelines and the Heart Rhythm Society. *J Am Coll Cardiol* 2013; **61**: e6.

20 Manotheepan, R., Saberniak, J., Danielsen, T.K. et al. Effects of individualized exercise training in patients with catecholaminergic polymorphic ventricular tachycardia type 1. *Am J Cardiol* 2014; **113**: 1829–33.

21 Viskin, S. The QT interval: too long, too short or just right? *Heart Rhythm* 2009; **1**: 587–91.

22 Heidbüchel, H., Corrado, D., Biffi, A. et al. Recommendations for participation in leisure-time physical activity and competitive sports of patients with arrhythmias and potentially arrhythmogenic conditions. Part II: ventricular arrhythmias, channelopathies and implantable defibrillators. *Eur J Cardiovasc Prev Rehabil* 2006; **13**: 676–86.

23 Prutkin, J.M., Reynolds, M.R., Bao, H. et al. Rates of and factors associated with infection in 200 909 Medicare implantable cardioverter-defibrillator implants. Results from the National Cardiovascular Data Registry. *Circulation* 2014; **130**: 1037–43.

24 Daubert, J.P., Zareba, W., Cannom, D.S. et al. Inappropriate implantable cardioverter-defibrillator shocks in MADIT II: frequency, mechanisms, predictors, and survival impact. *J Am Coll Cardiol* 2008; **51**: 1357–65.

25 Moss, A.J., Schuger, C., Beck, C.A. et al. Reduction in inappropriate therapy and mortality through ICD programming. *N Engl J Med* 2012; **367**: 2275–83.

26 Wilkoff, B.L., Williamson, B.D., Stern, R.S. et al. Strategic programming of detection and therapy parameters in implantable cardioverter-defibrillators reduces shocks in primary prevention patients results from the PREPARE (Primary Prevention Parameters Evaluation) Study. *J Am Coll Cardiol* 2008; **52**: 541–50.

27 Jacobs, I., Sunde, K., Deakin, C.D. et al. 2010 international consensus on cardiopulmonary resuscitation and emergency cardiovascular care science with treatment recommendations. Part 6: defibrillation. *Circulation* 2010; **122**: S325–37.

39 Management of Hypertension in Athletes

Maria-Carmen Adamuz

Department of Sports Medicine, ASPETAR, Qatar Orthopaedic and Sports Medicine Hospital, Doha, Qatar

Introduction and Epidemiology

Arterial hypertension is the most important preventable contributor to cardiovascular morbidity and mortality in the general population [1] and the most common cardiovascular condition in competitive athletes [2]. As in the general population, however, hypertension remains undetected or poorly treated in many young athletes [3]. In Western countries, the prevalence of hypertension ranges from 14.4% in men aged 20–29 years to 21.2% in those aged 30–39, with lower prevalence in females (6.2 and 9.9%, respectively) [4]. The exact prevalence in young athletes is unknown. A recent systematic review found no significant differences in blood pressure between athletes and nonathletes [5]. Other studies have found a higher prevalence of hypertension in young athletes compared to matched nonathletic populations. Karpinos et al. [6] reported a 19% prevalence of hypertension in young American football players, compared to 9.1% amongst men aged 20–34 years in the general US population.

In addition, there is growing evidence that a mildly elevated blood pressure is much more common in adolescents and young athletes than previously thought, with up to two-thirds of athletes exhibiting a mean blood pressure in the prehypertensive range [5]. This is important, as in young individuals prehypertension progresses to hypertension at an annual rate of 7%, so blood pressure abnormalities in young adulthood frequently translate into adult hypertension. The recognition of athletes at increased risk of early-life hypertension is important for three reasons: prompt diagnosis and treatment provide an important opportunity to reduce subsequent cardiovascular morbidity and mortality; assessment of global cardiovascular risk is mandatory for sports eligibility; and untreated hypertension may impair left ventricular diastolic filling, so recognition of risk ensures optimal cardiovascular performance and allows athletes to achieve their full potential.

Considerations Relating to Sports Participation and Blood Pressure in Athletes

Arterial blood pressure in athletes is influenced by a number of factors related to sports participation, including sporting discipline, type of training, level/intensity of training [5] and even position of play. Sports with different static and dynamic components [5] and training in different positions in the same sport may have distinct effects on the athlete's blood pressure, due to the varied physical demands and the nature of repetitive position-specific skills [7,8]. Additional factors that may contribute to elevated blood pressure in athletes are: competition-related stress [3], pain due to injuries, weight gain (aimed at enhancing performance) [7,8] and the use of drugs (e.g. nonsteroidal anti-inflammatory drugs (NSAIDs)) or performance-enhancing substances.

Both endurance [9] and resistance exercise [10], in moderation, are effective in reducing blood pressure in hypertensive subjects, but vigorous physical activity does not seem to reduce blood pressure in athletes when compared with controls [5]. Interestingly, aerobic endurance exercise significantly reduces daytime but not

IOC Manual of Sports Cardiology, First Edition. Edited by Mathew G. Wilson, Jonathan A. Drezner and Sanjay Sharma.
© 2017 International Olympic Committee. Published 2017 by John Wiley & Sons, Ltd.

night-time blood pressure [9]. Night-time hypertension is frequently observed when 'normotensive athletes' are assessed with ambulatory blood pressure monitoring (ABPM) [3] and has been associated with masked hypertension [3]. Mental and physical stress associated with competition may increase the sympathetic tone, which in turn will elevate the nocturnal blood pressure [3]. Other factors, such as endothelial dysfunction resulting from oxidative stress or the abnormal large artery compliance observed after months of intense resistance training, may also negatively influence the blood pressure in competitive athletes. Consequently, more rigorous blood pressure monitoring is desirable in athletes at risk, not only during the pre-season but also at different times during the season. Moreover, although it is not currently recommended, the widespread use of ABPM in the evaluation of apparently normotensive athletes would probably increase the detection of hypertensive athletes affected by masked hypertension [3].

Definition and Classification of Arterial Hypertension in Athletes

Hypertension in athletes is diagnosed and classified at the same cut-off values used in the nonathletic population. Definitions are based on office blood pressure measurements and differ from the cut-off values utilised when blood pressure is measured in other environments, such as the patient's home. *In athletes older than 18 years*, hypertension is diagnosed when systolic blood pressure (SBP) is ≥140 mmHg and/or diastolic blood pressure (DBP) is ≥90 mmHg. Hypertension is arbitrarily classified in different categories, with prognostic and therapeutic implications (Table 39.1) [11,12]. Observational studies show a linear relationship between blood pressure and cardiovascular morbidity/mortality, with a threshold of 115/75 mmHg [13]. Above 115/75 mmHg, for each increase of 20 mmHg in SBP or 10 mmHg in DBP, the risk of major cardiovascular events doubles.

In young athletes under 18 years, hypertension is defined and classified based on percentiles [14,15], according to age, height and gender (percentiles tables can be downloaded at: http://pediatrics.aappublications.org/content/114/Supplement_2/555.full.pdf+html?sid=50fa22ce-078e-46e7-b2e7-ef8db6d94d78). Normal blood pressure in this population is defined as SBP and DBP below the 90th percentile, whereas hypertension is defined as SBP and/or DBP persistently at or above the 95th percentile.

Challenges of Diagnosing Hypertension in Athletes

Isolated Systolic Hypertension

The diagnosis of *isolated systolic hypertension* (ISH), defined as SBP ≥140 mmHg and DBP <90 mmHg, is challenging in young athletes, as extreme pulse-pressure amplification between the aorta and brachial artery can induce 'spurious systolic hypertension' [16]. This mechanism may raise the recorded SBP by 20 mmHg and is mainly seen in young, male, tall individuals involved in sports activities. The differentiation between spurious systolic hypertension and true ISH in young athletes may be clinically relevant, but it requires the assessment of central blood pressure.

ASH/ISH category	ESC/ESH category	Systolic		Diastolic
Optimal		<120 mmHg	and	<80 mmHg
Pre-HTN	**Normal**	120–129 mmHg	and/or	80–84 mmHg
	High normal	130–139 mmHg		85–89 mmHg
Stage 1	**Grade 1**	140–159 mmHg	and/or	90–99 mmHg
Stage 2	**Grade 2**	160–179 mmHg	and/or	100–109 mmHg
	Grade 3	≥180 mmHg		≥110 mmHg
Isolated systolic hypertension		≥140 mmHg	and	<90 mmHg

Table 39.1 Definition and classification of blood pressure in adults [12,13]

The long-term significance of spurious systolic hypertension and ISH in athletes has not yet been established. The Framingham Study demonstrated that young individuals with ISH were not at increased cardiovascular risk [17]. Recent data from a 31-year prospective follow-up of more than 27 000 young adults (18–49 years of age) report a higher relative risk for cardiovascular disease (CVD) in young adults with ISH compared to those with normal blood pressure, however [18]. Currently, there is no consensus relating to the pharmacological treatment of athletes with ISH. Reasonable recommendations include evaluation of the athlete's individual risk and monitoring of their blood pressure.

White-Coat Hypertension and Masked Hypertension

Several studies have shown that complementary out-of-office methods of blood pressure measurement, such as ABPM or home blood pressure monitoring (HBPM), are more accurate in the evaluation of blood pressure than are office blood pressure measurements, and that they correlate better with cardiovascular morbidity and mortality, as well as with target organ damage [12]. The combined use of office and ambulatory blood pressure measurements has led to the identification of two groups of athletes:

1. Individuals with *white-coat hypertension* have elevated blood pressure in the office but normal blood pressure out of office. This condition has a prevalence of 15% in the general population [12] (its prevalence in athletes is unknown). White-coat hypertension should be suspected in young athletes with grade I hypertension in the office in the absence of a family history of hypertension or organ damage and where there is a low cardiovascular risk profile. Antihypertensive treatment is not currently recommended, although blood pressure monitoring is necessary.
2. Athletes with *masked hypertension* have normal office blood pressure measures but high out-of-office blood pressure measures. The prevalence of masked hypertension varies from 8 to 48% in the general population [19]. Its exact prevalence in athletes is unknown. A recent study reported masked hypertension in 35% of elite male football players [3], with night-time hypertension observed in 64% of those with normal blood pressure in office. Masked hypertension has been associated with excess cardiovascular morbidity/mortality and organ damage [19]. It should be suspected in athletes with normal–high blood pressure, in those with normal blood pressure in the office and high total cardiovascular risk, and in cases of asymptomatic organ damage. Masked hypertension has also been related to exercise-induced arterial hypertension (EIAH) [19].

How to Assess Blood Pressure in Athletes

The diagnosis of hypertension in competitive athletes requires a minimum of two office blood pressure measurements taken on separate occasions over a period of weeks or months [2,13]. Out-of-office blood pressure monitoring is recommended [2,12,13] to rule out white-coat hypertension and confirm the diagnosis, mainly in those with mildly elevated blood pressure.

Methodology for Office Blood Pressure Measurement

There are *five key recommendations for an accurate recording of blood pressure*. Adherence to these five points may be challenging in the setting of large screening projects at sporting venues, but every effort must be made to ensure the best possible conditions.

1. *General advice for the athlete before measurement*: Avoid caffeine intake and/or cigarette smoke 30 minutes before the measurement. Avoid high-intensity exercise the day of the measurement and do not exercise at all during the 30 minutes previous to the measurement. An empty bladder is essential to avoid the false-positive high blood pressure associated with a full bladder. Relax and do not talk during the measurement.
2. *Type of device*: Arm cuffs are preferred. Either an electronic device or a conventional sphygmomanometer can be used. An appropriately sized cuff should cover 80% of the athlete's upper arm (between the top

of the shoulder and the olecranon), encircling the arm completely. The standard cuff (12–13 cm wide and 35 cm long) is not recommended in thin or large arms (arm circumference >32 cm), since these can generate false blood pressure measurements [12].

3. *Preferred position*: For an accurate blood pressure recording, the athlete should be seated in the uncrossed position and should be at rest for at least for 5 minutes, with the arm supported at the level of the heart on a firm surface [13].

4. *Choice of arm*: At the initial evaluation, blood pressure should be measured on both arms; if the reading differs, the arm with the higher reading should be used for measurements thereafter [13]. A right-arm reading is suggested for evaluation of aortic coarctation, since the left one may give false low readings.

5. *Number of readings*: It is preferable to take two readings, 1–2 minutes apart, and to use the average of these measurements [12,13].

Methodology for Out-of-Office Blood Pressure Measurement

Out-of-office blood pressure measurements include HBPM and ABPM. Both modalities are useful for the diagnosis of hypertension and masked hypertension, exclusion of white-coat hypertension, evaluation of athletes with resistant hypertension, follow-up of athletes with normal–high blood pressure in the office and evaluation of the effects of therapeutic interventions.

Home Blood Pressure Monitoring

The cut-off values for the diagnosis of hypertension using HBPM are *SBP ≥135 mmHg* and/or *DBP ≥85 mmHg* [12,13]. Upper-arm electronic devices are preferable (the British Hypertension Society (BHS) provides a list of validated devices at http://www.bhsoc.org//index.php?cID=246). Wrist devices may be useful for athletes with large arms in whom the standard cuff sizes are not recommended. A number of mobile applications have become available in recent years, but none of them is currently recommended by the scientific societies. For an accurate blood pressure measurement, athletes must be instructed on the appropriate methodology, which is similar to that used in an office setting. Athletes must take at least two consecutive readings about 1–2 minutes apart twice daily (e.g. before breakfast and before the evening meal) for 5–7 days [12,13]. These measurements should be registered on a monitoring sheet. This method has the advantage of improving athletes' compliance with their own management, but the education and cooperation of the athlete are required for accurate measurement.

Ambulatory Blood Pressure Monitoring

One of the unique aspects of ABPM is its ability to record the diurnal variation of blood pressure. The normal pattern is a mean 10% decrease in average SBP or DBP at night compared with daytime, commonly referred to as 'dipping'. ABPM for 24 hours is considered the gold standard for out-of-office blood pressure measurement [12]. It has the additional advantage of providing information about the dipper status and blood pressure variability. Nocturnal hypertension is associated with sleep apnoea and masked hypertension in athletes [3]. The non-dipper status is related to higher cardiovascular mortality, and is more common in cases of secondary hypertension (mostly in hyperaldosteronism, hyperthyroidism, sleep apnoea and chronic kidney disease (CKD)) [13]. ABPM is also better at assessing the effectiveness of therapeutic interventions.

The definition of hypertension is based on the following ABPM cut-off values [12]:

- average SBP ≥130 mmHg and/or DB ≥80 mmHg;
- daytime (or awake) SBP ≥135 mmHg and/or DBP ≥85 mmHg;
- night-time (or asleep) SBP ≥120 mmHg and/or DBP ≥70 mmHg.

An abnormal, 'non-dipper' pattern is defined by a <10% decline in the SBP.

Assessment of the Blood Pressure Response to Exercise in Athletes

Hypertensive athletes should undergo maximal exercise testing as part of the clinical evaluation [20], which will provide valuable information about the blood pressure response during exercise and recovery and the functional capacity of the athlete. The utility of the exercise test for the diagnosis of congenital heart disease (CHD) in hypertensive athletes is beyond the scope of this chapter, but it is important to highlight that exercise-induced hypertension is frequently associated with abnormal ST-segment depression and false-positive exercise tests.

During exercise testing, systemic vascular resistance decreases and cardiac output increases. As a result, the SBP increases during exercise, whilst the DBP either does not change or decreases. *Defining hypertensive response to exercise or EIAH* in the presence of either normal or high blood pressure at rest is a complex issue. Whilst the exaggerated blood pressure response to exercise testing has been used to identify normotensive individuals at increased cardiovascular risk and at risk of developing hypertension [21] and target organ damage, there is lack of consensus regarding how to interpret and manage such individuals. Given that EIAH has been associated with masked hypertension [19,21], it would be reasonable to suggest that athletes with an abnormal blood pressure response during exercise undergo an ABPM [12].

Definition of EIAH at the Peak of Exercise

Different cut-off values for SBP at the peak of exercise have been proposed. Whilst an SBP ≥210 mmHg for men and ≥190 mmHg for women has been used in a number of studies [12], others consider a blood pressure over the 90th or 95th percentile of the reference population the most accurate parameter. There are no specific blood pressure reference values in athletic populations. It is well established that competitive endurance athletes reach a higher SBP at the peak of exercise and during heavier workouts, which could overestimate the incidence of EIAH in this population. It is also worth noting that it is challenging to obtain an accurate measure of blood pressure at peak exercise. Both these limitations are negated when assessing the blood pressure response to exercise at low or moderate loads.

Definition of EIAH at Submaximal Exercise

The evaluation of blood pressure through percentile curves of SBP and DBP at submaximal exercise provides a more accurate and comprehensive evaluation of the blood pressure response to exercise than does evaluation at peak exercise, and has been shown to identify individuals at risk of developing hypertension [21]. The percentile curves of SBP and DBP refer to the relative heart rate increases at different submaximal workloads, allowing for the comparison of individuals with varying levels of physical conditioning, related to gender, age and fitness level [21]. The heart rate, an index of exercise intensity, is expressed as a percentage of the maximal heart rate reserve (HRR).

HHR for a submaximal load (e.g. 100W) can be calculated by:

$$\frac{\textit{Heart rate at } 100W - \textit{basal heart rate}}{\textit{Predicted maximal heart rate} - \textit{basal heart rate}} \times 100 = HRR \qquad \text{(Equation 39.1)}$$

Figure 39.1 gives an example of how to use this method in the assessment of the blood pressure response during exercise in athletes.

A variant of this method using the mean artery pressure (MAP) instead of SBP and DBP has been recently been proposed [22]. Given that MAP is an index of the overall blood pressure and a marker of cardiovascular risk, this method may prove more useful in the cardiovascular risk stratification of athletes.

Abnormal Blood Pressure Response in Recovery

A blood pressure ≥140/90 mmHg measured after 5 minutes of recovery is considered abnormal. In addition, a ratio ≥0.9 between the SBP measured 3 minutes into recovery and the peak SBP has been associated with CAD.

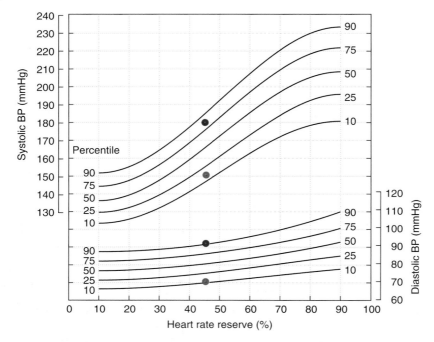

Figure 39.1 Percentile curves of SBP and DBP responses by HRR during ergometric testing at 100 W in normotensive men. Plotted in red and blue dots are the SBP and DBP of the calculated HRR in the following examples: Red: A normotensive 20-year-old football player underwent an exercise test on a bike with the following parameters: basal heart rate = 50 beats.min⁻¹; heart rate at 100 W = 120 beats.min⁻¹; blood pressure at 100 W = 150/70 mmHg. The calculated HRR at 100 W is: (120 − 50/200 − 50) × 100 = 46 beats. min⁻¹. His SBP and DBP for the calculated HRR (46 beats.min⁻¹) at 100 W fall in the lower percentile. Blue: Suppose that the blood pressure in the previous example was 180/95 mmHg at 100 W. The calculated HRR would be the same, but both SBP and DBP would fall within a very high percentile. As the incidence of hypertension increases progressively with higher percentiles of SBP and DBP response, the athlete represented in the blue plots is at increased risk of developing hypertension (*Source:* Miyai et al. [21]. Reprinted with permission)

Diagnostic Evaluation of the Hypertensive Athlete

Once hypertension is confirmed by several office blood pressure recordings and/or out-of-office methods, athletes should undergo a detailed medical history, physical examination and complementary investigations to assess aetiology (primary or secondary hypertension) and cardiovascular risk stratification, based on the evaluation of the presence of additional *cardiovascular risk factors, associated clinical conditions and target organ damage* [12,13].

Although echocardiography and exercise tests are not always recommended in the nonathletic population, the European Society of Cardiology (ESC) recommends that athletes with hypertension undergo both investigations as part of their clinical evaluation [20]. The 36th Bethesda guidelines [2] recommend the following investigations for hypertensive athletes:

- If hypertension is stage 1 (140–159/90–99 mmHg), the patient should undergo:
  ○ blood chemistry (glucose, creatinine or the corresponding estimated glomerular filtration rate, electrolytes and lipid profile), haematocrit, urine analysis (protein);
  ○ electrocardiogram (ECG).
- If hypertension is stage 2 (≥160/100 mmHg), the results of the initial tests are abnormal or features suggestive of secondary causes are noted by history or physical examination, the patient should be referred for additional investigations and therapy.

Medical History

Individual characteristics, such as family history, ethnicity, gender, age, weight and sporting discipline [12], must be evaluated. Hypertensive athletes warrant careful investigation for the use of external agents (drugs and/or performance-enhancing substances) that can raise the blood pressure [2,20].

Family History Hypertension is a heritable condition, and genes encoding the renin–angiotensin system seem to be involved in both exercise-induced cardiac remodelling and pathologic hypertension-induced remodelling. Studies have demonstrated that people with a heritable hypertensive predisposition may manifest signs of cardiovascular dysfunction before the onset of hypertension. It can be challenging, however, to differentiate these signs from the physiological cardiac remodelling induced by exercise training in athletes. Baggish et al. [23] demonstrated that physiological exercise-induced cardiac remodelling differs between normotensive athletes with and without family history of hypertension. Although both groups have increased left ventricular mass, athletes with no family history of hypertension demonstrate features of normal athlete's heart remodelling, with an eccentric pattern of left ventricular hypertrophy (LVH), normal diastolic function and greater left ventricular cavity length. Athletes with a positive family history, on the other hand, demonstrate concentric hypertrophy and abnormal diastolic function, which are common findings in hypertension-induced cardiac remodelling. *Parental hypertension* is therefore relevant not only when assessing blood pressure in athletes, but also when evaluating and interpretating the athlete's echocardiogram, even in normotensive subjects. If secondary hypertension is suspected, the family history of phaeochromocytoma and/or CKD (e.g. polycystic kidneys) is also relevant [12].

Ethnicity Hypertension is more prevalent, occurs at a younger age and is often more severe in terms of blood pressure levels in black individuals [13]. *This is relevant for the screening and follow-up of hypertension in black athletes.* Black ethnicity is also more sensitive to the blood pressure-raising effects of dietary salt, has a different blood pressure response to different antihypertensive drugs and is more vulnerable to stroke and kidney disease [13].

Gender, Age, Weight and Sporting Discipline The prevalence of hypertension is higher in male than in female athletes [5], and increases with age and weight [5]. Consideration must be given to athletes competing in sports, or specific positions, requiring a high body mass index (BMI) and in which a body mass increase during the season is likely to enhance performance, placing them at higher risk of hypertension [8].

Drugs Associated with Hypertension in Athletes

A number of external agents are associated with elevated blood pressure in athletes, some of which are included in the World Anti-Doping Agency (WADA) list of prohibited substances (denoted by an asterisk in the following list). These include:

- Stimulants (energy drinks, caffeine drinks, caffeine supplements, amphetamines,* ephedrine,* Ma Huang (ephedra*) – pseudoephedrin*), tobacco, alcohol, herbal supplements, guarana and liquorice. Cocaine* consumption is associated with acute but not chronic hypertension.
- Treatment NSAIDs; these may increase the SBP by 4–5 mmHg. *Acetaminophen has less of an impact on blood pressure and is the preferred analgesic treatment in hypertensive athletes.*
- Drugs such as glucocorticoids,* antidepressant agents, diet pills and decongestants. Adolescent females should be questioned about oral contraceptive use, given that about 5% develop elevated blood pressure over a 5-year period [24].
- Performance-enhancing drugs such as growth hormone,* erythropoietin* and anabolic steroids.*

Hypertension in Paralympic Athletes with Spinal Cord Injuries

Athletes with spinal cord injuries above T6 level may exhibit severe episodic hypertension as a result of self-induced autonomic dysreflexia (commonly known as 'boosting') and high sympathetic discharge induced by nociceptive stimuli. Experimental evidence indicates that self-induced boosting can improve performance by 10% in elite wheelchair marathon racers. Given its detrimental effects on health, the International Paralympic Committee (IPC) has banned athletes from voluntarily inducing boosting during competition [25].

Physical Examination of the Hypertensive Athlete

The following parameters and signs should be evaluated at the first visit: weight, height, BMI, waist circumference, pallor (anaemia in CKD), heart rate (relative tachycardia in hyperthyroidism, phaeochromocytoma) peripheral pulse, interscapular murmur and peripheral pulses (aortic coarctation), abdominal bruits (renal artery stenosis), exophthalmos (hyperthyroidism) and signs of heart failure [12,13].

Cardiovascular Risk Stratification of the Hypertensive Athlete

The evaluation of additional cardiovascular risk factors, associated conditions and target organ damage is highly relevant for the management and prognostic evaluation of hypertensive athletes (Table 39.2).

Cardiovascular Risk Factors

Young athletes with hypertension usually have a low or moderate cardiovascular risk. Master and recreational athletes may be at higher risk. There are several scores for cardiovascular risk stratification: the *Framingham score estimates the absolute 10-year risk of CVD*, whilst the *Systematic Coronary Risk Evaluation (SCORE) estimates the risk of dying from CVD over 10 years*. The SCORE underestimates the risk in black individuals, those with family history of premature CVD and those with diabetes mellitus or CKD.

Target Organ Damage

Hypertensive athletes should be examined to assess asymptomatic target organ damage. Target organ damage is a determinant of overall cardiovascular risk and can predict cardiovascular mortality independently of cardiovascular risk stratification. The key markers for organ damage are microalbuminuria, increased left ventricular mass with concentric LVH, increased pulse-wave velocity of the peripheral vasculature, retinopathy and carotid plaques. Ophthalmology assessment is recommended in young individuals with mild to moderate hypertension and should always be carried out in those with diabetes and severe or refractory hypertension. Peripheral artery disease and carotid plaques are commonly observed in older populations and are less relevant when assessing young athletes, in whom the heart and kidney are more commonly affected.

The assessment of LVH secondary to hypertension is challenging in athletes, due to the ECG and echocardiography findings related to the physiological remodelling of the athlete's heart. In the athletic population, ECG criteria for LVH relating to the size of the QRS complexes are common training-related findings. Although athletes can have an increased left ventricular mass, assessed by echocardiograph (left ventricular

Other risk factors, organ damage or associated condition	Grade 1 HT SBP 140–159 or DBP 90–99	Grade 2 HT SBP 160–179 or DBP 100–109	Grade 3 HT SBP ≥180 or DBP ≥110
0 risk factors	**Low risk** Allow all sports	**Moderate risk** Restriction from IIIC	**High risk** Restriction from IIIA–IIIC
1–2 risk factors	**Moderate risk** Restriction from IIIC	**Moderate to high risk** Restriction from IIIC, possible restriction from IIIA and IIIB	**High risk** Restriction from IIIA–IIIC
≥3 risk factors, organ damage, CKD stage 3 or diabetes mellitus	**High risk** Restriction from IIIC, possible restriction from IIIA and IIIB	**High risk** Restriction from IIIA–IIIC	**Very high risk** Only IA and IB allowed
CVD, CKD stage 4 or diabetes and organ damage/risk factors	**Very high risk** Only IA and IB allowed	**Very high risk** Only IA and IB allowed	**Very high risk** Only IA and IB allowed

Table 39.2 Stratification of total cardiovascular risk into categories of low, moderate, high and very high according to SBP and DBP and prevalence of risk factors (male gender, age >55 years in men and >45 in women, smoking, dyslipidaemia, abdominal obesity, first-degree family history of premature CVD, asymptomatic organ damage, diabetes, CKD or CVD), as per the ESC [12] and the Bethesda guidelines [2,20]

mass index: men $>115\,g.m^{-2}$; women $>95\,g.m^{-2}$ body surface area (BSA)), as a result of the athletic remodelling, other parameters such as relative wall thickness can be used for the differential diagnosis between normal athlete's heart and hypertensive cardiomyopathy (HCM): physiological athletic remodelling is associated with *eccentric remodelling* (relative wall thickness <0.41) *with normal diastolic function*, whilst hypertension induces concentric remodelling and may be associated with diastolic dysfunction.

Novel echocardiographic techniques may also be useful in differentiating physiological and pathological hypertrophy in hypertensive athletes. Hypertensive subjects with LVH have significantly lower longitudinal strain, peak systolic strain rate and peak early diastolic strain rate than normotensive athletes with nonpathological LVH [26].

Aetiology Assessment: Primary versus Secondary Hypertension

Secondary hypertension is defined as hypertension due to an identifiable cause. It has a prevalence of 5–10% in the general population, but its prevalence in athletes is unknown. Young athletes under 30 years of age without family history or other risk factors for hypertension should undergo screening for secondary forms. The majority of young athletes with secondary hypertension respond to specific treatment, so early detection and treatment are important to minimising irreversible organ damage.

Clinical characteristics suggestive of secondary hypertension are resistant hypertension ($>140/90\,mmHg$) despite three antihypertensive drugs, severe hypertension ($>180/110\,mmHg$), a sudden increase of blood pressure in a previously controlled patient, non-dipping or reverse dipping during ABPM and target organ damage.

Management of Hypertension in Athletes

The management of hypertensive athletes encompasses tailored nonpharmacological and pharmacological treatment, decisions relating to eligibility for sports competition and long-term follow up with re-evaluation of the blood pressure and other cardiovascular risk factors.

Nonpharmacological Treatment

Lifestyle changes, such us a change in diet, weight control and restriction of tobacco, caffeine, alcohol, stimulants, drugs and performance-enhancing substances, are the preferred first-line treatment. Education of the athlete plays an important role in long-term adherence to healthy habits.

The Mediterranean diet and DASH-style diet (Dietary Approach to Stop Hypertension) are associated with lower blood pressure. Salt restriction is recommended, although this is probably more effective in black athletes, in communities with a high-salt diet and in diabetic athletes. Athletes should be taught about available sources of dietary potassium [13].

Changes in the training routine may also be helpful. In a recent meta-analysis, Cornelissen and Smart [27] examined the effects of endurance, dynamic resistance, combined endurance and resistance and isometric resistance training on resting blood pressure in adults. They found that *endurance training* decreased blood pressure more than dynamic resistance and combined training in *hypertensive* participants, whilst *dynamic resistance training* might be superior to endurance and combined training in *prehypertensive* participants. Furthermore, *in contrast with previous observations* [9], *isometric resistance training resulted in larger reductions in SBP and a trend towards lower DBP compared with the other exercise modalities* in normotensive, prehypertensive and hypertensive participants. The generalisability of these results may be premature as data were available from only four trials.

Pharmacological Treatment

Pharmacological treatment is indicated in addition to nonpharmacological measures in those athletes with hypertension in stage 2 or 3, or in those with hypertension in stage 1 if there is high total cardiovascular risk or organ damage [2]. Athletes with low cardiovascular risk, no organ damage and stage 1 hypertension should be treated with nonpharmacological measures, but close follow-up is necessary to ensure the effectiveness of these interventions. When nonpharmacological treatment is not sufficient to achieve the target blood pressure, pharmacological treatment should be considered [2]. It is a reasonable approach to individualise the waiting time before the start of pharmacological treatment in these cases, as some sub-groups of athletes (those with a family history of hypertension, black athletes, those with EIAH, resistance athletes) would probably benefit from prompt pharmacological intervention.

Choice of Antihypertensive Drug

The selection of the appropriate antihypertensive treatment in athletes is based primarily on data derived from the general population. As in the general population, drug therapy is influenced by the athlete's welfare, demographics, associated comorbidities and the presence of target organ damage. Participation in competitive sports poses additional challenges, however, as certain drugs may affect the athlete's performance or infringe anti-doping rules.

Ethnicity In non-black athletes, angiotensin receptor blocker (ARB), angiotensin-converting enzyme (ACE) inhibitors and dihydropyridine calcium antagonists are the drugs of choice for the treatment of hypertension. Blockers of the renin–angiotensin system can be combined with calcium-channel blockers when one drug is insufficient for optimum blood pressure control. Diuretics should be reserved as third-line treatment: preferably thiazides or loop diuretics in conjunction with a potassium-sparing diuretic, in case of hypokalaemia.

Black individuals exhibit reduced response to ARBs, ACE inhibitors and beta blockers compared with their white counterparts. The preferred first-line treatment in black athletes is thus dihydropyridine calcium-antagonists [1]. ARBs are recommended as second-line treatment, as angioedema is a more common complication when using ACE inhibitors in the black population [13].

Gender ACE inhibitors and ARBs should be avoided in young females during their reproductive years, as these medications are contraindicated during pregnancy. Pregnant females can be treated safely with the calcium antagonist nifedipine, whilst the beta-blocker labetalol and methyldopa can be used as second-line treatment.

Age Young-adolescent athletes may be treated safely with ARBs, ACE inhibitors, calcium antagonists, diuretics and beta blockers following a similar approach to that taken in adult athletes, under paediatric advice.

Athlete-Specific Considerations
- *WADA prohibited list (*https://www.wada-ama.org/en/what-we-do/prohibited-list*)*: Diuretics are banned in all cases, as they can mask the use of other performance-enhancing drugs and have been used to rapidly reduce weight in sports in which the competition categories are weight-related. Beta blockers are prohibited during competition in motor sports, billiards, darts, golf, skiing and snowboarding (in some subspecialties) and in some underwater sports, and are prohibited even during out-of-competition periods in archery and shooting. Therapeutic use exemption (TUE) should be requested from the appropriate governing bodies if prescription of these drugs is deemed necessary to safeguard the athlete's well being.
- *Influence of antihypertensives on the athlete's performance*: Beta blockers and diuretics can affect the athlete's performance. Beta blockers have negative chronotropic and inotropic effects and affect the muscle blood flow, increasing the perception of exertion and negatively affecting the energy metabolism (lipolysis and glycogenolysis inhibition). Diuretics can affect performance through their hypovolemic effects during the first weeks of treatment.
- *Specific risks associated with some antihypertensive drugs in athletes: Diuretics* may increase the risk of dehydration and electrolyte imbalance, which increases the risk of arrhythmic events, especially when training/competing in hot/wet environments. Both diuretics and beta blockers may affect thermoregulatory function. Beta blockers may also cause hypoglycaemia in diabetic athletes.

Although current recommendations advocate office blood pressure monitoring annually in most athletes and every 6 months in those at very high risk [20], a more frequent follow-up (every 2–4 months, or even more often if indicated) will allow closer monitoring during the pre-season, season and off season for most athletes, resulting in an improved rate of detection and control of hypertension (Figure 39.2).

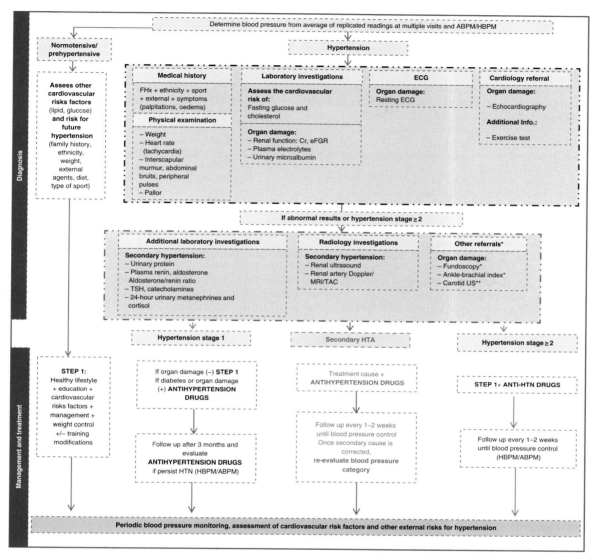

Figure 39.2 Flow chart showing the proposed diagnostic procedures in hypertensive athletes and appropriate management of fulminant hepatic failure. *Recommended in athletes with severe or refractory hypertension as complementary organ damage assessment. **Not recommended in young athletes; may be necessary in master and veteran athletes

Eligibility for Sports Participation in Hypertensive Athletes

According to the current recommendations [2], prehypertensive athletes should be encouraged to modify their lifestyle but should not be restricted from competitive sport. In case of sustained hypertension, the athlete should be evaluated with echocardiography to assess organ damage. If an abnormal pattern of LVH is found (high added risk), athletes should be commenced on antihypertensive drug therapy, and in addition should be restricted from competitive sport with a high static component (classes IIIA–IIIC) until the blood pressure normalises. Athletes with stage 1 hypertension, low cardiovascular risk and no organ damage can compete without restriction. In those with more severe hypertension (stages 2 and 3), sports participation should be restricted (particularly high-static sports: classes IIIA–IIIC) until blood pressure is well controlled [2]. Current recommendations for competitive sport participation in athletes with hypertension, in accordance with their risk classification [20], are shown in Table 39.2. Finally, when hypertension coexists with another CVD, decisions concerning eligibility for sports participation should be based on the restrictions associated with the type and severity of the relevant condition.

References

1 James, P.A., Oparil, S., Carter, B.L. et al. 2014 evidence-based guideline for management of high blood pressure in adults. Report from the panel members appointed to the Eight Joint National Committee (JNC 8). *JAMA* 2014; **311**(5): 507–20.

2 Maron, B.J. and Zipes, D.P. 36th Bethesda Conference eligibility recommendations for competitive athletes with cardiovascular abnormalities. *J Am Coll Cardiol* 2005; **45**: 1311–75.

3 Berge, H.M., Andersen, T.E., Solberg, E.E. and Steine, K. High ambulatory blood pressure in male professional football players. *Br J Sports Med* 2013; **4**: 521–5.

4 Kerney, P.M., Whelton, M., Reynolds, K. et al. Global burden of hypertension: analysis of worldwide data. *Lancet* 2005; **365**: 217–23.

5 Berge, H.M., Isern, C.B. and Berge, E. Blood pressure and hypertension in athletes: a systematic review. *Br J Sports Med* 2015; **49**(11): 716–23.

6 Karpinos, A.R., Roumie, C.L., Nian, H. et al. High prevalence of hypertension among collegiate football athletes. *Circ Cardiovasc Qual Outcomes* 2013; **6**: 716–23.

7 Balady, G.J. and Drezner, J.A. Tackling cardiovascular health risks in college football players. *Circulation* 2013; **128**: 477–80.

8 Weiner, R.B., Wang, F., Isaacs, S.K. et al. Blood pressure and left ventricular hypertrophy during american-style football participation. *Circulation* 2013; **128**: 524–31.

9 Corneliseen, V.A., Buys, R. and Smart, N.A. Endurance exercise beneficially affects ambulatory blood pressure: a systematic review and meta-analysis. *J Hypertens* 2013; **31**(4): 639–48.

10 Cornelissen, V.A., Fagard, R.H., Coeckelberghs, E. and Vanhees, L. Impact of resistance training on blood pressure and other cardiovascular risk factors. A meta-analysis of randomized, controlled trials. *Hypertension* 2011; **58**: 1–9.

11 Mancia, G., Fagard, R., Narkiewicz, N. et al. 2013 ESH/ESC guidelines for the management of arterial hypertension. The Task Force for the Management of Arterial Hypertension of the European Society of Hypertension (ESH) and of the European Society of Cardiology (ESC). *Eur Heart J* 2013; **34**: 2159–219.

12 Weber, M.A., Schiffrin, E.L., White, W.B. et al. Clinical practice guidelines for the management of hypertension in the community. A statement by the American Society of Hypertension and the International Society of Hypertension. *J Clin Hypertens* 2014; **16**(1): 14–26.

13 Lewington, S., Clarke, R., Qizilbash, N. et al. Age-specific relevance of usual blood pressure to vascular mortality: a meta-analysis of individual data for one million adults in 61 prospective studies. Prospective Studies Collaboration. *Lancet* 2002; **360**: 1903–13.

14 National High Blood Pressure Education Program Working Group on High Blood Pressure in Children and Adolescents. The fourth report on the diagnosis, evaluation, and treatment of high blood pressure in children and adolescents. *Pediatrics* 2004; **114**(2 Suppl. 4th report): 555–76.

15 Lurbe, E., Cifkova, R., Cruickshank, J.K. et al. Management of high blood pressure in children and adolescents: recommendations of the European Society of Hypertension. *J Hypertens* 2009; **27**: 1719–42.

16 Mahmud, A. and Feely, J. Spurious systolic hypertension of youth: fit young men with elastic arteries. *Am J Hypertens* 2003; **16**: 229–32.

17 Franklin, S.S., Larson, M.G., Khan, S.A. et al. Does the relation of blood pressure to coronary heart disease risk change with aging? The Framingham Heart Study. *Circulation* 2001; **103**: 1245–9.

18 Yano, Y., Stamler, J., Garside, D.B. et al. Isolated systolic hypertension in young and middle-aged adults and 31-year risk for cardiovascular mortality. *J Am Coll Cardiol* 2015; **65**(4): 327–35.

19 Bobrie, G., Clerson, P., Menard, J. et al. Masked hypertension: a systematic review. *J Hypertens* 2008; **26**: 1715–25.

20 Pellicia, A., Fagardg, R., Bjørnstad, H.H. et al. Recommendations for competitive sports participation in athletes with cardiovascular disease. A consensus document from the Study Group of Sports Cardiology of the Working Group of Cardiac Rehabilitation and Exercise Physiology and the Working Group of Myocardial and Pericardial Diseases of the European Society of Cardiology. *Eur Heart J* 2005; **26**: 1422–45.

21 Miyai, N., Arito, M., Miyashita, K. et al. Blood pressure response to heart rate during exercise test and risk of future hypertension. *Hypertension* 2002; **39**: 761–6.

22 Miyai, N., Shiozaki, M., Yabu, M. et al. Increased mean arterial pressure response to dynamic exercise in normotensive subjects with multiple metabolic risk factors. *Hypertens Res* 2013; **36**: 534–9.

23 Baggish, A.L., Weiner, R.B., Yared, K. et al. Impact of family hypertension on exercise-induced cardiac remodeling. *Am J Cardiol* 2009; **104**: 101–6.

24 Leddy, J.J. and Izzo, J. Hypertension in athletes. *J Clin Hypertens* 2009; **11**: 226–33.

25 Bhambhani, Y. Physiology of wheelchair racing in athletes with spinal cord injury. *Sports Med* 2002; **32**(1): 23–51.

26 Saghir, M., Areces, M. and Makan, M. Strain rate imaging differentiates hypertensive cardiac hypertrophy from physiologic cardiac hypertrophy (athlete's heart). *J Am Soc Echocardiogr* 2007; **20**(2): 151–7.

27 Cornelissen, V.A. and Smart, N.A. Exercise training for blood pressure: a systematic review and metaanalysis. *J Am Heart Assoc* 2013; **2**: e004473.

Part 5
Conundrums in Sports Cardiology

40 Distinguishing Physiological Left Ventricular Hypertrophy from Hypertrophic Cardiomyopathy in Athletes

Aneil Malhotra and Sanjay Sharma

Department of Cardiovascular Sciences, St George's University of London, London, UK

Introduction

The single most common cause of sudden cardiac death (SCD) in young athletes (<35 years old) is hypertrophic cardiomyopathy (HCM). Since the phenotypic expression of HCM is variable and some individuals exhibit only mild left ventricular hypertrophy (LVH), the differentiation between HCM and physiological LVH consistent with the 'athlete's heart' can be challenging. Correct distinction between the two entities is critical given that HCM accounts for nearly a third of exercise-related SCD in young athletes [1] and false reassurance may jeopardise a young life. Conversely, an erroneous diagnosis of HCM in a young athlete can lead to unnecessary disqualification and curtailment of a potentially lucrative career, as well as causing psychological distress.

This chapter discusses current noninvasive clinical strategies that differentiate physiological LVH as a result of sustained, regular physical activity from HCM. Although most data have traditionally been derived from cross-sectional studies comparing athletes with LVH to sedentary HCM patients [2,3], more recent studies have focused on direct comparisons between athletes with LVH and athletes with HCM [4,5], as the latter group demonstrate a greater functional capacity than sedentary HCM patients and may exhibit a differing set of parameters. In all cases, the differentiation between physiological LVH and HCM relies on a combination of history and familial evaluation, echocardiographic parameters, electrocardiography (ECG), echocardiography, cardiac magnetic resonance (CMR), cardiopulmonary exercise testing (CPEX), ambulatory ECG monitoring, family screening or genetic analysis and, occasionally, establishing the effects of de-training on the magnitude of LVH (Figure 40.1). It is prudent to emphasise that the results of these investigations should be used in conjunction with one another.

Establishing the 'Grey Zone'

Physiological LVH in athletes has long been established as a normal adaptive response to regular and intense bouts of exercise, with athletes demonstrating a 10–20% increase in left ventricular wall thickness (LVWT) measurements compared to sedentary controls [6]. Studies in large cohorts of athletes have revealed that the vast majority demonstrate a maximal LVWT ≤12 mm, which is considered within normal limits for the

---

IOC Manual of Sports Cardiology, First Edition. Edited by Mathew G. Wilson, Jonathan A. Drezner and Sanjay Sharma.

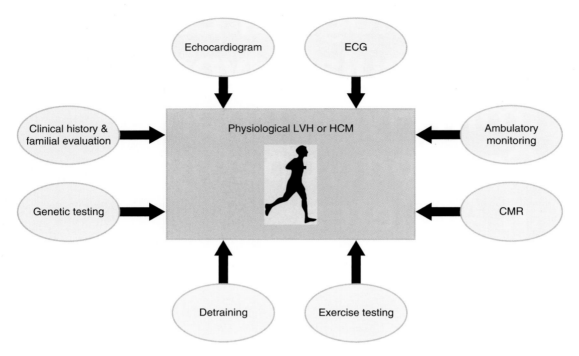

Figure 40.1 Assessment tools for differentiating physiological LVH from mild HCM

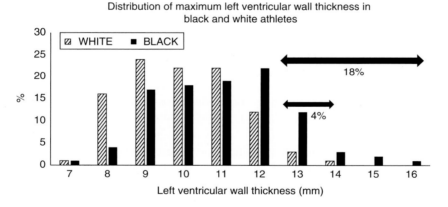

Figure 40.2 Bar chart showing the distribution of maximum LVWT in black and white athletes. Over four times as many black athletes (18%) exhibited a maximum LVWT >12 mm compared with white athletes (4%) (*Data source*: Basavarajaiah et al. [8])

general population. However, in a small proportion of athletes, the LVWT exceeds 12 mm and overlaps with morphologically mild HCM. An Italian study of nearly 1000 Olympians showed that most revealed a normal LVWT ranging between 7 and 12 mm but a small minority (1.7%) exhibited an LVWT >12 mm [7], with the greatest increases observed in elite rowers, cross-country skiers, cyclists and swimmers. A British study revealed a similar proportion of athletes with an LVWT >12 mm in cohort of 3500 [8]. Whilst both studies were based primarily on Caucasian (white) athletes, the latter group conducted a separate study evaluating the impact of ethnicity on LVH in athletes. The results demonstrated that Afro-Caribbean (black) athletes have greater magnitudes of LVH than Caucasians [8]. In this study, 18% of 300 black athletes exhibited an LVWT >12 mm, with 3% ≥15 mm. In contrast, none of the Caucasians showed an LVWT ≥15 mm (Figure 40.2). In all studies discussed, the maximal value was 16 mm; beyond this limit, LVH in an athlete is now considered pathological.

Therefore, a small minority of Caucasian athletes and up to one-fifth of black athletes reveal LVWT measurements of 13–16 mm, which overlap with up to 15% of individuals with HCM. This spectrum of

LVWT measurements forms the conventional grey zone between physiological LVH and morphologically mild HCM. The vast majority of patients with HCM cannot augment stroke volume for prolonged periods and have a relatively low functional capacity. However, the heterogeneous nature of HCM is such that some affected individuals have an excellent exercise capacity and are capable of competing at regional or national level.

History and Familial Evaluation

Symptoms such as chest pain, dyspnoea that is disproportionate to the amount of exercise, palpitations or unheralded loss of consciousness should raise concern when evaluating an athlete with LVH, especially if they occur during or immediately after exercise. Given the autosomal-dominant nature of HCM, a positive family history for sudden or unexplained deaths, particularly in first-degree relatives less than 40 years old, should raise the suspicion of an inherited cardiac condition. This issue becomes especially pertinent if there is already a confirmed diagnosis of HCM in the family, or if a first-degree relative expresses an abnormal ECG or echocardiography consistent with HCM.

A number of demographic factors need also to be accounted for when determining whether LVH is likely to be physiological. In general, physiological LVH >12 mm is confined to large Caucasian, adult male athletes competing in endurance sports and black males competing in both endurance sports and activities with a start–stop nature, such as football or basketball. Caucasian females do not show an LVWT >11 mm and only a very small minority of adult black female athletes reveal an LVWT >12 mm (see Chapter 5).

Echocardiography

Echocardiography is the most widely available cardiac imaging modality. It has the ability to visualise the magnitude and pattern of LVH, measure chamber dimensions and assess both systolic and diastolic function. Hitherto, most data establishing normal parameters in athletes have been derived from observational studies using echocardiography as the only imaging modality.

Pattern of LVH

Athletes with physiological LVH exhibit a homogenous and symmetrical increase in LVWT. In HCM, by contrast, several patterns are observed, including asymmetrical, septal and apical hypertrophy. Our experience has demonstrated that most athletes with HCM exhibit the apical variant, compared with sedentary individuals with HCM [4].

Dynamic Left Ventricular Outflow Tract Obstruction

Systolic anterior motion (SAM) of the mitral valve against the interventricular septum causing dynamic left ventricular outflow tract (LVOT) obstruction is present in approximately 25% of HCM individuals and up to 70% of cases during exercise. Such features are not present in athletes with physiological LVH.

Left Ventricular Cavity Size

The vast majority of athletes with physiological LVH demonstrate concomitant left ventricular cavity enlargement ranging between 55 and 65 mm. In contrast, individuals with HCM generally have a reduced left ventricular cavity size of <50 mm. In this regard, the relative wall thickness (RWT), which is the sum of the interventricular septum and the posterior wall thickness in end diastole divided by left ventricular end-diastolic diameter, is a useful parameter in differentiating between physiological LVH and HCM. Athletes generally have a RWT <0.45. Recently, a study comparing athletes with LVH with HCM controls found that a left ventricular cavity size <54 mm distinguished pathology from physiology with a sensitivity and specificity of 100% [9]. A large left ventricular cavity (>54 mm) is rare in HCM and is usually a marker of end-stage disease, with decreased left ventricular function and a marked reduction in functional capacity.

Tissue Doppler Imaging and Global Longitudinal Function

Whilst ejection fraction (EF) and fractional shortening of the left ventricle may be increased as a result of hyperdynamic left ventricular function in HCM patients, tissue Doppler imaging (TDI) reveals a reduction in longitudinal systolic function in athletes with HCM compared to those with physiological LVH. Diastolic function is also reduced in HCM individuals, due to impaired myocardial relaxation caused by myofibre disarray, fibrosis and impaired sarcoplasmic calcium kinetics. TDI at the mitral valve level has demonstrated that subjects with mild obstructive HCM exhibit lower early diastolic velocities (E′ <9 cm.s^{-1} with a sensitivity of nearly 90%) compared to physiological LVH athletes [3]. However, our experience of comparing 19 athletes with physiological LVH with 37 athletes (rather than sedentary subjects) with mild HCM without obstruction demonstrates that TDI indices of longitudinal systolic and diastolic function have poor sensitivity for the detection of disease in HCM [5]. Cut-off values of S′ <9 cm.s^{-1}, E′ <9 cm.s^{-1}, E/E′ >12 and E/A <1 had sensitivities of 43, 35, 14 and 5%, respectively. However, the specificity of these markers was high (84, 100, 100 and 95, respectively), suggesting that in the context of LVH, the presence of any of these parameters is indicative of disease. Importantly, the absence of these markers did not exclude the presence of disease in an athlete with LVH, as they all had negative predictive values (NPVs) below 44%.

Two-dimensional strain (2DS) is a relatively novel method that can measure strain from standard two-dimensional (2D) echocardiography images using speckle tracking, which is less angle-dependent and more reproducible that conventional Doppler-derived strain. A global longitudinal strain (GLS) of more than −10% results in a sensitivity of 87% and specificity of 95% for the diagnosis of HCM, although these results come from a study comparing sedentary individuals with HCM to athletes [10]. In an athlete, a GLS of more than −15% is thought to suggest pathology.

Electrocardiography

In many instances, certain repolarisation patterns and specific anomalies may facilitate the diagnosis of HCM in an athlete with LVH. Pure voltage criteria for LVH alone are observed in up to 60% of male athletes and are not accompanied by ST-segment depression or T-wave inversion (Figure 40.3). In contrast, pure or isolated criteria for LVH are uncommon in individuals with HCM. ECG anomalies favouring a diagnosis of

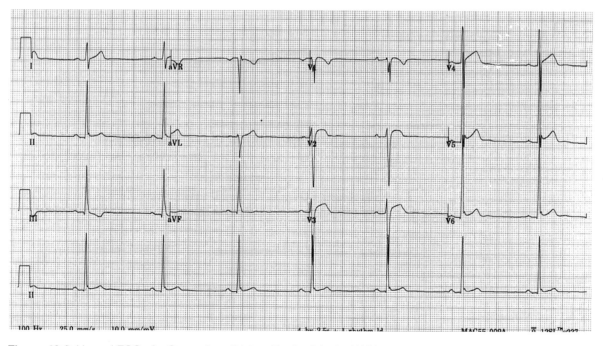

Figure 40.3 Normal ECG of a Caucasian athlete with physiological LVH, demonstrating a resting bradycardia, early repolarisation with convex ST-segment elevation across the precordial leads and isolated QRS voltage criteria for LVH

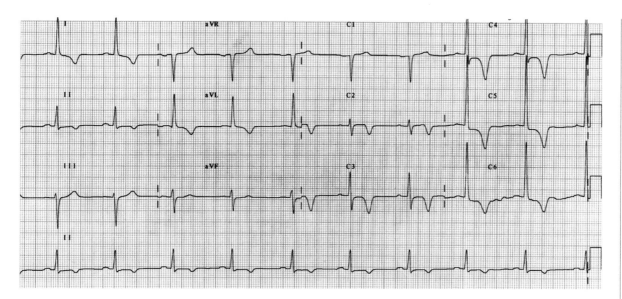

Figure 40.4 Abnormal ECG of an athlete with HCM and a maximum LVWT of 15 mm. There is marked T-wave inversion extending across the precordial leads to the lateral leads (V5–V6, aVL), with concomitant ST depression and left-axis deviation. These findings are highly abnormal and warrant further investigation

HCM include deep T-wave inversions in the inferior and/or lateral leads (Figure 40.4), left bundle branch block (LBBB), pathological Q-waves and ST-segment depression (above −0.2 mV). In a recent study of 155 athletes with pathological T-wave inversion, the inversion was mainly confined to the lateral leads, with 80% exhibiting concomitant ST-segment depression laterally. Nearly half of the athletes were diagnosed with cardiac disease at initial evaluation or within a follow-up period of 1 year. HCM accounted for 81% of all conditions diagnosed and was detected in over a third of all athletes with T-wave inversion [11].

Consideration of Ethnicity with ECG Interpretation

T-wave inversion is a recognised manifestation of HCM and is detected in over 90% of patients. T-wave inversion in leads other than III, aVR or V1–V2 is considered abnormal in an adult Caucasian athlete but is common in black athletes, where it is present in as many as 25% of adults and adolescents. T-wave inversion that is preceded by convex ST elevation in leads V1–V4 is considered a normal variant [12]. The significance of inferior T-wave inversion in isolation is unknown; however, longitudinal follow-up studies have revealed an association between lateral T-wave inversions and sudden death or a subsequent diagnosis of HCM [11,13].

Cardiac Magnetic Resonance

Having emerged as a useful adjunctive modality to echocardiography, CMR has now become the gold standard for HCM imaging. CMR provides optimum visualisation of the myocardium, with more accurate and reproducible measurements of the LVWT and its distribution [14]. CMR is unique in its high spatial and temporal resolution and excellent contrast between blood pool and myocardium, without limitation of either imaging window or plane. It is generally reserved for athletes with a LVWT >12 mm with a non-dilated left ventricle or for those with marked repolarisation changes, including ST depression and T-wave inversion. It is superior to echocardiography in detecting apical HCM and LVH confined to the lateral wall. Techniques such as gadolinium administration can reveal underlying fibrosis within the myocardium, which is indicative of HCM rather than physiological LVH [15]. Stress perfusion is another technique that can be implemented to identify widespread areas of subendocardial ischaemia, typical for HCM rather than physiological LVH [16].

Similar to LVWT/cavity ratio, the measurement of a diastolic left ventricular wall to left ventricular volume ratio >0.15 mm × m^2.ml^{-1} has >90% specificity for a diagnosis of HCM [17].

The metabolic response to pharmacologically mediated increases in heart rate during CMR may also facilitate the differentiation between physiological LVH and HCM. Studies have characterised the metabolic response to vasodilator stress in athletes, patients with phenotypic HCM and patients with disease causing mutations without LVH. Perfusion and oxygenation were normal in athletes and impaired in patients with HCM, whilst only oxygenation was impaired in mutation carriers without LVH [18]. This has important future implications for our understanding of the metabolic responses in athletes, which is playing an increasing role in the assessment of this group.

More recent developments in CMR with T1 mapping and extracellular volume (ECV) content measurement has the potential of differentiating physiological LVH from mild HCM in athletes. Current data reveal that patients with HCM demonstrate high T1 signals and in increased ECV due to extracellular fibrosis and inflammation. In contrast physiological LVH is due to an increase in cell size and a relative decrease in the ECV. A study of 30 endurance athletes and 15 sedentary patients revealed that the ECV component of LV mass was similar between athletes and controls, yet athletes showed a significantly higher indexed cellular mass compared to controls [19]. Furthermore the highest performing athletes (peak oxygen consumption, VO2 max > 60mls/min/kg) had the lowest ECV.

Another study by the same group investigated 16 patients with HCM and 10 athletes with physiological LVH. The HCM group had a higher ECV compared to athletes and also demonstrated a string correlation between ECV and wall thickness. An ECV of 22.5% differentiated physiological LVH from HCM with a sensitivity of 100% and specificity of 90%.

Cardiopulmonary Exercise Testing

The physiological response to exercise is somewhat ironically a powerful discriminator of physiology from pathology in athletes with LVH. Almost 25% of individuals with HCM demonstrate an attenuated blood pressure response during exercise, due to abnormal vascular tone, small-vessel ischaemia or exertional LVOT obstruction [16]. ST-segment depression, T-wave inversion or ventricular arrhythmias may be observed in individuals with HCM.

Measurement of peak oxygen consumption (VO_{2max}) has been shown to help as a discriminator between HCM and physiological LVH in athletes [20]. Individuals with HCM may be affected by impaired diastolic function, small left ventricular cavity size, dynamic LVOT obstruction and microcirculatory coronary disease leading to a reduction in subendocardial flow. The net effect is a reduced ability of the myocardium to augment stroke volume as exercise progresses, resulting in a relatively low cardiac output and low VO_{2max}.

Athletes with physiological LVH, especially those competing in endurance sports, generally have an enlarged left ventricular cavity and enhanced left ventricular filling in diastole, enabling them to generate and maintain a large stroke volume and cardiac output throughout exercise. A VO_{2max} >50 ml.kg^{-1}.min^{-1}, or >120% of age-predicted value, was been used to differentiate physiological LVH from disease. However, this cut-off is based primarily on Caucasian male athletes. As with echocardiography and ECG interpretation, VO_{2max} variations for African/Afro-Caribbean athletes and those with HCM are yet to be validated, as 50 ml.kg^{-1}.min^{-1} as a discriminator may not be applicable to this group.

Ambulatory ECG Monitoring

The presence of multiple (>2000) ventricular extrasystoles arising from the left ventricle or of runs of non-sustained ventricular tachycardia (NSVT) during 24–48-hour Holter monitoring in an athlete with LVH is suggestive of underlying pathology.

Genetics

The past 2 decades have witnessed a tremendous unravelling of the molecular genetics of HCM: 12 genes and over 1400 sarcomeric mutations accounting for the HCM phenotype have been identified. However, given the heterogeneity of the condition, the diagnostic yield is currently 60%, leaving a significant proportion of individuals without a definitive result. It is our practice to offer screening of first-degree relatives in an athlete who continues to pose a diagnostic dilemma despite comprehensive investigation. We offer genetic testing after informed consent according to ethical guidelines when we do not have access to family members or if family screening is normal. Genetic testing is currently not widely available and sample analysis may take months, and the expense needs to be considered. We permit the athlete to continue participation pending the results of the analysis.

De-training

The cessation of exercise for 6–8 weeks often reverses the structural and electrical changes of the athlete's heart, with normalisation of ECG repolarisation changes and regression of physiological LVH [21]. An athlete with HCM will show a persistent pathological phenotype [22]. Whilst this approach appears highly practical, persuading an athlete to de-train is a difficult task, as they will often strive to maintain their fitness level, position within a team or earnings through ongoing participation. The usual mode of de-training generally occurs when an athlete is injured and therefore has a forced period of rest during which the reversal of physiological changes can be observed.

Potential Role of Biomarkers

There are emerging data to show that certain biomarkers may be elevated by the pathological processes of cardiomyocyte hypertrophy, sarcomeric disarray and fibrosis, resulting in myocardial remodelling in HCM. High-sensitivity cardiac troponin T (hs-cTnT) and B-type natriuretic peptide (BNP) have been proposed as biomarkers of fibrosis in HCM patients [23]. Furthermore, several studies have demonstrated a functional role of the signalling nanomolecule, microribonucleic acid (miRNA), in myocardial hypertrophy and fibrosis [24]. Whilst research intensifies in this field, the current clinical significance of such biomarkers is yet to be fully validated.

Conclusion

Whilst the majority of athletes exhibit LVH that falls within the normal range, a small proportion have a maximum LVWT in the grey zone between 13 and 16 mm. A variety of noninvasive methods (summarised in Figure 40.5) based on current evidence are available to facilitate the differentiation between physiological LVH and morphologically mild HCM in this group.

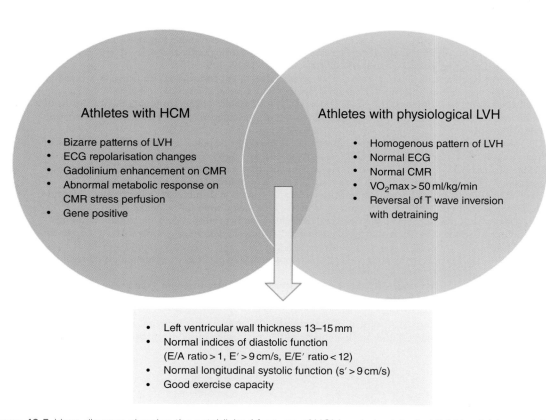

Figure 40.5 Venn diagram showing the established features of HCM and physiological LVH in athletes and the 'grey zone' overlap between the two

References

1 Maron, B.J. Hypertrophic cardiomyopathy and other causes of sudden cardiac death in young competitive athletes, with considerations for preparticipation screening and criteria for disqualification. *Cardiol Clin* 2007; **25**: 399–414.

2 Sharma, S., Maron, B.J., Whyte, G. et al. Physiologic limits of left ventricular hypertrophy in elite junior athletes: relevance to differential diagnosis of athlete's heart and hypertrophic cardiomyopathy. *J Am Coll Cardiol* 2002; **40**(8): 1431–6.

3 Vinereanu, D., Florescu, N., Sculthorpe, N. et al. Differentiation between pathologic and physiologic left ventricular hypertrophy by tissue doppler assessment of long-axis function in patients with hypertrophic cardiomyopathy or systemic hypertension and in athletes. *Am J Cardiol* 2001; **88**(1): 53–8.

4 Sheikh, N., Papadakis, M., Ghani, S. et al. Comparison of electrocardiographic criteria for the detection of cardiac abnormalities in elite black and white athletes. *Circulation* 2013; **129**(16): 1637–49.

5 Malhotra, A., Sheikh, N., Dhutia, H. et al. Differentiating physiological left ventricular hypertrophy from hypertrophic cardiomyopathy in athletes: proposed echocardiographic protocol. *Heart* 2014; **100**(Suppl. 3): A52.

6 Maron, B. Structural features of the athlete heart as defined by echocardiography. *JACC* 1986; **7**(1): 190–203.

7 Pelliccia, A., Maron, B.J., Spataro, A. et al. The upper limit of physiologic cardiac hypertrophy in highly trained elite athletes. *N Engl J Med* 1991; **324**(5): 295–301.

8 Basavarajaiah, S., Boraita, A., Whyte, G. et al. Ethnic differences in left ventricular remodeling in highly-trained athletes relevance to differentiating physiologic left ventricular hypertrophy from hypertrophic cardiomyopathy. *J Am Coll Cardiol* 2008; **51**(23): 2256–62.

9 Caselli, S., Maron, M.S., Urbano-Moral, J.A. et al. Differentiating left ventricular hypertrophy in athletes from that in patients with hypertrophic cardiomyopathy. *Am J Cardiol* 2014; **114**(9): 1383–9.

10 Butz, T., van Buuren, F., Mellwig, K.P. et al. Two-dimensional strain analysis of the global and regional myocardial function for the differentiation of pathologic and physiologic left ventricular hypertrophy: a study in athletes and in patients with hypertrophic cardiomyopathy. *Int J Cardiovasc Imaging* 2011; **27**(1): 91–100.

11 Schnell, F., Riding, N., O'Hanlon, R. et al. Recognition and significance of pathological T-wave inversions in athletes. *Circulation* 2015; **131**(2): 165–73.

12 Sheikh, N., Papadakis, M., Carre, F. et al. Cardiac adaptation to exercise in adolescent athletes of African ethnicity: an emergent elite athletic population. *Br J Sports Med* 2013; **47**(9): 585–92.

13 Papadakis, M., Carre, F., Kervio, G. et al. The prevalence, distribution, and clinical outcomes of electrocardiographic repolarization patterns in male athletes of African/Afro-Caribbean origin. *Eur Heart J* 2011; **32**(18): 2304–13.

14 Moon, J., Fisher, N.G., McKenna, W.J. and Pennell, D.J. Detection of apical hypertrophic cardiomyopathy by cardiovascular magnetic resonance in patients with non-diagnostic echocardiography. *Heart* 2004; **90**(6): 645–9.

15 Popović, Z.B., Kwon, D.H., Mishra, M. et al. Association between regional ventricular function and myocardial fibrosis in hypertrophic cardiomyopathy assessed by speckle tracking echocardiography and delayed hyperenhancement magnetic resonance imaging. *J Am Soc Echocardiogr* 2008; **21**(12): 1299–305.

16 Kawasaki, T., Azuma, A., Kuribayashi, T. et al. Vagal enhancement due to subendocardial ischemia as a cause of abnormal blood pressure response in hypertrophic cardiomyopathy. *Int J Cardiol* 2008; **129**(1): 59–64.

17 Petersen, S.E., Selvanayagam, J.B., Francis, J.M. et al. Differentiation of athlete's heart from pathological forms of cardiac hypertrophy by means of geometric indices derived from cardiovascular magnetic resonance. *J Cardiovasc Magn Reson* 2005; **7**(3): 551–8.

18 Karamitsos, T.D., Dass, S., Suttie, J. et al. Blunted myocardial oxygenation response during vasodilator stress in patients with hypertrophic cardiomyopathy. *J Am Coll Cardiol* 2013; **61**(11): 1169–76.

19 Swoboda, P.P., McDiarmid, A.K., Erhayiem, B. et al. Assessing myocardial extracellular volume by T1 mapping to distinguish hypertrophic cardiomyopathy from athlete's heart. *J Am Coll Cardiol* 2016; **67**(18): 2189–90.

20 Sharma, S., Elliott, P.M., Whyte, G. et al. Utility of metabolic exercise testing in distinguishing hypertrophic cardiomyopathy from physiologic left ventricular hypertrophy in athletes. *J Am Coll Cardiol* 2000; **36**(3): 864–70.

21 Basavarajaiah, S., Wilson, M., Junagde, S. et al. Physiological left ventricular hypertrophy or hypertrophic cardiomyopathy in an elite adolescent athlete: role of detraining in resolving the clinical dilemma. *Br J Sports Med 2006*; **40**(8): 727–9, disc. 729.

22 Pelliccia, A., Maron, B.J., De Luca, R. et al. Remodeling of left ventricular hypertrophy in elite athletes after long-term deconditioning. *Circulation* 2002; **105**(8): 944–9.

23 Kawasaki, T., Sakai, C., Harimoto, K. et al. Usefulness of high-sensitivity cardiac troponin T and brain natriuretic peptide as biomarkers of myocardial fibrosis in patients with hypertrophic cardiomyopathy. *Am J Cardiol* 2013; **112**(6): 867–72.

24 Roncarati, R., Viviani Anselmi, C., Losi, M.A. et al. Circulating miR-29a, among other up-regulated microRNAs, is the only biomarker for both hypertrophy and fibrosis in patients with hypertrophic cardiomyopathy. *J Am Coll Cardiol* 2014; **63**(9): 920–7.

41 Screening for Cardiovascular Disease in the Older Athlete

Mats Börjesson

Åstrand Laboratory, Swedish School of Sport and Exercise Sciences (GIH) and Department of Cardiology, Karolinska University Hospital, Stockholm, Sweden

Introduction

In parallel with a surge in the prevalence of obesity and its associated cardiovascular risks, the past 2 decades have also witnesssed an increase in the number of middle-aged and older individuals engaging in competitive sports and mass exercise events, such as marathon-running [1]. Such trends invariably mean that a greater proportion of individuals participating in high-intensity sport have a higher risk profile.

The rationale for screening the older athlete for cardiovascular disease (CVD) is to minimise the inherent risks of sports/physical activity whilst achieving the well-established benefits of regular physical activity, as shown in Table 41.1 [2–6]. The older athlete is traditionally defined as aged >35 years of age and is frequently referred to as a 'master or senior athlete' [7,8]. The causes of exercise-related sudden cardiac death (SCD) in this group differ considerably from those in younger athletes. This chapter also encompasses seniors who want to participate in leisure-time sports.

Coronary artery disease (CAD) is by far the most common cause of SCD in senior athletes [9], accounting for >75% of all cardiac deaths during exercise [10]. CAD is a progressive disease. It may not cause symptoms for many, but individuals at the highest risk of SCD can be identified using conventional methods for detecting myocardial ischaemia.

Risk–Benefit of Physical Activity

Most existing recommendations concerning the effect of physical activity on health primarily recommend moderate-intensity aerobic activity, corresponding to at least 150 minutes a week [11]. This level of activity has been shown to provide significant and established health effects, including a 50% reduction in adverse cardiac events due to CAD [3] and reduced mortality [12,13]. It is noteworthy that this level of physical activity is recommended in addition to daily life activites, and that more intense activity may lead to further health benefits [14].

Studies have shown that high-intensity activity produces a greater reduction in blood lipid concentration [15]. In addition, high-intensity aerobic activity leads to a superior maximal oxygen uptake (VO_{2max}) [16], which is an independent risk factor for future morbidity and death. Conversely, the risk of cardiac events is increased 2–56 times during exercise in individuals with CAD [17,18]. Although regular physical activity has multiple health benefits during the disease process and its complications, in individuals with CAD, the risk–benefit ratio of exercise will vary greatly between individuals. Generally, those who have been previously sedentary, have multiple risk factors and are taking part in high-intensity activity are considered at highest risk. Both the American Heart Association (AHA) [8] and the European Society of Cardiology (ESC) [7] have proposed recommendations for the evaluation of seniors before their participation in sports. Both organisations propose a practical approach, using initial self-assessment to identify at-risk patients who are deemed appropriate for further cardiac assessment by specialists.

IOC Manual of Sports Cardiology, First Edition. Edited by Mathew G. Wilson, Jonathan A. Drezner and Sanjay Sharma.
© 2017 International Olympic Committee. Published 2017 by John Wiley & Sons, Ltd.

Effect on coronary artery disease (CAD) risk factors

- Increased serum high-density lipoprotein (HDL) cholesterol levels
- Reduced serum triglyceride and low-density lipoprotein (LDL) cholesterol levels
- Reduced obesity
- Reduced blood pressure
- Improved insulin sensitivity and glucose balance
- Improved endothelial function
- Reduced stress

Effects on blood and circulation

- Decreased haematocrit and blood viscosity
- Expanded blood plasma volume (BPV)
- Increased red blood cell (RBC) deformability and tissue perfusion
- Increased circulatory fibrinolytic activity
- Increased coronary flow reserve
- Increased coronary collateral circulation
- Increased tolerance of ischaemia
- Increased myocardial capillary density
- Increased ventricular fibrillation thresholds
- Reduced atherosclerosis
- Reduced major morbidity and mortality

Table 41.1 Positive effects of physical activity (*Source*: Lavie et al. [4]. Reproduced with permission of Elsevier)

Coronary Artery Disease: Pathogenesis

Atherosclerosis is a progressive arterial disease that is responsible for a large proportion of deaths worldwide, predominantly from CAD and cerebrovascular accidents [19]. Risk factors for atherosclerosis include smoking, diabetes, hypertension, hyperlipidaemia and lack of physical activity. There has been a global increase in the incidence of CAD over the past 5 decades, due to the establishment of a sedentary lifestyle combined, inadequate dietary habits and the prevalence of smoking.

Atherosclerosis is a complex process, involving a number of factors and inflammatory cells, which typically interact throughout life [19,20]. The atherosclerotic process is initiated when circulating plasma low-density lipoprotein (LDL) enters the subendothelial space of the blood vessel. The oxidation of LDL is associated with an inflammatory process which upregulates adhesion molecules on the endothelium and induces the expression of chemotactic agents in endothelial cells. The activated endothelium attracts coagulation proteins, whilst the upregulation of adhesion molecules leads to recruitment of monocytes and T-lymphocytes within the vessel wall. Chemokines and cytokines such as interferon gamma (IFN-γ), tumour necrosis factor alpha (TNF-α) and interleukin 6 (IL-6) are thus expressed. In response to these factors, smooth-muscle cells migrate from the tunica media into the intimal or subendothelial space and the typical atherosclerotic fibrous cap is gradually built [20].

The inflammatory cells within the plaque also produce angiogenic factors, which result in plaque growth and possibly haemorrhage and thrombosis. The focal thickening of the vessel, caused by the growing atherosclerotic plaque, may subsequently occlude the blood flow and cause ischaemia. Rupture of the fibrous cap exposes subendothelial and thrombotic factors to the blood, causing an immediate aggregation of platelets and thrombus formation, which is the key mechanism responsible for myocardial infarction (MI) or stroke [19].

Importantly, the coronary atheriosoclerotic process may begin in early adulthood in individuals with high risk factors, whilst disease progression may take several years. Physical activity may influence several key factors in the atherosclerotic process [20], and thereby the progression of the disease, as well as the risk of acute events (Table 41.1).

SCD due to CAD in Senior Athletes

Whilst SCD in younger athletes is often attributable to inherited/congenital cardiac diseases, CAD is by far the most common cause in athletes over 35 years of age [10,18]. CAD may be asymptomatic and first manifest as sudden death.

The risk of SCD during exercise increases in parallel with the intensity of physical activity. Physical activity itself is a trigger, and increases the risk of cardiac events and sudden death considerably [17,18]. The principal mechanisms of sudden death in an individual with underlying CAD associated with sports include malignant ventricular arrhythmia associated with myocardial ischaemia, arterial vasoconstriction and platelet aggregation induced by exercise [18], possibly exaggerated by environmental factors such as stress, high altitude, dehydration, electrolyte imbalance and performance-enhancing agents (PEAs).

The risk of sudden death during exercise increases with age, particulalry in those with underlying CAD [21]. Indeed, recent studies have shown that CAD may be the most common cause of heart-related sudden death from 25 years of age onwards. In a study from King County, WA, 43% of deaths in young 25–35 year olds were attributed to CAD [22].

Clinical Presentation of CAD

As coronary artheriosclerosis progresses, some individuals begin to experience anginal pain, whilst others remain asymptomatic [23]. Importantly, in some patients, myocardial ischaemia manifests as dyspnoea on exertion ('angina equivalent') or as capacity impairment. This is particularly so in well-trained older athletes (personal perspective).

It is important to recognise that angina is a visceral pain and is therefore typically accompanied by autonomous efferent activity, such as pilorection, sweating and nausea. Referred pain, typically to the left arm, the jaw or the back, is caused by the spreading of afferent fibres from the heart several segments up and down, at spinal level through the layers of Lissauer, making it difficult for the brain to ascertain the origin of the pain stimuli. The convergence of afferents, for instance from the left arm, with afferents originating from the heart, may lead to anginal pain being perceived as coming 'from the left arm' [24]. Failure to recognise the symptoms of stable angina will increase the risk of SCD during activity.

Whilst a resting elecrocardiogram (ECG) may show ischaemic ST changes at rest, during unstable angina in the acute setting the resting ECG of an individual with stable CAD is usually normal [8]. This means that the 12-lead resting ECG, which is essential in the cardiac screening of younger athletes, has a limited role in screening of older athletes, where CAD is the most common underlying disease. The diagnostic yield of CAD is increased by performance of a stress test (cycle ergometer, treadmill or other pharmaceutical stress testing), revealing symptoms or ECG features of myocardial ischaemia [25].

Positive Effects of Physical Activity

To compare the impact of different sports on the individual athlete, a classification system has been created, where sporting activities can be characterised regarding their degree of static versus dynamic component [26]. This classification also specifies the intensity of the activity, traditionally as absolute intensity in metabolic equivalents (METs, where 1 MET is equivalent to resting energy expenditure). Various activities can then be expressed in absolute terms in METs, regardless of who performs them. When using this classification, the clinician must account and correct for this, using the concept of 'relative intensity' [27].

A given absolute activity, such as walking or playing golf, can be of different relative intensity for different individuals, depending on their current oxygen uptake (VO_{2max}, fitness). Thus, for example, golf can be a low-intensity activity for a fit individual, a moderate-intensity activity for the little less well trained and a high-intensity activity for the older individual or the younger, untrained individual. This is especially important to consider when evaluating sporting participation in a patient with underlying cardiac disease [27]. Middle-aged men, post-cardiac event, may have a severely reduced oxygen uptake ability (VO_{2max} ~20 ml.min^{-1}.kg^{-1}) [28]. In these individuals, walking on level ground may be the equivalent to high-intensity activity.

To assess the relative intensity of a given exercise or sporting activity in clinical practice, it is recommended that self-assessed rate of perceived exertion (RPE) be used, which is associated with percentage maximal heart rate [25]. Alternatively, the actual heart rate can be measured (e.g. using a sports watch). The disadvantage of this is that to accurately assess the relative intensity, the individual's maximal heart rate must be known.

Evaluation of Older Individuals before Participation in Sports

The rationale for cardiac screening of older individuals who plan to take part in sporting activity (older athletes) is to identify those at higher risk of cardiovascular events and to provide them with advice on suitable activities. The existing recommendations from the major cardiac scientific societies [7,8] aim to be pragmatic and practical and to encourage safe participation in sports, without adding unnecessary obstacles to particpation.

Current Recommendations from the American Heart Assocation

The AHA Science Advisory Committee recommends preparticipation screening for all master athletes (defined as >40 years old and participating in competitive events) [8]. This screening comprises 12 relevant points as defined by the AHA, including:

- family history (premature death and heart disease);
- personal history (effort-related symptoms and earlier cardiac disease);
- physical examination (heart auscultation, femoral pulses, stigmata of Marfan syndrome and blood pressure).

Resting ECG is considered of limited diagnostic value for detecting CAD in asymptomatic master athletes. Instead, in the presence of at least one major risk factor, men >40 and women >50 years of age are advised to undergo a maximal exercise test [8]. Likewise, exercise testing is warranted in any master athlete with symptoms suggestive of underlying CAD and in all master athletes >65 years of age, regardless of risk factors and symptoms.

The use of exercise testing for the detection of CAD in asymptomatic individuals (and in middle-aged runners) has been debated, mainly due to the risk of false-negative results [29]. However, several studies have shown that if an exercise test is abnormal in an individual with coronary risk factors, the prognosis is worse [30]; thus, the potential use of exercise testing is greater, as the risk profile increases. In addition, it has to be acknowledged that the vast majority of exercise tests in this population may be falsely positive (95%) [31].

Current Recommendations from the European Association for Cardiac Prevention and Rehabilitation

The rationale for the existing European Association for Cardiac Prevention and Rehabilitation (EACPR) recommendations [7] is that the extent of the cardiovascular evaluation needed in middle-aged/senior individuals before commencement of sporting activity depends on three parameters:

1. the individual risk profile;
2. the habitual level of physical activity;
3. the type of sport intended (level of physical activity).

The *individual risk profile* should be estimated from the burden of the recognised cardiovascular risk factors, in combination with the current level of fitness or habitual physical activity of the individual. The identification of risk factors for CAD can be achieved in several ways. In the current recommendations, the first line of risk evaluation is self-assessment (by the individual or by non-physician health professionals) using validated questionnaires, such as the AHA Preparticipation Questionnaire or the Physical Activity Readiness Questionnaire (PAR-Q) (Table 41.2) [32]. This method of self-assessment can be applied for large groups of individuals, minimising obstacles to exercise.

If an individual provides a 'positive' answer to any of the questions on the PAR-Q, they should be assessed more thoroughly by a qualified physician, using traditional risk scores, such as the ESC Systematic Coronary Risk Evaluation (SCORE) [11]. In the SCORE, the presence and degree of five traditional risk factors (age, gender, blood pressure, serum cholesterol and smoking) provide an estimate of the predicted 10-year mortality risk (from 0 to 50%) [11]. As not all risk factors are part of the ESC/Framingham risk scores, consideration must also be given to additional major risk factors, such as family history, diabetes and individual fitness level.

Because individuals with underlying CAD may often be asymptomatic (silent CAD), it is very important to assess family history (asking about early-onset CAD, unexplained death and inherited diseases, such as familiar hypercholesterolaemia) and the total risk factor profile (risk factors, inactivity) [7,8]. This may assist

1. Has a doctor ever said that you have a heart condition and recommended only medically supervised activity? Yes/No
2. Do you have chest pain brought on by physical activity? Yes/No
3. Have you developed chest pain in the past month? Yes/No
4. Have you on 1 or more occasions lost consciousness or fallen over as a result of dizziness? Yes/No
5. Do you have a bone or joint problem that could be aggravated by the proposed physical activity? Yes/No
6. Has a doctor ever recommended medication for your blood pressure or a heart condition? Yes/No
7. Are you aware, through your own experience or a doctor's advice, of any other physical reason that would prohibit you from exercising without medical supervision? Yes/No

Table 41.2 Revised Physical Activity Readiness Questionnaire (PAR-Q) (*Source*: Thomas et al. [32]. Reproduced with permission of Taylor and Francis)

in deciding the proper evaluation of the older individual (e.g. whether they are suitable for further evaluation by stress testing).

Assessment of the *habitual level of physical activity* can be achieved by several methods, including pedometers, accelerometers and questionnaires, depending on availability and need for accuracy. Studies have shown that an individual with a low habitual physical activity level may be at a considerably higher risk than shown by the Framingham score alone [33], where the physical activity level is not considered per se. For instance, it has been shown that a sedentary, lean woman may have a higher cardiovascular risk than a physically active, overweight women [34]. Also, habitual exercise reduces the triggering effect of intensive exercise [35]. Thus, the EACPR divides its recommendations according to the level of habitual physical activity.

Evaluation of Sedentary Older Individuals

Apparently healthy older (>35 years) individuals who wish to engage in low-intensity physical activity (<3 METs) are considered eligible without further evaluation [7]. However, before engaging in regular medium- to high-intensity exercise (3–6 METs), sedentary older individuals should also have a maximal exercise test, as part of the physician's evaluation. Individuals with a normal test are eligible for moderate- or even high-intensity exercise training, although cardiovascular evaluation should be repeated on an individual basis. An abnormal exercise test (e.g. showing inducible ischaemia, malignant arrhythmias, an abnormal blood pressure response or severely decreased physical capacity) warrants further evaluation by a cardiologist.

Evaluation of Physically Active Older Individuals

Physically active individuals have a statistically lower risk for cardiovascular complications during sports compared with sedentary individuals with the same ESC/Framingham risk score classification. Therefore, asymptomatic active individuals aged over 35 years do not require cardiovascular evaluation in order to participate in low-intensity activity.

Physically active individuals who wish to participate in moderate-intensity (3–6 METs) physical activity, or to continue being active at that level, should be evaluated by self-assessment questionnaire (e.g. PAR-Q), as already described. Individuals with symptoms or a history of CVD on self-assessment should be further evaluated by a physician. This traditional risk assessment should include reassessment of the personal and family history, physical examination, SCORE and a 12-lead resting ECG (Figure 41.1).

All physically active individuals >35 years of age who are contemplating or are already engaged in high-intensity (>6 METs) activity are recommended to undergo a similarly detailed evaluation by a qualified physician. This applies even in the absence of symptoms or other known risk factors for CAD. Furthermore, these individuals are recommended to undergo additional maximal exercise testing. If the exercise test is normal, they are eligible for moderate/high-intensity sports In clinical practice, this comprises a large group of older athletes taking part in master competitions, including long-distance running, skiing and cycling.

With greater numbers of older and less fit individuals expected to take part in competitive races in the future, the number of older athletes with underlying subclinical CAD is expected to rise, as is the number of older athletes with positive exercise tests.

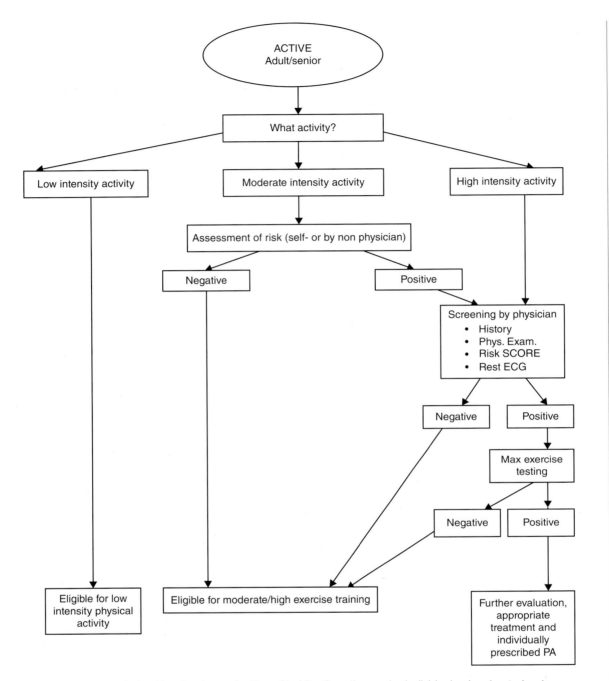

Figure 41.1 Proposed algorithm for the evaluation of habitually active senior individuals planning to begin sporting activity (*Source*: Borjesson et al. [7]. Reproduced with permission from Springer)

In the event of a positive exercise test, further evaluation is necessary to confirm or refute the presence of CAD or another underlying cardiovascular abnormality. If the results are unequivocal, further stress testing and assessment may be necessary, including pharmacological stress echocardiography, single-photon emission computed tomography (SPECT) and myocardial scintigraphy. If there are signs of inducible myocardial ischaemia, coronary angiography is recommended [25]. Additional coronary imaging, including cardiac magnetic resonance (CMR), echocardiography, Holter monitoring and biochemichal and other markers (troponin-T, high-sensitivity C-reactive protein (CRP), coronary calcium score [36]), could add valuable information but must not delay coronary angiography, when indicated.

Follow-Up/Reassessment

A regular reassessment of the risk factor profile, on an individual basis, is recommended by the EACPR [7]. The exercise test remains an important tool, providing information on cardiorespiratory fitness, blood pressure responses and exercise-related arrhythmias. Exercise testing also offers guidance on the optimal individual intensity of physical activity. Regular reassessment of the cardiorespiratory fitness level, using a suitable evaluation method, should therefore be part of the regular follow-up of these individuals. Older patients may have comorbidities, potentially affecting the ability to reach an adequate level of activity, mainly due to musculoskeletal or orthopedic problems. In addition, the use of cardiac medications can affect the ability to reach maximal pulse (e.g. beta blockers, diuretics).

If underlying CAD is confirmed, the patient should be treated according to international standards. Advice on their ability to engage in sports should follow AHA [37] and/or ESC-recommendations [38].

Conclusion

CAD is by far the most common cause of SCD in older athletes. Whilst it may progress slowly and remain asymptomatic over many years, it can potentially be identified by testing, most readily in at-risk patients.

References

1 Aagaard, P., Sahlén, A. and Braunschweig, F. Performance trends and cardiac biomarkers in a 30-km cross-country race, 1993–2007. *Med Sci Sports Exerc* 2012; **44**: 894–9.
2 Hambrecht, R., Wolf, A., Gielen, S. et al. Effect of exercise on coronary endothelial function in patients with coronary artery disease. *N Engl J Med* 2000; **342**: 454–60.
3 Blair, S.N. and Morris, J.N. Healthy hearts and the beneficial effect of being physically active. *Ann Epidemiol* 2009; **19**: 253–6.
4 Lavie, C.J., Thomas, R.J., Squires, R.W. et al. Exercise training and cardiac rehabilitation in primary and secondary prevention of coronary heart disease. *Mayo Clin Proc* 2009; **84**: 373–83.
5 Hamer, M., Ingle, L., Carroll, S. and Stamatakis, E. Physical activity and cardiovascular mortality risk: possible protective mechanisms? *Med Sci Sports Exerc* 2012; **44**: 84–8.
6 Cornelissen, V.A. and Smart, N.A. Exercise training for blood pressre: a systematic review and meta-analysis. *J Am Heart Assoc* 2013; **2**: e004473.
7 Börjesson, M., Urhausen, A., Kouidi, E. et al. Cardiovascular evaluation of middle-aged/senior individuals engaged in leisure-time sport activities: position stand from the section of exercise physiology and sports cardiology of the European Association of Cardiovascular Prevention and Rehabilitation. *Eur J Cardiovasc Prev Rehabil* 2011; **18**: 446–58.
8 Maron, B.J., Araujo, C.G., Thompson, P.D. et al. Recommendations for preparticipation screening and the assessment of cardiovascular disease in masters athletes: an advisory for healthcare professionals from the working groups of the World Heart Federation, the International Federation of Sports Medicine, and the American Heart Association Committee on Exercise, Cardiac Rehabilitation, and Prevention. *Circulation* 2001; **103**: 327–34.
9 Börjesson, M. and Pelliccia, A. Incidence and aetiology of sudden cardiac death in young athletes: an international perspective. *Br J Sports Med* 2009; **43**: 644–8.
10 Chugh, S.S. and Weiss, J.B. Sudden cardiac death in the older athlete. *J Am Coll Cardiol* 2015; **65**: 493–502.
11 Perk, J., Debacker, G., Gohlke, H. et al. European guidelines on cardiovascular disease prevention in clinical practice (version 2012). The Fifth Joint Task Force of the European Society of Cardiology and other Societies on Cardiovascular Disease Prevention in Clinical Practice. *Eur J Prev Cardiol* 2012; **19**: 585–667.
12 Anderson, L.B., Schnor, P., Schroll, M. and Hein, H.O. All-cause mortality associated with physical activity during leisure-time, work, sports and cycling to work. *Arch Intern Med* 2000; **160**: 1621–8.
13 Talbot, L.A., Morrell, C.H., Fleg, J.L. and Metter, E.J. Changes in leisure-time physical activity and risk of all-cause mortality in men and women: the Baltimore longitudinal study of aging. *Prev Med* 2007; **45**: 169–76.
14 Swain, D.P. and Franklin, B.A. Comparison of cardiorespiratory benefits of vigorous versus moderate intensity aerobic activity. *Am J Cadiol* 2006; **97**: 141–7.
15 Kraus, W.E., Houmard, J.A., Duscha, B.D. et al. Effects of the amount and intensity of exercise on plasma lipoproteins. *N Engl J Med* 2002; **347**: 1483–92.
16 Munk, P., Staal, E., Butt, N. et al. High-intensity interval training may reduce in-stent restenosis following percutaneous coronary intervention with stent implantation. *Am Heart J* 2009; **158**: 734–41.
17 Albert, C.M., Mittleman, M.A., Chae, C.U. et al. Triggering of sudden death from cardiac causes by vigorous exertion. *N Engl J Med* 2000; **343**: 1355–61.
18 Thompson, P.D., Franklin, B.A., Balady, G.J. et al. Exercise and acute cardiovascular events. Placing the risks into perspective. A scientific statement from the American Heart Association Council on Nutrition, Physical Activity, and Metabolism and the Council on Clinical Cardiology. *Circulation* 2007; **115**: 2358–68.
19 Lusis, A.J. *Atherosclerosis. Nature* 2000; **407**: 233–41.

20 Palmefors, H., Dutta-Roy, S., Rundqvist, B. and Börjesson, M. The effect of physical activity or exercise on key biomarkers in atherosclerosis – a systematic review. *Athersoclerosis* 2014; **235**: 150–61.

21 Vanhees, L., Rauch, B., Piepoli, M. et al. Importance of characteristics and modalities of physical activity and exercise in the management of cardiovascular health in individuals with cardiovascular disease (part III). *Eur J Prev Cardiol* 2012; **19**: 1333–56.

22 Meyer, L., Stubbs, B., Fahrenbruch, C. et al. Incidence, causes and survival trends from cardiovascular-related sudden cardiac arrest in children and young adults 0 to 35 years of age: a 30-year review. *Circulation* 2012; **126**: 1363–72.

23 Maseri, A., Crea, F., Kaski, J.C. and Davies, G. Mechanisms and significance of cardiac ischemic pain. *Prog Cardiovasc Dis* 1992; **35**: 1–18.

24 Börjesson, M. and Mannheimer, C. Chest pain: an update. *Curr Opin Anaesthesiol* 2002; **15**: 569–74.

25 Börjesson, M., Assanelli, D., Carré, F. et al. ESC Study Group of Sports Cardiology: recommendations for participation in leisure-time physical activity and competitive sports for patients with iscaemic heart disease. *Eur J Cardiovasc Prev Rehabil* 2006; **13**: 137–49.

26 Mitchell, J.H., Haskell, W., Snell, P., Van Camp, S.P. Task Force 8: classification of sports. *J Am Coll Cardiol* 2005; **45**: 1364–7.

27 Lee, I.M., Sesso, H.D., Oguma, Y. and Paffenbarger, R.S. Relative intensity of physical activity and risk of coronary heart disease. *Circulation* 2003; **107**: 1110–16.

28 Ades, P.A., Savage, P.D., Brawner, C.A.J. et al. Aerobic capacity in patients entering cardiac rehabilitation. *Circulation* 2006; **113**: 2706–12.

29 Siscovick, D.S., Ekelund, L.G. and Johnson, J.L. Sensitivity of exercise electrocardiography for acute cardiac events during moderate and strenuous physical activity. The lipid research clinics coronary primary prevention trial. *Arch Intern Med* 1991; **151**: 325–30.

30 Leon, A.S. and Connett, J. Physical activity and 10.5 year mortality in the Multiple Risk Factor Intervention Trial (MRFIT). *Int J Epidemiol* 1991; **20**: 690–7.

31 van de Sande, D.A., Hoogeveen, A., Hoogsteen, J. and Kemps, H.M. The diagnostic accuracy of exercise electrocardiography in asymptomatic recreational and competitive athletes. *Scand J Med Sci Sports* 2016; **26**(2); 214–20.

32 Thomas, S., Reading, J. and Shephard, R.J. Revision of the Physical Activity Readiness Questionnaire (PAR-Q). *Can J Sports Sci* 1992; **17**: 338–45.

33 Mora, S., Redberg, R.F., Sharnett, R. and Blumenthal, R.S. Enhanced risk assessment in asymptomatic individuals with exercise testing and Framingham Risk Scores. *Circulation* 2005; **112**: 1566–72.

34 Farrell, S.W., Braun, L.A., Barlow, C.E. et al. The relation of body mass index, cardiorespiratory fitness and all cause mortality in women. *Obes Res* 2002; **10**: 417–23.

35 Mittleman, M.A., Maclure, M., Tofler, G.H. et al. Triggering of acute myocardial infarction by heavy physical exertion. Protection against triggering by regular exercise. *N Engl J Med* 1993; **329**: 1677–83.

36 Braber, T.L., Mosterd, A., Prakken, N.H.J. et al. Rationale and the design of the Measuring Athlete's Risk of Cardiovascular Events (MARC) study. *Neth Heart J* 2015; **23**: 133–8.

37 Thompson, P.D., Myerburg, R.J., Levine, B.D. et al. Eligibility and disqualification recommendations for competitive athletes with cardiovascular abnormalities: Task Force 8: coronary artery disease: a scientific statement from the American Heart Association and American College of Cardiology. *J Am Coll Cardiol* 2015; **66**(21): 2406–11.

38 Pelliccia, A., Fagard, R., Bjornstad, H. et al. Recommendations for competitive sports participation in athletes with cardiovascular disease: a consensus document from the Study Group of Sports Cardiology of the Working Group of Cardiac Rehabilitation and Exercise Physiology and the Working Group of Myocardial and Pericardial Diseases of the European Society of Cardiology. *Eur Heart J* 2005; **26**: 1422–45.

42   Is Ultra-Endurance Exercise Damaging to the Right Ventricle?

Guido Claessen[1] and Hein Heidbuchel[2]

[1] Department of Cardiovascular Medicine, University Hospitals Leuven, Leuven, Belgium
[2] Hasselt University and Heart Center, Jessa Hospital, Hasselt, Belgium

Introduction

The health benefits of exercise, on both cardiovascular and noncardiovascular mortality, have been widely established. These benefits can be achieved with relatively low doses of exercise and provide the evidence supporting current recommendations of at least 30 minutes of moderate-intensity exercise on most days to prevent cardiovascular disease (CVD). Despite the undeniable benefits of exercise, particularly when faced with the modern inactivity pandemic, there has been very limited study of the upper ranges of the exercise dose–response relationship. Over the past few decades, we have witnessed an increasing proportion of society engaging in ultra-endurance events well in excess of the usual exercise recommendations. Although it is recognised that prolonged intense exercise is associated with an increased risk of development of musculoskeletal injuries, the concept that too much exercise could also result in cardiac fatigue/injury is rarely entertained.

To date, there have been no prospective studies assessing the health effects of intense prolonged exercise. Some studies suggest that well-trained athletes have greater life expectancy than the general population [1,2]. On the other hand, there are also data suggesting an increased prevalence of arrhythmias and chronic structural remodelling of the athlete's heart. Perhaps the most compelling evidence for this is provided by a number of studies which have demonstrated a consistent association between long-term endurance exercise and atrial fibrillation and atrial flutter [3]. The evidence that intense endurance exercise can promote arrhythmogenic remodelling of the ventricles is less definitive. Indeed, ventricular arrhythmias in athletes are rare. However, in athletes presenting with complex ventricular arrhythmias, the arrhythmias tend to originate from the right ventricle [4]. During intense exercise, the right ventricle has to withstand a greater haemodynamic load than the left [5], resulting in dysfunction of the right ventricle at the end of [6] and immediately after [7–9] several hours of intense endurance exercise. Therefore, it has been suggested that intense endurance activities may lead to right ventricular alterations due to a particularly high strain on the right ventricle, promoting an arrhythmogenic substrate in some individuals, even in the absence of an underlying identifiable genetic abnormality [9].

In this chapter, we will review the evidence showing that vigorous prolonged exercise may result in atrial and ventricular arrhythomogenic remodelling. We will detail how intense exercise places a disproportionate physiological stress on the right ventricle, which over time may lead to a proarrhythmogenic state resembling arrhythmogenic right ventricular cardiomyopathy (ARVC). This is distinctly different from the load imposed by exercise on the left ventricle, due to the greater capacity for reductions in systemic afterload. Luckily, real life-threatening damage is the exception rather than the rule, but this does not mean the sports cardiologist should not be vigilant or should not make use of the available evaluation tools in order to differentiate pathological from physiological right ventricular remodelling.

From Physiological to Pathological Remodelling in Athletes: the Atrial Example

It is well known that regular, intensive endurance training induces a combination of electrical, structural and functional cardiac alterations, commonly referred to as 'athlete's heart'. Cardiac alterations are particularly profound in those engaged in high-intensity endurance activities that are of long duration and combine endurance and power (e.g. cycling, triathlon, rowing, cross-country skiing). Cardiac dilation is generally accepted as one of the main mechanisms underpinning the athlete's superior sporting performance, as evidenced by data showing that maximal oxygen consumption during exercise correlates strongly with the extent of eccentric cardiac remodelling (Figure 42.1). The question arises as to whether there is an upper limit defining normal versus 'excessive' cardiac dilation. Profound cardiac remodelling and dilatation are linked to an increased risk of arrhythmias at the atrial and ventricular level in virtually all clinical settings.

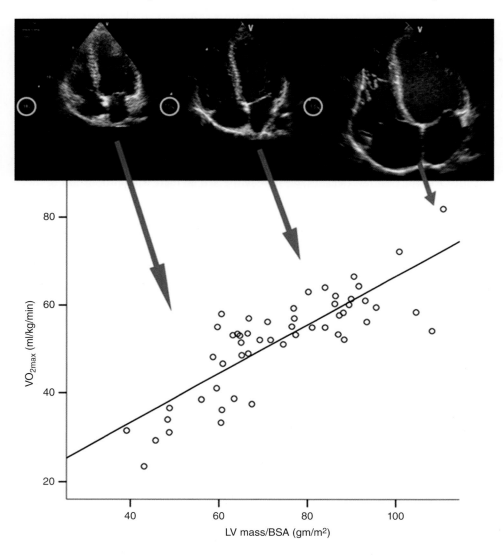

Figure 42.1 Relationship between cardiac remodelling and exercise capacity (VO_{2max}). Data derived from a mixed cohort of athletes and nonathletes demonstrates a strong correlation ($r = 0.79$, $p < 0.0001$) between left ventricular mass measured by cardiac magnetic resonance (CMR, x-axis) and maximal oxygen uptake at maximal exercise intensity (VO_{2max}, y-axis). Above the graph are representative examples of a 23-year-old nonathlete with average cardiac dimensions and VO_2 (left) a 23-year-old international footballer with a modest increase in cardiac size and VO_{2max} (middle) and an elite cyclist with a markedly increased left ventricular mass and a VO_{2max} in excess of 80 ml. $min^{-1}.kg^{-1}$ (right). BSA, body surface area (*Source:* La Gerche and Heidbuchel [10]. Reproduced with permission of Wolters Kluwer Health)

However, there is reluctance to consider this possibility when it comes to the heart of a well-trained athlete. Most likely, there is no real black-or-white border: physiological dilatation may create a progressive propensity for developing arrhythmias.

The best evidenced example of gradual conversion from exercise-induced benefit to development of an arrhythmogenic substrate is the U-shaped incidence of atrial fibrillation or flutter amongst endurance athletes. Atrial enlargement and autonomic changes are part of the cardiac adaptations of athlete's heart, modestly increasing the risk for atrial fibrillation at the extremes of exercise. In a meta-analysis of smaller studies mainly looking at endurance athletes, a 5.3-fold increase of atrial fibrillation was noted [3]. Later data from three much larger studies investigating the interaction between exercise and atrial fibrillation point to a U-shaped pattern of the exercise dose–response curve, whereby regular mild to moderate exercise provides strong protection from atrial fibrillation, whilst long-term intensive endurance exercise constitutes a risk factor, albeit a small one [11–13].

From Physiologic to Pathologic Remodelling in Athletes: and the Ventricles?

The evidence that long-term endurance exercise may also predispose to ventricular pathological remodelling and/or arrhythmias is less resolute. Fortunately, ventricular arrhythmias in athletes are rare events, but by nature they may be life-threatening. Evaluation of the possible association between exercise and occurrence of ventricular arrhythmias is challenging due to the low prevalence of ventricular tachycardia amongst athletes, making it difficult to adequately power epidemiological studies. Biffi et al. [14] reported that a greater proportion of athletes have ventricular premature beats (VPBs) on 12-lead ECG than is found in the nonathletic population. Studies indicate that VPBs are not related to cardiac events and should be considered benign in athletes in the absence of structural heart disease [14]. On the other hand, about 30% of athletes with >2000 VPBs per 24 hours have underlying structural abnormalities.

In 2003, Heidbuchel et al. [4] reported on 46 endurance athletes presenting with ventricular arrhythmias who were evaluated in the context of nonspecific symptoms like palpitations and dizziness. Despite the seemingly mild clinical presentation, 18 athletes had a major arrhythmic event during follow-up, and 9 (not treated with an implantable cardioverter-defibrillator, ICD) died suddenly. Evaluation of these athletes showed that the majority had structural, functional and/or electric abnormalities of the right but not the left ventricle. According to the 1994 task force criteria for ARVC [15], 59% of the athletes had manifest ARVC and an additional 30% had probable ARVC. However, in contrast to what would be expected with familial ARVC, evidence of familial disease was uncommon (only 1 of 46 athletes had a familial history). Thus, the clinical presentation was indistinguishable from ARVC except for the fact that the predisposing factor seemed to be the environment (i.e. intense endurance exercise) rather than genetic predisposition. In a follow-up study, La Gerche et al. [16] showed that only a small minority (<13%) of athletes with an ARVC phenotype had desmosomal mutations, an observation later confirmed by US investigators [17]. Heidbuchel et al. [4] coined the term 'exercise-induced right ventricular cardiomyopathy', whilst the American investigators referred to 'gene-elusive ARVC' [17].

The premise that the exercise dose–response curve has a U-shaped pattern and that sustained vigorous exercise constitutes a risk factor would seem to be at odds with studies describing a greater life expectancy amongst well trained athletes compared to reference groups (military recruits or the general population) [1,2]. These studies provide reassurance, but they need to be interpreted with caution, because the reference groups differ substantially from the athletes in many aspects other than just the amount of exercise performed. Indeed, the athletes' longer life expectancy may not be attributable to exercise training per se, but may just reflect the fact that former athletes continue to lead a healthier lifestyle and smoke less than the general population. Also, it is possible that high doses of exercise do decrease all-cause cardiovascular mortality, but only at the expense of a concomitant increase in CVDs of lesser prevalence or lesser lethality, such as arrhythmias. Thus, high doses of exercise may have beneficial effects on some aspects of the cardiovascular system and negative effects on others.

Why is the Right Ventricle Affected?

From these observations, the intriguing question arises as to why the right ventricle (and not the left) would undergo proarrhythmic structural changes in endurance athletes. We have previously put forward the hypothesis that the disproportionately greater right ventricular wall stress during intense exercise provides a plausible link between the haemodynamic stressors of exercise and subsequent proarrhythmic remodelling of the right ventricle [10,18]. There are differences between the right and left ventricles in the arterial load imposed by exercise and in the ventricular capacity to counter that load (i.e. maintain ventricular arterial coupling). At rest, the left ventricle contracts against a systemic circulation with moderate resistance and compliance as compared with the low-resistance and high-compliance pulmonary circulation. As a result, right ventricular function is relatively unimportant in the healthy circulation at rest, when little work is required to generate flow across the pulmonary circulation. During exercise, cardiac output augmentation will increase vascular pressures unless sufficiently counterbalanced by decreases in resistance and increases in compliance. However, the pulmonary vascular bed has a limited capacity for further decreases in resistance, in contrast with much more profound reductions in systemic vascular resistance. As a result, vascular (systolic) pressures increase, but more so in the pulmonary circulation than in the systemic circulation. Thus, the harder the exercise, the greater the right ventricular pressure demands and the larger the proportional difference between the demands placed on the right and left ventricles (Figure 42.2).

This increase in afterload during exercise demands an increase in right ventricular contractility if normal ventricular–arterial coupling is to be maintained and stroke volume is to increase during exercise. Despite the disproportionate haemodynamic load on the right ventricle during exercise, current evidence suggest that the right ventricular contractile reserve is sufficient to generate the increased work required to preserve right ventricular–arterial coupling during short-duration exercise. Using multiple echocardiographic surrogates of right ventricular contractility, we have previously shown that right ventricular contractile reserve is similar between athletes and nonathletes, although the former attain much higher pulmonary artery pressures at peak exercise as they are able to generate higher maximal COs [9]. However, whilst the right ventricle can maintain function against the disproportionate increase in vascular load during exercise of short duration, data from previous studies suggest that there is a point at which the right ventricle fatigues. Studies in relatively amateur marathon runners [7], well-trained ultra-endurance runners [8] and triathletes [9] have consistently demonstrated significant decrements in right ventricular function during [6] and immediately following endurance exercise, but preserved left ventricular function. In a study of 40 athletes evaluated after different endurance events (from marathon to ultra-endurance triathlon, 3–11 hours in duration), we reported an overall reduction in end-diastolic and end-systolic left ventricular volumes immediately after races, in sharp contrast to dilation of the right ventricle [9]. Moreover, right ventricular ejection fraction (EF) decreased immediately after the events, recovering to normal after 1 week. This contrasted with unchanged left ventricular EFs throughout the evaluation. Intriguingly, the degree of transient right ventricular dysfunction was significantly related to the duration of the endurance event. Moreover, B-type natriuretic peptide (BNP) and cardiac troponin-I increases correlated with reductions in right ventricular EF ($r = 0.52$, $p = 0.001$ and $r = 0.49$, $p = 0.002$, respectively), but not left ventricular EF [9].

As a result of this disproportionate haemodynamic stress and bouts of right ventricular dysfunction, some data suggest that, in the longer term, endurance athletes develop slightly greater right than left ventricular remodelling [5]. In keeping with this hypothesis, Arbab-Zadeh et al. [19], led by Levine, elegantly demonstrated that both ventricles respond differently to endurance training. Left ventricular volumes did not change significantly during the first 6–9 months after commencement of endurance training (depending on the duration and intensity of exercise), whereas right ventricular volumes increased progressively from the outset at all levels of training [19]. Similarly, using cardiac magnetic resonance (CMR) to evaluate biventricular function *during* intense endurance exercise, we demonstrated that a bout of endurance exercise (150 km cycling race) resulted in acute right ventricular dilation and reduced right ventricular EF but left left ventricular volumes and function unaltered [6].

Although the haemodynamic impact of endurance exercise on the right ventricle is more profound than that on the left, there is insufficient evidence to definitively draw a link between the acute effects of endurance exercise and development of right ventricular proarrhythmic remodelling in the long term. Nevertheless, the observation that increases in both troponin and BNP correlate with reductions in right ventricular EF following endurance exercise, whilst changes in left ventricular function do not [9], suggests that the right ventricle (and not the left) represents a source of injury following prolonged endurance exercise, probably because its work requirements and imposed mechanical stress are far greater than those of the left ventricle. This would support our 2003 hypothesis that endurance events lead to right ventricular insults (reflected in enzyme rise and slight dysfunction), recovering after a single bout, but that excessive, repetitive wall stress (training that is too intense and/or recovery that is too short) causes disruption of normal desmosomes, eventually resulting in ARVC (Figure 42.3). In other words, there may be a limit to what is healthy for the

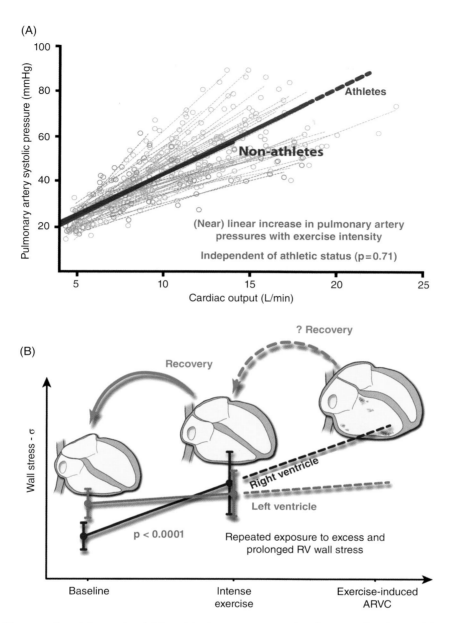

Figure 42.2 Disproportionately greater right ventricular pressures and wall stress give rise to right ventricular remodelling. (A) There is a near-linear increase in pulmonary artery pressures during exercise with cardiac output. This relationship is similar for athletes (brown) and nonathletes (green). In healthy subjects, greater exercise capacity predicts higher pulmonary artery pressures, with well-trained athletes generating the highest pressures of all. (B) Relative increases in wall stress are greater for the right than for the left ventricle during intense exercise, the result of which is healthy cardiac remodelling with a very slight right ventricular dominance, which diminishes with de-training. Repeated bouts of excessive and prolonged right ventricular wall stress may result in cumulative right ventricular damage, which may predispose to arrhythmias. The degree to which this adverse remodelling recovers with de-training is unclear (*Source:* Heidbuchel et al. [18]. Reproduced with permission of BMJ)

right ventricle. Further support for the concept of exercise-induced proarrhythmic remodelling of the right ventricle is the preclinical model of Benito et al. [20], in which endurance-trained rats have been shown to develop right ventricular inflammation, fibrosis and inducible right ventricular arrhythmias, with relative sparing of the left ventricle.

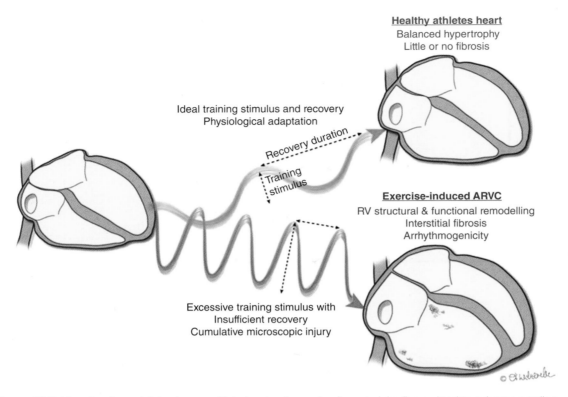

Figure 42.3 Hypothesis explaining how multiple bouts of exercise ('overtraining') may lead to adverse cardiac remodelling. Healthy training with balanced exercise and recovery results in physiological remodelling, promoting enhanced cardiac structure and function and leaving the heart better able to tolerate subsequent exercise loads. On the other hand, we hypothesise that excessive exercise (training that is too intense or recovery that is too short) may cause cardiac injury and proarrhythmic remodelling, which predominantly affects the right ventricle and atrium. LV, left ventricle; RV, right ventricle (*Source:* Heidbuchel et al. [18]. Reproduced with permission of BMJ)

Genetic Predisposition?

We have proposed the term 'exercise-induced arrhythmogenic right ventricular cardiomyopathy' (EI-ARVC) to reflect the fact that some endurance athletes have a propensity to develop right ventricular remodelling consisting of structural, functional and electrophysiological changes which predispose to right ventricular arrhythmias even in the absence of familial disease [16]. La Gerche et al. [16] systematically evaluated the five desmosomal genese for mutations in a cohort of 47 athletes, of whom 87% met criteria for a definite or probable diagnosis of ARVC. The proportion with desmosomal mutations was much lower than that described for familial ARVC (13 vs ~50%). If right ventricular arrhythmogenicity were the early expression of a latent underlying genetic (desmosomal) mutation, we would have expected at least a similar prevalence to that described in nonathletes with ARVC. Moreover, a familial history of ARVC was only present in 4% of athletes [16], which is very similar to the prevalence of 9% amongst patients with so-called 'gene-elusive ARVC' [17].

Nevertheless, it is evident that only a small minority of endurance athletes develops this phenotype without current predictors of who is most at risk. It is possible that susceptibility to this syndrome depends on combinations of low-penetrant variants in desmosomal or other genes. Thus, a spectrum of disease may exist (Figure 42.4), with genetic mutations of the desmosomal proteins explaining the majority of disease expression at one end (classical familial or 'desmosomal' ARVC) and increased mechanical stress through long-term endurance exercise proving the major factor at the other (EI-ARVC). In keeping with this hypothesis, Sawant et al. [17] showed that endurance exercise increases the risk of disease penetrance and clinical manifestation amongst patients with gene-elusive ARVC. Furthermore, the authors confirmed our previous observation that ARVC in gene-elusive patients is associated with a higher amount of cumulative endurance exercise than that in those with a similar phenotype due to desmosomal mutations [16,17].

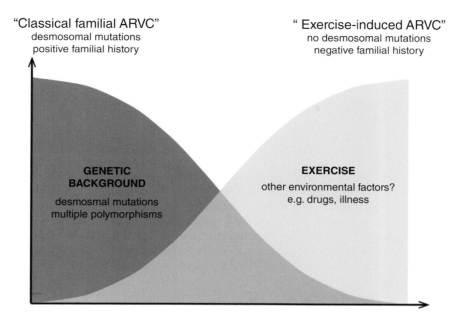

Figure 42.4 Potential overlap between classical 'desmosomal' and 'exercise-induced' ARVC. Pathogenesis of ARVC, with genes explaining the majority of disease expression at one end (classical familial ARVC) and exercise proving the major factor at the other (exercise-induced ARVC)

The debate about whether or not EI-ARVC is part of the spectrum of classical familial ARVC may be somewhat academic. Nevertheless, the notion that exercise plays an important role in the pathogenesis of ARVC has important clinical implications, as endurance sports by themselves may promote progression and clinical manifestation of the disease, and hence it is likely that they may also induce the phenotype.

Doping?

The usual suspect in explaining the many things that we do not understand about arrhythmias in athletes is performance-enhancing drugs. Indeed, doping agents are known to increase the risk of cardiac death, and they are more prevalent in high-level endurance sports due to the intense demands of this area of activity. There are limited data on the direct cardiopathic effects of doping, and it is unclear why they would selectively impact on the right ventricle. Therefore, despite reliable data on the use of illicit drugs, we have no indication that they are a direct cause of cardiopathic effects. Nevertheless, we cannot exclude that performance-enhancing measures (including illicit drugs) may indirectly promote EI-ARVC by allowing more and protracted volume/pressure overload through longer and more strenuous training and competition.

Who is at Risk?

Clinicians face the challenging tasks of working out who is at risk of life-threatening arrhythmias and distinguishing physiological from potentially pathological right ventricular adaptation. This can be a very difficult task, not just in asymptomatic athletes but even in those presenting with nonspecific symptoms such as lethargy, palpitations or presyncope. A number of considerations and investigations may help the clinician.

Type and Intensity of Sport Activity

In our original series of athletes with EI-ARVC, 80% were high-level cyclists or triathlon athletes [4,21]. It is well recognised that different types of sport have different impacts on the cardiovascular system. Cycling is a particular type of strain, even when compared with other endurance sports like running. Cyclists perform the most protracted exercise, working more hours per day and more days per year than any other athlete. Cyclists frequently sustain heart rates around 80% of maximum for prolonged periods. Their protracted aerobic exercise is regularly interrupted by intense anaerobic dashes, which are less common in other endurance athletes. Therefore, the right ventricular effects seem to be linked to high-intensity endurance activities, particularly those of long duration and those which combine endurance and power.

The question that arises is how much exercise is too much? Since the development of an arrhythmogenic substrate depends on a complex interplay between environmental, motivational and, perhaps, (poly)genetic factors involved in stress and repair, it is at present impossible to suggest a cut-off dose that defines 'too much exercise' – not in general terms, and certainly not at the individual level.

12-Lead ECG

The role of the ECG in the differentiation between physiological adaptations to endurance exercise and underlying right ventricular pathology cannot be underestimated. In accordance with the 2010 Task Force Criteria and Seattle criteria, T-wave inversion (TWI) in all the right precordial leads (V1–V3) should trigger comprehensive evaluation for ARVC (genetically dependent and/or due to the increased load of exercise) in Caucasian athletes [22]. In black athletes, convex ST-segment elevation with biphasic TWI in leads V1–V4 is a common finding and is considered benign [22]. However, symmetrical anterior TWI in V1–V3 preceded by isoelectric or downsloping ST segments is rare and should prompt further investigation to exclude ARVC [22].

ECG findings related to ARVC, particularly in early in the course of the disease, can be subtle and can overlap with those frequently observed in healthy endurance athletes. Around 1 in 7 highly trained endurance athletes has been observed to demonstrate inverted T-waves in right precordial leads, with 1 in 25 demonstrating biphasic TWI extending into lead V3, constituting a major criterion for the diagnosis of ARVC [23]. This suggests that these changes are not exclusively 'training unrelated', but in fact reflect increased structural and electrical right ventricular remodelling in these athletes: a continuum between physiology and pathology that we have already described. Nevertheless, early recognition of ECG features of ARVC is important because sports continuation in an athlete with ARVC may trigger life-threatening arrhythmias and cause progression of the arrhythmogenic substrate. Given the phenotypic overlap between ECG changes related to physiological remodelling and early ARVC, minor diagnostic ECG findings such as TWI in V1–V2 require extensive evaluation if accompanied by alarming symptoms (e.g. syncope) [22].

A large subset of ARVC patients have late potentials on the signal-averaged ECG. Nevertheless, the same overlap between physiology and pathology exists, as asymptomatic athletes – and particularly endurance athletes – also develop changes on the signal-averaged ECG, intermediate to those of controls and those of athletes with ventricular arrhythmias.

Cardiac Imaging Studies

A cornerstone of the diagnosis of ARVC is the occurrence of global and regional dysfunction and structural adaptations. However, differentiating between the enlarged right ventricle of a well-trained endurance athlete and right ventricular dilation related to ARVC can be challenging using imaging techniques such as echocardiography. Healthy endurance athletes display significantly larger right ventricular chamber dimensions than those described by 'normal ranges' [5]. Moreover, measures of right ventricular systolic function, such as right ventricular EF and strain/strain rate, are frequently reduced in endurance athletes when they are evaluated at rest [5]. On the other hand, in our experience, right ventricular systolic dysfunction in endurance athletes presenting with EI-ARVC is in general less pronounced than that seen in familial series of ARVC [21]. Detailed quantitative right ventricular angiographic evaluation in 22 high-level endurance athletes presenting with ventricular arrhythmias showed they had a right ventricular EF of $49.1 \pm 10.4\%$, compared to 63.7% in normal athletes and 67% in nonathletic controls ($p < 0.001$) [21].

It is important to emphasise that the imaging components of the ARVC diagnostic criteria need to be accompanied by wall-motion abnormalities. However, visual assessment of the latter using echocardiography is unreliable and may lead to false-positive results. In this regard, myocardial deformation imaging using speckle tracking may enable a better distinction between pathology and normal physiologic adaptation to endurance sports. Nevertheless, studies report that strain and strain rate are lower in the basal segments of the right ventricle in healthy athletes, particularly amongst those who are most trained and have the greatest dilation [24].

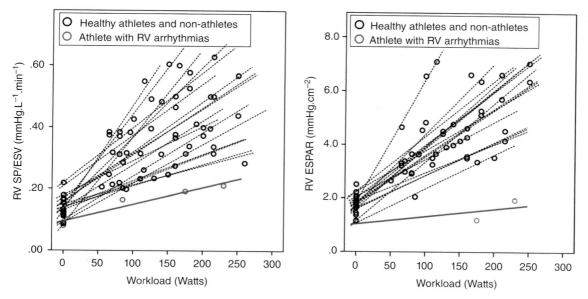

Figure 42.5 Reduced exercise right ventricular function in an athlete with ventricular arrhythmias, as compared with normal exercise right ventricular function in healthy endurance athletes and nonathletes. Right ventricular functional reserve can be measured as the exercise-induced change in the right ventricular end-systolic pressure/volume ratio (derived using exercise CMR with invasive pressure measurements) or as the change in the right ventricular end-systolic pressure/area ratio (using echocardiography), each of which is a surrogate for right ventricular function incorporating load (akin to contractility). During short intense exercise in healthy endurance athletes and nonathletes (black lines), right ventricular systolic pressure/end-systolic volume (SP/ESV) and right ventricular end-systolic pressure/area ratio (ESPAR) increase due to a progressive reduction in right ventricular end-systolic volume/area and concomitant increases in pulmonary artery pressures. In the endurance athlete with right ventricular arrhythmias (red line), right ventricular function is similar at rest, but fails to augment during exercise

Given that the contribution of right ventricular function to overall cardiac performance becomes relatively more important during exercise, it would seem more relevant to evaluate right ventricular function when its work requirements are most profound (i.e. during exercise) [5]. La Gerche et al. [24] demonstrated that endurance athletes have a comparable right ventricular contractile reserve during exercise to that in nonathletic controls, despite lower resting values, confirming that resting measures are a poor surrogate for right ventricular functional reserve. Therefore, assessment of right ventricular functional reserve during exercise may provide additional information beyond that provided by resting measures in distinguishing physiological right ventricular remodelling from right ventricular abnormalities in the context of EI-ARVC. This premise is supported by very recent data from our group [25]. Using echocardiographic and CMR measures of right ventricular function performed during exercise, we demonstrated that athletes with ventricular arrhythmias of right ventricular origin develop right ventricular dysfunction during exercise despite having very few abnormalities at rest (Figure 42.5). Importantly, although resting measures could not clearly distinguish athletes with complex arrhythmias from healthy subjects, exercise measures were much more distinctive.

Delayed Gadolinium Enhancement

The use of delayed gadolinium enhancement (DGE) imaging on inversion recovery magnetic resonance sequences provides information about the presence and location of myocardial fibrosis. However, whilst the detection of myocardial fibrosis raises the suspicion of underlying cardiac pathology, several studies have reported an increased prevalence of fibrosis in 12–50% of highly trained, asymptomatic, healthy endurance athletes [24,26]. Considering that DGE may be identified in at least 12% of healthy athletes, this would indicate that its positive predictive value (PPV) in identifying true pathology is poor. Also, care must be taken before extrapolating conclusions regarding prognosis from other clinical conditions in which DGE is associated with clinical events. For example, La Gerche et al. [24] described a particular pattern of focal DGE confined to the interventricular septum and right ventricular insertion points in highly trained endurance athletes, which is very similar to that observed in patients with pulmonary hypertension. Nevertheless, at present, there is no evidence that this pattern of DGE relates to prognosis or that it should influence clinical decision-making.

Intriguingly, the majority of athletes in our studies with EI-ARVC did not have overt fibrosis or adiposis on CMR, and only a minority showed histological fibroadiposis [4]. Thus, macrostructural fibroadiposis seems to be less a hallmark of EI-ARVC than of familial ARVC: one of the few ways in which EI-ARVC seems to differ from familial ARVC. This may be due to the fact that desmosomal mutations might have other molecular effects beyond cell rupture, which may be a common pathway in both EI-ARVC and desmosomal ARVC. This does not necessarily exclude diffuse intercellular fibrosis as a result of repair after myocyte disruption, which is beyond the limited resolution of CMR. Hence, it is possible that cardiac fibrosis may be underreported using current techniques that assess relative enhancement. Novel techniques which assess global fibrosis may be more informative regarding the degree to which extracellular matrix expansion contributes to the EI-ARVC syndrome.

Electrophysiology Study

As already outlined, it can be extremely difficult to determine the significance of palpitations, isolated ventricular extrasystoles or nonsustained ventricular tachycardia (NSVT) in athletes, particularly when extensive noninvasive electrical, morphological and functional evaluation is within the ranges considered normal for an endurance athlete. The inducibility of re-entrant arrhythmias during invasive electrophysiological testing has been shown to be predictive for later arrhythmic events (relative risk (RR) 3.4, $p = 0.02$) [4]. More evidence to support invasive assessment is provided by Dello Russo et al. [27], who assessed 57 athletes with frequent ventricular ectopy or NSVT, amongst a population of 1644 screened athletes in whom cardiac structure and function were ostensibly normal. Electroanatomical mapping and guided right ventricular biopsy were performed, revealing myocardial inflammation, fibrosis and/or fatty infiltrates in 13 of 17 athletes. The extent to which exercise played a causative or incidental role in this series is unclear, however. Given that ventricular ectopic beats and nonsustained arrhythmias are not uncommon amongst endurance athletes [14,27], invasive risk stratification using electrophysiological tests and biopsies in high-risk anatomical sites is not ideal. Therefore, there is a need for more studies investigating noninvasive imaging modalities, in order to differentiate athletes with complex ventricular arrhythmias from healthy athletes.

Conclusion

There is indisputable evidence that exercise, including endurance exercise, offers a plethora of health benefits to the general population. However, it is increasingly recognised that intense endurance exercise puts a strain on the heart. This is clearly the case at the atrial level, with increased propensity for atrial fibrillation in the highest quartile of athletics. Also, the right ventricle appears to be a potential 'Achilles' heel' for the exercising heart. It is subject to disproportionate increases in load during exercise and, as compared with the left ventricle, impairment in function develops earlier and more significantly when exercise is prolonged. We hypothesise that an imbalance between training-induced acute cardiac 'injury' (due to high wall stress leading to cell damage, as evidenced by BNP and cardiac enzyme rises) and the available time or capacity for regenerative recovery may result in chronic right ventricular remodelling. We have coined the term 'exercise-induced right ventricular cardiomyopathy' (EI-ARVC) for this ARVC-like phenotype when it occurs in the absence of desmosomal mutations. The exact determinants and individual predispositions (genetic or otherwise) of this condition require further research. What is clear now is that the syndrome is not benign. Although rare, athletes deserve the clinician's vigilance in its detection. This often requires a combination of tests, of which imaging during exercise (with echo or CMR) shows most promise for the immediate future.

References

1 Karvonen, M.J., Klemola, H., Virkajärvi, J. and Kekkonen, A. Longevity of endurance skiers. *Med Sci Sports* 1974; **6**(1): 49–51.

2 Marijon, E., Tafflet, M., Antero-Jacquemin, J. et al. Mortality of French participants in the Tour de France (1947–2012). *Eur Heart J* 2013; **34**(40): 3145–50.

3 Abdulla, J. and Nielsen, J.R. Is the risk of atrial fibrillation higher in athletes than in the general population? A systematic review and meta-analysis. *Europace* 2009; **11**(9): 1156–9.

4 Heidbuchel, H., Hoogsteen, J., Fagard, R. et al. High prevalence of right ventricular involvement in endurance athletes with ventricular arrhythmias. Role of an electrophysiologic study in risk stratification. *Eur Heart J* 2003; **24**(16): 1473–80.

5 La Gerche, A., Heidbüchel, H., Burns, A.T. et al. Disproportionate exercise load and remodeling of the athlete's right ventricle. *Med Sci Sports Exerc* 2011; **43**(6): 974–81.

6 Claessen, G., Claus, P., Ghysels, S. et al. Right ventricular fatigue developing during endurance exercise: an exercise cardiac magnetic resonance study. *Med Sci Sports Exerc* 2014; **46**(9): 1717–26.

7 Neilan, T.G., Januzzi, J.L., Lee-Lewandrowski, E. et al. Myocardial injury and ventricular dysfunction related to training levels among nonelite participants in the Boston marathon. *Circulation* 2006; **114**(22): 2325–33.

8 Oxborough, D., Shave, R., Warburton, D. et al. Dilatation and dysfunction of the right ventricle immediately after ultraendurance exercise: exploratory insights from conventional two-dimensional and speckle tracking echocardiography. *Circ Cardiovasc Imaging* 2011; **4**(3): 253–63.

9 La Gerche, A., Burns, A.T., Mooney, D.J. et al. Exercise-induced right ventricular dysfunction and structural remodelling in endurance athletes. *Eur Heart J* 2012; **33**(8): 998–1006.

10 La Gerche, A. and Heidbüchel, H. Can intensive exercise harm the heart? You can get too much of a good thing. *Circulation* 2014; **130**(12): 992–1002.

11 Mozaffarian, D., Furberg, C.D., Psaty, B.M. and Siscovick, D. Physical activity and incidence of atrial fibrillation in older adults: the cardiovascular health study. *Circulation* 2008; **118**(8): 800–7.

12 Aizer, A., Gaziano, J.M., Cook, N.R. et al. Relation of vigorous exercise to risk of atrial fibrillation. *Am J Cardiol* 2009; **103**(11): 1572–7.

13 Andersen, K., Farahmand, B., Ahlbom, A. et al. Risk of arrhythmias in 52 755 long-distance cross-country skiers: a cohort study. *Eur Heart J* 2013; **34**(47): 3624–31.

14 Biffi, A., Pelliccia, A., Verdile, L. et al. Long-term clinical significance of frequent and complex ventricular tachyarrhythmias in trained athletes. *J Am Coll Cardiol* 2002; **40**(3): 446–52.

15 McKenna, W.J., Thiene, G., Nava, A. et al. Diagnosis of arrhythmogenic right ventricular dysplasia cardiomyopathy. *Br Heart J* 1994; **71**: 215–18.

16 La Gerche, A., Robberecht, C., Kuiperi, C. et al. Lower than expected desmosomal gene mutation prevalence in endurance athletes with complex ventricular arrhythmias of right ventricular origin. *Heart* 2010; **96**(16): 1268–74.

17 Sawant, A.C., Bhonsale, A., te Riele, A.S. et al. Exercise has a disproportionate role in the pathogenesis of arrhythmogenic right ventricular dysplasia/cardiomyopathy in patients without desmosomal mutations. *J Am Heart Assoc* 2014; **3**(6): e001471.

18 Heidbüchel, H., Prior, D.L. and La Gerche, A. Ventricular arrhythmias associated with long-term endurance sports: what is the evidence? *Br J Sports Med* 2012; **46**(Suppl. 1): i44–50.

19 Arbab-Zadeh, A., Perhonen, M., Howden, E. et al. Cardiac remodeling in response to 1 year of intensive endurance training. *Circulation* 2014; **130**(24): 2152–61.

20 Benito, B., Gay-Jordi, G., Serrano-Mollar, A. et al. Cardiac arrhythmogenic remodeling in a rat model of long-term intensive exercise training. *Circulation* 2011; **123**(1): 13–22.

21 Ector, J., Ganame, J., van der Merwe, N. et al. Reduced right ventricular ejection fraction in endurance athletes presenting with ventricular arrhythmias: a quantitative angiographic assessment. *Eur Heart J* 2007; **28**(3): 345–53.

22 Drezner, J.A., Ashley, E., Baggish, A.L. et al. Abnormal electrocardiographic findings in athletes: recognising changes suggestive of cardiomyopathy. *Br J Sports Med* 2013; **47**(3): 137–52.

23 Brosnan, M., La Gerche, A., Kalman, J. et al. Comparison of frequency of significant electrocardiographic abnormalities in endurance versus nonendurance athletes. *Am J Cardiol* 2014; **113**(9): 1567–73.

24 La Gerche, A., Burns, A.T., D'Hooge, J. et al. Exercise strain rate imaging demonstrates normal right ventricular contractile reserve and clarifies ambiguous resting measures in endurance athletes. *J Am Soc Echocardiogr* 2012; **25**(3): 253–62.e1.

25 La Gerche, Claessen et al. Submitted.

26 Wilson, M., O'Hanlon, R., Prasad, S. et al. Diverse patterns of myocardial fibrosis in lifelong, veteran endurance athletes. *J Appl Physiol (1985)* 2011; **110**(6): 1622–6.

27 Dello Russo, A., Pieroni, M., Santangeli, P. et al. Concealed cardiomyopathies in competitive athletes with ventricular arrhythmias and an apparently normal heart: role of cardiac electroanatomical mapping and biopsy. *Heart Rhythm* 2011; **8**(12): 1915–22.

43 Clinical Implications of Performance-Enhancing Drugs for Cardiovascular Health

Peter J. Angell[1] and Yorck O. Schumacher[2]

[1]School of Health Sciences, Liverpool Hope University, Liverpool, UK
[2]Department of Sports Medicine, ASPETAR, Qatar Orthopaedic and Sports Medicine Hospital, Doha, Qatar

Introduction

Despite increased control of the use of performance-enhancing drugs both 'in' and 'out' of competition, as well as increasing punishments for those found contravening the rules, there remain many athletes who are willing to risk using substances to improve their performance and/or aid their recovery [1]. The World Anti-Doping Agency (WADA) strictly regulates the use of pharmaceutical products in competitive sport, producing and regularly updating the World Anti-Doping Code, which includes a prohibited drug list. This list dictates what is and is not acceptable, from a doping perspective, within sport (Table 43.1). In addition to promoting the Olympic ideal of free and fair competition, these restrictions also exist for the protection of athletes and to help prevent the negative health consequences associated with the use of many substances on the list. This chapter examines the impact of performance-enhancing drugs from a range of categories on cardiovascular health.

Anabolic Agents

According to WADA's 2012 report, anabolic agents still account for around 50% of adverse findings in athletes [3]. Consequently, it is important to fully understand the potential cardiovascular health consequences of these substances. Whilst the category of 'anabolic agents' covers a broad range of substances, they are all taken with the principal aim of increasing muscle mass. Anabolic androgenic steroids (AASs) are still the most commonly abused drug by athletes, but other agents such as human growth hormone (hGH), human chorionic gonadotropin (hCG), insulin-like growth factors and selective androgen receptor modulators (SARMS) are growing in popularity. The effect of AASs on cardiovascular health has been a subject of interest for some time, with greater media/public focus when an athlete fails a 'doping' test. Once the preserve of Olympic weightlifters and elite bodybuilders, AAS use has now permeated not only elite athletes but also recreational users, who use the drugs for both performance- and image-enhancement purposes [1]. There is a general belief amongst users that different agents promote different adaptations of muscular size and strength, whilst some may be better suited to promoting body fat loss, leading to simultaneous use of multiple AASs. Despite significant concerns about the possible cardiovascular consequences of AAS use outside of therapeutic prescription, the data are somewhat limited, and in parts controversial. Despite this ambiguity, AASs have been associated with a number of cardiovascular disease (CVD) end-points, as well as a number of cardiovascular risk factors (Table 43.2).

IOC Manual of Sports Cardiology, First Edition. Edited by Mathew G. Wilson, Jonathan A. Drezner and Sanjay Sharma.
© 2017 International Olympic Committee. Published 2017 by John Wiley & Sons, Ltd.

Group	Examples
Anabolic agents	Anabolic androgenic steroids (AASs)
Peptide hormones, growth factors and related substances	Erythropoietin (EPO), human chorionic gonadotropin (hCG), insulin and insulin-like growth factors
Beta-2 agonists	All except therapeutic doses of salbutamol, formoterol and salmeterol
Hormone and metabolic modulators	Aromatase inhibitors
Diuretics and other masking agents	Diuretics, dextran
Stimulants	Amphetamines, methamphetamines, cocaine

Table 43.1 WADA prohibited substance list (*Data source:* WADA [2])

Event/risk factor	Case study	Cohort study
Myocardial infarction (MI)	✓	×
Sudden death	✓	×
Stroke	✓	×
Thromboembolism	✓	×
Cardiac hypertrophy	✓	×
Endocarditis	✓	×
Cardiac arrhythmias	✓	×
Heart failure	✓	×
Subdural haematoma	✓	×
Elevated blood pressure	✓	✓
Decreased high-density lipoprotein (HDL)	✓	✓
C-reactive protein (CRP)	✓	✓

Table 43.2 Cardiovascular events and risk factors of anabolic steroid use (*Data source:* Angell et al. [4])

As illustrated by Table 43.2, many of the data regarding any association between AAS use and the presence of cardiovascular events or CVD are generated from case study reports. Whilst these provide a valuable insight into the possible effects of AAS use/abuse, they are by no means conclusive and do not allow for a causal relationship to be established. Self-reporting of substance use can be unreliable, and without independent confirmation of the quality of the products used, it is hard to determine the exact cause of an event [5].

A relatively small number of cohort studies have tried to elucidate the impact that AASs might have on cardiovascular risk by assessing independent risk factors for CVD/cardiovascular events, including hypertension and altered lipid profiles, as well as homocysteine and high-sensitivity C-reactive protein (hsCRP). In addition, studies have also tried to examine any structural and functional changes in the myocardium and vasculature through a range of noninvasive techniques.

Hypertension has long been identified as an important risk factor for future development of CVD. Whilst early studies reported significantly higher systolic blood pressure (SBP) in bodybuilders using anabolic steroids [6], more recent data have failed to report similar elevations in comparable groups [7]. Nevertheless, AAS use has been associated with a reduction in aortic elasticity, which may augment blood pressures in an AAS user [8]. It has been postulated that this could be caused by a direct effect of AAS on nitric oxide-mediated dilation.

Elevated total cholesterol, low high-density lipoproteins (HDLs) and high low-density lipoproteins (LDLs) have long been associated with increased cardiovascular risk. As with many areas of AAS research, reports from studies on total cholesterol, HDL and LDL have produced contradictory outcomes. Whilst most studies report little difference in total cholesterol, many have demonstrated significantly lower HDL in AAS users, with concomitant increases in LDL [4]. A negative alteration to blood lipid profiles increases the risk of arterial fat deposition, thereby increasing the risk of a thromboembolic event. A number of mechanisms have been postulated regarding how AASs impact blood lipid profiles: increased hepatic triglyceride lipase activity has been reported in a short-term study, and a possible impact on apolipoprotein has also been suggested, but the exact mechanisms still remain unclear [9].

A marker of cardiovascular inflammation, hsCRP, has been associated with acute myocardial infarctions (MIs) and stroke [10]. Measurement of hsCRP is not routinely performed by medical personnel and so has received limited attention in AAS users. However, elevated hsCRP has been reported in AAS users, demonstrating a possibility of both local and systemic cardiovascular inflammation. A further marker of endothelial damage is homocysteine, which has also been associated with an increase in cardiovascular risk. Whilst there are again conflicting data, it has been suggested that AASs may limit the absorption of certain B vitamins, leading to elevated haemoglobin levels and thereby promoting endothelial damage. This would help explain the finding of significantly elevated levels of haematocrit/haemoglobin in previous studies [4].

A number of case reports have demonstrated a possible effect of AAS use on cardiac electrical activity, such as sinus tachycardia and atrial fibrillation. Whilst some athletes have been shown to have a prolonged QT interval as a result of training, AAS use has been associated with a shortened QT interval. Testosterone use has been associated with myocardial rhythm disturbances through a possible facilitation of the expression of potassium channels shown to be implicit in ventricular repolarisation, which may in turn be the cause of any alteration in cardiac rhythm. Whilst this has not been confirmed in widespread studies, it does suggest a possible focal point for diagnosis of AAS abuse.

Cardiac structure has been the focus of investigation for a number of studies examining the impact of AAS abuse. A number of hypertrophic adaptations have been observed, with particular attention given to increases in left ventricular dimensions. Increases in left ventricular posterior wall thickness and septal wall thickness have been demonstrated on a number of occasions, with subsequent increases in the left ventricular wall thickness/diameter ratio and the left ventricular muscle mass/volume ratio [11]. In some studies, significant increases in internal left ventricular diameters at end diastole have also been observed. Whilst many of the data suggest an increase in absolute cardiac dimensions as a result of AAS abuse, it is important to consider the significantly greater body mass of AAS users. More recent data using cardiac magnetic resonance (CMR) show that when left ventricular mass is scaled according to fat free mass, any significance is removed [7]. AASs have been observed to have a direct effect on cardiac muscle protein metabolism through activation of cell-surface androgen receptors by modulation of gene transcription, suggesting a possible role of AASs in cardiac remodelling [12].

Whilst gross changes in cardiac structure have provided a useful insight into the effects of AAS use, it is also important to focus on the impact of cardiac function. Early studies observed little difference in measures of systolic function, but more recent data have suggested a possible reduction in ejection fraction (EF) in AAS users that would be considered clinically relevant [13]. However, this is still subject to significant debate. Right ventricular systolic function has received little attention, but a recent study demonstrated a significant effect of AAS use on right ventricular EF in the absence of any depression in left ventricular function [7]. Whilst this requires further investigation, it does highlight another possible role of AAS use in the onset of cardiac dysfunction. Measures of myocardial contractility have also provided conflicting data, with some finding reductions in peak strain and strain rates in the left ventricular posterior and septal walls [14,15]. The reasons for these contradictions remain unclear, but interindividual differences between participants (including dosage and substance variation) could help to explain the conflicting results. It had been postulated that a reduction in myocardial elastance through an increase in collagen cross-links and fibrosis might explain any reductions in systolic function in AAS users. More recent data show an absence of focal fibrosis in long-term AAS users, although this cannot rule out the possible presence of diffuse myocardial fibrosis in long-term users [7].

A significant amount of attention has been given to the possible impact of AAS use on left ventricular diastolic function, due to a potential link to concentric cardiac hypertrophy. Data are once again mixed, with conflicting reports often found. AAS use has been linked to reductions in early/late diastolic filling velocity ratios. often with a reduced early and/or an increased atrial contribution to ventricular diastolic filling [13]. Moreover, measures of diastolic tissue velocities have shown a similar pattern in alterations to diastolic cardiac function. as well as reductions in right ventricular diastolic function [16]. A reduction in early diastolic filling parameters suggests a negative effect of AAS use on early myocardial relaxation. Reduced myocardial elastance could explain the reduction in early relaxation indicative of a stiffer left ventricular. A number of cellular mechanisms have been suggested for any increased ventricular rigidity observed in AAS users. Androgenic effects of AAS on extracellular calcium channels have been proposed as having an apoptogenic effect on cardiac myocytes through an increase in mitochondrial permeability [17,18]. Whilst there are data to support these suggested mechanisms, they are still significantly limited in their scope and scale.

The effects of AAS use on vascular health have received little consideration despite the thromboembolic consequences associated with their use. Given the progression from endothelial dysfunction to atherosclerotic development in coronary arteries, it is pertinent to try to further understand the possible physiological underpinnings of any possible impact of AAS use. Flow-mediated dilation is a noninvasive method of assessing conduit artery function, with reduced values used as a predictor of cardiovascular events. Reductions in endothelial-independent dilation have been observed in AAS users, demonstrating a possible effect of AAS on vascular smooth-muscle function. It has also been suggested, however, that relatively short-term abstinence will see a reversal of these effects and that resistance training alone may have a negative impact on vascular function. A number of mechanisms have been suggested for an AAS-mediated role in a reduction in vascular function. This might include a direct effect on the downregulation of the nitric oxide dilator system, which could underpin an increase in arterial stiffness. It has also been suggested that AASs may directly impact endothelial proliferation and propagation, thereby causing an increase not only in vascular but also in myocardial stiffness [8]. Further, AASs have been associated with an increase in endothelial cell adhesion, as well as attenuating the effects of vasodilators whilst simultaneously enhancing the effects of vasoconstrictors [19,20].

Despite conflicting evidence with regards to the effect of AAS use on a range of cardiovascular risk factors and functional parameters, it is clear that there is a link between AAS use and the risk of CVD or a cardiovascular event that warrants further investigation. Whilst the preconception is that these types of performance enhancer are mainly used by those in strength/power-based sports, the continued high prevalence of use across a range of sports suggests that medical staff should be alert to their use in any athlete. There are a number of ways of detecting AAS use in an athlete. Aside from the obvious changes in appearance, look for significant increases in ventricular dimensions (accompanied by reductions in diastolic function) and the presence of cardiac arrhythmias (such as a shortened QT interval). It is also important to note that measures of ventricular structure and function will normalise following a period of abstinence, so transient changes may be evident in those cycling AASs.

Peptide Hormones, Growth Factors and Related Substances

The peptide hormone hGH possesses significant anabolic properties and has significant effects on metabolic processes. Many of the positive effects associated with hGH use stem from its regulation of insulin-like growth factor 1 (IGF-1) release, which mediates the increase in muscle protein synthesis and total body protein turnover. Whilst initially developed for therapeutic use as a treatment for growth deficiencies and for relief from excessive burns, since the late 1980s hGH has been used as an ergogenic agent. It has been shown to have a significant effect on muscle mass, body composition and cardiac output in those with growth hormone deficiencies. In contrast, little effect has been observed on muscle strength or protein synthesis in healthy individuals [21], although anecdotal and 'underground' reports offer an alternative perspective. Despite this apparent paradox, its use as a performance enhancer has continued (due in part to the difficulty of detecting it in the body and its ready availability), and it is considered by many to be the most widely abused performance-enhancing drug [21]. In light of this, it is important that any negative cardiac effects are fully understood. Unfortunately, a majority of the available data are generated from animal models, and there are few examining the effects of hGH use on the cardiovascular system of humans. Although some beneficial cardiac effects have been observed in patients who are deficient in hGH, there are few or no data examining the effects of hGH use on cardiac parameters in healthy individuals where there has been no concomitant use of other anabolic agents. However, as hGH is somewhat indiscriminate in terms of its target sites, it can be postulated that significant hGH use outside of therapeutic guidelines would increase the risk of ventricular hypertrophy and negative alterations to lipid profiles. Reports have also suggested that far from any cardiac hypertrophy occurring without a functional impact, its use can lead to an increase in collagen deposition, fibrosis and possible cellular infiltration and necrosis [19]. These negative consequences would also suggest an association with cardiac arrhythmias and possible development of heart failure.

Erythropoietin (EPO) is a naturally occurring hormone produced by the kidneys in response to low circulating oxygen levels. It is responsible for stimulating the production of red blood cells in bone marrow. For many endurance athletes, the stimulation of EPO release will enhance aerobic capacity, thereby leading to an improved performance. Since the development of the first clinically available EPO, it has been used by athletes as a replacement for the older, more established, 'blood doping'. This technique, involving the withdrawal of blood and subsequent transfusion some months later, was fraught with technical problems, as well as substantial health risks. The appeal of EPO is that its detection is particularly difficult and it can replicate the effects of alternative training methods, such as altitude training. Despite being somewhat safer than blood doping, EPO use still presents some inherent problems. Whilst somewhat dose-dependent, increased haematocrit – resulting in an increased blood viscosity – predisposes the individual to significant hypertension and an increased cardiac afterload, with an increase in thromboembolic event risk in some subgroups. It has also been suggested that the increased thromboembolic risk occurs due to greater platelet attachment to the endothelia [22].

Stimulants

Stimulants consist of a broad plethora of psychoactive substances that increase both physiological and psychological activity to varying degrees. This subgroup of drugs includes amphetamines, ephedrine and cocaine, as well as caffeine and nicotine. In the short term, stimulants increase mental alertness/focus and elicit a concurrent increase in heart rate and vasoconstriction. In addition, they can mask the effects of fatigue, thereby extending exercise time. Whilst affecting the central nervous system (CNS) and the cardiovascular system in an acute manner, they have also been associated with a number of cardiovascular events.

Amphetamines affect both the central and autonomic nervous systems, causing vasoconstriction and tachycardia as well as the aforementioned psychological effects. Their use has been associated with a number of adverse cardiovascular events, including acute MI, coronary artery vasospasm and sudden cardiac death (SCD). Prolonged use has also been linked with stroke, arterial and pulmonary hypertension, cardiomyopathy and a number of cardiac rhythm abnormalities [22]. It is thought that these arrhythmias stem from an increase in intracellular cyclic adenosine monophosphate (AMP) and sympathetic nervous tone, particularly in those with myocardial hypertrophy. Whilst many of these data come from case reports, making interpretation difficult, they nevertheless raise awareness of the possible side effects of both acute and chronic use.

Other stimulants include the sympathomimetic amines ephedrine and pseudoephedrine, which are commonly used as appetite suppressants and decongestants and can have potent effects on the cardiovascular system, including increasing heart rate and blood pressure through vasoconstriction. Aside from what could be considered minor side effects such as headaches and insomnia, ephedrine has been linked to a number of cardiovascular outcomes, including cardiomyopathy, stroke and MI [23]. Even over-the-counter products containing pseudoephedrine have been linked to cardiovascular events resulting in either death or disability. A confounding factor, however, is that many of the over-the-counter products also contain considerable amounts of caffeine, which is likely to enhance any cardiovascular effect. It is thought that the increase in catecholamines coupled with the blocking of adenosine receptors increases blood pressure through vasoconstriction and elevated heart rates, leading to hypertension and an increased cardiovascular risk [24]. It has also been suggested that the adverse effects may not be dose-dependent and that any toxicity may be exacerbated by dehydration and athletic training, with prolonged use at high levels possibly causing myocardial necrosis [24].

Despite its limited use as a performance enhancer, cocaine still accounts for a relatively high number of adverse findings in athletes [2]. The inhibition of norepinephrine reuptake in the sympathetic system leads to its overstimulation, tachycardia and an increase in blood pressure and myocardial oxygen demand. This can result in ischaemia, further compounded by coronary artery vasospasm. As with the other stimulants previously described, use of cocaine has been associated with a number of cardiovascular events, and its toxicity can have a direct action on the myocardium, leading to endocarditis and myocarditis, as well as dilated cardiomyopathy, aortic aneurysms and vascular thrombus [25]. Further to this, ventricular arrhythmias such as extended QT and PR intervals can be seen as a precursor for SCD.

Beta-2 Agonists

The use of beta-2 agonists, such as salbutamol, is allowed for the treatment of asthma and exercise-induced vasospasm in some athletes. Their possible uses as anabolic agents and to improve endurance have meant they are on the controlled substance list, however. Whilst the data have demonstrated few cardiovascular effects of inhaled beta-2 agonists, oral forms of the drug have been shown to have a significant cardiovascular effect. Their use has been found to increase cardiovascular risk through positive chronotropic and inotropic actions, increasing heart rate and strengthening cardiac systole [22]. This can lead to cardiac arrhythmias, such as a prolonged QT interval, and may precipitate myocardial ischaemia, leading to acute MI, congestive heart failure and even SCD in those taking high doses.

Masking Agents

A number of agents are used to try and mask the presence of other banned substances. Aromatase inhibitors, such as tamoxifen and hCG, are used to help stimulate endogenous testosterone production following AAS use, countering the effects that would constitute a positive test. Diuretics are also sometimes used to remove substances from the system before testing. They are also used as a method of inducing rapid weight loss, particularly amongst athletes in weight-category sports. This rapid weight drop through excessive fluid loss leads to dehydration and possible electrolyte disturbances [22], which in turn can lead to arrhythmias and haemodynamic disorders. An increase in blood viscosity coupled with an increase in haemodynamic loads can lead to significant cardiac events.

Conclusion

Despite an ever-increasing focus on the control of performance-enhancing drugs in sports, there continue to be those who are willing to risk their use in order to gain a competitive advantage, even despite the associated cardiovascular risk. Whilst it is clear that there are still some significant gaps in the literature regarding the scale of effects on markers of cardiovascular health and the long-term impact they might have, there is a growing body of evidence to suggest the danger of their use. The balance of data regarding AAS use demonstrates a possible role in reduced myocardial elastance and shows a possible negative impact on blood lipid profiles. It has also been suggested that AASs may directly impact vascular function through endothelial damage. The addition of other anabolic agents is becoming increasingly common. There are limited data regarding the use of hGH, but its concomitant use with AASs is known anecdotally, and this may have significant impact on measures of cardiovascular structure and function. The use of EPO can pose a cardiovascular risk for certain patient groups, and, again, its concomitant use with other agents may augment any risk already posed. Stimulants can present a potent training and performance aid, but they have also been shown to pose a possible increased cardiovascular risk through increased myocardial oxygen demand.

As this chapter has demonstrated, a number of performance-enhancing drugs have been linked to significant cardiovascular events and an increased cardiovascular risk. Whilst far from conclusive, it does highlight the risk of individual subgroups of drugs on the prohibited drugs list. What cannot be defined are the possible interactions that might occur as a result of combining different performance enhancers. It could be postulated that this might significantly increase cardiovascular risk, but the extent to which this is true is difficult to hypothesise and will depend on a number of factors, including the combinations of substances used and the dosages taken. It is clear, however, that there are a number of ways in which those who are using performance-enhancing drugs might be identified when confronted in a medical setting. Regular assessment of cardiac electrical activity and the use of noninvasive methods of cardiac and vascular imaging may help to identify those at an increased risk of CVD progression or of an acute cardiovascular event.

References

1 Yesalis, C.E. and Bahrke, M.S. History of doping in sport. *Int Sports Studies* 2003; **24**(1): 42–76.
2 WADA. List of Prohibited Substances and Methods. Available from: http://list.wada-ama.org/ (last accessed 24 May 2016).
3 WADA. 2012 Anti-Doping Testing Figures Report. Available from: https://www.nada.at/files/doc/Statistiken/WADA-Statistik-2012.pdf (last accessed 24 May 2016).
4 Angell, M.P., Chester, N., Green, D. et al. Anabolic steroids and cardiovascular risk. *Sports Med* 2012; **42**: 119–34.
5 Franke, W.W. and Berendonk, B. Hormonal doping and androgenization of athletes: a secret program of the German Democratic Republic government. *Clin Chem* 1997; **43**: 1262–79.
6 Riebe, D., Fernhall, B. and Thompson, P.D. The blood pressure response to exercise in anabolic steroid users. *Med Sci Sports Exerc* 1992; **24**: 633–7.
7 Angell, P.J., Ismail, T.F., Jabbour, A. et al. Ventricular structure, function, and focal fibrosis in anabolic steroid users: a CMR study. *Eur J Appl Physiol* 2014; **114**: 921–8.
8 Kasikcioglu, E., Oflaz, H., Arslan, A. et al. Aortic elastic properties in athletes using anabolic-androgenic steroids. *Int J Cardiol* 2007; **114**: 132–4.
9 Applebaum-Bowden, D., Mclean, P., Steinmetz, A. et al. Lipoprotein, apolipoprotein, and lipolytic enzyme changes following estrogen administration in postmenopausal women. *J Lipid Res* 1989; **30**: 1895–906.
10 Ridker, P.M., Rifai, N., Clearfield, M. et al. Measurement of C-reactive protein for the targeting of statin therapy in the primary prevention of acute coronary events. *N Engl J Med* 2001; **344**: 1959–65.
11 Sachtleben, T.R., Berg, K.E., Elias, B.A. et al. The effects of anabolic steroids on myocardial structure and cardiovascular fitness. *Med Sci Sports Exerc* 1993; **25**: 1240–5.

12 Marsh, J.D., Lehmann, M.H., Ritchie, R.H. et al. Androgen receptors mediate hypertrophy in cardiac myocytes. *Circulation* 1998; **98**: 256–61.

13 Baggish, A.L., Weiner, R.B., Kanayama, G. et al. Long-term anabolic-androgenic steroid use is associated with left ventricular dysfunction. *Circ Heart Fail* 2010; **3**: 472–6.

14 Nottin, S., Nguyen, L.D., Terbah, M. and Obert, P. Cardiovascular effects of androgenic anabolic steroids in male bodybuilders determined by tissue Doppler imaging. *Am J Cardiol* 2006; **97**: 912–15.

15 D'Andrea, A., Caso, P., Salerno, G. et al. Left ventricular early myocardial dysfunction after chronic misuse of anabolic androgenic steroids: a Doppler myocardial and strain imaging analysis. *Br J Sports Med* 2007; **41**: 149–55.

16 Kasikcioglu, E. Androgenic anabolic steroids also impair right ventricular function. *Int J Cardiol* 2009; **134**: 123–5.

17 Lieberherr, M. and Grosse, B. Androgens increase intracellular calcium concentration and inositol 1,4,5-triphosphate and diacyglycerol formation via pertussis toxin-sensitive G-protein. *J Biol Chem* 1994; **269**: 7.

18 Zaugg, M., Jamali, N.Z, Lucchinetti, E. et al. Anabolic-androgenic steroids induce apoptotic cell death in adult rat ventricular myocytes. *J Cell Biol* 2001; **187**: 6.

19 D'Ascenzo, S., Millimaggi, D., Di Massimo, C. et al. Detrimental effects of anabolic steroids on human endothelial cells. *Toxicol Lett* 2007; **169**: 129–36.

20 Ammar, E., Said, S.A. and Hassan, M.S. Enhanced vasoconstriction and reduced vasorelaxation induced by testosterone and nandrolone in hypercholesterolemic rabbits. *Pharmacol Res* 2004; **50**: 253–9.

21 Saugy, M., Robinson, N., Saudan, C. et al. Human growth hormone doping in sport. *Br J Sports Med* 2006; **40**(Suppl. 1): i35–9.

22 Deligiannis, A.P. and Kouidi, E.I. Cardiovascular adverse effects of doping in sports. *Hellenic J Cardiol* 2012; **53**: 447–57.

23 Powers, M.E. Ephedra and its application to sport performance: another concern for the athletic trainer? *J Athl Train* 2001; **36**: 420.

24 Dhar, R., Stout, C.W., Link, M.S. et al. Cardiovascular toxicities of performance-enhancing substances in sports. *Mayo Clin Proc* 2005; **80**: 1307–15.

25 Deligiannis, A., Björnstad, H., Carre, F. et al. ESC study group of sports cardiology position paper on adverse cardiovascular effects of doping in athletes. *Eur J Cardiovasc Prev Rehabil* 2006; **13**: 687–94.

44 Cardiovascular Concerns in the Paralympic Athlete

Cindy J. Chang[1] and Suzy Kim[2]

[1]Department of Orthopaedic Medicine, Divisions of Sports Medicine and Pediatric Orthopaedic Medicine, Department of Family and Community Medicine, University of California, San Francisco, CA, USA
[2]St. Jude Centers for Rehabilitation & Wellness, Brea, CA, USA

Introduction

The precursor to the Paralympic Games was an archery competition for paralysed Second World War veterans at the Stoke Mandeville Rehab Hospital in southeastern England, held on the opening day of the 1948 London Olympics. The 9th Stoke Mandeville Games (for 400 athletes with spinal cord injury (SCI) from 23 countries) were held in Rome just after the 1960 Olympic Games, and were later considered the first Paralympic Games.

The number of athletes with disabilities has grown rapidly, especially over the past 2 decades, with war veterans returning from Middle Eastern conflicts. Many of these veterans will be participating in the 2016 Summer Paralympic Games in Rio de Janeiro, where over 4350 athletes from 160 countries will be competing in 22 sports, with para-canoe and paratriathlon making their debut. In the 2014 Sochi Winter Paralympic Games, 547 athletes from 45 countries competed in 5 sports.

In parallel to the Olympics, the Paralympic competitions are open only to elite athletes who meet the qualifying standards in their sport for competition for gold, silver and bronze medals. Although not every sport allows for every impairment category, athletes with one of six impairment types can compete following sport-specific classification by type and degree of disability. The impairment types are amputation or limb deficiency, cerebral palsy, SCI, visual impairment, intellectual impairment and les autres (achondroplasia, multiple sclerosis). Although seemingly confusing at times, the sport-specific classifications are designed to ensure equitable competition.

As the number of athletes with disabilities increases, sports medicine physicians and cardiologists must be better prepared to provide cardiac support to Paralympic athletes who wish to participate in high-level sport. This chapter will discuss the impact of SCI upon the autonomic nervous system (ANS) and address cardiovascular concerns, including autonomic dysreflexia, hypertension, hypotension and the risk of deep venous thrombosis (DVT) and coronary heart disease (CHD).

Cardiovascular Concerns in Athletes with SCI

Athletes with SCI make up one of the largest impairment groups participating in the Paralympic Games [1]. In athletes with high thoracic and cervical SCI, supraspinal control of the ANS is impaired, leading to such concerns as autonomic dysreflexia, bradycardia and hypotension. Other concerns in those with SCI include DVT and long-term risk for CHD.

SCI interrupts the communication between the brain stem and the ANS, which is important for control of the cardiovascular system (Figure 44.1). Because segmental outflow of the ANS originates at specific spinal cord levels, there is variable reduction in cardiovascular function in SCI athletes. Therefore, both

IOC Manual of Sports Cardiology, First Edition. Edited by Mathew G. Wilson, Jonathan A. Drezner and Sanjay Sharma.
© 2017 International Olympic Committee. Published 2017 by John Wiley & Sons, Ltd.

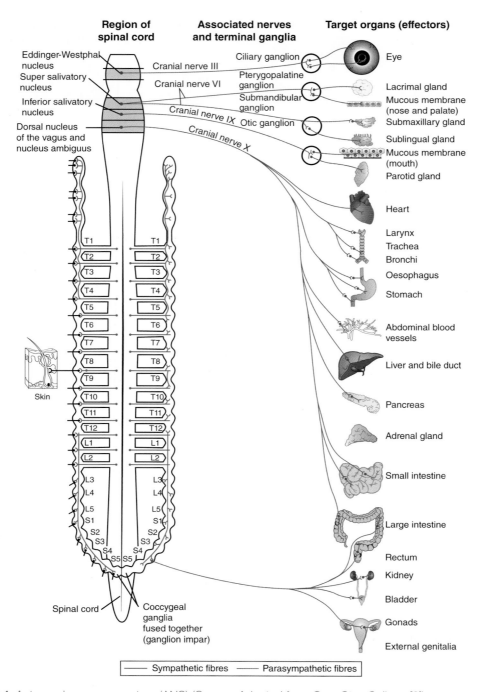

Region of spinal cord

Eddinger-Westphal nucleus
Super salivatory nucleus
Inferior salivatory nucleus
Dorsal nucleus of the vagus and nucleus ambiguus

Skin

Spinal cord
Coccygeal ganglia fused together (ganglion impar)

Associated nerves and terminal ganglia

Ciliary ganglion
Cranial nerve III
Pterygopalatine ganglion
Cranial nerve VI
Submandibular ganglion
Cranial nerve IX
Otic ganglion
Cranial nerve X

Target organs (effectors)

Eye
Lacrimal gland
Mucous membrane (nose and palate)
Submaxillary gland
Sublingual gland
Mucous membrane (mouth)
Parotid gland
Heart
Larynx
Trachea
Bronchi
Oesophagus
Stomach
Abdominal blood vessels
Liver and bile duct
Pancreas
Adrenal gland
Small intestine
Large intestine
Rectum
Kidney
Bladder
Gonads
External genitalia

——— Sympathetic fibres   ——— Parasympathetic fibres

Figure 44.1 Autonomic nervous system (ANS) (*Source:* Adapted from OpenStax College [2])

the level and the severity of SCI determine the degree of autonomic control in response to exercise. Sympathetic nervous system (SNS) neurons originate at the T1–L2 levels and control vasoconstriction and heart contractility. Specifically for aerobic capacity, the SNS innervates the heart from T1 to T5 level, limiting athletes with upper thoracic and cervical SCI, who have no ability to control most of their SNS function. Subsequently, with partial or complete denervation of the heart, athletes with cervical and high-level thoracic SCI have an impaired sympathetic response to exercise through attenuation of cardiac output. This phenomenon is often referred to as 'cardiac blunting' and is uniquely experienced by high-level SCI athletes.

Structurally, studies have found lower left ventricular wall stress with a smaller left atrium, left ventricle and vena cava in cervical SCI athletes [3]. Multiple physiologic consequences, including lower cardiac output and stroke volume, decreased cardiac preload, lower systolic blood pressure (SBP) and lower heart rate may explain these structural changes.

Autonomic Dysfunction

Athletes with SCI experience haemodynamic challenges during exercise due to impaired cardiovascular and autonomic control [4,5]. Specifically, wheelchair athletes with cervical and high-thoracic SCI have attenuated ability to elevate their heart rate and autoregulate blood pressure during training and competition. Blood-pressure lability from hypotension to episodic hypertension during autonomic dysreflexia further complicates the cardiovascular response to exercise in the wheelchair athlete.

Orthostatic Hypotension

The loss of neuroregulatory control after cervical and high-thoracic SCI results in baseline hypotension. Additionally, the loss of sympathetic-mediated vasomotor tone below the SCI level leads to blood pooling in the periphery and splanchnic vasculature. As a result, symptomatic orthostatic hypotension clinically presents as fatigue, lightheadedness, nausea, blurred vision and syncope, even in the wheelchair athlete. Management of orthostasis includes elastic stockings, an abdominal binder, adequate fluid intake, avoidance of diuretics (alcohol and caffeine) and small meals (to avoid postprandial hypotension). If an athlete experiences severe symptomatic orthostatic hypotension, they can be placed supine or in the Trendelenberg position, or given intravenous (IV) fluids or midodrine for blood pressure support. Caution is advised with the use of IV fluids and midodrine for emergent blood pressure support in Paralympians: midodrine, a stimulant, is prohibited in competition by the World Anti-Doping Agency (WADA), whilst IV infusion is prohibited if given outside of a hospital setting, and if given in an emergency, it may require an approved therapeutic use exemption (TUE).

Autonomic Dysreflexia

In contrast to orthostatic hypotension, athletes with SCI in T6 and above can experience episodic hypertension during a potentially life-threatening condition termed 'autonomic dysreflexia'. Autonomic dysreflexia presents as a syndrome caused by massive sympathetic output from uncontrolled spinal reflexes. Without prompt recognition, autonomic dysreflexia can result in extreme high blood pressure (>200/100), with case reports documenting intracranial haemorrhage, seizure, stroke and even death.

If a strong, often noxious stimulus is applied to an area below the T6 spinal cord level, the peripheral nerves attempt to send a signal via the spinal cord to the brain, but are blocked at the level of the spinal cord lesion (Figure 44.2). Simultaneously, a massive reflex sympathetic surge at the level of these SNS neurons from T1 to L2 is activated, resulting in vasoconstriction of the blood vessels and causing a rapid rise in blood pressure. Carotid and aortic baroreceptors detect this rise in blood pressure and send a signal to the brain, and the brain then tries to send inhibitory impulses to the sympathetic outflow levels in the thoracolumbar spine, but these impulses are blocked at the level of the SCI. Through the vagus nerve, part of the parasympathetic nervous system (PNS), the brain is able to signal the heart to slow the heart rate in an attempt to decrease the blood pressure. The blood vessels above the level of SCI are also able to vasodilate. However, in cases of autonomic dysreflexia, these measures are inadequate and the hypertension continues.

The higher the injury level, and the more complete the spinal injury, the greater the severity of autonomic dysreflexia. The T6 level is important because the greater splanchnic nerve (T5–T9) controls the splanchnic vascular bed, which is one of the body's largest reserves of circulatory volume. SCI at or above T6 allows the uninhibited sympathetic reflex to constrict the splanchnic vascular bed, causing systemic hypertension. SCI below T6 usually allows enough descending inhibitory parasympathetic control to modulate the tone of the splanchnic vascular bed and thus prevent hypertension. Common symptoms of autonomic dysreflexia reflect the dominance of the PNS above the level of the SCI, and the dominance of the SNS below it

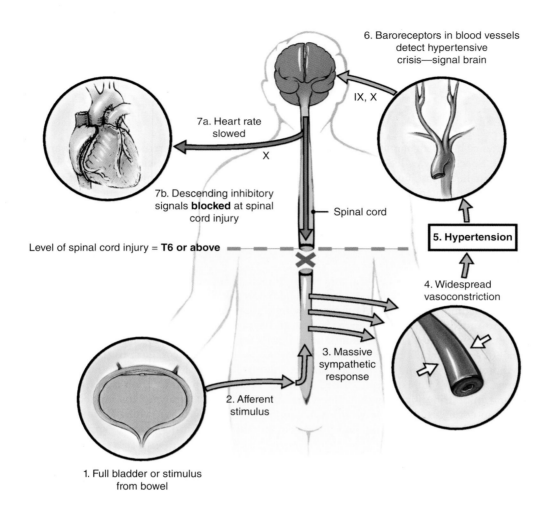

6. Baroreceptors in blood vessels detect hypertensive crisis—signal brain

IX, X

7a. Heart rate slowed

X

7b. Descending inhibitory signals **blocked** at spinal cord injury

Spinal cord

Level of spinal cord injury = **T6 or above**

5. Hypertension

4. Widespread vasoconstriction

3. Massive sympathetic response

2. Afferent stimulus

1. Full bladder or stimulus from bowel

Figure 44.2 Pathophysiology of autonomic dysreflexia (*Source*: Blackmer [6]. Reproduced with permission of the Canadian Medical Association)

Above the SCI level Parasympathetic responses	Below the SCI level Sympathetic responses
Flushing +/− red blotches on skin	Pale, cool clammy skin
Diaphoresis (sweating)	Piloerection (goose bumps)
Bradycardia	Headache (pounding sensation)
Pupillary constriction	Blurred vision
Nasal congestion	General apprehension, anxiety

Table 44.1 Symptoms and signs of autonomic dysreflexia

(Table 44.1). However, even with a significant increase in blood pressure, episodes of autonomic dysreflexia can be asymptomatic in athletes with cervical or high-thoracic injury.

Any inciting noxious event below the level of the SCI can trigger an episode of autonomic dysreflexia, with bladder and bowel conditions causing 90% of cases (Table 44.2). During athletic training and competition, many of the symptoms above the level of the SCI may appear as expected on vigorous exercise (facial flushing, sweating). Notably, autonomic dysreflexia is a syndrome and is best treated with an understanding of the presentation by the individual athlete. Generally, high-thoracic and cervical SCI athletes will not sweat above their level of injury, due to impaired thermoregulation. Therefore, sweating in a wheelchair

Bladder/bowel	Skin	Other
Overfilled bag/blocked catheter	Direct irritant (i.e. sharp object)	Deep venous thrombosis (DVT)
Urinary tract infection (UTI)	Pressure ulcers	Menstrual cramps
Constipation/impacted bowel	Ingrown toenails	Sitting on scrotum
Haemorrhoids/anal fissures	Thermal burns/sunburn	Acute abdominal issues
	Tight clothing	Occult fractures/heterotopic ossification

Table 44.2 Causes of autonomic dysreflexia

Place in upright position for potential orthostatic reduction of blood pressure	Use pharmacological intervention to lower blood pressure if no other method works (≥150 SBP in adults, ≥140 in adolescents, ≥130 in children 6–12 years old)
Check bladder first for distention (i.e. catheter drainage/drain collection bag), as it is the most likely cause	Apply topical nitrates to chest. Nitropaste can be wiped off once source is found
Check for bowel impaction using 1% lidocaine jelly, and gently disimpact if necessary	Nifedipine 10 mg sublingual (SL) (chew first then swallow) or captopril 25 mg SL followed by 5 mg nifedipine if still elevated 30 minutes later
Loosen tight clothing or constrictive devices	Check blood pressure every 5 minutes until resolution
Scan for and remove any irritating stimuli/pressure sores. Assess for new injuries	

Table 44.3 Management of autonomic dysreflexia

athlete with high-level SCI is usually pathologic and is most likely a symptom of autonomic dysreflexia. The initial management of this potential medical emergency is to identify and address the noxious stimulus in order to quickly lower the blood pressure and avoid the aforementioned life-threatening complications (Table 44.3).

After an episode of autonomic dysreflexia, blood pressure and pulse must return to normal resting levels, and ideally remain stable for 2 hours prior to return to sport. All symptoms, including headaches, also should be resolved before a return to training or competition. To prevent future episodes, all potential noxious stimuli should be removed from the athlete/wheelchair/field of play. If the athlete demonstrates predisposition to autonomic dysreflexia, alpha-1 adrenoceptor blockers (terazosin 1–10 mg adults or 1–2 mg children, or prazosin 0.5–1.0 mg 2–3 times per day) could be considered; these can be partially successful for prophylaxis [7]. With bladder and bowel distension as leading causes of autonomic dysreflexia, minimising urinary retention and constipation is highly recommended. Therefore, the medical staff should review optimal bladder programmes (e.g. clean intermittent catheterisation or timed voiding) and bowel regularity with SCI athletes prior to competition.

Boosting

Boosting is an intentional induction of autonomic dysreflexia prior to or during sports competition by competitive wheelchair athletes with cervical and high-thoracic SCI. Due to autonomic dysfunction, athletes with cervical and high-thoracic SCI may have limited cardiopulmonary exercise capacity, with an attenuated ability to increase cardiac output. Specifically for athletes with SCI in T6 and above, the loss of sympathetic innervation to the heart results in a maximal heart rate between 110 and 130 beats.min^{-1}.

To date, there has been no published documentation of an athlete experiencing a dangerous consequence from autonomic dysreflexia. However, anecdotal accounts of wheelchair athletes purposely inducing autonomic dysreflexia to enhance performance have been reported. This method of doping may result in a significant rise in blood pressure before or during competition to compensate for their physiologically blunted response. Athletes with cervical and high-level thoracic SCI commonly induce autonomic dysreflexia by intentionally distending their bladder (by consuming large amount of fluids or kinking their catheter), excessively tightening waist or leg straps or twisting or sitting on their scrotum.

In able-bodied athletes, the ability to exert supraspinal control of the autonomic system during exercise allows a balance between cardiac output and peripheral resistance in order to optimally redistribute blood volume to the working muscles. For athletes with cervical and high-thoracic SCI, the blood-pressure response to exercise is compromised by loss of chronotropic cardiac response and limited venous return. As a result, optimal blood redistribution to working muscles during exercise in SCI athletes may be severely compromised. Studies have shown that boosting the cardiovascular system can improve an athlete's physiologic response to exercise by increasing blood pressure, heart rate and catecholamine release. Burnham et al. [8] showed boosted wheelchair racers had 10% faster finishing times during a simulated 7.5 m marathon when compared to nonboosted athletes. Another study by Schmid et al. [9] found increased catecholamine release and improved exercise capacity during the boosted state.

As boosting to enhance athletic performance can have potentially catastrophic medical consequences, the International Paralympic Committee (IPC) has banned boosting as a method of performance enhancement. Recognition of self-induced autonomic dysreflexia by athletes mandates disqualification from Paralympic competitions. In an attempt to deter this dangerous method, the IPC Medical Committee initiated an Operational Management Plan to document boosting at three major international competitions: the 2008 Beijing Paralympic Games, the 2011 ParaPan American Games and the 2012 London Paralympic Games. During these events, Blauwet et al. [10] randomly tested a total of 78 wheelchair track racers and handcyclists whose functional classification identified their high level of SCI. For purposes of testing, boosting was defined as autonomic dysreflexia within 2 hours of the start of competition. A positive test was determined by two sequential recordings of SBP >180 mmHg. Since the implementation of the current IPC testing protocol at these three competitions, no athlete has tested positive or been withdrawn from competition. In April 2016, the IPC Medical Committee further refined the SBP threshold from 180 mm Hg to 160 mm Hg. The new protocol will be tested on appropriate athletes at the 2016 Rio Paralympic Games.

Other Important Considerations for the Team Physician

The Periodic Health Evaluation in the Paralympic Athlete

The 2009 International Olympic Committee (IOC) Consensus Statement on Periodic Health Evaluation (PHE) of Elite Athletes recommends that 'a 12-lead ECG [electrocardiogram]…be recorded on a non-training day, during rest, according to best clinical practice' [11].

The IPC Medical Code, approved December 2011, states that 'prior to engaging in competitive sport, and preferably with regular intervals throughout their athletic career, athletes should undergo pre-participation evaluation' [12]. There is no mention of screening ECGs. Yet recent studies indicate that more attention should be paid to the cardiac evaluations of Paralympians during the PHE.

During the acute phase of SCI, the absence of sympathetic tone can lead to severe bradycardia, atrioventricular (AV) block and even cardiac arrest [13]. However, Clayton et al. [14] found that healthy subjects with chronic traumatic SCI lasting >1 year were not at increased risk of cardiac arrhythmias during or after exercise, although there is evidence that SCI athletes are prone to arrhythmia during episodes of autonomic dysreflexia and are at increased risk of cardiovascular mortality compared to the able-bodied population [15].

Since 1982, it has been a national law requirement in Italy that every subject engaged in competitive sports undergo a clinical evaluation, including a 12-lead resting ECG and, in adult and senior competitive athletes, exercise ECG testing. For Olympians and Paralympians, the screening protocol adds exercise ECG testing and echocardiography.

Of the 2300 Italian Olympians screened over a recent 10-year period, 6% were identified with cardiovascular abnormalities, both structural and electrical. From a selected population of Paralympic athletes, 267 were screened over an 8-year period, 11% of whom were identified with cardiovascular abnormalities: 8% had structural cardiovascular abnormalities and 3% had major supraventricular or ventricular tachyarrhythmias (see Chapter 8).

These data from Italy demonstrate that a screening ECG will help identify Paralympic athletes with cardiac disorders associated with sudden death or other tachyarrhythmias. It is anticipated that the IPC will develop a consensus statement on the periodic health evaluation of elite Paralympic athletes, which will closely parallel the 2009 IOC Statement recommending a 12-lead ECG. Routine use of stress testing and echocardiography in the PHE of Paralympic athletes requires more research to understand its potential role in the cardiovascular evaluation of athletes.

Deep Venous Thrombosis

It is recognised that extensive travel lasting >8 hours, especially in confined spaces, such as on an aeroplane, is associated with an increased risk of DVT. Other risk factors include taking a combined oral contraceptive pill (OCP), smoking and a strong family history of DVT (e.g. with inherited hypercoagulable conditions such as factor V Leiden mutation or antithrombin III deficiency). Paralympians with SCI who have partial or complete loss of innervation from the SNS have diminished reflexive control of blood flow, decreased cardiac output, a tendency towards blood pooling in the lower extremities and thus theoretically an increased risk of DVT. Those who are wheelchair users also have venous stasis secondary to muscle paralysis and lower-extremity disuse.

The incidence of DVT within 3 months of an acute paralytic SCI is 38%, and the frequency of pulmonary embolus (PE) approximately 5% [16]. After 3–6 months, the risk of thromboembolic disease approaches that of the general population. Although not completely understood, some of the changes associated with chronic paralysis may be involved, including the development of collateral veins around older, subclinical venous thrombi.

There are few published reports in the medical literature of DVT in SCI and wheelchair-using Paralympic athletes. In the most recent epidemiological reports of injuries and illnesses in Paralympic athletes at the 2012 London Paralympic Games, there are no reports of thrombotic events [1,17]. No athlete with a clinical presentation suspicious for DVT presented for medical imaging services during the 2012 Paralympic Games [18]. In a retrospective analysis of the use of sonography at the 2008 Beijing Olympic and Paralympic Games, two cases of lower-extremity DVT were found in the Olympic Village (but it was not clear if these were in athletes or coaches/officials/volunteers), and two cases were discovered in Paralympic athletes [19].

Recommendations for the wheelchair athlete during a long flight or multiple flights over several days include adequate hydration, graduated use of compression stockings or 'flight socks' to minimise dependent oedema and frequent active or passive leg movement. Similarly, for athletes with lower-extremity amputations, strategies to minimise dependent oedema are necessary for long travel. Anecdotal experiences have led to the wearing of slightly smaller shrinkers, if tolerated, to minimise dependent oedema of the residual limb during flight. Additionally, if an amputee athlete removes their prosthesis during flight, the enlarged residual limb will make it challenging to don the prosthesis on arrival and increase the risk of skin breakdown. Evidence for prevention of DVT in chronic SCI and amputee athletes, as well as the use of low-dose aspirin, remains limited.

Coronary Heart Disease

CHD is more common and is seen at earlier ages in individuals with SCI than in those without SCI. The literature supports that SCI individuals have an increased risk of metabolic disorders compared to the general population, largely due to greatly reduced activity levels and an increased risk of obesity [20]. However, habitual high-level physical activity in those with SCI can maintain metabolic outcomes to the same level as sedentary able-bodied individuals, and perhaps even improve insulin sensitivity and high-density lipoprotein (HDL) cholesterol levels compared to able-bodied controls [21]. Paralympic athletes also tend to be older than their Olympic counterparts. Cardiac stress testing may be considered, depending on the athlete's age and risk factors for CHD. Because CHD may be asymptomatic in individuals with SCI due to decreased sensory feedback of angina, better recognition of CHD health risks may help reduce morbidity and mortality in these athletes.

In amputees, most deaths are from cardiac causes. Whilst coronary artery calcification scores (CACS) have been shown to be very high in dysvascular amputees (those who became amputees due to vascular conditions), they are even higher in traumatic amputees [22]. Post-traumatic lower-limb amputees have an increased morbidity and mortality from cardiovascular disease (CVD), with proximal leg amputation a greater risk than distal, and bilateral a greater risk than unilateral. There are hypothetical haemodynamic arterial abnormalities proximal to the site of amputation, with shear stress and circumferential strain causing degenerative conditions and arterial remodelling throughout the vascular system. Unilateral blood flow interruption also causes an asymmetric flow pattern at the aortic bifurcation, and perhaps an increased risk of developing abdominal aortic aneurysms [23]. The metabolic syndrome is prevalent in traumatic leg amputees, and high-level physical activity in Paralympic athletes may help mitigate this risk.

Conclusion

This chapter has reviewed the unique cardiovascular concerns of athletes with disabilities. Sports medicine physicians and cardiologists who are involved with elite able-bodied athletes should also feel comfortable providing cardiovascular support to Paralympic athletes. As the number of athletes with disabilities increase, so will research opportunities to work with this population, and our scientific knowledge about these cardiovascular conditions and other medical challenges facing our Paralympic athletes will continue to grow.

References

1 Derman, W., Schwellnus, M. and Jordaan, E. Clinical characteristics of 385 illnesses of athletes with impairment reported on the WEB-IISS system during the London 2012 Paralympic Games. *PM&R* 2014; **6**: S23–30.
2 OpenStax College. Anatomy & physiology. Available from: http://cnx.org/content/col11496/1.6/(last accessed 24 May 2016).
3 deGroot, P.C., van Dijk, A., Dijk, E. and Hopman, M.T. Preserved cardiac function after chronic spinal cord injury. *Arch Phys Med Rehabil* 2006; **87**: 1195–200.
4 Krassioukov, A. and West, C. The role of autonomic function on sport performance in athletes with spinal cord injury. *PM&R* 2014; **6**: S58–65.
5 Theisen, D. Cardiovascular determinants of exercise capacity in the Paralympic athlete with spinal cord injury. *Exp Physiol* 2012; **97**: 319–24.
6 Blackmer, J. Rehabilitation medicine: 1. Autonomic dysreflexia. *CMAJ* 2003; **169**: 931–5.
7 Krassioukov, A., Warburton, D.E., Teasell, R. and Eng, J.J. A systematic review of the management of autonomic dysreflexia after spinal cord injury. *Arch Phys Med Rehabil* 2009; **90**: 682–95.
8 Burnham, R., Wheeler, G., Bhambhani, Y. et al. Intentional induction of autonomic dysreflexia among quadriplegic athletes for performance enhancement: efficacy, safety, and mechanism of action. *Clin J Sports Med* 1994; **4**: 1–10.
9 Schmid, A., Schmidt-Trucksäú, A., Huonker, M. et al. Catecholamine response of high performance wheelchair athletes at rest and during exercise with autonomic dysreflexia. *Int J Sports Med* 2001; **22**: 2–7.
10 Blauwet, C., Benjamin-Laing, H., Stomphorst, J. et al. Testing for boosting at the Paralympic games: policies, results and future directions. *Br J Sports Med* 2013; **47**: 832–7.
11 Ljungqvist, A., Jenoure, P., Engebretsen, L. et al. The International Olympic Committee (IOC) consensus statement on periodic health evaluation of elite athletes. *Br J Sports Med* 2009; **43**: 631–43.
12 International Paralympic Committee (IPC) Medical Code. Available from: http://www.paralympic.org/sites/default/files/document/120131082554885_ipc+medical+code_final.pdf (last accessed 24 May 2016).
13 Myers, J., Lee, M. and Kiratli, J. Cardiovascular disease in spinal cord injury: an overview of prevalence, risk, evaluation, and management. *Am J Phys Med Rehabil* 2007; **86**: 1–11.
14 Claydon, V.E., Hol, A.T., Eng, J.J. and Krassioukov, A.V. Cardiovascular responses and postexercise hypotension after arm cycling exercise in subjects with spinal cord injury. *Arch Phys Med Rehabil* 2006; **8**: 1106–14.
15 Wan, D. and Krassioukov, A.V. Life-threatening outcomes associated with autonomic dysreflexia: a clinical review. *J Spinal Cord Med* 2014; **37**: 2–10.
16 Anderson, F.A. and Spencer F.A. Risk factors for venous thromboembolism. *Circulation* 2003; **107**: I9–16.
17 Willick, S.E., Webborn, N., Emery, C. et al. The epidemiology of injuries at the London 2012 Paralympic Games. *Br J Sports Med* 2013; **47**: 426–32.
18 Bethapudi, S., Campbell, R.S.D., Budgett, R. et al. Imaging services at the Paralympic Games London 2012: analysis of demand and distribution of workload. *Br J Sports Med* 2015; **49**: 20–4.
19 He, W., Xiang, D. and Dai, J. Sonography in the 29th Olympic and Paralympic Games: a retrospective analysis. *Clinical Imaging* 2011; **35**: 143–7.
20 Myers, J. Cardiovascular disease after SCI: prevalence, instigators, and risk clusters. *Topics Spinal Cord Injury Rehabil* 2009; **14**: 1–14.
21 Mojtahedi, M.C., Valentine, R.J., Arngrímsson S.A. et al. The association between regional body composition and metabolic outcomes in athletes with spinal cord injury. *Spinal Cord* 2008; **46**: 192–7.
22 Nallegowda, M., Lee, E., Brandstater, M. et al. Amputation and cardiac comorbidity: analysis of severity of cardiac risk. *PM&R* 2012; **4**: 657–66.
23 Naschitz, J.E. and Lenger, R. Why traumatic leg amputees are at increased risk for cardiovascular diseases. *Q J Med* 2008; **101**: 251–9.

Part 6
Emergency Cardiac Care

45 Emergency Cardiac Care in the Athletic Setting: From School Sports to the Olympic Arena

Efraim Kramer and Martin Botha

Division of Emergency Medicine, Faculty of Health Sciences, University of the Witwatersrand, Johannesburg, South Africa

Introduction

It is acknowledged best practice that health care providers at sporting events are able to competently care for cardiac emergencies [1]. Optimal outcomes are achieved via comprehensive emergency planning that ensures prompt and appropriate care. Diversity in athletic venues, sporting codes, age and competition level present challenges to the provision of emergency care in sport. An efficient and coordinated medical response to cardiac emergencies requires an established emergency medical plan, training of skilled responders in cardiopulmonary resuscitation (CPR) and the use of an automated external defibrillator (AED), access to emergency equipment and coordination of communication and transportation systems [1]. Prompt recognition, immediate CPR and early defibrillation are critical benchmarks in the management of patients suffering sudden cardiac arrest (SCA) [2]. This chapter reviews the principles of emergency cardiac care in sport at every level from an event held at a small school to the Olympic setting, focussing specifically on care of the athlete and not on spectator or mass-gathering issues.

Epidemiology

SCA is the leading cause of death in athletes during sport [1,3]. Sudden cardiac death (SCD) in athletes occurs approximately once every 3 days in the US [4]. A recent review reported rates varying from 1 in 3000 to 1 in 917 000, with data from higher-quality studies suggesting incidence rates of 1 in 40 000 to 1 in 80 000 [5]. The aetiology of SCA varies with age: in athletes younger than 35 years, SCA is primarily the result of genetic or functional structural and electrical cardiac disorders, acquired illnesses (such as myocarditis) or trauma (commotio cordis) [1].

SCA is also prevalent in the school sport milieu. In a prospective study of 2149 high schools in the US [6], 59 cases of SCA occurred, including 26 (44%) in students and 33 (56%) in adults; 39 (66%) cases occurred at an athletic facility during training or competition, whilst 55 (93%) cases were witnessed and 54 (92%) received prompt CPR. A defibrillator was applied in 50 (85%) cases and a shock delivered onsite in 39 (66%). Overall, 42 of 59 (71%) SCA victims and 16 of 18 (89%) student athletes with SCA survived to hospital discharge. Other studies have also demonstrated a survival benefit in high schools with onsite AED programmes, a high rate of bystander CPR and prompt emergency care [7].

IOC Manual of Sports Cardiology, First Edition. Edited by Mathew G. Wilson, Jonathan A. Drezner and Sanjay Sharma.
© 2017 International Olympic Committee. Published 2017 by John Wiley & Sons, Ltd.

Planning

A comprehensive Sport Emergency Cardiac Care (SECC) plan is a critical tool in facilitating emergency medical management of an event and in delivering efficient and effective emergency care.

All the elements of the SCA chain of survival need to be planned in detail, so as to make the SECC practical, effective and efficient, irrespective of the sports setting. The SECC plan should always encompass the following:

1. *Clear written procedures, policies and protocols.* The plan should have a contribution and consensus from all relevant stakeholders, and should be communicated to the same once finalised. A copy of the final, functional SECC plan – including a simple diagram and steps for doing CPR, use of the AED, access and egress routes for emergency medical services (EMS) and local emergency contact numbers – should be kept with the AED and emergency kits.
2. *Regular rehearsal, with debriefings to highlight, correct or improve any deficiencies* [8,9]. CPR and AED skills should be taught to all locally resident faculty, staff, coaches and other personnel who have regular contact with and supervisory responsibilities to the athletes. The plan should ensure there is always at least one competent person available for perform CPR at all sporting events, in order to enact the plan expeditiously. The larger the event, the more likely it is to have a designated professional emergency medical team onsite from a specific time before it begins until a specific time after it ends [9].
3. *An effective communication system to alert all persons onsite* – particularly first-responders – to immediately respond to the site of the collapse, with simultaneous or sequential retrieval of the AED from its known location.
4. *A checklist that includes the location of all onsite AEDs and a readiness check* prior to the event to ensure proper functioning of emergency equipment.

Training

Training is vital to implementation of the SECC. To be effective, instruction must be regular, targeted and simple. The programme should aim for skill proficiency and should include practice on manikins. Training and rehearsal should include all chain-of-survival points, including awareness and recognition of SCA, activation of the first-responder team and EMS (by calling the next tier in the system), initiation of CPR, retrieval and use of AEDs and use of checklists to enhance care and ensure adherence to procedure and protocol. All potential first-responders should practice the SECC plan at least once annually, and on-duty teams should review the SECC plan prior to events. Innovative training opportunities, such as the CPR 11 Smartphone Application [10], should be exploited as platforms for the training of CPR and use of AEDs, especially for events with a large number of volunteers. For example, thousands of volunteers were taught basic life-saving skills inside a stadium using large-screen technology as part of their duties at the 2012 London Olympic Games [11].

Personnel

The life-threatening nature of an SCA demands urgent recognition and expeditious management by a range of persons extending from members of the lay public to qualified and experienced health care professionals.

The incorporation of Public Access Defibrillation (PAD) protocols into SECC planning necessitates prompt recognition of SCA onsite within the sports environment and immediate summoning of assistance and activation of the SECC plan. This plan should include an easily accessible and simple-to-use AED with accompanying CPR instructions that can be followed by lay rescuers and health care providers alike. Use of the public as potential responders within the sports environment may in some cases allow the timely initiation of CPR and AED use in SECC incidents.

Immediate activation of the SECC response should be followed by basic life support, including hands-only CPR, standard CPR with rescue breathing and use of the AED. Spinal immobilisation techniques in SCA and transfer protocols for CPR within the sports environment may also be required [12,13].

Although SCA in the sports environment can be adequately managed at a basic life-support level, the presence of advanced life support (ALS) medical and paramedical personnel onsite may facilitate advanced airway procedures, automated mechanical or manual self-inflating bag ventilation, intravenous access, appropriate emergency medication administration and various other invasive resuscitative procedures that might be clinically indicated by the primary aetiology or the evolvement of the SCA.

The decision regarding what level and capacity of medical care is considered appropriate for a particular sporting event will be made by the capacity of the sporting and spectator mass present at the event, the medical (noncardiac) risk classification of the sporting event and other generic factors germane to the principles and practice of mass-gathering medicine.

Regarding SECC specifically, the capacity and capability of onsite medical care is determined by the mandatory requirement for on-duty medical and/or paramedical professionals to reach an athlete in SCA within 1 minute of noncontact collapse, enabling external initiation of chest compression within 1–2 minutes and application and use of an AED (when indicated) within 3 minutes from time of collapse.

For athletes in any setting, the proximity of the AED and other medical equipment should allow these critical-time standards to be realised.

Equipment

Efficient SCA management depends on the immediate onsite availability of well-maintained, fully functional, life-saving medical equipment. The higher the level of professional medical education, training and national registration, the more advanced and more invasive the clinically indicated medical management may become [9].

Whatever the capacity or location of the sporting event, type of sport(s) or prevailing local environmental conditions, the basic minimum SECC items of equipment that should be available, maintained, easy to access, clearly signposted and visible include the following:

- An *AED* with attached nonexpired adult or child defibrillation pads (whichever is appropriate).
- *AED accessory items:* Scissors to expose the bare chest for pad application, a razor for removal of excessive chest hair and a towelling cloth to wipe excessive moisture/sweat from the chest. A set of foam-type pads for knee protection during external chest compression can also be considered.
- *Manual rescue breathing barrier device:* A one-way, easy-to-use, transparent face mask device that allows efficient mouth-to-device manual rescue breathing. The size of the breathing device(s) should be appropriate for the expected age(s) of the sporting and spectator mass present, in order to ensure full functionality when required.
- *Personal protective equipment:* A set of small/medium/large nonsterile gloves for use by rescuers, if required. The provision of non-latex gloves should be considered. An alcohol-based, packaged antiseptic swab is advisable.
- *CPR instruction card:* A laminated card with simple, clear diagrammatic and written instructions for effective CPR, including the need to summon EMS assistance, the local EMS telephone number and, if necessary, the location of the nearest telephone. At large international, multilingual events, instructions should ideally be available in all relevant languages and should graphically illustrate the steps to follow.
- *SECC container/cabinet:* Dust- and waterproof, and appropriately sized to contain all of the necessary items for SECC. The container must be situated in a highly visible, adequately accessible location, so that people working at and frequenting the venue are aware of its presence. The outer face of the container should be transparent, so that the AED is always visible – including the AED window, which indicates whether or not the AED is fully functional. Due to the cost of AEDs, the security of the SECC container must be weighed against accessibility. Options include an alarm that is activated once the container door is opened or a secured container front that must be smashed to allow access. Whatever method is chosen, the AED must be functionally and publicly accessible to prevent delays and allow for swift defibrillation [14]. At school sports events, the AED may have to be temporarily relocated to the sporting venue from the main school building using a portable AED case.

This is the basic minimum equipment that any institution hosting sporting events should have available for use in the event of an SCA on the field of play in order to facilitate early PAD. If an event is sufficiently large and there are sufficient resources, the services of a commercial or voluntary event medical services team may be sought. At larger, more established sports venues, resident medical teams and infrastructure may already be in place. Under these circumstances, additional items of SECC equipment are recommended, elevating the basic minimum level of SECC to that of trained basic life support. These additional items permit:

- Timely activation of SECC within recommended critical time limits.
- Oropharyngeal airway insertion, to maintain an open airway.
- Ventilation via manual bag-valve-mask resuscitator. Use of the resuscitator must be practised for it to be effective. The mask can be held by one rescuer and the bag squeezed by another.
- Full spinal immobilisation, allowing for appropriate transfer of the SCA athlete from the field of play without interruption of chest compressions. SCA in the sporting environment is associated with noncontact, unprotected collapse of the athlete to the ground (unless in water), with potential risk of injury to the spine and neck. This necessitates that all movements of the SCA athlete be undertaken carefully and gently. Therefore, the SCA athlete must be transferred from the field of play whilst under full spinal immobilisation, protecting the spine and neck and allowing for effective chest compression on a hard surface. A long spinal trauma board, scoop stretcher, Stokes-type rescue basket or equivalent device must be available, together with accompanying head-immobilisation blocks and straps, not only for traditional transfer of the injured athlete from the field of play for orthopaedic injuries, but as part of the mandatory SECC equipment.

In large international sports events, such as the Olympics, the medical mandate for the host country is the provision of basic life support by experienced and fully equipped ALS pre-hospital personnel, elevating the onsite level of SECC to full ALS, as recommended by the International Liaison Committee on Resuscitation (ILCOR). This ALS level of care encompasses the necessary expertise and equipment to recognise, interpret and acutely manage not only nonperfusing cardiac arrhythmias (e.g. SCA) but also life-threatening perfusing cardiac arrhythmias. The range of medical equipment required for effective and efficient recognition and acute management of cardiac ALS includes primarily:

- An electrocardiogram (ECG) monitor/defibrillator (manual and AED functionality), includeing 3-lead ECG monitoring and, ideally, 12-lead diagnostic ECG capability, synchronised cardioversion and external transcutaneous pacing functions, with noninvasive blood-pressure, oxygen-saturation and end-tidal carbon dioxide monitoring multifunctionality.
- Advanced airway capability for the normal, difficult and failed airway.
- Central and peripheral venous access capability.
- A comprehensive range of emergency medications for intravenous administration.

This hierarchy of SECC is built on PAD and CPR, with basic life support (BLS) and then ALS serving as supplementary levels.

Communications

Activation and coordination of the SECC plan and eventual transfer and transport of the SCA athlete require effective and efficient communication between the various strategic role-players.

SCA requires activation and implementation of the SECC plan. In the absence of official on-duty health care providers, as in a school setting, a specific, easy-to-use, functional and regularly rehearsed form of communication must be triggered to efficiently notify previously identified persons/systems, local officials and EMS. Whatever form of communication is considered, it must be pratical and appropriate to the specific location, and therefore it may differ from location to location, nationally and internationally.

In a larger sporting event, where official on-duty health care providers are available and are constantly in sight of the athletic activity, they will be expected to instantly recognise a collapsed athlete, and to respond immediately. In this case, communication is required to activate internal and/or external medical assistance and backup, for treatment and/or transfer, as applicable. However, in those sporting events which are held over extended locations (e.g. marathon or cross-country events), multiple observers will be required, located strategically across the area to identify any athletic collapse and immediately activate the SECC plan. In these settings, more trained first-responders with AED capacity are recommended.

In all of these situations, effective and efficient forms of communication are imperative, using whatever mobile, logistically relevant, appropriate technology is locally available (e.g. two-way radios, mobile phones, radio-paging, global positioning technology, etc.).

Onsite Emergency Cardiac Care Protocol

Recognition of SCA

Prompt recognition of SCA in an athlete is the first step in the SECC treatment plan. SCA is the primary and presumptive diagnosis in any athlete who presents with the following signs:

1. *Noncontact collapse.* Any athlete who collapses without contact with another athlete or obstacle is to be regarded as SCA with immediate response. Similarly, collapse with unconsciousness following blunt trauma to the chest (possible commotio cordis) should elicit the same urgent response.
2. *Lack of response to any verbal or painful stimuli (unconsciousness).* Removal of sport-specific protective gear may be necessary to fully assess a collapsed athlete and initiate resuscitative efforts.
3. *Absence of normal breathing.* Initial normal breathing may occasionally be present for a very short period, deteriorating rapidly into gasping and/or slow agonal respirations and then total cessation of breathing (apnoea).
4. *Brief seizure-like activity presenting as involuntary arm and leg movements.* This is reported in approximately half of young athletes with SCA. Any collapsed and unresponsive athlete who is not breathing normally or who has seizure-like activity must be regarded as an SCA and must *not* be mistaken as a seizure.

Onsite Treatment of SCA

Onsite treatment of SCA within the sporting environment involves six steps:

Early recognition of a noncontact collapse: Any athlete who collapses to the ground (excluding water sports) without having had any forceful contact with another athlete or obstacle and who appears unresponsive is to be regarded as an SCA. Collapse following a blow to the chest (possible commotio cordis) should be treated the same way.

1. *Immediate response to the site of collapse:* Due to the critical nature of this medical condition, response should not be delayed by the rules of the sport, which may put the athlete's life at risk. Delayed response and cardiac resuscitation cannot wait for endorsement from officials, unless other safety factors necessitate this.
2. *Immediate evaluation and commencement of CPR:* Once the signs of SCA have been identified in the collapsed athlete, immediate CPR should be initiated. It is not critical whether *hands-only chest-compression CPR* or *standard compression–ventilation CPR* is undertaken initially, as long as effective chest compressions are immediately commenced: pushing hard, pushing fast with minimal interruption (less than 10 seconds). The type of manual rescue ventilation instituted will depend on the qualification and expertise of the initial responders and backup health care providers and on attendant medical equipment, including supplemental oxygenation.
3. *Application and use of AED:* The most common form of lethal cardiac arrhythmia in collapsed athletes is ventricular fibrillation, making expeditious availability of an AED paramount to survival. In smaller locations, initial SECC may require a two-pronged response to SCA: response to the collapsed athlete's side, with immediate initiation of CPR, and response to retrieve the AED, if it has not been located within the immediate sporting environment. During preparation and application of the AED, chest compressions should ideally not be interrupted, and certainly not for more than 10 seconds. The exception to this is when the AED instructs personnel to stand clear from the SCA victim for rhythm identification, charging and recommended defibrillation shock. Compressions should be resumed immediately post-shock.
4. *Activation of the EMS or summoning of onsite medical services to the site of the SCA collapse, whichever is relevant*: It may be necessary to activate the EMS for resuscitative assistance and transfer or for transfer assistance only if there are adequate onsite health care providers on duty. In the unfortunate case that an AED is not available onsite, the local EMS will need to be activated. This situation prolongs the time before effective AED use, resulting in decreased athlete survival. If this situation is relevant, the SECC plan must ensure that immediate CPR and EMS activation are incorporated and rehearsed in tandem.

5. *Transfer of the SCA athlete from the site of collapse to the athlete medical centre or to the nearest, most appropriate emergency department or cardiac catheterisation unit:* Once CPR and AED resuscitative measures have been established, a decision must be made whether to transfer the SCA athlete to a medical centre for definitive diagnosis and treatment. For this to occur safely and effectively, the athlete in SCA must be appropriately transferred, via coordinated logroll or a similar transfer method, on to a long trauma board or equivalent, and adequately immobilised so that the immobilising device, SCA athlete and AED are immobilised as one unit. This process is undertaken to ensure high-quality uninterrupted CPR en route. Once this has been achieved, a decision must be made as to whether the EMS ambulance can be brought to the site of collapse or whether the immobilised SCA athlete should be transferred to the waiting ambulance. If the athlete is to be taken to an ambulance, CPR must *not* be interrupted for more than any single 10-second period. Ideally, CPR will be continued whilst the athlete is moved towards the ambulance. This may require someone to ride on top of the stretcher or cart during transport. In circumstances where this is not possible, the transfer team should count 10 seconds and halt transfer, place the athlete on the ground (still trapped and immobilised) and commence external chest compressions for at least 2 minutes. The AED will automatically advise a reanalysis when it is due, at which point the team must pause compressions to allow the analysis. After any required AED shock, compressions should be resumed immediately for at least 60 seconds, after which the transfer team may begin their next set of 10-second transfer towards the ambulance. This sequence must be repeated with team leader-controlled discipline and attention to detail, always with the awareness that during cessation of chest compressions, the SCA athlete is without necessary perfusion, until the athlete is securely inside the ambulance.

Transport

All athletes with SCA, whether still in cardiac arrest and receiving active CPR/AED or returned to spontaneous rhythm, must be transferred to the nearest, most appropriate medical facility.

It is important to note that current internationally recommended Out-of-Hospital Cardiac Arrest (OHCA) CPR protocols, which recommend that a patient without return of spontaneous circulation (ROSC) not be transferred by ambulance to hospital, *do not apply* to resuscitation of the unexpected SCA athlete. This means that once CPR and AED defibrillation have been commenced onsite in the sports environment, they must be continued (if medically indicated) en route to the medical facility. Transfer should be by either air or road ambulance, with personnel who have been adequately trained in performing CPR (manual chest compressions/positive-pressure ventilation/defibrillation/drug administration) inside a moving ambulance, in order that the quality of the CPR is never compromised and interruptions are absolutely minimised. The use of automated external chest compression devices is to be encouraged if resources allow it.

Definitive Cardiac Critical Care

Definitive cardiac critical care may require invasive cardiac catheterisation, coronary artery device insertion, therapeutic post-cardiac arrest hypothermia, ventilation, internal defibrillator device insertion and a number of other related pharmacological or surgical interventions that can only be adequately undertaken in an appropriately staffed and equipped facility. Currently, good clinical practice mandates that patients with ROSC post-cardiac arrest be transferred to a facility that can provide post-arrest cardiac critical care, if and whenever possible. Patients in refractory cardiac arrest would also benefit from this definitive care.

Therefore, during SECC planning, the availability and location of adequate and appropriate cardiac facilities should be identified and pre-event preparatory arrangements should be made with the administrative and clinical personnel necessary to expedite any emergency cardiac admission during the event. This pre-emergency event planning should be undertaken whatever the size, capacity or location of the sporting event, from a small school event to the Olympic Games.

Post-SCA Debrief

The occurrence of SCA on the sports field in a fit and healthy sportsperson may generate an emotional response locally, nationally and internationally. For those who are intimately involved in the recognition, response, onsite treatment and related transport, it can be a very emotional and disturbing event, particularly if it involves someone known to the rescuers or when the rescue is undertaken in full view of a large spectator mass and attendant media.

It is therefore important, after the conclusion of the SCA resuscitation, for all those involved to be adequately and professionally debriefed as soon as possible. The entire event should be systematically reviewed. Both good performance and areas for improvement should be identified, inherent errors should be acknowledged and psychological counselling should be offered to responders, where needed. Family counselling, including the need for extended family screening once the SCA athlete's pathological process has been analysed and defined, should be undertaken. The aim should be continuous improvement within a constructive atmosphere, encouraging those involved to plan, train and maintain their current level of expertise with confidence and optimism, in preparation for the next SCA event.

Conclusion

Although many cases of SCA in athletes are potentially preventable if cardiac abnormalities are diagnosed through screening before training or competition, life-threatening cardiovascular emergencies will nevertheless still occur. The presence of a well-structured, regularly rehearsed SECC plan, put together and undertaken by motivated and adequately skilled CPR-trained personnel, using highly visible, easily accessible, well-maintained and fully functional AEDs, enhances the potential for survival of a SCA event. Whether the sporting activity is located at a school, college, university, premium-league sport stadium or the Olympics, the necessity for effective and efficient emergency medical planning, preparation, practice and provision remains the same. This will enable rescuers to recognise, respond to and resuscitate an athlete in SCA in a time-critical manner.

References

1 Toresdahl, B., Courson, R., Börjesson, M. et al. Emergency cardiac care in the athletic setting: from schools to the Olympics. *Br J Sports Med* 2012; **46**(Suppl. I): i85–90.
2 Koster, R.W., Sayre, M.R., Botha, M. et al. Part 5: adult basic life support: 2010 International Consensus on Cardiopulmonary Resuscitation and Emergency Cardiovascular Care Science With Treatment Recommendations. *Circulation* 2010; **122**(Suppl. 2): S298–324.
3 Drezner, J.A., Roberts, W.O., Mosesso, V.N. et al. Inter-association task force recommendations on emergency preparedness and management of sudden cardiac arrest in high school and college athletic programs: a consensus statement. *J Athl Train* 2007; **42**(1): 143–58.
4 Harmon, K.G. Update on sideline and event preparation for management of sudden cardiac arrest in athletes. *Curr Sports Med Rep* 2007; **6**(3): 170–6.
5 Harmon, K.G., Drezner, J.A., Wilson, M.G. et al. Incidence of sudden cardiac death in athletes: a state-of-the-art review. *Heart* 2014; **100**(16): 1227–34.
6 Drezner, J.A., Toresdahl, B., Rao, A.L. et al. Outcomes from sudden cardiac arrest in US high schools: a 2-year prospective study from the National Registry for AED Use in Sports. *Br J Sports Med* 2013; **47**(18): 1179–83.
7 Drezner, J.A., Rao, A.L., Heistand, J. et al. Effectiveness of emergency response planning for sudden cardiac arrest in United States high schools with automated external defibrillators. *Circulation* 2009; **120**(6): 518–25.
8 Drezner, J.A., Dvorak, J., Kramer, E.B. et al. The FIFA® 11 Steps to prevent sudden cardiac death during football games. *Eur Heart J* 2013; **34**(47): 3594–5.
9 Dvorak, J., Kramer, E.B., Schmied, C.M. et al. The FIFA medical emergency bag and FIFA 11 steps to prevent sudden cardiac death: setting a global standard and promoting consistent football field emergency care. *Br J Sports Med* 2013; **47**(18): 1199–202.
10 FIFA. New app hoping to help prevent Sudden Cardiac Death. Available from: http://www.fifa.com/development/news/y=2014/m=12/news=new-app-hoping-to-help-prevent-sudden-cardiac-death-2487197.html (last accessed 24 May 2016).
11 BBC. Olympics volunteers 'taught life-saving CPR skills'. Available from: http://www.bbc.com/news/health-18414183 (last accessed 24 May 2016).
12 Kramer, E.B., Botha, M., Drezner, J. et al. Practical management of sudden cardiac arrest on the football field. *Br J Sports Med* 2012; **46**(16): 1094–6.
13 Kramer, E., Dvorak, J. and Kloeck, W. Review of the management of sudden cardiac arrest on the football field. *Br J Sports Med* 2010; **44**(8): 540–5.
14 Cronin, O., Jordan, J., Quigley, F. et al. Prepared for sudden cardiac arrest? A cross-sectional study of automated external defibrillators in amateur sport. *Br J Sports Med* 2013; **47**: 1171–4.

Part 7
Sports Cardiology Training

46 Recommendations for Sports Cardiology Training for the Sports Medicine Physician

Irfan M. Asif[1] and Jonathan A. Drezner[2]

[1] Department of Family Medicine, Greenville Health System, University of South Carolina Greenville School of Medicine, Greenville, SC, USA
[2] Department of Family Medicine, University of Washington, Seattle, WA, USA

Introduction

Sports medicine physicians are an essential part of an athletic health care team responsible for the cardiovascular safety of athletes. Sports medicine training requirements vary by country and by training programme. Currently, no universal standard for sports cardiology training exists for the sports medicine physician. This chapter provides the rationale and recommendations for fundamental sports cardiology training for the sports medicine physician.

The Need for a Sports Cardiology Curriculum

The role of sports cardiology in the care of athletes and physically active individuals of all ages has become increasingly evident, especially with growing efforts towards the prevention of sudden death in athletes. Exercise recommendations also transcend efforts to combat the obesity epidemic and decrease cardiovascular morbidity and mortality in order to promote a healthier population. The ultimate goal of sports cardiology is to delineate safe exercise recommendations for all individuals in order to maximise the benefits of physical activity and organised sport, whilst minimising potential adverse outcomes.

Although the European Society of Cardiology (ESC) has defined a core curriculum for sports cardiology qualification for physicians with formal cardiology training, in the US cardiology training programmes fail to define core competencies in sports cardiology or to provide any organised or required training in athlete cardiovascular care [1,2].

Unfortunately, medical curricula addressing preventative medicine and the proper diagnosis and management of cardiovascular disorders in athletes are also absent from sports medicine training programmes. Whilst educational programmes differ worldwide, the goal of a sports cardiology curriculum is to provide the training, assessment and competencies needed to develop sports medicine physicians capable of providing broad and high-quality cardiovascular care for the athlete, in conjunction with cardiovascular specialists.

A sports cardiology training programme can be divided into three main sections:

1. A sports cardiology curriculum that defines the medical knowledge and skills required to properly deliver cardiovascular care of both competitive and recreational athletes.
2. Guidelines for the training environment and infrastructure.
3. Strategies for the learning and assessment needed to evaluate a trainee in sports cardiology.

Sports Cardiology Curriculum

The following curricular recommendations may be used as a framework for international training programmes that wish to educate sports medicine physicians in this evolving field. The most crucial aspects of sports cardiology training and practice for a sports medicine physician involve:

1. The promotion of healthy lifestyles through physical activity.
2. Knowledge of the physiologic cardiovascular adaptations to regular exercise.
3. A comprehensive understanding of the various cardiovascular conditions associated with sudden cardiac death (SCD) in athletes of different ages, as well as the disorders causing long-term morbidity.
4. Pre-participation cardiovascular screening and guidance for safe athletic activity.
5. Evaluation of cardiovascular-related symptoms in athletes.
6. Coordinated emergency action planning for sideline care or mass-participation events and the management of exercise-related cardiovascular emergencies.

Healthy Lifestyle through Physical Activity

Chronic diseases are a major cause of morbidity and mortality worldwide, and lead to excessive health care spending in many countries. Regular exercise and other healthy lifestyle choices are critical to preventing and treating obesity, hypertension, hyperlipidaemia, diabetes, coronary artery disease (CAD), peripheral vascular disease, osteoarthritis, cancer, chronic obstructive pulmonary disease (COPD) and many other disabling conditions [3].

Sports medicine physicians with expertise in sports cardiology can play a pivotal role in improving individual and population health through the promotion of physical activity (see Chapter 6). They should be competent in addressing traditional cardiovascular risk factors and providing exercise prescriptions for athletes of all ages. In older athletes with risk factors, screening for CAD through exercise stress testing should be considered (see Chapter 41).

Physiologic Cardiovascular Adaptations to Regular Exercise

Regular and long-term participation in intensive exercise is associated with physiologic cardiac remodelling, which results in increased vagal tone and enlarged cardiac chamber size. These cardiac adaptations cause unique electrical manifestations that are considered normal physiologic changes to regular exercise and do not require further evaluation. A comprehensive understanding of changes in the athlete's heart is required for the accurate interpretation of screening or diagnostic testing in athletes (see Chapters 4 and 5). Nonetheless, distinguishing physiologic from pathologic cardiac alterations can remain challenging and requires careful consideration (see Chapter 40).

Causes of Cardiovascular Mortality and Morbidity

SCD is caused by a variety of structural and electrical cardiovascular conditions, which are largely genetic in nature. Sports medicine physicians should have a thorough knowledge of the disorders that place young athletes at risk during sports participation. The cardiomyopathies represent a heterogeneous group of heart muscle diseases and are responsible for a significant proportion of SCD in athletes (see Chapters 19–21). Primary electrical diseases such as ion channelopathies and ventricular pre-excitation are also important causes of cardiac fatalities in young athletes (see Chapters 26–29). Other important structural cardiac disorders associated with SCD include coronary artery anomalies and connective-tissue disorders affecting the aorta (see Chapters 22 and 25). Acquired cardiac disorders such as myocarditis or congenital heart disease and valvular disorders also place athletes at risk of SCD and have long-term implications (see Chapters 23, 24 and 32). Additionally, management of traditional cardiovascular risk factors, such as hypertension and hyperlipidaemia, including the choice of pharmacotherapy, has nuances unique to the treatment of competitive athletes and requires specific knowledge by the sports medicine physician (see Chapter 39).

Pre-Participation Cardiovascular Screening

Pre-participation screening of young athletes and medical clearance prior to participation in competitive sport are recommended by major medical and sporting societies. Controversy exists regarding the most suitable approach to screening. Nevertheless, sports medicine physicians are chiefly responsible for conducting pre-participation screening as a means of ensuring athletes' safety. The primary objective of pre-participation cardiovascular screening is to prospectively identify or raise suspicion of previously unrecognised and largely genetic/congenital cardiovascular diseases (CVDs) known to cause sudden cardiac arrest (SCA) and sudden death in young people [4]. As such, the pre-participation evaluation is a crucial aspect of sports cardiology, and sports medicine physicians should be knowledgeable about both the physiologic adaptations to regular exercise and the conditions associated with SCD.

Most screening protocols include at minimum a personal medical history, a family history and a physical examination. Whilst the sensitivity of history and physical examination alone to detect potentially lethal cardiac conditions is limited [5], it is critical that sports medicine physicians utilise standardised questionnaires when performing a pre-participation screening in young athletes. Guidelines exist to assist sports medicine physicians in developing a differential diagnosis, asking follow-up questions to positive history responses and understanding the role of and indications for additional diagnostic testing and consultation with a cardiovascular specialist [6]. Sports medicine physicians should be aware of the limitations of a history- and symptom-based protocol, in that most cases of SCA occur in individuals with no antecedent symptoms and a normal cardiovascular examination. Importantly, screening should address a family history of premature SCA or SCD before the age of 40, which is associated with a significant risk of an inherited pathologic cardiac disorder [7].

The addition of a resting 12-lead electrocardiogram (ECG) to pre-participation screening increases the sensitivity to detect CVDs (e.g. cardiomyopathy, myocarditis, ion-channel disorders, ventricular pre-excitation). Many countries, however, do not have the physician infrastructure to engage in large-scale, high-quality screening efforts. Nevertheless, accurate interpretation of an ECG in an athlete is a critical skill for the sports medicine physician. Physicians responsible for the cardiovascular care of athletes must learn ECG interpretation standards that distinguish normal ECG findings in athletes from ECG abnormalities requiring additional evaluation for conditions associated with SCD [8,9]. Free online training programmes (http://learning.bmj.com/ECGathlete) are available to improve physician education in ECG interpretation and guide secondary testing for ECG abnormalities. Efforts are ongoing to further refine standardised ECG interpretation criteria in order to improve specificity without compromising sensitivity, using the latest scientific evidence (see Chapters 10–12).

Athletes identified as having a serious cardiac disorder should be managed in collaboration with a cardiovascular specialist. Sports medicine physicians should remain actively involved in eligibility decisions and recommendations for safe sports and physical activities (see Chapter 34).

Evaluation of Cardiovascular-Related Symptoms

Cardiovascular symptoms in athletes are often vague and overlap considerably with the normal, physical response to strenuous exercise, creating a considerable challenge for the sports medicine physician in determining which complaints require comprehensive testing. Potential warning signs or symptoms of a serious cardiovascular condition include exertional chest pain, excessive shortness of breath, exertional syncope, heart palpitations, unexplained seizure-like activity and new-onset exertional intolerance and fatigue (see Chapter 35).

Syncope occurring during exercise remains an ominous sign of a serious cardiovascular condition and necessitates a comprehensive assessment for both structural and electrical conditions associated with SCD [10]. The sports medicine physician should be able to distinguish benign from malignant presentations of syncope. Premonitory symptoms prior to collapse are common in neurally mediated (vasovagal) syncope; they include lightheadedness, dizziness, diaphoresis, nausea and tunnel vision. In contrast, individuals with syncope from a cardiac disorder at risk for SCD usually have an abrupt collapse without warning, due to the onset of a potentially lethal ventricular arrhythmia.

Emergency Action Planning and Management of SCA

No screening programme offers absolute protection against SCA. As such, every school, club and organisation that sponsors an athletic event must be prepared to respond to a collapsed athlete through a well-developed emergency action plan (EAP) [11,12]. Treatment of SCA should begin with immediate recognition, early cardiopulmonary resuscitation and prompt application of a defibrillator, with a goal of less than 3 minutes from collapse to first shock. In young athletes with SCA, rapid emergency care and use of an automated external defibrillator (AED) have demonstrated survival rates over 80% [13]. Thus, SCD in athletes is largely preventable with proper emergency preparations, and the sports medicine physician must be prepared to lead an efficient and rehearsed resuscitation effort in cases of suspected SCA. The details of proper emergency planning will vary depending on the sporting event, venue and location, and require coordination with event organisers, administrators, local emergency medical services and potential on-site responders (see Chapter 45).

Training Environment and Infrastructure

Beyond a core curriculum, a comprehensive sports cardiology training programme will define the requirements of the teaching institution and for education of the trainee. Multiple sites can be used to provide formal education in sports cardiology through direct observation, supervised patient care, lectures and mentorship. Ideally, the training programme should have a dedicated core faculty with expertise in sports cardiology, including members with backgrounds in sports medicine and paediatric/adult cardiology.

The training programme should provide exposure to and opportunities in exercise physiology, pre-participation screening, medical coverage of sporting/mass-participation events and cardiology, ideally including inherited disease clinics. Trainees should attend multidisciplinary rounds to review sports cardiology topics, discuss interesting cases and diagnostic dilemmas, critically examine peer-reviewed journal articles and analyse case information and advanced imaging/testing with specialists involved in comanagement of the athlete.

Strategies for Learning and Assessment

The educational experience that sports medicine physicians receive during their training can include lectures and coursework, supervised clinical experiences and procedural training, mentored research, attendance at scientific meetings and feedback through regular assessment and evaluation of their progress.

Lectures and Coursework

Didactic instruction may occur through a dedicated lecture series within the sports medicine training programme or via formal sports cardiology courses. These sessions should be coupled with critical appraisal of sports cardiology chapters, contemporary review articles and peer-reviewed manuscripts.

BMJ Learning provides a free online education course on ECG Interpretation in Athletes (http://learning. bmj.com/ECGathlete). Developed by international experts in sports cardiology, this course provides a solid foundation in understanding the aetiology of CVDs predisposing to SCD in athletes, as well as ECG interpretation standards and the rationale for secondary testing of ECG abnormalities. As such, this course should be a compulsory piece of sports cardiology training for the sports medicine physician.

Learning objective	Knowledge, skills and practice
1. Characterise the role of the sports medicine physician in the athlete' health care team	• Coordinate care of athletes within a multidisciplinary team • Build rapport with athletes and ensure proper physician–patient confidentiality • Appropriately counsel athletes regarding safe sports participation, screening and management of CVD, including potential effects on mental health
2. Describe the structural and functional cardiac adaptations associated with regular exercise, including the influence of sport, age, gender and race	• Recognise the physiologic adaptations associated with regular vigorous exercise (athlete's heart) and distinguish these changes from underlying cardiac pathology • Classify the effects of sports and training regimens on cardiovascular adaptation (endurance vs strength, dynamic vs static, aerobic vs anaerobic) • Understand the relationship between athletic activity and atrial abnormalities, such as atrial fibrillation
3. Define the cardiovascular and general health benefits of habitual physical activity	• Counsel patients on lifestyle recommendations and the benefits of regular physical activity in order to reduce cardiovascular morbidity and mortality • Counsel patients regarding screening and risk stratification of those with cardiovascular risk factors, such as hypertension, hypercholesterolaemia, diabetes, smoking, obesity or a significant family history • Write an exercise prescription specifying frequency, intensity, timing and type of exercise, and modify it based on the individual patient's progress and goals
4. Understand the structural, electrical and acquired aetiologies of SCD in athletes	• Describe the incidence of SCA/SCD in athletes, including differences based on age, race, gender and sport • Define the causes and prevalences of disorders associated with SCA/SCD in athletes • Recognise noncardiac causes of sudden death in sport, such as heat stroke and exertional collapse related to sickle-cell trait
5. Conduct comprehensive pre-participation cardiovascular screening in competitive athletes	• Define the advantages and limitations of pre-participation screening modalities, such as medical history, physical examination and ECG • Recognise the differences in screening practices recommended by the American Heart Association (AHA), European Society of Cardiology (ESC), Fédération Internationale de Football Association (FIFA), Union of European Football Associations (UEFA), International Olympic Committee (IOC) and other sports governing or medical organisations • Correctly interpret cardiovascular symptoms and physical examination findings during a pre-participation screening evaluation • Understand the major considerations in the use of a resting ECG in the cardiovascular screening of athletes, such as the need for athlete-specific interpretation standards, sensitivity, specificity, cost-effectiveness, infrastructure development and adequate cardiology resources • Describe the evaluation of athletes with screening abnormalities and the role of advanced cardiac testing/imaging, such as echocardiogram, ambulatory ECG, stress ECG, cardiac magnetic resonance (CMR), cardiac computed tomography (CT), cardiopulmonary exercise testing and electrophysiology (EP) study
6. Demonstrate accurate ECG interpretation in athletes and the proper distinction of physiologic findings from ECG abnormalities suggestive of an underlying cardiac disorder	• Complete the British Medical Journal (*BMJ*) ECG Interpretation in Athletes module (http://learning.bmj.com/ECGathlete) • Understand the importance of proper lead placement in performing an athlete's ECG • Differentiate ECG findings suggestive of physiologic cardiovascular adaptations from abnormalities consistent with disorders predisposing to SCA/SCD

Table 46.1 Core learning objectives in sports cardiology for the sports medicine physician

Learning objective	Knowledge, skills and practice
7. Participate in the evaluation and management of CVD in athletes, in collaboration with a cardiologist	• Describe the follow-up evaluation and management of acquired CVDs (e.g. hypertension, hyperlipidaemia, atrial fibrillation) and inherited cardiovascular disorders (e.g. cardiomyopathies, ion channelopathies) • Define the role of familial testing, including genetic analysis, in athletes diagnosed with inherited cardiac disease • Provide guidelines on safe sports participation for individuals identified with underlying cardiac disease • Understand the indications, potential complications and ethical considerations of implantable cardioverter-defibrillators (ICDs) • Counsel patients with cardiac disease on safe physical activity recommendations, including competitive sports eligibility considerations, and manage the psychological impact of a cardiac diagnosis
8. Outline the essential elements of an emergency action plan (EAP) for SCA at sporting events, as well as specific considerations based on the type of event, number of participants and environmental factors	• Describe the importance of an EAP and the role of AEDs in the prevention of SCD in athletes • Coordinate the EAP with on-site first responders, emergency medical services personnel and the athlete health care team • Tailor an EAP based on type of event (mass-participation vs single-venue), number of participants and environmental factors (e.g. climate, terrain, altitude)
9. Describe the cardiovascular effects of medications, substances and doping	• Understand the side-effect profile and potential impact on exercise performance of common medications used in the management of CVDs such as hypertension and hypercholesterolaemia • Recognise the practices and potential adverse effects of banned substances in sports • Define the role of and criteria for therapeutic use exemptions
10. Characterise the ethical and legal considerations – as well as diagnostic conundrums – associated with the cardiovascular care of athletes, including issues surrounding sports eligibility and participation with an identified cardiovascular disorder	• Recognise the ethical implications of screening in athletes and the diagnosis of cardiac disease • Describe the ethical and legal ramifications of disqualification from competitive sports participation • Balance medical recommendations with the athlete's desire to participate and excel in sport

Table 46.1 (Continued)

Procedure	Minimum to attend/observe	Target to actively perform/interpret
ECG interpretation	100	500
Exercise prescription	10	25
Exercise treadmill testing	10	50
Cardiopulmonary exercise testing	10	50
Pre-participation cardiovascular screening	50	100
Medical coverage of sporting events and competitions	20	50
Medical director or codirector for a mass-participation event	1	1

Table 46.2 Targeted skills and procedural training in sports cardiology for the sports medicine physician

Supervised Clinical Experiences and Procedural Training

Physician education is founded on direct observation and supervision, with increasing autonomy as the trainee becomes more proficient. The key areas of clinical focus for sports cardiology training are captured through the core learning objectives listed in Table 46.1, whilst Table 46.2 provides a list of target skills and procedural training. Importantly, the training emphasis should be on mastering *competency*, and not solely on the number of encounters. Procedures should be recorded in a detailed log to assist with future hospital credentialing.

Mentored Research

Research can enhance the overall training of a sports medicine physician, and trainees may conduct basic, clinical or translational research related to sports cardiology. Ideally, each trainee should be given a focused investigation with an appropriate scope and timeline for completion. Presentation and publication of the research is encouraged.

Scientific Meetings

Scientific conferences provide an additional means of sports cardiology education. Sports medicine trainees should participate in and attend at least one national/international meeting with dedicated sessions in sports cardiology. A training programme should reinforce the need for ongoing learning and education in sports cardiology.

Assessment and Evaluation of Progress

Trainees should be assessed using standard competencies consistent with the normal practice of the teaching programme. Assessment methods should include a mixture of formative and summative evaluations, including evaluations from supervising faculty. Programme directors should review the evaluations and provide regular feedback so that trainees can adjust learning strategies if adequate progress is not being made.

Conclusion

Sports cardiology is a rapidly evolving field, and the cardiovascular care of athletes represents a major responsibility of the sports medicine physician. Safe sports and exercise participation for athletes of all ages is a primary objective, which requires fundamental knowledge of the disorders associated with SCD, their diagnosis through screening and secondary testing and their distinction from physiologic cardiac adaptations to regular exercise. The exponential rise in knowledge in this discipline and the demand for expertise dictate the need for formal training and curricula dedicated to the field that can be incorporated into a sports medicine training programme. This curriculum outlines a framework for sports medicine physicians who wish to gain the requisite training needed to comprehensively care for the cardiovascular needs of the athlete in conjunction with cardiology specialists and should be incorporated into sports medicine training programmes.

References

1 Heidbuchel, H., Papadakis, M., Panhuyzen-Goedkoop, N. et al. Position paper: proposal for a core curriculum for a European Sports Cardiology qualification. *Eur J Prev Cardiol* 2013; **20**: 889–903.

2 Lawless, C.E., Olshansky, B., Washington, R.L. et al. Sports and exercise cardiology in the United States: cardiovascular specialists as members of the athlete healthcare team. *J Am Coll Cardiol* 2014; **63**: 1461–72.

3 Shiroma, E.J. and Lee, I.M. Physical activity and cardiovascular health: lessons learned from epidemiological studies across age, gender, and race/ethnicity. *Circulation* 2010; **122**: 743–52.

4 Maron, B.J., Friedman, R.A., Kligfield, P. et al. Assessment of the 12-lead electrocardiogram as a screening test for detection of cardiovascular disease in healthy general populations of young people (12–25 years of age): a scientific statement from the American Heart Association and the American College of Cardiology. *J Am Coll Cardiol* 2014; **64**: 1479–514.

5 Harmon, K.G., Zigman, M. and Drezner, J.A. The effectiveness of screening history, physical exam, and ECG to detect potentially lethal cardiac disorders in athletes: a systematic review/meta-analysis. *J Electrocardiol* 2015; **48**: 329–38.

6 Asif, I.M., Roberts, W.O., Fredericson, M. and Froelicher, V. The cardiovascular preparticipation evaluation (ppe) for the primary care and sports medicine physician, part I. *Curr Sports Med Rep* 2015; **14**: 246–67.

7 Ranthe, M.F., Winkel, B.G., Andersen, E.W. et al. Risk of cardiovascular disease in family members of young sudden cardiac death victims. *Eur Heart J* 2013; **34**: 503–11.

8 Drezner, J.A., Ackerman, M.J., Anderson, J. et al. Electrocardiographic interpretation in athletes: the 'Seattle Criteria'. *Br J Sports Med* 2013; **47**: 122–4.

9 Sheikh, N., Papadakis, M., Ghani, S. et al. Comparison of electrocardiographic criteria for the detection of cardiac abnormalities in elite black and white athletes. *Circulation* 2014; **129**: 1637–49.

10 Colivicchi, F., Ammirati, F. and Santini, M. Epidemiology and prognostic implications of syncope in young competing athletes. *Eur Heart J* 2004; **25**: 1749–53.

11 Drezner, J.A., Courson, R.W., Roberts, W.O. et al. Inter-association task force recommendations on emergency preparedness and management of sudden cardiac arrest in high school and college athletic programs: a consensus statement. *Heart Rhythm* 2007; **4**: 549–65.

12 Toresdahl, B., Courson, R., Börjesson, M. et al. Emergency cardiac care in the athletic setting: from schools to the Olympics. *Br J Sports Med* 2012; **46**(Suppl. 1): i85–9.

13 Drezner, J., Toresdahl, B., Rao, A. et al. Outcomes from sudden cardiac arrest in US high schools: a 2-year prospective study from the National Registry for AED Use in Sports. *Br J Sports Med* 2013; **47**: 1179–83.

Index

IOC Manual of Sports Cardiology, First Edition. Edited by Mathew G. Wilson, Jonathan A. Drezner and Sanjay Sharma.
© 2017 International Olympic Committee. Published 2017 by John Wiley & Sons, Ltd.